Essentials of
# Mucosal
# Immunology

# Essentials of

# Mucosal

# Immunology

EDITED BY

## Martin F. Kagnoff

*Department of Medicine*
*University of California, San Diego*
*La Jolla, California*

## Hiroshi Kiyono

*University of Alabama at Birmingham*
*Birmingham, Alabama and Oskaka University*
*Oskaka, Japan*

**ACADEMIC PRESS**

*San Diego   New York   Boston   London   Sydney   Tokyo   Toronto*

Copyright © 1996 by ACADEMIC PRESS

Academic Press, Inc.
525 B Street, Suite 1900, San Diego, California 92101-4495, USA
http://www.apnet.com

Academic Press Limited
24-28 Oval Road, London NW1 7DX, UK
http://www.hbuk.co.uk/ap/

Library of Congress Cataloging-in-Publication Data

Essentials of mucosal immunology / edited by Martin F. Kagnoff, Hiroshi
   Kiyono.
            p.        cm.
   Expanded and reviewed papers presented at the 8th International
Congress of Mucosal Immunology.
   Includes bibliographical references and index.
   ISBN 0-12-394330-2 (alk. paper)
   1. Mucous membrane--Immunology--Congresses.   I. Kagnoff, M. F.
(Martin F.)   II. Kiyono, H. (Hiroshi)
   [DNLM: 1. Mucous Membrane--immunology--congresses.   QS 532.5.M8
E78   1996]
QR185.9.M83E87   1996
616.07'9--dc20
DNLM/DLC
for Library of Congress                                    96-14720
                                                           CIP

Printed and bound in the United Kingdom
Transferred to Digital Printing, 2011

# Contents

## *part*
# I

## ANTIGEN PROCESSING AND PRESENTATION IN MUCOSAL-ASSOCIATED TISSUE

v

CHAPTER 3

## Toward an *in Vitro* Model for Microorganism Transport and Antigen Sampling through the Epithelial Digestive Barrier 37

*Eric Pringault*

CHAPTER 4

## Role of Dendritic Cells, Macrophages, and $\gamma\delta$ T Cells, in Antigen Processing and Presentation in the Respiratory Mucosa 47

*P. G. Holt, D. J. Nelson, A. S. McWilliam, D. Cooper, D. Strickland, and J. W. Upham*

CHAPTER 5

## Nonprofessional Antigen Presentation: New Rules and Regulations 55

*L. Mayer, X. Y. Yio, A. Panja, and N. Campbell*

# part
# II

## ROLE OF EPITHELIAL CELLS IN MUCOSAL IMMUNITY

CHAPTER 9

# Regulatory Peptides and Integration of the Intestinal Epithelium in Mucosal Responses

**101**

*Daniel K. Podolsky*

CHAPTER 10

# Role of Stromal–Epithelial Cell Interactions and of Basement Membrane Molecules in the Onset and Maintenance of Epithelial Integrity

**111**

*M. Kedinger, C. Fritsch, G. S. Evans, A. De Arcangelis, V. Orian-Rousseau, and P. Simon-Assmann*

CHAPTER 11

# Neuroendocrine Regulation of Mucosal Immune Responses

**125**

*Hiroshi Nagura, Mitsuru Kubota, and Noriko Kimura*

## CHAPTER 12
## New Insights into Epithelial Cell Function in Mucosal Immunity: Neutralization of Intracellular Pathogens and Excretion of Antigens by IgA                               141

*Michael E. Lamm, John G. Nedrud, Charlotte S. Kaetzel, and Mary B. Mazanec*

## CHAPTER 13
## Structure and Function of the Polymeric Immunoglobulin Receptor in Epithelial Cells                                           151

*James E. Casanova*

*part*
# III

### MUCOSAL T LYMPHOCYTES AND LYMPHOCTYE MIGRATION

## CHAPTER 14
## Ligand Recognition by $\gamma\delta$ T Cells                                            169

*Yueh-hsiu Chien*

CHAPTER 15

## Development of Intestinal Intraepithelial Lymphocytes     183

*Leo Lefrançois, Barbara Fuller, Sara Olson, and Lynn Puddington*

CHAPTER 16

## Intraepithelial $\gamma\delta$ T Cells and Epithelial Cell Interactions in the Mucosal Immune System     195

*Hiroshi Kiyono, Kohtaro Fujihashi, Masafumi Yamamoto, Takachika Hiroi, Michel Coste, Shigetada Kawabata, Prosper Boyaka, and Jerry R. McGhee*

CHAPTER 17

# Lymphocyte–Epithelial Cross-Talk in the Intestine: Do Nonclassical Class I Molecules Have a Big Part in the Dialogue?        205

*Beate C. Sydora, Richard Aranda, Shabnam Tangri, Hilda R. Holcombe, Victoria Camerini, A. Raul Castaño, Jeffrey E. W. Miller, Susanna Cardell, William D. Huse, Per A. Peterson, Hilde Cheroutre, and Mitchell Kronenberg*

CHAPTER 18

# Lamina Propria Lymphocytes: A Unique Population of Mucosal Lymphocytes        227

*Maria T. Abreu-Martin and Stephan R. Targan*

CHAPTER 19

# Cytokine Gene Knockout Mice—Lessons for Mucosal B-Cell Development        247

*Alistair J. Ramsay, Shisan Bao, Kenneth W. Beagley, Sarah J. Dunstan, Alan J. Husband, Manfred Kopf, Klaus I. Matthaei, Ian A. Ramshaw, Richard A. Strugnell, Ian G. Young, and Xiaoyun Tan*

CHAPTER 20

## Adhesion Molecules on Mucosal T Lymphocytes                                                  263

*Alexandre Benmerah, Natacha Patey, and Nadine Cerf-Bensussan*

CHAPTER 21

## Intestinal Epithelial Cell-Derived Interleukin-7 as a Regulatory Factor for Intestinal Mucosal Lymphocytes    279

*Mamoru Watanabe, Yoshitaka Ueno, and Toshifumi Hibi*

CHAPTER 22

## Defects in T-Cell Regulation: Lessons for Inflammatory Bowel Disease    291

*Stephen J. Simpson, Georg A. Holländer, Emiko Mizoguchi, Atul K. Bhan, Baoping Wang, and Cox Terhorst*

*part*
# IV

## MUCOSAL INFLAMMATION

CHAPTER 25

## Mast Cell Heterogeneity and Functions in Mucosal Defenses and Pathogenesis    341

*A. Dean Befus*

CHAPTER 26

## Hepatocellular Autoantigens    355

*Michael Peter Manns, Christian Straßburg, Maria Gracia Clemente, and Petra Obermayer-Straub*

*part*

# V

## MUCOSAL INFECTION

## CHAPTER 30

## Mucosal HIV Infection: A Paradigm for Dysregulation of the Mucosal Immune System     421

*Martin Zeitz, Thomas Schneider, and Reiner Ullrich*

## CHAPTER 31

## Genital and Rectal Mucosal Immunity against Transmission of SIV/HIV     437

*T. Lehner, L. A. Bergmeier, R. Brookes, L. Hussain, L. Klavinskis, E. Mitchell, and L. Tao*

## CHAPTER 32

## Beneficial and Harmful Immune Responses in the Respiratory Tract     449

*Peter J. M. Openshaw, Lindsay C. Spender, and Tracy Hussell*

# *part*
# VI

## MUCOSAL VACCINES

CHAPTER 39

Oral Tolerance: Immunologic Mechanisms and Treatment of
Autoimmune Diseases 555

*Howard L. Weiner*

CHAPTER 40

A Molecular Approach to the Construction of an Effective
Mucosal Vaccine Adjuvant: Studies Based on Cholera Toxin
ADP-Ribosylation and Cell Targeting 563

*Nils Lycke*

# Contributors

*Numbers in parentheses indicate the pages on which the authors' contributions begin.*

MARIA T. ABREU-MARTIN (227), Inflammatory Bowel Disease Center, Cedars-Sinai Medical Center, Los Angeles, California 90048

WILLIAM AGACE (73), Department of Medical Microbiology, Division of Clinical Immunology, Lund University, 22362 Lund, Sweden

RICHARD ARANDA (205), Molecular Biology Institute, Los Angeles, California 90095 and Department of Medicine, Division of Digestive Diseases, UCLA School of Medicine, Los Angeles, California 90095

STEVEN P. BALK (85), Hematology-Oncology Division, Beth Israel Hospital, Harvard Medical School, Boston, Massachusetts 02115

ELISABETH BAN (461), Departments of Microbiology and Oral Biology, Immunobiology Vaccine Center, University of Alabama at Birmingham Medical Center, Birmingham, Alabama 35294

JACQUES BANCHEREAU (477), Laboratory of Immunology Research, Schering-Plough Corp., 69571 Dardilly, France

SHISAN BAO (247), Department of Veterinary Pathology, University of Sydney, Sydney, Australia 2006

KENNETH W. BEAGLEY (247), Discipline of Pathology, University of Newcastle, Newcastle, Australia 2300

A. DEAN BEFUS (341), Pulmonary Research Group, Department of Medicine, University of Alberta, Edmonton, Alberta, Canada T6G 2S2

ALEXANDRE BENMERAH (263), Développement Normal et Pathologique du Système Immunitaire, INSERM U429, Hôpital Necker-Enfants Malades, 75743 Paris, France

L. A. BERGMEIER (437), Department of Immunology, United Medical and Dental Schools at Guy's Hospital, London Bridge, London SE1 9RT, England

ATUL K. BHAN (291), Department of Pathology, Massachusetts General Hospital, Harvard Medical School, Boston, Massachusetts 02115

MARTIN J. BLASER (377), Department of Medicine and Department of Microbiology and Immunology, Division of Infectious Diseases, Vanderbilt University School of Medicine, Nashville, Tennessee 37232

RICHARD S. BLUMBERG (85), Gastroenterology Division, Brigham and Women's Hospital, Harvard Medical School, Boston, Massachusetts 02115

KENNETH L. BOST (513), Department of Microbiology and Immunology, Tulane University School of Medicine, New Orleans, Louisiana 70112

PROSPER BOYAKA (195), Departments of Oral Biology and Microbiology, Immunobiology Vaccine Center, University of Alabama at Birmingham Medical Center, Birmingham, Alabama 35294; and Department of Mucosal Immunology, Research Institute for Microbial Diseases, Osaka University, Suita, Osaka 565, Japan

R. BROOKES (437), Department of Immunology, United Medical and Dental Schools at Guy's Hospital, London Bridge, London SE1 9RT, England

EUGENE BUTCHER (477), Department of Pathology, Stanford University School of Medicine, Palo Alto, California 94305

VICTORIA CAMERINI (205), Molecular Biology Institute, University of California, Los Angeles, California 90095; and Department of Pediatrics, Division of Neonatology, UCLA School of Medicine, Los Angeles, California 90095

N. CAMPBELL (55), Division of Clinical Immunology, The Mount Sinai Medical Center, New York, New York 10029

SUSANNA CARDELL (205), Institut de Génétique et Biologie Moléculaire et Cellulaire, INSERM-CNRS, Université Louis Pasteur, 67085 Strasbourg, France

JAMES E. CASANOVA (151), Pediatric Gastroenterology, Massachusetts General Hospital East, Charlestown, Massachusetts 02129

A. RAUL CASTAÑO (3, 205), The R. W. Johnson Pharmaceutical Research Institute at The Scripps Research Institute, La Jolla, California 92037

NADINE CERF-BENSUSSAN (263), Développement Normal et Pathologique du Système Immunitaire, INSERM U429, Hôpital Necker-Enfants Malades, 75743 Paris, France

HILDE CHEROUTRE (205), Department of Microbiology and Immunology and Molecular Biology Institute, University of California at Los Angeles, Los Angeles, California 90095

YUEH-HSIU CHIEN (169), Department of Microbiology and Immunology, Stanford University, Stanford, California 94305

CELESTE CHONG (513), Department of Microbiology and Immunology, Tulane University School of Medicine, New Orleans, Louisiana 70112

ANDREAS D. CHRIST (85), Gastroenterology Division, Brigham and Women's Hospital, Harvard Medical School, Boston, Massachusetts 02115

MARIA GRACIA CLEMENTE (355), Division of Gastroenterology and Hepatology, Medizinische Hochschule Hannover, D-30623 Hannover, Germany

JOHN D. CLEMENTS (513), Department of Microbiology and Immunology, Tulane University School of Medicine, New Orleans, Louisiana 70112

SEAN P. COLGAN (85), Department of Anesthesia, Brigham and Women's Hospital, Harvard Medical School, Boston, Massachusetts 02115

D. COOPER (47), TVW Telethon Institute for Child Health Research, West Perth, Western Australia, Australia 6872

MICHEL COSTE (195), Departments of Oral Biology and Microbiology, Immunobiology Vaccine Center, University of Alabama at Birmingham Medical Center, Birmingham, Alabama 35294; and Department of Mucosal Immunology, Research Institute for Microbial Diseases, Osaka University, Suita, Osaka 565, Japan

ROY CURTISS III (499), Department of Biology, Washington University, St. Louis, Missouri 63130

CECIL CZERKINSKY (477, 489), Department of Medical Microbiology and Immunology, University of Göteborg, S-413 46 Göteborg, Sweden; and INSERM Unit 80, 69437 Lyon, France

STEVEN J. CZINN (391), Division of Pediatric Gastroenterology and Nutrition, Rainbow Babies and Childrens Hospital, and Institute of Pathology, Case Western Reserve University, Cleveland, Ohio 44106

A. DE ARCANGELIS (111), INSERM Research Unit 381, Ontogenesis and Pathology of the Digestive Tract, 67200 Strasbourg, France

TERESA DOGGETT (499), Department of Biology, Washington University, St. Louis, Missouri 63130

SARAH J. DUNSTAN (247), Department of Microbiology, University of Melbourne, Melbourne, Australia 3052

LARS ECKMANN (63), Department of Medicine, University of California, San Diego, La Jolla, California 92093

CHARLES O. ELSON (543), Department of Medicine, University of Alabama at Birmingham, Birmingham, Alabama 35294

KRISTINA ERIKSSON (477), Department of Medical Microbiology and Immunology, University of Göteborg, S-413 46 Göteborg, Sweden

G. S. EVANS (111), Department of Pediatrics, University of Sheffield, The Sheffield Children's Hospital, Sheffield S10 2TH, England

JOSHUA FIERER (63), Department of Medicine, University of California, San Diego, La Jolla, California 92093

C. FRITSCH (111), INSERM Research Unit 381, Ontogenesis and Pathology of the Digestive Tract, 67200 Strasbourg, France

KOHTARO FUJIHASHI (195), Departments of Oral Biology and Microbiology, Immunobiology Vaccine Center, University of Alabama at Birmingham Medical Center, Birmingham, Alabama 35294; and Department of Mucosal Immunology, Research Institute for Microbial Diseases, Osaka University, Suita, Osaka 565, Japan

BARBARA FULLER (183), Department of Medicine, University of Connecticut Health Center, Farmington, Connecticut 06030

ROBERTO GAROFALO (405), Department of Pediatrics, University of Texas Medical Branch, Galveston, Texas 77555

SPENCER HEDGES (73), Department of Medical Microbiology, Division of Clinical Immunology, Lund University, 22362 Lund, Sweden

MARIA HEDLUND (73), Department of Medical Microbiology, Division of Clinical Immunology, Lund University, 22362 Lund, Sweden

TOSHIFUMI HIBI (279), Department of Internal Medicine, School of Medicine, Keio University, Tokyo 160, Japan; and Keio Cancer Center, Tokyo 160, Japan

TAKACHIKA HIROI (195), Departments of Oral Biology and Microbiology, Immunobiology Vaccine Center, University of Alabama at Birmingham Medical Center, Birmingham, Alabama 35294; and Department of Mucosal Immunology, Research Institute for Microbial Diseases, Osaka University, Suita, Osaka 565, Japan

HILDA R. HOLCOMBE (205), Department of Microbiology and Immunology and Molecular Biology Institute, University of California at Los Angeles, Los Angeles, California 90095

GEORG A. HOLLÄNDER (291), Division of Pediatric Oncology, Dana Farber Cancer Institute, Harvard Medical School, Boston, Massachusetts 02115

JAN HOLMGREN (477, 489), Department of Medical Microbiology and Immunology, University of Göteborg, S-413 46 Göteborg, Sweden

P. G. HOLT (47), TVW Telethon Institute for Child Health Research, West Perth, Western Australia 6872, Australia

GEORGE HUANG (63), Department of Medicine, University of California, San Diego, La Jolla, California 92093

ALAN J. HUSBAND (247), Department of Veterinary Pathology, University of Sydney, Sydney, Australia 2006

WILLIAM D. HUSE (205), Ixsys Corporation, La Jolla, California 92037

L. HUSSAIN (437), Department of Immunology, United Medical and Dental Schools at Guy's Hospital, London Bridge, London SE1 9RT, England

TRACY HUSSELL (449), Respiratory Medicine, St. Mary's Hospital Medical School, Imperial College of Science, Technology and Medicine, London W2 1PG, United Kingdom

ESTHER J. ISRAEL (85), Division of Pediatric Gastroenterology and Nutrition, Massachusetts General Hospital, Harvard Medical School, Boston, Massachusetts 02115

RAYMOND J. JACKSON (461), Departments of Microbiology and Oral Biology, Immunobiology Vaccine Center, University of Alabama at Birmingham Medical Center, Birmingham, Alabama 35294

HYUN C. JUNG (63), Department of Medicine, University of California, San Diego, La Jolla, California 92093

CHARLOTTE S. KAETZEL (141), Department of Pathology and Laboratory Medicine, Markey Cancer Center, University of Kentucky, Lexington, Kentucky 40536

MARTIN F. KAGNOFF (63), Department of Medicine, University of California, San Diego, La Jolla, California 92093

LARS KARLSSON (3), The R. W. Johnson Pharmaceutical Research Institute at The Scripps Research Institute, La Jolla, California 92037

SHIGETADA KAWABATA (195), Departments of Oral Biology and Microbiology, Immunobiology Vaccine Center, University of Alabama at Birmingham Medical Center, Birmingham, Alabama 35294; and Department of Mucosal Immunology, Research Institute for Microbial Diseases, Osaka University, Suita, Osaka 565, Japan

M. KEDINGER (111), INSERM Research Unit 381, Ontogenesis and Pathology of the Digestive Tract, 67200 Strasbourg, France

NORIKO KIMURA (125), Department of Pathology, Tohoku University School of Medicine, Sendai 980-77, Japan

HIROSHI KIYONO (195, 461), Departments of Oral Biology and Microbiology, Immunobiology Vaccine Center, University of Alabama at Birmingham Medical Center, Birmingham, Alabama 35294; and Department of Mucosal Immunology, Research Institute for Microbial Diseases, Osaka University, Osaka 565, Japan

L. KLAVINSKIS (437), Department of Immunology, United Medical and Dental Schools at Guy's Hospital, London Bridge, London SE1 9RT, England

MANFRED KOPF (247), Basel Institute for Immunology, CH-4005 Basel, Switzerland

JEAN-PIERRE KRAEHENBUHL (29), Swiss Institute for Experimental Cancer Research and Institute of Biochemistry, University of Lausanne, CH-1066 Epalinges-Lausanne, Switzerland

MITCHELL KRONENBERG (205), Department of Microbiology and Immunology and Molecular Biology Institute, University of California at Los Angeles, Los Angeles, California 90095

MITSURU KUBOTA (125), Department of Pathology, Tohoku University School of Medicine, Sendai 980-77, Japan

MEKURIA LAKEW (477), Department of Medical Microbiology and Immunology, University of Göteborg, S-413 46 Göteborg, Sweden

MICHAEL E. LAMM (141), Department of Pathology, Case Western Reserve University, Cleveland, Ohio 44106

ANDREW LAZAROVITS (477), Department of Medicine, University of Western Ontario, London, Ontario, Canada N6A 5C1

MICHAEL LEBENS (489), Department of Medical Microbiology and Immunology, Göteborg University, S-413 46 Göteborg, Sweden

LEO LEFRANÇOIS (183), Department of Medicine, University of Connecticut Health Center, Farmington, Connecticut 06030

T. LEHNER (437), Department of Immunology, United Medical and Dental Schools at Guy's Hospital, London Bridge, London SE1 9RT, England

MARIANNE LINDBLAD (489), Department of Medical Microbiology and Immunology, Göteborg University, S-413 46 Göteborg, Sweden

NILS LYCKE (563), Department of Medical Microbiology and Immunology, University of Göteborg, S-413 46 Göteborg, Sweden

RICHARD P. MACDERMOTT (321), Section of Gastroenterology, Lahey Hitchcock Medical Center, Burlington, Massachusetts 01805; and Department of Immunology, Massachusetts General Hospital, Boston, Massachusetts 02115; and Harvard Medical School, Boston, Massachusetts 02115

MICHAEL PETER MANNS (355), Division of Gastroenterology and Hepatology, Medizinische Hochschule Hannover, D-30623 Hannover, Germany

MARIAROSARIA MARINARO (461), Departments of Microbiology and Oral Biology, Immunobiology Vaccine Center, University of Alabama at Birmingham Medical Center, Birmingham, Alabama 35294

KLAUS I. MATTHAEI (247), The John Curtin School of Medical Research, The Australian National University, Canberra, Australia 0200

L. MAYER (55), Division of Clinical Immunology, The Mount Sinai Medical Center, New York, New York 10029

MARY B. MAZANEC (141), Department of Medicine, Case Western Reserve University, Cleveland, Ohio 44106

JERRY R. MCGHEE (195, 461), Departments of Oral Biology and Microbiology, Immunobiology Vaccine Center, University of Alabama at Birmingham Medical Center, Birmingham, Alabama 35294; and Department of Mucosal Immunology, Research Institute for Microbial Diseases, Osaka University, Osaka 565, Japan

A. S. MCWILLIAM (47), TVW Telethon Institute for Child Health Research, West Perth, Western Australia 6872, Australia

JEFFREY E. W. MILLER (205), Ixsys Corporation, La Jolla, California 92037

E. MITCHELL (437), Department of Immunology, United Medical and Dental Schools at Guy's Hospital, London Bridge, London SE1 9RT, England

EMIKO MIZOGUCHI (291), Department of Pathology, Massachusetts General Hospital, Harvard Medical School, Boston, Massachusetts 02115

HIROSHI NAGURA (125), Department of Pathology, Tohoku University School of Medicine, Sendai 980-77, Japan

AMIYA NAYAK (499), Department of Biology, Washington University, St. Louis, Missouri 63130

JOHN G. NEDRUD (141, 391), Division of Pediatric Gastroenterology and Nutrition, Rainbow Babies and Childrens Hospital, and Institute of Pathology, Case Western Reserve University, Cleveland, Ohio 44106

D. J. NELSON (47), TVW Telethon Institute for Child Health Research, West Perth, Western Australia 6872, Australia

MARIAN R. NEUTRA (29), Department of Pediatrics, Harvard Medical School and GI Cell Biology Laboratory, Children's Hospital, Boston, Massachusetts 02115

PETRA OBERMAYER-STRAUB (355), Division of Gastroenterology and Hepatology, Medizinische Hochschule Hannover, D-30623 Hannover, Germany

PEARAY L. OGRA (405), Department of Pediatrics, University of Texas Medical Branch, Galveston, Texas 77555

NOBUO OKAHASHI (461), Departments of Microbiology and Oral Biology, Immunobiology Vaccine Center, University of Alabama at Birmingham Medical Center, Birmingham, Alabama 35294

SARA OLSON (183), Department of Medicine, University of Connecticut Health Center, Farmington, Connecticut 06030

PETER J. M. OPENSHAW (449), Respiratory Medicine, St. Mary's Hospital Medical School, Imperial College of Science, Technology and Medicine, London W2 1PG, United Kingdom

V. ORIAN-ROUSSEAU (111), INSERM Research Unit 381, Ontogenesis and Pathology of the Digestive Tract, 67200 Strasbourg, France

A. PANJA (55), Division of Clinical Immunology, The Mount Sinai Medical Center, New York, New York 10029

DAVID W. PASCUAL (461), Departments of Microbiology and Oral Biology, Immunobiology Vaccine Center, University of Alabama at Birmingham Medical Center, Birmingham, Alabama 35294

NATACHA PATEY (263), Department of Pathology, Hôpital Necker-Enfants Malades, 75743 Paris, France

PER A. PETERSON (3, 205), The R. W. Johnson Pharmaceutical Research Institute at The Scripps Research Institute, La Jolla, California 92037

DANIEL K. PODOLSKY (101), Department of Medicine, Gastrointestinal Unit and Center for the Study of Inflammatory Bowel Disease, Massachusetts General Hospital at Harvard Medical School, Boston, Massachusetts 02114

ERIC PRINGAULT (37), Swiss Institute for Experimental Cancer Research and Institute of Biochemistry, University of Lausanne, CH-1066 Epalinges-Lausanne, Switzerland, and Pasteur Institute, 75015 Paris, France

LYNN PUDDINGTON (183), Department of Medicine, University of Connecticut Health Center, Farmington, Connecticut 06030

MARIANNE QUIDING-JÄRNBRINK (477), Department of Medical Microbiology and Immunology, University of Göteborg, S-413 46 Göteborg, Sweden

ALISTAIR J. RAMSAY (247), The John Curtin School of Medical Research, The Australian National University, Canberra, Australia 0200

IAN A. RAMSHAW (247), The John Curtin School of Medical Research, The Australian National University, Canberra, Australia 0200

SHARON L. REED (63), Department of Medicine, University of California, San Diego, La Jolla, California 92093

R. BALFOUR SARTOR (307), Division of Digestive Diseases, University of North Carolina at Chapel Hill, Chapel Hill, North Carolina 27599

THOMAS SCHNEIDER (421), Medical Clinic II, University of the Saarland, 66421 Homburg/Saar, Germany

NEIL SIMISTER (85), Rosensteil Center for Basic Biomedical Research, Brandeis University, Waltham, Massachusetts 02254

P. SIMON-ASSMANN (111), INSERM Research Unit 381, Ontogenesis and Pathology of the Digestive Tract, 67200 Strasbourg, France

STEPHEN J. SIMPSON (291), Division of Immunology, Beth Israel Hospital, Harvard Medical School, Boston, Massachusetts 02115

LINDSAY C. SPENDER (449), Respiratory Medicine, St. Mary's Hospital Medical School, Imperial College of Science, Technology and Medicine, London W2 1PG, United Kingdom

JAY SRINIVASAN (499), Department of Biology, Washington University, St. Louis, Missouri 63130

HERMAN F. STAATS (461), Center for AIDS Research, Department of Medicine, Duke University Medical Center, Durham, North Carolina 27710

CHRISTIAN STRAßBURG (355), Division of Gastroenterology and Hepatology, Medizinische Hochschule Hannover, D-30623 Hannover, Germany

D. STRICKLAND (47), TVW Telethon Institute for Child Health Research, West Perth, Western Australia 6872, Australia

RICHARD A. STRUGNELL (247), Department of Microbiology, University of Melbourne, Melbourne, Australia 3052

JIA-BIN SUN (489), Department of Medical Microbiology and Immunology, Göteborg University, S-413 46 Göteborg, Sweden

CATHARINA SVANBORG (73), Department of Medical Microbiology, Division of Clinical Immunology, Lund University, 22362 Lund, Sweden

ANN-MARIE SVENNERHOLM (489), Department of Medical Microbiology and Immunology, Göteborg University, S-413 46 Göteborg, Sweden

MAJLIS SVENSSON (73), Department of Medical Microbiology, Division of Clinical Immunology, Lund University, 223362 Lund, Sweden

BEATE C. SYDORA (205), Department of Microbiology and Immunology and Molecular Biology Institute, University of California, Los Angeles, California 90095

XIAOYUN TAN (247), The John Curtin School of Medical Research, The Australian National University, Canberra, Australia 0200

SHABNAM TANGRI (205), Department of Microbiology and Immunology, and Molecular Biology Institute, University of California, Los Angeles, California 90095; and Department of Medicine, Division of Digestive Diseases, UCLA School of Medicine, Los Angeles, California 90095

L. TAO (437), Department of Immunology, United Medical and Dental Schools at Guy's Hospital, London Bridge, London SE1 9RT, England

STEPHAN R. TARGAN (227), Inflammatory Bowel Disease Center, Cedars-Sinai Medical Center, Los Angeles, California 90048

COX TERHORST (291), Division of Immunology, Beth Israel Hospital, Harvard Medical School, Boston, Massachusetts 02115

YOSHITAKA UENO (279), Department of Internal Medicine, School of Medicine, Keio University, Tokyo 160, Japan

REINER ULLRICH (421), Department of Gastroenterology, Medical Clinic, Klinikum Benjamin Franklin, Free University of Berlin, 12200 Berlin, Germany

J. W. UPHAM (47), TVW Telethon Institute for Child Health Research, West Perth, Western Australia 6872, Australia

FREDERIK W. VAN GINKEL (461), Departments of Microbiology and Oral Biology, Immunobiology Vaccine Center, University of Alabama at Birmingham Medical Center, Birmingham, Alabama 35294

JOHN L. VANCOTT (461), Departments of Microbiology and Oral Biology, Immunobiology Vaccine Center, University of Alabama at Birmingham Medical Center, Birmingham, Alabama 35294

**BAOPING WANG** (291), Division of Immunology, Beth Israel Hospital, Harvard Medical School, Boston, Massachusetts 02115

**MAMORU WATANABE** (279), Department of Internal Medicine, School of Medicine, Keio University, Tokyo 160, Japan

**HOWARD L. WEINER** (555), Center for Neurologic Diseases, Brigham and Women's Hospital and Harvard Medical School, Boston, Massachusetts 02115

**MASAFUMI YAMAMOTO** (195), Departments of Oral Biology and Microbiology, Immunobiology Vaccine Center, University of Alabama at Birmingham Medical Center, Birmingham, Alabama 35294; and Department of Mucosal Immunology, Research Institute for Microbial Diseases, Osaka University, Suita, Osaka 565, Japan

**SUK-KYUN YANG** (63), Department of Medicine, University of California, San Diego, La Jolla, California 92093

**X. Y. YIO** (55), Division of Clinical Immunology, The Mount Sinai Medical Center, New York, New York 10029

**IAN G. YOUNG** (247), The John Curtin School of Medical Research, The Australian National University, Canberra, Australia 0200

**MARTIN ZEITZ** (421), Medical Clinic II, University of the Saarland, 66421 Homburg/Saar, Germany

**JAN ZIVNY** (543), Department of Medicine, University of Alabama at Birmingham, Birmingham, Alabama 35294

# *Preface*

The mucosal immune system is considered by many to be a "new world" in the area of immunology and has numerous unique features compared to the classical systemic immune compartment. For example, the mucosal immune system consists of specialized IgA inductive and effector sites, as well as unique cell trafficking patterns that underlie the common mucosal immune system (CMIS). Secretory IgA is the major antibody produced at mucosal surfaces and plays an important role in recognition and protection against non-self antigens in those sites. The polyimmunoglobulin receptor that transports IgA across epithelial cells has become a basis for the study of membrane receptor trafficking by cell biologists and immunologists alike. $\alpha\beta$ and $\gamma\delta$ T cells reside within the mucosal epithelial layer (i.e., intraepithelial lymphocytes) as well as in the lamina propria region of the mucosa, where they represent a key arm of the cellular immune system. These specialized T cells participate in the induction and regulation of antigen-specific IgA B-cell and effector T-cell responses. Furthermore, epithelial cells that line mucosal surfaces are themselves an integrated component of the mucosal immune system and provide signals important for initiation of the mucosal inflammatory response and key cell–cell communication between epithelial cells and mucosal lymphoid cells. The concept of the CMIS has provided a rational basis for the clinical development of mucosal vaccines for the prevention of infectious diseases, and mucosally induced tolerance has provided a therapeutic basis for the prevention and treatment of autoimmune disease and tissue rejection in organ transplantation. Thus, mucosal immunology is an exciting area for both basic and clinical scientists interested in the field of immunology.

*Martin F. Kagnoff*
*Hiroshi Kiyono*

# Acknowledgments

The National Institutes of Health

**Patron**
Japanese Society of Digestive Organs and Immunology

**Donors**
The American Digestive Health Foundation and the
American Gastroenterological Association
Crohn's & Colitis Foundation of America, Inc.
Lederle-Praxis Biologicals
The Procter & Gamble Company

**Sponsors**
Falk Foundation, e.V.
Glaxo, Inc.

**Supporters**
Abbott Laboratories
Amgen, Inc.
B. Braun Medical, Inc.
Connaught Laboratories Limited
Kissei Pharmaceuticals Co., Ltd.
Merck & Co., Inc.
Nestec Ltd. Research Centre
Nippon Glaxo, Ltd.
OraVax, Inc.
PharMingen
Sandoz Pharmaceuticals Corporation
Schering-Plough Pharmaceuticals
SmithKline-Beecham Pharma GmbH
Virus Research Institute, Inc.

The organizations, agencies, and corporations listed above provided generous financial support for the 8th International Congress of Mucosal Immunology. We express our appreciation to Ms. Debbie Lundemo, San Diego, and Ms. Wendy Jackson, Birmingham, who devoted their time and energy to assisting in the organization of the Congress and the preparation of the book. We also thank Dr. Jasna Markovac and Ms. Charlotte Brabants at Academic Press, who assisted in the publication of this work. Finally, we acknowledge our families, Marcia Kagnoff and Momoyo and Erika Kiyono, for their support and understanding during the organization of the congress and this book.

*part*

# I

# ANTIGEN PROCESSING AND PRESENTATION IN MUCOSAL-ASSOCIATED TISSUE

part

I

ANTIGEN PROCESSING AND
PRESENTATION IN
MUCOSA-ASSOCIATED TISSUE

# *Chapter 1*

# Principles of Antigen Processing and Presentation

Lars Karlsson, A. Raul Castaño, and Per A. Peterson

*The R. W. Johnson Pharmaceutical Research Institute at The Scripps Research Institute, La Jolla, California 92037*

## I. INTRODUCTION

The major function of the immune system is to rid the host of invading pathogens. This task is formidable considering the wide variety of pathogenic organisms and their ability to rapidly mutate when put under evolutionary selection. A number of different cell types, both antigen-independent and antigen-specific, have evolved to detect and neutralize invading organisms. T cells, which have a central role in regulating immune responses, have antigen-specific receptors with extensive primary sequence homology to immunoglobulins of B cells, but despite this homology the receptors of B and T cells recognize antigens in different ways. While the B cell receptor recognizes structural epitopes in proteins, T-cell receptors recognize antigens in the form of peptides associated with class I or class II molecules encoded in the major histocompatibility complex (MHC). Antigen processing is the process of peptide generation from antigenic proteins and the association of these peptides with MHC molecules. It is of crucial importance for T cell function and thus for the function of the immune system.

Though MHC class I or class II molecules are similar in three-dimensional structure, they are expressed in different cell types, activate different subsets of T cells, and present peptides derived from different subcellular compartments. The existence of two distinct but related systems is a reflection of how parasites invade and replicate in higher organisms. Viruses use the cellular machinery for replication as they utilize the host's synthetic machinery to manufacture the components of the virion. In the case where a cell is virus-infected, the viral polypeptides will be presented by MHC class I molecules which sample the newly synthesized proteins within a cell and report this information at cell surface. Extracellular pathogens, for example bacteria, are self-sufficient and can replicate within an organism without penetrating the host cells. Presentation of antigens from such pathogens requires that the pathogen is taken up from the extracellular space into the endosomal system, where they can be degraded and become associated with MHC class II molecules, which samples this pool of degradation products and displays them at the cell surface. Different types of T cells recognize the class I and class II molecules, respectively. Thus, cytotoxic T cells represent the major line of defense against viral infection, eliminating infected cells as a consequence of MHC class I–peptide complexes interacting with T cell receptors on CD8-positive T cells. CD4-positive helper T cells, which recognize peptides in association with MHC class II molecules, have a more regulatory role in that they provide help to anti-body-producing B cells and cytotoxic T cells, which in turn lead to neutralization of bacteria and improved detection of virus-infected cells.

The differences between the class I and class II antigen-presenting molecules are a reflection of the intracellular trafficking of these molecules and the compart-ments where they encounter peptides (Teyton and Peterson, 1992). While both class I and class II molecules assemble in the endoplasmic reticulum (ER) only class I molecules acquire peptides in this compartment. The peptides loaded onto class I are generated in the cytoplasm and transported into the ER. Newly synthe-sized class II molecules, in contrast, associate with an additional protein in the ER, the invariant chain (Kvist *et al.,* 1982), which prevents peptide binding (Teyton *et al.;* 1990, Roche and Cresswell, 1990). The invariant chain guides the class II molecules to the endosomal system where, after removal of the invariant chain, class II becomes associated with peptides derived mainly from extracellular pro-teins. Only after they have acquired peptides in the endosomes do class II mole-cules accumulate at the cell surface.

In addition to the normal class I and class II molecules, a number of class I-like molecules have been described. The function of these molecules is only now being elucidated, but several of them appear to have a role in antigen presentation.

In this article we summarize the present knowledge of the cell biology of MHC class I and class II antigen processing and presentation, as well as the current understanding of the biology and function of nonclassical class I molecules.

## II. Antigen Processing and Presentation by MHC Class I Molecules

The class I presenting pathway is outlined in Fig. 1. Class I molecules at the cell surface are composed of three subunits, class I heavy chain, $\beta2$-microglobulin, and peptide (Björkman *et al.,* 1987a). This trimeric complex is assembled in the endoplasmic reticulum (ER) and only correctly assembled complexes are trans-ported efficiently to the cell surface (Jackson and Peterson, 1993). While class I heavy chain and $\beta2$-microglobulin are targeted to the ER by virtue of their signal sequences, peptides are generated mainly in the cytosol and need to be transported into the lumen of the ER (Townsend and Trowsdale, 1993). The generation of peptides is thought to be mediated by the proteasome, a large catalytic complex which has essential housekeeping functions in addition to its role in generating

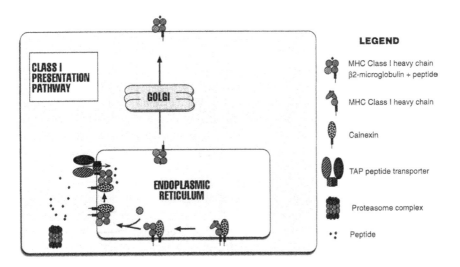

LEGEND

MHC Class I heavy chain
β2-microglobulin + peptide

MHC Class I heavy chain

Calnexin

TAP peptide transporter

Proteasome complex

Peptide

*FIGURE 1.* A schematic model of the class I antigen presentation pathway is shown. Antigens are degraded in the cytosol by the multicatalytic proteasome complex. Peptides are subsequently transported across the ER membrane by the TAP1–TAP2 (transporter associated with antigen processing) complex. Within the ER, class I molecules composed of a transmembrane heavy chain and a soluble β2-microglobulin bind the peptides and the trimolecular complex is then transported out of the ER to the cell surface via the exocytic pathway for inspection by T cells.

peptides for MHC class I (Goldberg and Rock, 1992). The mechanism by which antigen is unfolded and subsequently degraded by the proteasome is still poorly understood, but proteins destined for degradation by the proteasome are often initially modified by addition of ubiquitin, a highly conserved 8.5-kDa protein (Ciechanover, 1994). Ubiquitination appears to be essential for efficient processing of antigen for presentation by class I, since cell lines with temperature-sensitive defects in ubiquitination were incapable of presenting antigens to class I-restricted T cells (Michaelek *et al.,* 1993), thus providing the strongest evidence that the ubiquitin/proteasome system is actually responsible for generation of peptides associated with class I.

In order to be able to associate with the class I chains in the ER, peptides need to be translocated across the ER membrane. Studies of mutant cell lines and inbred rat strains defective in class I antigen presentation suggested that the genes responsible for this peptide transport were located in the class II region of the MHC (Livingstone *et al.,* 1989; Salter and Cresswell, 1986). Subsequently two genes were found in this region with homologies to ATP binding cassette (ABC) transporters, suggesting that the two resulting polypeptides, TAP1 and TAP2, were involved in translocating cytosolically produced peptides into the ER (Deverson *et al.,* 1990; Monaco *et al.,* 1990; Spies *et al.,* 1990; Trowsdale *et al.,* 1990). TAP1 and TAP2 form a heterodimer, and both genes are essential for peptide transport.

A number of studies have analyzed the function of the transporter complexes, using *in vitro* systems (Androlewicz *et al.,* 1993; Momburg *et al.,* 1994a,b; Neefjes *et al.,* 1993; Schumacher *et al.,* 1994; Shepherd *et al.,* 1993). The TAP complexes display preference for peptide substrates longer than 7 or 8 amino acids and can transport peptides of up to 40 amino acids, but transport rates are highest for peptides with lengths of 8–13 amino acids, which correlates well with the binding preferences of class I molecules (Momburg *et al.,* 1994a; Schumacher *et al.,* 1994). The transporter complexes do not transport all peptides equally well, but have some sequence specificities which appear to be correlated with the binding preferences of class I molecules, suggesting that the TAPs and class I molecules have coevolved (Heemels *et al.,* 1993; Momburg *et al.,* 1994b).

During the peptide loading process, class I appears to be physically associated with the TAP complex (Ortmann *et al.,* 1994; Suh *et al.,* 1994). This association is released when class I binds peptide; it appears that peptide transport and class I loading are closely linked events. Studies in transfected insect cells show that TAP1 and TAP2 are the only proteins necessary for peptide transport into the ER (Meyer *et al.,* 1994), but several other unknown proteins seem to be associated with the TAP–class I complexes in normal cell lines (Ortmann *et al.,* 1994), suggesting that they may be involved in the loading of transported peptides onto class I.

In the lumen of the ER, folding and assembly of class I heavy chain and $\beta$2-microglobulin is assisted by molecular chaperones. In the absence of $\beta$2-microglobulin, class I heavy chains remain associated with BiP and calnexin and only a small amount of free heavy chains leave the ER (Degen and Williams, 1991; Nossner and Parham, 1995). When peptide delivery into the ER is deficient, heavy chain and $\beta$2-microglobulin associate to form "empty" class I molecules, but these are only poorly transported out of the ER (Baas *et al.,* 1992; Ljunggren *et al.,* 1990; Van Kaer *et al.,* 1992). It is unclear what keeps empty class I molecules from leaving the ER, but association with both calnexin and TAPs has been implicated (Degen and Williams, 1991; Ortmann *et al.,* 1994; Suh *et al.,* 1994). However, also in cell lines lacking calnexin or TAPs class I is retained in the ER and thus it appears that other molecules may be involved in this retention (Baas *et al.,* 1992; Scott and Dawson, 1995). Empty class I molecules that do leave the ER are thermolabile and are rapidly degraded at or before they reach the cell surface, ensuring that exogenous peptides are not picked up at the cell surface (Jackson *et al.,* 1992; Ljunggren *et al.,* 1990).

## III. ANTIGEN PROCESSING AND PRESENTATION BY MHC CLASS II MOLECULES

A schematic model of the class II antigen-processing pathway and the main molecules involved in this process is outlined in Fig. 2.

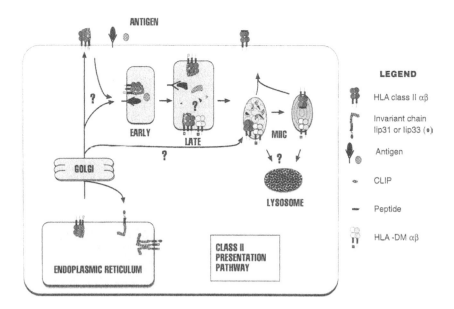

*FIGURE 2.* Schematic model of antigen processing for class II molecules. Invariant chain (Iip31 and Iip33) is synthesized in excess over class II in the endoplasmic reticulum. They associate to form a complex which is transported to endosomal compartments, either directly from the trans-Golgi network or via the cell surface. Antigen is taken up from the cell surface either by fluid-phase uptake or by receptor-mediated endocytosis. Proteases in the endosomal system degrade the antigen to peptide fragments. HLA-DM, which is an endosomal resident, mediates exchange of peptides so that CLIP peptide bound to class II is exchanged for antigen-derived peptides. The exact location of the loading process is unknown, but may occur in the MIIC (MHC class II compartment), class II-rich multivesicular or multilamellar structures with lysosomal characteristics. Peptide-containing class II is subsequently delivered to the cell surface for presentation to T cells.

## A. Assembly of Class II Molecules and the Function of the Invariant Chain

In comparison to the class I antigen-processing and presentation pathway, the processing and binding of peptides to class II molecules is still relatively poorly understood. Class II molecules at the cell surface are heterotrimeric complexes consisting of peptides bound to $\alpha\beta$ heterodimers; like class I molecules, the $\alpha$ and $\beta$ chains of class II assemble in the lumen of the ER. In contrast to class I, however, they do not bind peptides in this location, and instead they immediately become associated with a third chain, the invariant chain (Ii) (Kvist *et al.,* 1982). Invariant chain is produced in excess over class II and in normal cells it is impossible to detect any newly synthesized class II $\alpha\beta$ heterodimers not associated with invariant chain (Lamb and Cresswell, 1992; Nijenhuis and Neefjes, 1994). The invariant chain has three well-described properties: it blocks binding of peptides to class II, it facilitates class II transport out of the ER, and it directs class II to endosomes where peptide loading occurs (reviewed in Cresswell, 1994; Germain, 1994).

Despite the fact that class I molecules acquire peptides in the ER it is not clear to what extent the ER contains peptides accessible for binding to class II molecules. The data showing inhibition of peptide binding to class II by invariant chain are generated *in vitro* with purified molecules (Roche and Cresswell, 1990; Teyton *et al.*, 1990), and *in vivo* it appears that the main function of the invariant chain in the ER is to protect against binding of newly synthesized and partly folded proteins (Busch *et al.*, 1995; Dodi *et al.*, 1994; Aichinger *et al.*, manuscript in preparation). In the absence of invariant chain class II forms large, high-molecular-weight complexes and only small amounts of class II exit the ER (Bikoff *et al.*, 1993; Bonnerot *et al.*, 1994; Viville *et al.*, 1993). The class II that does leave the ER appears to be associated with proteins rather than peptides, and though some of this material appears to be present at the cell surface (Bikoff *et al.*, 1993; Viville *et al.*, 1993) other data suggest that the class II–protein complexes can be internalized into endosomal compartments where the bound proteins are trimmed down to form class II–peptide complexes (Aichinger *et al.*, manuscript in preparation).

Invariant chain has been reported to function as a chaperone for class II, facilitating transport out of the ER (Anderson and Miller, 1992), and it is also known to induce a change in the reactivity of class II with certain monoclonal antibodies, indicating that it influences the conformation of class II (Peterson and Miller, 1990). Protection from protein binding may also be part of the explanation why the invariant chain facilitates class II transport out of the ER.

Though genetically nonpolymorphic, several forms of invariant chain are synthesized (Strubin *et al.*, 1986). All are type II transmembrane proteins (i.e., they have the N-terminus located in the cytoplasm and the N-terminus located on the lumenal side) and appear to bind class II with similar efficiency. In man, two different initiation codons give rise to two different isoforms, Iip33 and Iip31 (Strubin *et al.*, 1986). The latter form is synthesized in larger amounts and is the main transported form of invariant chain. In contrast, Iip33, which has a 16-amino acid N-terminal extension, is an ER resident if expressed in the absence of class II (Lamb and Cresswell, 1992; Lotteau *et al.*, 1990). Mutational analysis has demonstrated that the N-terminal extension contains an arginine-rich ER retrieval motif reminiscent of the C-terminal KKXX retrieval motif present in many resident type I proteins (Jackson *et al.*, 1990; Schutze *et al.*, 1994). The function of Iip33 is not clear, but it may serve to increase the concentration of invariant chain in the ER, thus ensuring that class II molecules bind to invariant chain rather than to newly synthesized unfolded or partially folded proteins. Iip33 bound to class II does acquire carbohydrate modifications and thus it appears able to leave the ER to some extent (Newcomb and Cresswell, 1993). How class II induces transport of Iip33 is unknown, but it is possible that the arginine retrieval motif is being physically covered by the class II molecules similar to what has been described for the human high-affinity IgE receptor (Letourneur *et al.*, 1995). Alternatively, class II binding may result in conformational change or post-translational modification of the Iip33 tail, thus making it invisible to the retrieval machinery. Iip31 is also transported poorly out of the ER in the absence of class II (though it is not actively retrieved) (Lamb and Cresswell, 1992; Lotteau *et al.*, 1990) and it is possible that this is due to the formation of larger invariant chain complexes in the ER. Class II binding would in that case release invariant chain from the complexes for transport out of the ER.

In addition to the p31 and p33 forms of invariant chain, alternative splicing gives rise to two longer forms, Iip41 and Iip43. These forms of Ii result from the insertion of an additional exon in the lumenal domains of p31 and p33, respectively (Strubin *et al.*, 1986). Iip41 has been reported to improve the presentation of some antigens (Peterson and Miller, 1992), but does not appear to be essential in most cases. Interestingly, the peptide encoded by the inserted exon has been found naturally associated with the lysosomal protease cathepsin L and appears to inhibit and stabilize the enzyme (Ogrinc *et al.*, 1993). It is possible to speculate that Iip41 is somehow decreasing the proteolytic activity during antigen processing, thus modifying the spectrum of antigenic peptides available for binding to class II. The actual specific functions of the different forms of invariant chain are uncertain, however, and more experimental work is required to elucidate them.

## B. Endosomal Targeting by the Invariant Chain

Invariant chain–class II complexes are thought to leave the ER as nonamers (Lamb and Cresswell, 1992; Roche *et al.*, 1991), consisting of a core made up of three invariant chain residues with a class II $\alpha\beta$ heterodimer attached to each invariant chain residue. The complexes are transported through the Golgi complex where both class II and invariant chain acquire carbohydrate modifications. In contrast to most other cell surface proteins, including class I, which travel through the secretory pathway to the plasma membrane, the class II–invariant chain complexes are removed from the default pathway and instead are transported to endosomal compartments. It is not clear whether the endosomal sorting operation occurs mainly in the trans-Golgi network or at the cell surface, but very few invariant chain–class II complexes are present at the cell surface, indicating that sorting of these complexes is rapid and efficient (Neefjes *et al.*, 1990; Roche *et al.*, 1993). Deletion mutagenesis initially demonstrated that the N-terminal cytoplasmic tail of invariant chain p31 is responsible for the endosomal sorting (Bakke and Dobberstein, 1990; Lotteau *et al.*, 1990) and further analysis by several groups has revealed the importance of two di-leucine-like motifs in this sequence (Bremnes *et al.*, 1994; Odorizzi *et al.*, 1994; Pieters *et al.*, 1993; Pond *et al.*, 1995). Di-leucine-based endocytosis motifs were originally described in the T-cell receptor-associated CD3 complex (Letourneur and Klausner, 1992) and has subsequently been reported in a number of different proteins located in the endosomal–lysosomal system (reviewed by Sandoval and Bakke, 1994). Either of the two motifs in invariant chain appears to be sufficient for endosomal targeting, and it is not obvious that two motifs are more efficient than one motif. Detailed analysis of the invariant chain tail has revealed the importance of an acidic residue 3 or 4 residues N-terminal to each di-leucine motif (Pond *et al.*, 1995). Interestingly, internalization of invariant chain from the cell surface was unaffected if the acidic residues were mutated, but the morphology of invariant chain-containing endosomal compartments was changed. When overexpressed in the absence of class II, invariant chain has a tendency to form large perinuclear vesicular structures of endosomal origin (Lotteau *et al.*, 1990; Romagnoli *et al.*, 1993). These structures were not formed in cells transfected with invariant chain constructs lacking the acidic residues, and instead invariant chain was found in smaller vesicles. It is not clear that the targeting motif of invariant chain is able to direct it to a unique location, since similar motifs derived from other endosomal proteins, which themselves have a different localization, can also target invariant chain in a way similar to that of the wild-type tail. Thus, while the targeting motifs in the invariant chain tail are important for its endosomal location, other parts of the molecule must be involved in determining its final destination in the endosomal system.

## C. Peptide Loading of Class II

Class II molecules at the cell surface contain peptides generated from proteins in the endocytic pathway of either exogenous or endogenous origin. In contrast to the peptides loaded onto class I, which are generated in the cytosol making transport across the ER membrane necessary, the class II binding peptides are produced in the lumen of the endosomal system by lysosomal proteases (Blum and Cresswell, 1988; Neefjes and Ploegh, 1992). These proteases are only active in acidic pH, and agents that increase endosomal pH efficiently block antigen presentation by class II (Machamer and Cresswell, 1984; Ziegler and Unanue, 1982). Several studies have tried to use protease inhibitors to determine the importance of different proteases for generation of antigenic peptides (Bennett *et al.*, 1992; Falo *et al.*, 1992; Morton *et al.*, 1995), but the relatively broad specificity of these inhibitors makes it difficult to draw firm conclusions. It is also not clear whether class II molecules initially bind actual peptides or whether they bind to denatured and partially degraded proteins which are subsequently trimmed down by exoproteases to form peptides. Some support for the latter theory comes from the fact that class II-associated peptides have rugged ends and do not appear to be preferentially generated in relation to any specific protease cleavage sites (Barber and Parham, 1993).

Removal of invariant chain from class II occurs after the invariant chain–class II complexes have reached the endosomal system, and its removal is essential for presentation of antigen. The dissociation from class II can partly be inhibited by the serine protease inhibitor leupeptin (Blum and Cresswell, 1988; Newcomb and Cresswell, 1993), and thus it appears that invariant chain, at least in leupeptin-treated cells, is proteolytically degraded while bound to class II. In the absence of protease inhibitors it is difficult to demonstrate class II associated with invariant chain degradation products (other than CLIP, see below), and it cannot be totally excluded that the invariant chain fragments seen bound to class II in leupeptin-treated cells represent rebinding to class II rather than incomplete removal of invariant chain from class II.

An MHC class II-encoded molecule, HLA-DM (DM) has been found to be essential for efficient peptide–class II association (Fling et al., 1994; Morris et al., 1994). Human B cell lines lacking HLA-DM have been shown to be deficient in presentation of whole protein antigens, despite the fact that they can present exogenously added peptide antigens and contain normal class II and invariant chain genes (Ceman et al., 1992; Mellins et al., 1990; Riberdy et al., 1992). Reintroduction into these cell lines of the HLA-DM $\alpha$ and $\beta$ chains (or the equivalent mouse molecule, H2-M), by transfection, restored antigen presentation ability (Denzin et al., 1994; Fling et al., 1994; Morris et al., 1994). Several lines of evidence indicated that the class II molecules of the DM-deficient cell lines had an abnormal peptide content. First, certain conformation-specific monoclonal antibodies react poorly with the class II molecules expressed by the mutant cell lines, despite the fact that class II can be detected with other antibodies (Mellins et al., 1990). Second, class II molecules from normal B cell lines containing well-fitting peptides often migrate as heterodimers in SDS–PAGE gels, as long as the samples are not heated (Sadegh-Nasseri and Germain, 1991; Stern and Wiley, 1992). Class II molecules derived from the mutant cell lines, in contrast, were unstable is SDS. Third, class II-derived from the mutant cell lines, in contrast, were unstable is SDS. Third, class II-derived peptides eluted from cell lines lacking HLA-DM were found to consist mainly of invariant chain peptides, derived from the CLIP (class II-associated invariant chain peptides) region of invariant chain (Mellins et al., 1994; Riberdy et al., 1992). These peptides can also be found associated with class II from normal cell lines, but to a much smaller extent. Recent reports have described in vitro experiments where purified or recombinant HLA-DM has been shown to induce peptide exchange in purified HLA-DR molecules, including the removal of CLIP (Denzin and Cresswell, 1995; Sloan et al., 1995). The fact that CLIP is binding in the peptide-binding groove of class II molecules derived from cells lacking DM (Wolf and Ploegh, 1995) suggests that the CLIP region of the intact invariant chain is binding to the peptide binding groove of class II and that the CLIP fragment is protected from proteolysis by its binding to class II. Loading of other peptides requires the removal of the CLIP fragment and it appears that DM is directly responsible for removing CLIP. In vivo, however, it is not clear that class II containing CLIP is the only substrate for DM, since DM can remove larger invariant chain fragments as well. Intact invariant chain, in contrast, has been reported not to be removed by DM (Denzin and Cresswell, 1995).

## D. Compartments for Peptide Loading

Where does invariant chain deliver class II and where does class II acquire peptides? Electron microscopy has revealed the existence of morphological class II-rich compartments in B cells, called MIIC (MHC class II compartment) (Peters *et al.*, 1991). These compartments have multivesicular or multilamellar appearance and beside class II they contain lysosomal markers, including lysosomal proteases and lysosome-associated membrane proteins (lamps). Similar structures (without class II) have been described previously in other cell types as prelysosomes (Griffiths *et al.*, 1988), and it appears that the MIIC is closely related to these structures. Interestingly, expression of only class II $\alpha$ and $\beta$ chains appears to induce MIIC formation in transfected human kidney cells (Calafat *et al.*, 1994). Morphologic studies cannot prove, however, whether the MIIC are involved in class II peptide loading; a number of groups have used different subcellular fractionation methods in order to characterize biochemically the compartments where class II molecules acquire peptides (Amigorena *et al.*, 1994; Castellino and Germain, 1995; Qiu *et al.*, 1994; Tulp *et al.*, 1994; West *et al.*, 1994). The results of these studies do not give a clear answer, and it appears that different cell types and different separation techniques may influence the conclusions reached. Thus, while several studies have indicated dense lysosome-like compartments, possibly MIIC, to be responsible for peptide loading in different cell lines (Qiu *et al.*, 1994; Tulp *et al.*, 1994; West *et al.*, 1994), two studies using the same murine B lymphoma, A20, but different methodologies, both found markers for early endosomes in the assigned loading compartments (Amigorena *et al.*, 1994; Barnes and Mitchell, 1995). Electron microscopy confirmed that the isolated compartments were not MIIC in this case (Amigorena *et al.*, 1994). Castellino and Germain (1995) come to the conclusion that there is no distinct loading compartment, but that class II can acquire peptides throughout the endocytic pathway. Their experiments are difficult to interpret, though, since they were made with spleen cells containing a mixture of different cell types and cells in different stages of activation. The data from West *et al.* (1994) suggest that a portion of the class II which does become loaded with peptide in dense compartments never reaches the cell surface, but instead remains in dense intracellular compartments, raising the possibility that the MIIC or part of the MIIC population is a biosynthetic dead end. An indication that a peptide loading compartment is likely to be a relatively minor modification of existing endosomal compartments also comes from our finding that HeLa cells transiently transfected with class II, invariant chain, and H2-M are able to produce peptide-loaded class II molecules (Karlsson *et al.*, 1994). These data implicate that, in mammalian cells, class II, invariant chain, and H2-M are the minimally required specialized components necessary for efficient class II–peptide association. They do not exclude, however, that other molecules may be involved in modulating the peptide loading process, but do question the requirements for a specialized compartment of the endosomal–lysosomal pathway for class II loading.

Both H2-M and HLA-DM are largely absent from the cell surface; immuno-fluorescence microscopy has shown that H2-M is located mainly to lysosome-like structures when transfected by itself or with invariant chain, while electron microscopy has confirmed that HLA-DM is located to MIIC in B cell lines (Karls-son *et al.*, 1994; Sanderson *et al.*, 1994). Both HLA-DM$\beta$ and H2-M$\beta$ contain sequences in their cytoplasmic tails resembling the tyrosine-based endosomal tar-geting sequences seen in many other endosomal and lysosomal resident proteins (Trowbridge *et al.*, 1993); mutation of this tyrosine residue to an alanine resulted in surface expression of the H2-M mutant (Lindstedt *et al.*, 1995). Surprisingly, both endosomal localization and ability to induce peptide loading were restored in transfected cells expressing the truncated form of H2-M together with normal in-variant chain. In contrast to what has been reported for HLA-DM, we found that H2-M does associate with invariant chain, and it appears that the invariant chain targeting motif is sufficient to direct class II and truncated H2-M to compartments where class II loading can occur.

In conclusion, it is presently not clear where class II acquires peptides or whether all class II molecules get their peptides in the same compartment. Differ-ent antigens are likely to have different sensitivity to proteases and are probably degraded with unequal efficiency. Class II molecules may be able to bind sensitive antigens in early compartments, thus protecting them from further degradation, or these antigens will have to be protected and delivered to a specific class II loading compartment by other transport molecules. Alternatively, only relatively protease-resistant parts of antigens will survive long enough to reach a class II loading compartment, thus explaining why certain epitopes of a given antigen are more efficiently presented than other epitopes, despite the fact that peptides derived from both epitopes are equally capable of binding class II *in vitro*. Definite proof of where class II acquires peptides and how these are selected will require the establishment of *in vitro* systems where the delivery of loaded class II molecules to the cell surface from different isolated compartments can be monitored.

## IV. ANTIGEN PRESENTATION BY NONCLASSICAL CLASS I MOLECULES

A number of proteins have been found to be class I-related by virtue of their domain organization, structural homology, and association with $\beta$2-microglobulin. They are less polymorphic than class I molecules and are expressed at lower lev-els, and often display limited tissue distribution (Stroynowski and Fischer-Lindahl, 1994). They are called nonclassical class I molecules or class Ib, and although their function as antigen-presenting molecules has been widely suggested, it is far from certain in most cases. Though it can be argued that the large number of class I-like molecules encoded inside and outside the MHC are irrelevant as presenting molecules as most of the T cell reactivity in peripheral compartments is clearly restricted by normal class I and class II molecules, their importance could come from their potential involvement in antigen presentation in specific localizations, presentation of specific pathogens or peptides, or presentation of ligands other than the normal peptide antigens with which class I and II molecules deal. In this chapter, we will try to update what it is known about antigen presentation by nonclassical class I molecules from a molecular point of view. We will focus on the mouse system, as very little information is available regarding presentation and recognition of human nonclassical molecules. We will not discuss other molecules with structural homology to class I which are known not to be presenting antigen.

## A. Molecules Derived from the *Qa* Region of the MHC

Of the several molecules from the *Qa* region of the mouse, only Qa-2, encoded by the *Q6–Q9* genes, has been studied extensively. Expression of the membrane-bound isoform of Qa-2 is partially dependent on TAP proteins, which suggests that Qa-2 could require peptides derived from the class I processing pathway for its stable expression. Biochemical analysis of acid extracts from purified Qa-2[a] antigens encoded by genes *Q7* and *Q9* showed the presence of bound peptides, suggesting that Qa-2 is functionally similar to class I molecules (Rötzschke *et al.*, 1993). Protein sequencing of pooled, eluted peptides suggested that these were nonamers with main anchor residues at positions 7 and 9 with several auxiliary anchor residues. This analysis was corroborated by the study of a soluble isoform, Q7[b], which was also shown to be associated mostly with nonameric peptides (Joyce *et al.*, 1994). The number of different peptides bound to Qa-2 was estimated to be at least 200, thus in a range similar to that for class I molecules (200–1000) (Hunt *et al.*, 1992). All identified peptides derived from known sequences corresponded to endogenous proteins of cytosolic localization, which again suggests that Qa-2 acquires peptides by the normal class I processing pathway. Surprisingly, no T cell responses restricted by Qa-2 have been described.

## B. Molecules Derived from the *Tla* Region of the MHC

A variable number of genes are encoded in the *Tla* region of the mouse MHC depending on the strain analyzed, but no human equivalents have been found. *Tla* genes range from pseudogenes and genes which are transcriptionally silent or where the RNA transcripts are poorly spliced to genes with a restricted pattern of expression (the TL antigen, encoded by the *T3[d]/T18[d]* gene pair) and genes transcribed in most tissues (represented by *T10/T22*) (Eghtesady *et al.*, 1992).

Although T-cell responses to *Tla* products have been reported (Bonneville *et al.*, 1989; Ito *et al.*, 1990) and TL binds CD8, the accessory molecule involved in class I recognition (Teitell *et al.*, 1991), the presenting properties of *Tla* antigens are debatable and have been proved only in a few cases.

The putative peptide-presenting properties of TL antigen (*T3[d]*) have been studied biochemically. Analysis of acid-extracted material from purified TL molecules expressed in transfected cell lines did not contain any identifiable peptides (H. R. Holcombe, unpublished). Screening of peptide display phage libraries with soluble TL, a technique that has proved useful for analyzing peptide binding properties of other classical and nonclassical class I and class II molecules (Castaño et al., 1995; Hammer et al., 1992, 1993; Miller et al., manuscript in preparation) failed to select any specific phage clones, which questions the peptide binding capacity of TL (A. R. Castaño and J. E. W. Miller, unpublished). Furthermore, TL is transported out of the ER in the absence of TAP proteins, indicating that TL is not loaded with cytosolic peptides (Holcombe et al., 1995). It is conceivable that the complex of TL and $\beta$2-microglobulin could acquire peptides from a distinct processing pathway. This does not seem to be the case, however, as peptide-free TL/$\beta$2-microglobulin complexes expressed in *Drosophila melanogaster* are stable to thermal denaturation at physiological temperatures, which would allow their transport and expression at the cell surface without the requirement for peptide binding. Recognition by T cells expressing $\gamma\delta$ T cell receptors of the *Tla* gene product T22 was similarly independent of TAP and seemed not to be affected by the absence of conventional antigenic peptides (Schild et al., 1994; Weintraub et al., 1994).

The only well-characterized example of antigen presentation by a *Tla* product is the presentation by the $T23^b$ gene product. This gene encodes the inappropriately named Qa-1$^b$ (Qa-1.2) antigen (Wolf and Cook, 1990), to which a number of T-cell responses have been described. Aldrich et al., (1994) have demonstrated that about 30% of the Qa-1 determinants defined by allogeneic T cells are due to the presentation by Qa-1 of a nonamer peptide derived from the signal sequence of the $D^d$ or $L^d$ class I antigens. Peptide presentation by Qa-1 displays features similar to normal class I presentation not only regarding the length of the peptide, but also in its dependence on the TAP transporters.

In summary, although recognition of *Tla* gene products by T cells has been documented, peptide presentation ability seems doubtful for some antigens, such as TL and T10/T22, while other *Tla*-encoded molecules seem to bind and present a small repertoire of peptides. Nonpeptide antigens have been reported to be presented to T cells, and it is an open question whether *Tla*-derived molecules are the presenting elements in some of these cases (Morita et al., 1994; Beckman et al., 1994; Constant et al., 1994).

## C. The H2–M3 Molecule

Telomeric to the *Qa–Tla* region lies the *H2–M* region (which is not identical with the H2-M region involved in class II presentation), which harbors at least eight genes, four of which are pseudogenes (*M4*, *M6*, *M7*, and *M8*), and two of which (*M1* and *M5*) have not been shown to be transcribed. *M2* is transcribed at low levels in the thymus and *M3* is well expressed in many tissues (Wang and Fischer-Lindahl, 1993). *H2–M3* encodes the presenting molecule of the maternally transmitted factor (Wang *et al.*, 1991), an N-formylated peptide derived from the ND1 subunit of the NADH mitochondrial dehydrogenase (Loveland *et al.*, 1990; Shawar *et al.*, 1990), which constitutes the maternally transmitted antigen (Mta) defined by cytotoxic T cells (Fischer-Lindahl *et al.*, 1986). Subsequent analysis of the presenting capabilities of the M3 molecule showed a unique specificity for formylated peptides (Vyas *et al.*, 1992). The 13 proteins encoded in the mitochondrial genome, ND1 being one of them, are the only mammalian proteins containing N-formyl methionine, while formyl-methionine is the amino acid used to initiate protein synthesis in prokaryotes, suggesting a putative role for M3 in presenting bacterial antigens to cytotoxic T cells. Such a role has been demonstrated by the presentation of formylated peptides of bacterial origin to specific cytotoxic T cells after infection with *Listeria monocytogenes* (Kurlander *et al.*, 1992; Pamer *et al.*, 1992). Thus, M3 constitute the first example of an MHC molecule specifically adapted to deal with specific pathogens. The molecular basis for that specific function has been shown with the determination of the three-dimensional structure of a complex between M3 and a ND1-derived peptide (see below) (Wang *et al.*, 1995). Little is known about the processing pathway for formylated peptides, but the low level of M3 reactivity in RMA-S, a cell line which lacks functional peptide transporters, suggests that peptide binding occurs in the ER and that peptides are translocated by the TAPs (Hermel *et al.*, 1991).

## D. CD1 Molecules

CD1 comprise a heterogeneous group of nonpolymorphic molecules encoded outside the MHC. Two CD1 genes on mouse chromosome 3 and five CD1 genes on human chromosome 1 encode two groups of proteins remotely homologous to both class I and class II MHC molecules. Several reports have described T cell lines (using either $\alpha\beta$ or $\gamma\delta$ receptors) reacting to different CD1 molecules (Balk *et al.*, 1991; Porcelli *et al.*, 1989). In one case a human CD1 molecule (CD1b) was able to present antigens from *Mycobacterium tuberculosis* extracts to $\alpha\beta$ T cells (Porcelli *et al.*, 1992). Surprisingly, the antigen recognized by this T cell line seems to be a processed form of mycolic acid, a lipid exclusive to the cell wall of mycobacteria (Beckman *et al.*, 1994), suggesting that CD1b could bind and present lipids, as class I molecules present peptides. Other T cell lines have subsequently been shown to recognize metabolites from another mycobacterial glycolipid, lipoarabinomannan, in the context of CD1b (Sieling *et al.*, 1995). The structures of the mycobacterial compounds are quite different and it remains to be elucidated which are the specific structures actually bound and presented by CD1b. We have used random peptide phage display technique and synthetic peptides to analyze the peptide-binding capacity of murine CD1, which is less than 40% homologous in its $\alpha1\alpha2$ domains to human CD1b. We found that murine CD1 is able to bind peptides with similar characteristics to MHC class I and class II molecules (see below) (Castaño *et al.*, 1995). Furthermore, we were able to generate peptide-specific CD1-restricted T-cell responses, indicating the immunological relevance of the peptide binding and establishing that murine CD1 can indeed be an antigen-presenting molecule which can present a unique set of peptides with hydrophobic characteristics. It is presently not known whether the human CD1 molecules, especially CD1d, the human counterpart of murine CD1, are able to present peptides or if mouse CD1, besides binding peptides, is also able to bind lipids. Little is known about the antigen-processing pathway for CD1 presentation, but it appears that lysosomal acidification is required for presentation by CD1b (Sieling et al., 1995), as is the case for class II presentation. CD1 expression is also independent of the TAP transporters (Hanau et al., 1994; Teitell et al., 1995) and does probably not require binding of peptides, as the complex of CD1 and $\beta$2-microglobulin is intrinsically stable to thermal denaturation at physiological temperatures (A. R. Castaño, unpublished).

## V. PEPTIDE BINDING BY CLASS I, CLASS II, AND NONCLASSICAL CLASS I MOLECULES

Considering their overall similarity, it is not surprising that the peptide binding grooves of class I and class II molecules are similar to each other (Figs. 3A and 3B). Closer analysis, made possible by the availability of several class I crystal structures and one class II crystal structure, does reveal distinct differences, however, regarding both the shape of the grooves and the way peptides are anchored in them (Björkman et al., 1987a,b; Brown et al., 1993; Fremont et al., 1992; Madden et al., 1992, 1993; Matsumura et al., 1992; Stern et al., 1994).

The peptide binding site of class I molecules is formed by the $\alpha 1$ and $\alpha 2$ domains of the heavy chain, which fold to form a base of $\beta$ sheets with two $\alpha$ helices located on top. Peptides bind to the groove formed between these two helices. In class I molecules the groove is closed at both ends, in one end by the formation of a salt bridge between the two helices and a ring of conserved tyrosine residues which bind to the N-terminus of the peptide, and in the other end of the groove by a conserved triad of amino acids which bind the C-terminus of the peptide (Fremont et al., 1992). The fact that the groove is closed explains why short peptides, between 8 and 10 amino acids, are preferred for class I binding. Some length differences can be accommodated by the peptide bulging out in the middle (Fremont et al., 1992; Guo et al., 1992), but distinctly longer peptides can only bind by extending out of the pocket (Collins et al., 1994). In general this is less favorable and is thought to occur infrequently, except in certain class I molecules. Peptide binding specificity is achieved by pockets in the peptide binding groove with geometrical and chemical complementary for some of the side chains of the peptide. The location and specificity of the pockets explain the differences in binding specificity for different class I molecules. Some of the pockets are highly specific, and peptide residues that fit in these pockets (i.e., anchor residues) are important for peptide binding. They do not constitute an absolute requirement

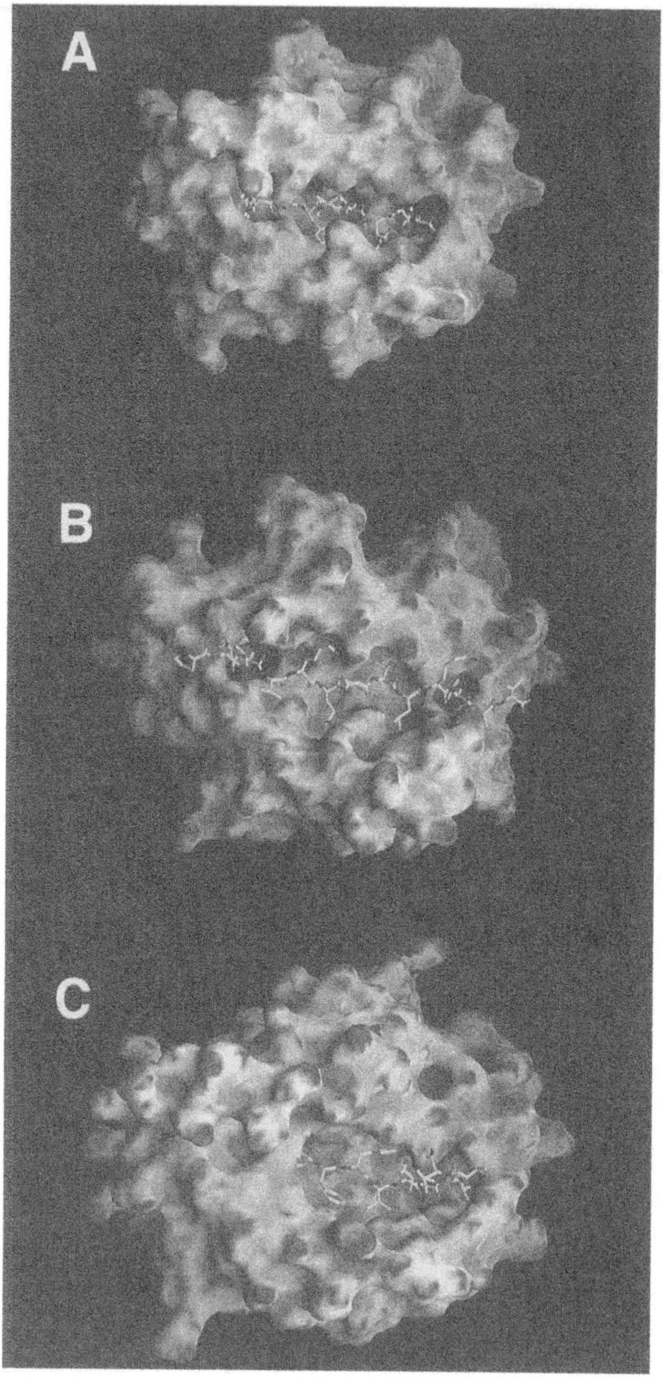
A
B
C

for binding, however, as peptides without anchor residues can occasionally bind with strong affinity. In addition to the specific anchor residues, the N- and C-termini of the peptides are important for binding to the class I molecule and they normally also are buried in binding pockets (Matsamura *et al.,* 1992). Crystal structures of the same class I molecule associated with different peptides have revealed that a relatively small part of the peptide protrudes from the surface of the class I molecule, but also that binding of different peptides induces structural differences in the class I molecules themselves (Fremont *et al.,* 1992). The combined surface created by a particular class I–peptide combination, rather than only the peptide, is therefore likely to be what the T-cell receptor recognizes.

The binding site in class II molecules is derived from the $\alpha 1$ and $\beta 1$ domains of the class II molecule and, like the site in class I molecules, it is formed by two helices on top of a $\beta$ sheet. In contrast to the situation in class I, however, the class II groove is not closed off at the ends and instead the peptides bound to class II can extend out of the pocket at both ends (Brown *et al.,* 1993; Rudensky *et al.,* 1991; Stern *et al.,* 1994). This means that there are no strict size limitations on the peptides bound to class II and that longer peptides or even small proteins can bind (Sette *et al.,* 1989). The fact that the peptide protrudes out of the binding pocket can also allow for *in situ* trimming of the ends by exoproteases, or in the case of invariant chain removal, for degradation of the invariant chain while the CLIP region remains protected by its location in the peptide binding groove.

The class II molecule for which the crystal structure has been determined (HLA-DR1) has only one highly specific binding pocket, while several other shallow pockets contribute to the binding specificity (Stern *et al.,* 1994). Since the N- and C-termini are not anchored, they do not contribute to the binding affinity and peptide binding to class II is instead determined by a single anchor position and a large number of sequence-independent interactions with the backbone of the peptide. Class II proteins can therefore accommodate a large number of different peptides by compensating for unfavorable interaction in one or more shallow pockets with favorable interactions elsewhere along the peptide.

Peptide binding by class Ib molecules most likely cannot be enclosed in a common category, since different molecules have different properties, but two molecules have been analyzed with enough detail to be discussed here.

The three-dimensional structure of the M3 molecule, in association with a peptide derived from ND1, shows that the pocket which accommodates the N-terminus of the peptide in class I molecules is occluded by a general rearrangement of

---

FIGURE 3. Three-dimensional structures of MHC molecules/peptide complexes. (A) H2–K$^b$ class I molecule with a vesicular stomatitis virus peptide (Fremont *et al.,* 1992); (B) HLA–DR1 class II molecule with an influenza virus peptide (Stern *et al.,* 1994); (C) H2–M3 class Ib molecule with the fND1 peptide (Wang *et al.,* 1995). The view is from the top of the molecules showing the molecular surface of the MHC-presenting molecule and the C$\alpha$ and side-chain atoms of the specific bound peptides.

the side chains of the amino acids in the wall of the pocket (compare Fig. 3A with Fig. 3C). Instead, the formylated N-terminus is accommodated in a pocket more centrally located in the groove, where the formyl group is held by a network of hydrogen bonds involving five amino acid residues and a water molecule. The methionine side chain is completely buried in the same pocket (Wang *et al.*, 1995). The other end of the groove accommodates peptides of different lengths, as opposed to class I molecules, and the C-terminus extends out of the groove. The first four residues of the peptide contribute most to the binding affinity, which explains why short peptides are able to bind (Vyas *et al.*, 1995). No specificity besides the N-formyl methionine seems to be required for peptide binding by M3, but aromatic residues are preferred in position 2 (A. R. Castaño and J. E. W. Miller, unpublished) and hydrophobic residues are favored in general as the peptide binding groove is significantly more hydrophobic than the class I binding groove.

Peptide binding to murine CD1 has been characterized biochemically. This molecule is able to bind peptides containing a stringent motif consisting of an aromatic residue in position 1, a long aliphatic residue in position 4, and a tryptophan in position 7 (Castaño *et al.*, 1995). Peptide binding is similar to binding by class II molecules in that long peptides are required, with both N and C termini hanging out from the peptide binding groove. Resemblance to peptide binding by class I comes from the selectivity of the three anchor positions, mutations of which highly impair binding to CD1, as is the case with class I–peptide interactions. Therefore, peptide binding to mouse CD1 seems to have distinct characteristics with features of peptide binding both to class I and class II, in concordance with its similar level of homology to both MHC molecules.

## VI. Conclusions

The antigen-processing pathways for class I and class II are surprisingly different considering that T cells expressing the same type of T cell receptors (but different coreceptor molecules) can react either with peptide–class I complexes or with peptide–class II complexes. The processing pathway for class I molecules is presently better understood, partly due to the fact that most of the major events occur in the ER which is better known and easier to access than the endosomal system where class II antigen processing occurs. Class II processing is intensely studied, however; several recent reports have made progress in trying to define where class II molecules acquire peptides and which molecules are involved in this process. The coming years will undoubtedly reveal more details on how class I, class II, and nonclassical class I molecules acquire their ligands and how these are presented to T cells.

## Acknowledgments

We thank M. Jackson and Z. Zeng for help with graphics.

## REFERENCES

Aldrich, C. J., DeCloux, A., Woods, A. S., Cotter, R. J., Soloski, M. J., and Forman, J. (1994). Identification of a tap-dependent leader peptide recognized by alloreactive T cells specific for a class Ib antigen. *Cell (Cambridge, Mass.)* **79,** 649–658.

Amigorena, S., Drake, J. R., Webster, P., and Mellman, I. (1994). Transient accumulation of new class II MHC molecules in a novel endocytic compartment in B lymphocytes. *Nature (London)* **369,** 113–120.

Anderson, M. S., and Miller, J. (1992). Invariant chain can function as a chaperone protein for class II major histocompatibility complex molecules. *Proc. Natl. Acad. Sci. U.S.A.* **89,** 2282–2286.

Androlewicz, M. J., Anderson, K. S., and Cresswell, P. (1993). Evidence that transporters associated with antigen processing translocate a major histocompatibility complex class I-binding peptide into the endoplasmic reticulum in an ATP-dependent manner. *Proc. Natl. Acad. Sci. U.S.A.* **90,** 9130–9134.

Baas, E. J., van Santen, H. M., Kleijmeer, M. J., Geuze, H. J., Peters, P. J., and Ploegh, H. L. (1992). Peptide-induced stabilization and intracellular localization of empty HLA class I complexes. *J. Exp. Med.* **176,** 147–156.

Bakke, O., and Dobberstein, B. (1990). MHC class II-associated invariant chain contains a sorting signal for endosomal compartments. *Cell (Cambridge, Mass.)* **63,** 707–716.

Balk, S. P., Ebert, E. C., Blumenthal, R. L., McDermott, F. V., Wucherpfenning, K. W., Landau, S. B., and Blumberg, R. S. (1991). Oligoclonal expansion and CD1 recognition by human intestinal intraepithelial lymphocytes. *Science* **253,** 1411–1414.

Barber, L. D., and Parham, P. (1993). Peptide binding to major histocompatibility complex molecules. *Annu. Rev. Cell Biol.* **9,** 163–206.

Barnes, K. A., and Mitchell, R. N. (1995). Detection of functional class II-associated antigen: Role of a low density endosomal compartment in antigen processing. *J. Exp. Med.* **181,** 1715–1727.

Beckman, E. M., Porcelli, S. A., Morita, C. T., Behar, S. M., Furlong, S. T., and Brenner, M. B. (1994). Recognition of a lipid antigen by CD1-restricted $\alpha\beta^+$ T cells. *Nature (London)* **372,** 691–694.

Bennett, K., Levine, T., Ellis, J. S., Peanasky, R. J., Samloff, I. M., Kay, J., and Chain, B. M. (1992). Antigen processing for presentation by class II major histocompatibility complex requires cleavage by cathepsin E. *Eur. J. Immunol.* **22,** 1519–1524.

Bikoff, E. K., Huang, L. Y., Episkopou, V., van Meerwijk, J., Germain, R. N., and Robertson, E. J. (1993). Defective major histocompatibility complex class II assembly, transport, peptide acquisition, and $CD4^+$ T cell selection in mice lacking invariant chain expression. *J. Exp. Med.* **177,** 1699–1712.

Björkman, P. J., Saper, M. A., Samraoui, B., Bennett, W. S., Strominger, J. S., and Wiley, D. (1987a). Structure of the human class I antigen, HLA-A2. *Nature (London)* **329,** 506–512.

Björkman, P. J., Saper, M. A., Samraoui, B., Bennett, W. S., Strominger, J. S., and Wiley, D. (1987b). The foreign antigen binding site and T cell recognition regions of class I histocompatibility antigens. *Nature (London)* **329,** 512–518.

Blum, J. S., and Cresswell, P. (1988). Role for intracellular proteases in the processing and transport of class II HLA antigens. *Proc. Natl. Acad. Sci. U.S.A.* **85,** 3975–3979.

Bonnerot, C., Marks, M. S., Cosson, P., Robertson, E. J., Bikoff, E. K., Germain, R. N., and Bonifacino, J. S. (1994). Association with BiP and aggregation of class II MHC molecules synthesized in the absence of invariant chain. *EMBO J.* **13,** 934–944.

Bonneville, M., Ito, K., Krecko, E. G., Itohara, S., Kappes, D., Ishida, I., Kanawa, O., Jaeway, C. A., Jr., Murphy, D. B., and Tonegawa, S. (1989). Recognition of a self major histocompatibility complex TL region product by $\gamma\delta$ T-cell receptors. *Proc. Natl. Acad. Sci. U.S.A.* **86,** 5928–5932.

Bremnes, B., Madsen, T., Gedde-Dahl, M., and Bakke, O. (1994). An LI and ML motif in the cytoplasmic tail of the MHC-associated invariant chain mediate rapid internalization. *J. Cell Sci.* **107,** 2021–2032.

Brown, J. H., Jardetzky, T. S., Gorga, J. C., Stern, L. J., Urban, R. G., Strominger, J. L., and Wiley, D. C. (1993). Three-dimensional structure of the human class II histocompatibility antigen HLA-DR1. *Nature (London)* **364**, 33–39.

Busch, R., Vturina, I. Y., Drexler, J., Momburg, F., and Hämmerling, G. J. (1995). Poor loading of major histocompatibility complex class II molecules with endogenously synthesized short peptides in the absence of invariant chain. *Eur. J. Immunol.* **25**, 48–53.

Calafat, J., Nijenhuis, M., Janssen, H., Tulp, A., Dusselje, S., Wubbolts, R., and Neefjes, J. (1994). Major histocompatibility complex class II molecules induce the formation of endocytic MIIC-like structures. *J. Cell Biol.* **126**, 967–977.

Castaño, A. R., Tangri, S., Miller, J. E. W., Holcombe, H. R., Jackson, M. R., Huse, W. D., Kronenberg, M., and Peterson, P. A. (1995). Peptide binding and presentation by mouse CD1. *Science* **269**, 223–226.

Castellino, F., and Germain, R. N. (1995). Extensive trafficking of MHC class II-invariant chain complexes in the endocytic pathway and appearance of peptide-loaded class II in multiple compartments. *Immunity* **2**, 73–88.

Ceman, S., Rudersdorf, R., Long, E. O., and Demars, R. (1992). MHC class II deletion mutant expresses normal levels of transgene encoded class II molecules that have abnormal conformation and impaired antigen presentation ability. *J. Immunol.* **149**, 754–761.

Ciechanover, A. (1994). The ubiquitin–proteasome proteolytic pathway. *Cell (Cambridge, Mass.)* **79**, 13–21.

Collins, E. J., Garboczi, D. N., and Wiley, D. C. (1994). Three-dimensional structure of a peptide extending from one end of a class I binding site. *Nature (London)* **371**, 626–629.

Constant, P., Davodeu, F., Peyrat, M. A., Poquet, Y., Puzo, G., Bonneville, M., and Fournié, J.J. (1994). Stimulation of human γδ T cells by nonpeptidic mycobacterial ligands. *Science* **264**, 267–270.

Cresswell, P. (1994). Assembly, transport, and function of MHC class II molecules. *Annu. Rev. Immunol.* **12**, 259–293.

Degen, E., and Williams, D. B. (1991). Participation of a novel 88-kD protein in the biogenesis of murine class I histocompatibility molecules. *J. Cell Biol.* **112**, 1099–1115.

Denzin, L. K., and Cresswell, P. (1995). HLA-DM induces CLIP dissociation from MHC class II αβ dimers and facilitates peptide loading. *Cell (Cambridge, Mass.)* **82**, 155–165.

Denzin, L. K., Robbins, N. F., Carboy-Newcomb, C., and Cresswell, P. (1994). Assembly and intracellular transport of HLA-DM and correction of the class II antigen processing defect in T2 cells. *Immunity* **1**, 595–606.

Deverson, E. V., Gow, I. R., Coadwell, W. J., Monaco, J. J., Butcher, G. W., and Howard, J. C. (1990). MHC class II region encoding proteins related to the multidrug resistance family of transmembrane transporters. *Nature (London)* **348**, 738–741.

Dodi, A. I., Brett, S., Nordeng, T., Sidhu, S., Batchelor, R. J., Lombardi, G., Bakke, O., and Lechler, R. I. (1994). The invariant chain inhibits presentation of endogenous antigens by a human fibroblast cell line. *Eur. J. Immunol.* **24**, 1632–1639.

Eghtesady, P., Brorson, K. A., Cheroutre, H., Tigelaar, R. E., Hood, L., and Kronenberg, M. (1992). Expression of mouse *Tla* region class I genes in tissues enriched for gammadelta cells. *Immunogenetics*, 377–388.

Falo, L., Jr., Colarusso, L. J., Benacerraf, B., Rock, K. L., Rock, K. L., Couderc, J., Mouton, D., and Benacerral, B. (1992). Serum proteases alter the antigenicity of peptides presented by class I major histocompatibility complex molecules. Processing and presentation of ovalbumin in mice genetically selected for antibody response. Diversity in MHC class II ovalbumin T cell epitopes generated by distinct proteases. *J. Immunol.* **149**, 8347–8350.

Fischer-Lindahl, K., Hausmann, B., Robinson, P. J., Guenet, J. L., Wharton, D. C., and Winking, H. (1986). Mta, the maternally transmitted antigen, is determined jointly by chromosomal *Hmt* and the extrachromosomal *Mtf* genes. *J. Exp. Med.* **163**, 334–346.

Fling, S. P., Arp, B., and Pious, D. (1994). *HLA-DMA* and *-DMB* genes are both required for MHC class II/peptide complex formation in antigen-presenting cells. *Nature (London)* **368**, 554–558.

Fremont, D. H., Matsumura, M., Stura, E. A., Peterson, P. A., and Wilson, I. A. (1992). Crystal structures of two viral peptides in complex with murine MHC class I H-2Kb. *Science* **257**, 919–927.

Germain, R. N. (1994). MHC-dependent antigen processing and peptide presentation: Providing ligands for T lymphocyte activation. *Cell (Cambridge, Mass.)* **76**, 287–299.

Goldberg, A. L., and Rock, K. L. (1992). Proteolysis, proteasomes and antigen presentation. *Nature (London)* **357**, 375–379.

Griffiths, G., Hoflack, B., Simons, K., Mellman, I., and Kornfeld, S. (1988). The mannose 6-phosphate receptor and the biogenesis of lysosomes. *Cell (Cambridge, Mass.)* **52**, 329–341.

Guo, H. C., Jardetzky, T. S., Garrett, T. P., Lane, W. S., Strominger, J. L., and Wiley, D. C. (1992). Different length peptides bind to HLA-Aw68 similarly at their ends but bulge out in the middle. *Nature (London)* **360**, 364–366.

Hammer, J., Takacs, B., and Sinigaglia, F. (1992). Identification of a motif for HLA-DR1 binding peptides using M13 display libraries. *J. Exp. Med.* **176**, 1007–1013.

Hammer, J., Valsasnini, P., Tolba, K., Bolin, D., Higelin, J., Takacs, B., and Sinigaglia, F. (1993). Promiscuous and allele-specific anchors in HLA-DR-binding peptides. *Cell (Cambridge, Mass.)* **74**, 197–203.

Hanau, D., Fricker, D., Bieber, T., Esposito-Farese, M. E., Bausinger, H., Cazenave, J. P., Donato, L., Tongio, M. M., and De la Salle, H. (1994). CD1 expression is not affected by human peptide transporter deficiency. *Hum. Immunol.* **41**, 61–68.

Heemels, M. T., Schumacher, T. N., Wonigeit, K., and Ploegh, H. L. (1993). Peptide translocation by variants of the transporter associated with antigen processing. *Science* **262**, 2059–2063.

Hermel, E., Grigorenko, E., and Fischer-Lindahl, K. (1991). Expression of medial class I histocompatibility antigens on RMA-S mutant cells. *Int. Immunol.* **3**, 407–412.

Holcombe, H. R., Castaño, A. R., Cheroutre, H., Teitell, M., Maher, J. K., Peterson, P. A., and Kronenberg, M. (1995). Nonclassical behaviour of the thymus leukemia antigen, peptide transporter-independent expression of a nonclassical class I molecule. *J. Exp. Med.* **181**, 1433–1443.

Hunt, D. F., Henderson, R. A., Shabanowitz, J., Sakaguchi, K., Michel, H., Sevilir, N., Cox, A. L., Apella, E., and Engelhard, V. (1992). Characterization of peptides bound to the class I MHC molecule HLA-A2.1 by mass spectrometry. *Science* **255**, 1261–1263.

Ito, K., Van Kaer, L., Bonneville, M., Hsu, S., Murphy, D. B., and Tonegawa, S. (1990). Recognition of the product of a novel MHC TL region gene (27b) by a mouse $\gamma\delta$ T cell receptor. *Cell (Cambridge, Mass.)* **62**, 549–561.

Jackson, M. R., and Peterson, P. A. (1993). Assembly and intracellular transport of MHC class I molecules. *Annu. Rev. Cell Biol.* **9**, 207–235.

Jackson, M. R., Nilsson, T., and Peterson, P. A. (1990). Identification of a consensus motif for retention of transmembrane proteins in the endoplasmic reticulum. *EMBO J.* **9**, 3153–3162.

Jackson, M. R., Song, E. S., Yang, Y., and Peterson, P. A. (1992). Empty and peptide-containing conformers of class I major histocompatibility complex molecules expressed in *Drosophila melanogaster* cells. *Proc. Natl. Acad. Sci. U.S.A.* **89**, 12117–12121.

Joyce, S., Tabaczewski, P., Angeletti, R. H., Nathenson, S. G., and Stroynowski, I. (1994). A nonpolymorphic major histocompatibility complex class Ib molecule binds a large array of diverse self-peptides. *J. Exp. Med.* **179**, 579–588.

Karlsson, L., Péléraux, A., Lindstedt, R., Liljedahl, M., and Peterson, P. A. (1994). Reconstitution of an operational MHC class II compartment in nonantigen-presenting cells. *Science* **266**, 1569–1573.

Kurlander, R. J., Shawar, S. M., Brown, M. L., and Rich, R. R. (1992). Specialized role for a murine class I-b MHC molecule in prokaryotic host defenses. *Science* **257**, 678–679.

Kvist, S., Wiman, K., Claesson, L., Peterson, P. A., and Dobberstein, B. (1982). Membrane insertion and oligomeric assembly of HLA-DR histocompatibility antigens. *Cell (Cambridge, Mass.)* **29**, 61–69.

Lamb, C. A., and Cresswell, P. (1992). Assembly and transport properties of invariant chain trimers and HLA-DR-invariant chain complexes. *J. Immunol.* **148,** 3478–3482.

Letourneur, F., and Klausner, R. D. (1992). A novel di-leucine motif and a tyrosine-based motif independently mediate lysosomal targeting and endocytosis of CD3 chains. *Cell (Cambridge, Mass.)* **69,** 1143–1157.

Letourneur, F., Hennecke, S., Demolliere, C., and Cosson, P. (1995). Steric masking of a dilysine endoplasmic reticulum retention motif during assembly of the human high affinity receptor for immunoglobulin E. *J. Cell Biol.* **129,** 971–978.

Lindstedt, R., Liljedahl, M., Péléraux, A., Peterson, P. A., and Karlsson, L. (1995). The MHC class II molecule H-2M is targeted to an endosomal compartment by a tyrosine-based targeting motif. Submitted.

Livingstone, A. M., Powis, S. J., Diamond, A. G., Butcher, G. W., and Howard, J. C. (1989). A transacting major histocompatibility complex-linked gene whose alleles determine gain and loss changes in the antigenic structure of a classical class I molecule. *J. Exp. Med.* **170,** 777–795.

Ljunggren, H. G., Stam, N. J., Ohlen, C., Neefjes, J. J., Hoglund, P., Heemels, M. T., Bastin, J., Schumacher, T. N., Townsend, A., and Kärre, K. (1990). Empty MHC class I molecules come out in the cold. *Nature (London)* **346,** 476–480.

Lotteau, V., Teyton, L., Peleraux, A., Nilsson, T., Karlsson, L., Schmid, S. L., Quaranta, V., and Peterson, P. A. (1990). Intracellular transport of class II MHC molecules directed by invariant chain. *Nature (London)* **348,** 600–605.

Loveland, B., Wang, C.-R., Yonekawa, H., Hermel, E., and Fischer-Lindahl, K. (1990). Maternally transmitted histocompatibility antigen of mice, a hydrophobic peptide of a mitochondrially encoded protein. *Cell (Cambridge, Mass.)* **60,** 971–980.

Machamer, C. E., and Cresswell, P. (1984). Monensin prevents terminal glycosylation of the N- and O-linked oligosaccharides of the HLA-DR-associated invariant chain and inhibits its dissociation from the alpha–beta chain complex. *Proc. Natl. Acad. Sci. U.S.A.* **81,** 1287–1291.

Madden, D. R., Gorga, J. C., Strominger, J. L., and Wiley, D. C. (1992). The three-dimensional structure of HLA-B27 at 2.1 A resolution suggests a general mechanism for tight peptide binding to MHC. *Cell (Cambridge, Mass.)* **70,** 1035–1048.

Madden, D. R., Garboczi, D. N., and Wiley, D. C. (1993). The antigenic identity of peptide-MHC complexes: A comparison of the conformations of five viral peptides presented by HLA-A2. *Cell (Cambridge, Mass.)* **75,** 693–708.

Matsumura, M., Fremont, D. H., Peterson, P. A., and Wilson, I. A. (1992). Emerging principles for the recognition of peptide antigens by class I molecules. *Science* **257,** 927–934.

Mellins, E., Smith, L., Arp, B., Cotner, T., Celis, E., and Pious, D. (1990). Defective processing and presentation of exogenous antigens in mutants with normal HLA class II genes. *Nature (London)* **343,** 71–74.

Mellins, E., Cameron, P., Amaya, M., Goodman, S., Pious, D., Smith, L., and Arp, B. (1994). A mutant human histocompatibility leukocyte antigen DR molecule associated with invariant chain peptides. *J. Exp. Med.* **179,** 541–549.

Meyer, T. H., van Endert, P. M., Uebel, S., Ehring, B., and Tampe, R. (1994). Functional expression and purification of the ABC transporter complex associated with antigen processing (TAP) in insect cells. *Febs Lett.* **351,** 443–447.

Michaelek, M. T., Grant, E. P., Gramm, C., Goldberg, A. L., and Rock, K. L. (1993). A role for the ubiquitin dependent proteolytic pathway in MHC class I-restricted antigen presentation. *Nature (London)* **363,** 552–554.

Momburg, F., Roelse, J., Hammerling, G. J., and Neefjes, J. J. (1994a). Peptide size selection by the major histocompatibility complex-encoded peptide transporter. *J. Exp. Med.* **179,** 1613–1623.

Momburg, F., Roelse, J., Howard, J. C., Butcher, G. W., Hammerling, G. J., and Neefjes, J. J. (1994b). Selectivity of MHC-encoded peptide transporters from human, mouse and rat. *Nature (London)* **367,** 648–651.

Monaco, J. J., Cho, S., and Attaya, M. (1990). Transport protein genes in the murine MHC: Possible implications for antigen processing. *Science* **250,** 1723–1726.

Morita, A., Takahashi, T., Stockert, E., Nakayama, E., Tsuji, T., Matsudaira, Y., Old, L. J., and Obata, Y. (1994). TL antigen as a transplantation antigen recognized by TL-restricted cytotoxic T cells. *J. Exp. Med.* **179,** 777–784.

Morris, P., Shaman, J., Attaya, M., Amaya, M., Goodman, S., Bergman, C., Monaco, J. J., and Mellins, E. (1994). An essential role for HLA-DM in antigen presentation by class II major histocompatibility molecules. *Nature (London)* **368,** 551–554.

Morton, P. A., Zacheis, M. L., Giacoletto, K. S., Manning, J. A., and Schwartz, B. D. (1995). Delivery of nascent MHC class II-invariant chain complexes to lysosomal compartments and proteolysis of invariant chain by cysteine proteases precedes peptide binding in B-lymphoblastoid cells. *J. Immunol.* **154,** 137–150.

Neefjes, J. J., and Ploegh, H. L. (1992). Inhibition of endosomal proteolytic activity by leupeptin blocks surface expression of MHC class II molecules and their conversion to SDS resistance alpha beta heterodimers in endosomes. *EMBO J.* **11,** 411–416.

Neefjes, J. J., Stollorz, V., Peters, P. J., Geuze, H. J., and Ploegh, H. L. (1990). The biosynthetic pathway of MHC class II but not class I molecules intersects the endocytic route. *Cell (Cambridge, Mass.)* **61,** 171–183.

Neefjes, J. J., Momburg, F., and Hammerling, G. J. (1993). Selective and ATP-dependent translocation of peptides by the MHC-encoded transporter. *Science* **261,** 769–771.

Newcomb, J. R., and Cresswell, P. (1993). Structural analysis of proteolytic products of MHC class II-invariant chain complexes generated *in vivo. J. Immunol.* **151,** 4153–4163.

Nijenhuis, M., and Neefjes, J. (1994). Early events in the assembly of major histocompatibility complex class II heterotrimers from their free subunits. *Eur. J. Immunol.* **24,** 247–256.

Nossner, E., and Parham, P. (1995). Species-specific differences in chaperone interaction of human and mouse major histocompatibility complex class I molecules. *J. Exp. Med.* **181,** 327–337.

Odorizzi, C. G., Trowbridge, I. S., Xue, L., Hopkins, C. R., Davis, C. D., and Collawn, J. F. (1994). Sorting signals in the MHC class II invariant chain cytoplasmic tail and transmembrane region determine trafficking to an endocytic processing compartment. *J. Cell Biol.* **126,** 317–330.

Ogrinc, T., Dolenc, I., Ritonja, A., and Turk, V. (1993). Purification of a complex of cathepsin L and the MHC class II-associated invariant chain fragment from human kidney. *Febs Lett.* **336,** 555–559.

Ortmann, B., Androlewicz, M. J., and Cresswell, P. (1994). MHC class I/beta 2-microglobulin complexes associate with TAP transporters before peptide binding. *Nature (London)* **368,** 864–867.

Pamer, E. G., Wang, C.-R., Fischer Lindahl, K., and Bevan, M. J. (1992). H-2M3 presents a *Listeria monocytogenes* peptide to cytotoxic T lymphocytes. *Cell (Cambridge, Mass.)* **70,** 215–223.

Peters, P. J., Neefjes, J. J., Oorschot, V., Ploegh, H. L., and Geuze, H. J. (1991). Segregation of MHC class II molecules from MHC class I molecules in the Golgi complex for transport to lysosomal compartments. *Nature (London)* **349,** 669–676.

Peterson, M., and Miller, J. (1990). Invariant chain influences the immunological recognition of MHC class II molecules. *Nature (London)* **345,** 172–174.

Peterson, M., and Miller, J. (1992). Antigen presentation enhanced by the alternatively spliced invariant chain gene product p41. *Nature (London)* **357,** 596–598.

Pieters, J., Bakke, O., and Dobberstein, B. (1993). The MHC class II-associated invariant chain contains two endosomal targeting signals within its cytoplasmic tail. *J. Cell Sci.* **106,** 831–846.

Pond, L., Kuhn, L. A., Teyton, L., Schutze, M.-P., Tainer, J. A., Jackson, M. R., and Peterson, P. A. (1995). A role for acidic residues in di-leucine motif-based targeting to the endocytic pathway. *J. Biol. Chem.* **270,** 19989–19997.

Porcelli, S., Brenner, M. B., Greenstein, J. L., Balk, S. P., Terhorst, C., and Bleicher, P. A. (1989).

Recognition of cluster of differentiation 1 antigens by human CD4⁻CD8⁻ cytolytic T lymphocytes. *Nature (London)* **341,** 447–450.

Porcelli, S., Morita, C. T., and Brenner, M. B. (1992). CD1b restricts the response of human CD4⁻CD8⁻T lymphocytes to a microbial antigen. *Nature (London)* **360,** 593–597.

Qiu, Y., Xu, X., Wandinger-Ness, A., Dalke, D. P., and Pierce, S. K. (1994). Separation of subcellular compartments containing distinct functional forms of MHC class II. *J. Cell Biol.* **125,** 595–605.

Riberdy, J. M., Newcomb, J. R., Surman, M. J., Barbosa, J. A., and Cresswell, P. (1992). HLA-DR molecules from an antigen-processing mutant cell line are associated with invariant chain peptides. *Nature (London)* **360,** 474–477.

Roche, P. A., and Cresswell, P. (1990). Invariant chain association with HLA-DR molecules inhibits immunogenic peptide binding. *Nature (London)* **345,** 615–618.

Roche, P. A., Marks, M. S., and Cresswell, P. (1991). Formation of a nine-subunit complex by HLA class II glycoproteins and the invariant chain. *Nature (London)* **354,** 392–394.

Roche, P. A., Teletski, C. L., Stang, E., Bakke, O., and Long, E. O. (1993). Cell surface HLA-DR-invariant chain complexes are targeted to endosomes by rapid internalization. *Proc. Natl. Acad. Sci. U.S.A.* **90,** 8581–8585.

Romagnoli, P., Layet, C., Yewdell, J., Bakke, O., and Germain, R. N. (1993). Relationship between invariant chain expression and major histocompatibility complex class II transport into early and late endocytic compartments. *J. Exp. Med.* **177,** 583–596.

Rötzschke, O., Falk, K., Stevanovic, S., Grahovac, B., Soloski, M. J., Jung, G., and Rammensee, H. G. (1993). Qa-2 molecules are peptide receptors of higher stringency than ordinary class I molecules. *Nature (London)* **361,** 642–644.

Rudensky, A. Y., Preston-Hurlburt, P., Hong, S.-C., Barlow, A., and Janeway, Jr., C. A. (1991). Sequence analysis of peptides bound to MHC class II molecules. *Nature (London)* **353,** 622–628.

Sadegh-Nasseri, S., and Germain, R. N. (1991). A role for peptide in determining MHC class II structure. *Nature (London)* **353,** 167–170.

Salter, R. D., and Cresswell, P. (1986). Impaired assembly and transport of HLA-A and -B antigens in a mutant TxB cell hybrid. *EMBO J.* **5,** 943–949.

Sanderson, F., Kleijmeer, M. J., Kelly, A., Verwoerd, D., Tulp, A., Neefjes, J. J., Geuze, H. J., and Trowsdale, J. (1994). Accumulation of HLA-DM, a regulator of antigen presentation, in MHC class II compartments. *Science* **266,** 1566–1569.

Sandoval, I. V., and Bakke, O. (1994). Targeting of membrane proteins to endosomes and lysosomes. *Trends Cell Biol.* **4,** 292–297.

Schild, H., Mavaddat, N., Litzenberger, C., Ehrich, E. W., Davis, M. M., Bluestone, J. A., Matis, L., Draper, R. K., and Chien, Y. (1994). The nature of major histocompatibility complex recognition by gammadelta T cells. *Cell (Cambridge, Mass.)* **76,** 29–37.

Schumacher, T. N., Kantesaria, D. V., Heemels, M. T., Ashton-Rickardt, P. G., Shepherd, J. C., Fruh, K., Yang, Y., Peterson, P. A., Tonegawa, S., and Ploegh, H. L. (1994). Peptide length and sequence specificity of the mouse TAP1/TAP2 translocator. *J. Exp. Med.* **179,** 533–540.

Schutze, M. P., Peterson, P. A., and Jackson, M. R. (1994). An N-terminal double-arginine motif maintains type II membrane proteins in the endoplasmic reticulum. *EMBO J.* **13,** 1696–1705.

Scott, J. E., and Dawson, J. R. (1995). MHC class I expression and transport in a calnexin deficient cell line. *J. Immunol.* **155,** 143–148.

Sette, A., Adorini, L., Colon, S. M., Buus, S., and Grey, H. M. (1989). Capacity of intact proteins to bind to MHC class II molecules. *J. Immunol.* **143,** 1265–1267.

Shawar, S. M., Vyas, J. M., Rodgers, J. R., Cook, R. G., and Rich, R. R. (1990). Specialized functions of MHC class I molecules. II. Hmt binds N-formylated peptides of mitochondrial and prokaryotic origin. *J. Exp. Med.* **174,** 941–944.

Shepherd, J. C., Schumacher, T. N., Ashton-Rickardt, P. G., Imaeda, S., Ploegh, H. L., Janeway, C., Jr., and Tonegawa, S. (1993). TAP1-dependent peptide translocation *in vitro* is ATP dependent and peptide selective. *Cell (Cambridge, Mass.)* **74,** 577–584.

Sieling, P. A., Chatterjee, D., Porcelli, S. A., Prigozy, T. I., Mazzaccaro, R. J., Soriano, T., Bloom, B. R., Brenner, M. B., Kronenberg, M., Brennan, P. J., and Modlin, R. L. (1995). CD1-restricted T cell recognition of microbial lipoglycan antigens. *Science* **269**, 227–230.

Sloan, V. S., Cameron, P., Porter, G., Gammon, M., Amaya, M., Mellins, E., and Zaller, D. M. (1995). Mediation by HLA-DM of dissociation of peptides from HLA-DR. *Nature (London)* **375**, 802–806.

Spies, T., Bresnahan, M., Bahram, S., Arnold, D., Blanck, G., Mellins, E., Pious, D., and DeMars, R. (1990). A gene in the human major histocompatibility complex class II region controlling the class I antigen presentation pathway. *Nature (London)* **348**, 744–747.

Stern, L. J., and Wiley, D. C. (1992). The human class II MHC protein HLA-DR1 assembles as empty alpha beta heterodimers in the absence of antigenic peptide. *Cell (Cambridge, Mass.)* **68**, 465–477.

Stern, L. J., Brown, J. H., Jardetzky, T. S., Gorga, J. C., Urban, R. G., Strominger, J. L., and Wiley, D. C. (1994). Crystal structure of the human class II MHC protein HLA-DR1 complexed with an influenza virus peptide. *Nature (London)* **368**, 215–221.

Stroynowski, I., and Fischer-Lindahl, K. (1994). Antigen presentation by non-classical class I molecules. *Curr. Opin. Immunol.* **6**, 38–44.

Strubin, M., Berte, C., and Mach, B. (1986). Alternative splicing and alternative initiation of translation explain the four forms of the Ia antigen-associated invariant chain. *EMBO J.* **5**, 3483–3488.

Strubin, M., Long, E. O., and Mach, B. (1986). Two forms of the Ia antigen-associated invariant chain result from alternative initiations at two in-phase AUGs. *Cell (Cambridge, Mass.)* **47**, 619–625.

Suh, W. K., Cohen-Doyle, M. F., Fruh, K., Wang, K., Peterson, P. A., and Williams, D. B. (1994). Interaction of MHC class I molecules with the transporter associated with antigen processing. *Science* **264**, 1322–1326.

Teitell, M., Mescher, M. F., Olson, C. A., Littman, D. R., and Kronenberg, M. (1991). The thymus leukemia antigen binds human and mouse CD8. *J. Exp. Med.* **174**, 1131–1138.

Teitell, M., Holcombe, H. R., Jackson, M. R., Pond, L., Balk, S. P., Terhorst, C., Peterson, P. A., and Kronenberg, M. (1995). Nonclassical behavior of the mouse CD1 class-I-like molecule. submitted.

Teyton, L., and Peterson, P. A. (1992). Assembly and transport of MHC Class II Molecules. *New Biol.*, **4**, 441–447.

Teyton, L., O'Sullivan, D., Dickson, P. W., Lotteau, V., Sette, A., Fink, P., and Peterson, P. A. (1990). Invariant chain distinguishes between the exogenous and endogenous antigen presentation pathways. *Nature (London)* **348**, 39–44.

Townsend, A., and Trowsdale, J. (1993). The transporters associated with antigen presentation. *Semin. Cell Biol.* **4**, 53–61.

Trowbridge, I. S., Collawn, J. F., and Hopkins, C. R. (1993). Signal-dependent membrane protein trafficking in the endocytic pathway. *Annu. Rev. Cell Biol.* **9**, 129–161.

Trowsdale, J., Hanson, I., Mockridge, I., Beck, S., Townsend, A., and Kelly, A. (1990). Sequences encoded in the class II region of the MHC related to the 'ABC' superfamily of transporters. *Nature (London)* **348**, 741–744.

Tulp, A., Verwoerd, D., Dobberstein, B., Ploegh, H. L., and Pieters, J. (1994). Isolation and characterization of the intracellular MHC class II compartment. *Nature (London)* **369**, 120–126.

Van Kaer, L., Ashton-Rickardt, P. G., Ploegh, H. L., and Tonegawa, S. (1992). TAP1 mutant mice are deficient in antigen presentation, surface class I molecules, and CD4-8+ T cells. *Cell (Cambridge, Mass.)* **71**, 1205–1214.

Vidovic, D., Mihovil, R., McKune, K., Guerder, S., MacKay, C., and Dembic, Z. (1989). Qa-1 restricted recognition of foreign antigen by a γδ T cell hybridoma. *Nature (London)* **340**, 646–649.

Viville, S., Neefjes, J., Lotteau, V., Dierich, A., Lemeur, M., Ploegh, H., Benoist, C., and Mathis, D. (1993). Mice lacking the MHC class II-associated invariant chain. *Cell (Cambridge, Mass.)* **72**, 635–648.

Vyas, J. M., Shawar, S. M., Rodgers, J. R., Cook, R. G., and Rich, R. R. (1992). Biochemical specificity of H-2M3a. Stereospecificity and space-filling requirements at position 1 maintain N-formyl peptide binding. *J. Immunol.* **149**, 3605–3611.

Vyas, J. M., Rodgers, J. R., and Rich, R. R. (1995). H-2M3a violates the paradigm for major histocompatibility complex class I peptide binding. *J. Exp. Med.* **181,** 1817–1825.

Wang, C.-R., and Fischer-Lindahl, K. (1993). Organization and structure of the *H-2M4-M8* class I
genes in the mouse major histocompatibility complex. *Immunogenetics* **38,** 258–271.

Wang, C.-R., Loveland, B. E., and Fischer-Lindahl, K. (1991). *H-2M3* encodes the MHC class I molecule presenting the maternally transmitted antigen of the mouse. *Cell (Cambridge, Mass.)* **66,** 335–
345.

Wang, C.-R., Castaño, A. R., Peterson, P. A., Slaughter, C., Fischer Lindahl, K., and Deisenhofer, J.
(1995). Nonclassical binding of formylated peptide in crystal structure of MHC class Ib molecule,
H2-M3. *Cell (Cambridge, Mass.)* **82,** 655–664.

Weintraub, B. C., Jackson, M. R., and Hedrick, S. M. (1994). $\gamma\delta$ T cells can recognize nonclassical
MHC in the absence of conventional antigenic peptides. *J. Immunol.* **153,** 3051–3058.

West, M. A., Lucocq, J. M., and Watts, C. (1994). Antigen processing and class II MHC peptide-
loading compartments in human B-lymphoblastoid cells. *Nature* **369,** 147–151.

Wolf, P. R., and Cook, R. G. (1990). The *TL* region gene *37* encodes a Qa-1 antigen. *J. Exp. Med.*
**172,** 1795–1804.

Wolf, P. R., and Ploegh, H. L. (1995). DM exchange mechanism. *Nature (London)* **376,** 464–465.

Ziegler, H. K., and Unanue, E. R. (1982). Decrease in macrophage antigen catabolism caused by
ammonia and chloroquine is associated with inhibition of antigen presentation to T cells. *Proc.
Natl. Acad. Sci. U.S.A.* **79,** 175–178.

# *Chapter 2*

# M Cells as a Pathway for Antigen Uptake and Processing

Marian R. Neutra* and Jean-Pierre Krachenbuhl†

*Department of Pediatrics, Harvard Medical School and GI Cell Biology Laboratory,
Children's Hospital, Boston, Massachusetts 02115;
and †Swiss Institute for Experimental Cancer Research and Institute of Biochemistry,
University of Lausanne, CH-1066 Epalinges-Lausanne, Switzerland

## I. Introduction

Design of effective mucosal vaccines requires information about the cellular and molecular mechanisms that operate during sampling of antigens across mucosal barriers, and about the strategies that pathogens use to exploit these sampling systems. The vast mucosal surfaces of the gastrointestinal and respiratory tracts are lined largely by a single layer of epithelial cells sealed by tight junctions. In the intestine, this barrier is generally effective in excluding peptides and macromolecules with antigenic potential (Madara *et al.*, 1990). Uptake of macromolecules, particulate antigens, and microorganisms across intestinal epithelia can occur only by active transepithelial vesicular transport, and this is restricted by multiple mechanisms including local secretions containing mucins and secretory IgA antibodies (Neutra *et al.*, 1994a), rigid, closely packed microvilli (Mooseker, 1985), the "glycocalyx" which is a thick (400–500 nm) layer of membrane-anchored glycoproteins (Ito, 1974; Maury *et al.*, 1995), and adsorbed pancreatic enzymes and stalked glycoprotein enzymes responsible for terminal digestion (Semenza, 1986). The glycocalyx of enterocytes is both a highly degradative microenvironment and a diffusion barrier, impeding the access of macromolecular aggregates, particles, viruses, and bacteria, and preventing direct contact with the microvillus membrane (Amerongen *et al.*, 1991; Apter *et al.*, 1993). Although enterocytes can endocytose intact proteins, the combined digestive activities of the enterocyte surface and the lysosomes tends to discourage transport of intact antigens across the epithelial barrier.

*Essentials of Mucosal Immunology*

## II. THE FOLLICLE-ASSOCIATED EPITHELIUM AND M CELLS

The cardinal feature of the follicle-associated epithelium (FAE) is the presence of M cells that provide functional openings in the epithelial barrier through vesicular transport activity (review: Neutra and Kraehenbuhl, 1992; Neutra et al., 1994b). In M cells, unlike most epithelial cells, transepithelial vesicular transport is the major pathway for endocytosed materials. The M-cell basolateral surface is deeply invaginated to form a large intraepithelial "pocket," a structural modification that shortens the distance from apical to basolateral surface and ensures that transcytosis is rapid and efficient. Transcytosed particles and macromolecules are delivered primarily to the intraepithelial pocket.

Multiple types of immigrant cells have been identified in M-cell pockets by immunolabeling of rodent, rabbit, and human Peyer's patches (Ermak and Owen, 1986; Jarry et al., 1989; Ermak et al., 1990; Farstad et al., 1994). In all species, both B and T cells were present along with a small number of macrophages. The phenotypes of these cells suggest that T cells can interact with antigen-presenting B cells in the pocket and that B lymphoblast traffic into the M-cell pocket allows continued antigen exposure, and extension and diversification of the immune response (Farstad et al., 1994). Below the epithelium of the dome lies an extensive network of dendritic cells and macrophages intermingled with $CD4^+$ T cells and B cells from the underlying follicle (Ermak and Owen, 1986; Farstad et al., 1994). Viruses and bacteria that use the M cell as an invasion route can infect and destroy M cells and local macrophages.

The M-cell apical surface differs from that of intestinal absorptive cells in the increased accessibility of the plasma membrane, and the predominance of endocytic domains that function in endocytosis of macromolecules, particles, and microbes (Neutra et al., 1988). The organization of the apical cytoskeleton in M cells is distinct: they generally lack typical brush borders with uniform microvilli, and the actin-associated protein villin that is confined to microvillar cores in enterocytes is diffusely distributed in M cells (Kerneis, S., Bogdanova, A., Colucci-Guyon, E., Kraehenbuhl, J. P., and Pringault, E., submitted), reflecting their modified apical organization and perhaps their ability to respond to adherence of microorganisms with ruffling and phagocytosis.

## III. M-CELL MEMBRANES

Most (but not all) M cells lack the uniform thick glycocalyx seen on enterocytes, but their apical membranes do display abundant glycoconjugates in a cell coat that varies widely in thickness and density (Bye et al., 1984). In several species M cells have been shown to have specific glycosylation patterns that distinguish them from their epithelial neighbors (Clark et al., 1993; Falk et al., 1994; Giannasca et al., 1994). These lectin binding sites are found not only on M-cell apical membranes but also on intracellular vesicles and basolateral membranes, including the pocket domain, and on basal processes that extend 10 $\mu$m or more into the underlying lymphoid tissue (Giannasca et al., 1994). These extensions could make direct contact with lymphoid or antigen-presenting cells in the subepithelial tissue and might play a role either in the induction of the unique M-cell phenotype or in the processing and presentation of antigens after M-cell transport. In addition, there is diversity in the glycosylation patterns of individual M cells within a single FAE that might expand the possible microbial lectin–M-cell surface carbohydrate interactions of the local M-cell population (Giannasca et al., 1994; Neutra et al., 1996).

Adherent macromolecules or particles bound to the apical plasma membranes of M cells are efficiently endocytosed or phagocytosed (Neutra et al., 1987). It follows that pathogens or vaccines that can bind selectively to M cells would be most effective in mucosal invasion and induction of mucosal immune responses, and this assumption underlies many of the current approaches to vaccine design. Rapid binding and uptake of polystyrene or latex beads that adhere to M cells (Pappo and Ermak, 1989), along with the lectin binding studies described above, suggest that particles or microorganisms with hydrophobic surfaces as well as those with appropriate lectin-like adhesins could interact with M-cell surfaces. Lectins that fail to recognize mucins and other cells could be highly M-cell-selective, whereas hydrophobic particles would also interact with mucus and the glycocalyx of enterocytes on villi and this would tend to reduce the efficiency of M-cell uptake.

M-cell membranes contain the glycolipid GM1 and bind cholera toxin. Cholera toxin B subunit (CT-B), the nontoxic pentameric portion of the toxin responsible for binding to the membrane glycolipid GM1, can enhance mucosal immune responses when coupled directly to antigen, and this is thought to be due in part to the ability of CT-B to enhance mucosal adherence and uptake (Dertzbaugh and Elson, 1991; Nedrud and Lamm, 1991). Although soluble CT-B binds to apical membrames of all intestinal cells, EM studies showed that cholera toxin or its B subunit adsorbed to colloidal gold particles lost the ability to bind to enterocyte brush borders (presumably due to the diffusion barrier created by the thick enterocyte glycocalyx) but still adhered to a subpopulation of M cells. This suggested that adding CT-B to the surfaces of particulate vaccine vectors or carriers (such as copolymer microspheres) would enhance M-cell transport. However, when CT-B was immobilized on the surfaces of 1-$\mu$m particles, they failed to adhere either to enterocytes or to M cells. The inability of 1-$\mu$m particles to bind to M cells via the glycolipid receptor was shown to be due to the molecular barrier to large particles provided by the M-cell glycocalyx (A. Frey, W. Lencer, K. Giannasca, R. Weltzin, and M. Neutra, unpublished data). Thus, the M-cell targeting ability of CT-B may be limited to relatively small macromolecular complexes or particles. This has important implications for its use in targeting of oral vaccines to the mucosal immune system.

## IV. LOCAL ANTIGEN UPTAKE AND REGIONAL
## IMMUNE RESPONSES

There are regional differences in M-cell surface glycoconjugates that must be taken into account when using live vectors as mucosal vaccines for region-specific pathogens. It is now clear that the location in which M-cell transport and inductive events occur has a profound influence on the subsequent regional distribution of specific IgA plasma cells and IgA secretion (Mestecky *et al.*, 1994). This was demonstrated in human studies using poliovirus and the polio vaccine: a secretory immune response against poliovirus was demonstrated in colon but not in nasopharynx following immunization of distal colon (Ogra and Karzon, 1969). Similarly, secretory immune responses to Sendai virus were concentrated in either the digestive tract or the airways, when administration of antigen was carefully restricted either to the stomach or the trachea (Nedrud *et al.*, 1987). Similarly, CT instilled into proximal intestine, distal intestine, or colon evoked highest levels of specific anti-toxin secretory IgA in the segment of antigen exposure (Pierce and Cray, 1982). We have quantitatively analyzed local IgA responses using "wicks" made of an absorbent filter material for direct retrieval of secretions associated with mucosal surfaces of the gastrointestinal system and vagina of mice (Haneberg *et al.*, 1994). After immunization of mice via different mucosal routes with cholera toxin (Haneberg *et al.*, 1994) or with recombinant Salmonella vector expressing a foreign antigen (Hopkins *et al.*, 1995), only the rectal immunization route produced high levels of specific sIgA in the mucus coating the rectum and distal colon. Lymphoid follicles with M cells are particularly numerous in the distal colonic and rectal mucosa of humans (O'Leary and Sweeney, 1986; Langman and Rowland, 1986). This and other alternative mucosal immunization sites are currently being tested in experimental animals and humans, and the information gained will be important for future design of mucosal vaccines against HIV.

## V. INTERACTIONS OF MICROORGANISMS WITH M CELLS

As noted above, M-cell membrane surfaces display distinct oligosaccharides that may be important determinants in selective M-cell adherence of certain enteric pathogens. However, the microbial surface molecules that mediate adherence of bacteria or viruses to M cells have not been identified. M-cell recognition and transport of pathogens is an important first step in initiation of antimicrobial immune responses, but this carries the risk of infection and disease since microorganisms can initiate mucosal and/or systemic disease by crossing the epithelial barrier (review Neutra *et al.*, 1996). A wide range of gram-negative bacteria bind selectively to M cells, including *Vibrio cholerae* (Owen *et al.*, 1986; Winner *et al.*, 1991; Neutra *et al.*, 1994b), some strains of *Escherichia coli* (Inman and Cantey, 1983; Uchida, 1987), *Salmonella typhi* (Kohbata *et al.*, 1986), *Salmonella typhimurium* (Jones *et al.*, 1994), *Shigella flexneri* (Wassef *et al.*, 1989), *Yersinia enter-*

*ocolitica* (Grutzkau *et al.*, 1990), *Yersinia pseudotuberculosis* (Fujimura *et al.*, 1992), and *Campylobacter jejuni* (Walker *et al.*, 1988). Viruses that use M cells as a route of entry include reovirus (Wolf *et al.*, 1981), poliovirus (Sicinski *et al.*, 1990), and possibly HIV (Amerongen *et al.*, 1991).

Viruses are relatively simple molecular packages that rely on adherence to exploit the normal endocytic and transport activities of M cells (Nibert *et al.*, 1991; Amerongen *et al.*, 1994). Bacteria, in contrast, use more complex strategies: for example they can enzymatically alter the host cell surface, initiate signal transduction events that promote internalization, and recruit inflammatory cells which in turn alter the epithelial barrier (Sansonetti, 1991; Pace *et al.*, 1993; Bliska *et al.*, 1993). M-cell adherence and uptake of bacteria is likely to involve a sequence of events including initial recognition (perhaps via a lectin–carbohydrate interaction) followed by more intimate associations that could require expression of additional bacterial genes, processing of M-cell surface molecules, activation of intracellular signalling pathways, and recruitment of integral or submembrane M-cell proteins to the interaction site. Recognition and adherence to M cells is a prerequisite, and current studies are aimed at identifying the M-cell surface components that serve as receptors and determining the accessibility of these receptors to specific viral or bacterial ligands.

## VI. Conclusion

Information about the mechanisms underlying the interactions of microorganisms, toxins, and particles with M cells will be useful for design of new mucosal immunization strategies. Our goal is shared by many research groups: to enhance delivery of attenuated bacterial vaccine strains, live viral and bacterial vectors containing recombinant proteins or genes, and nonliving, particulate immunogens to the mucosal immune system.

## Acknowledgments

The important contributions of the current and former members of our laboratories are gratefully acknowledged. The Neutra laboratory is supported by NIH Research Grants HD17557 and AI34757 and NIH Center Grant DK34854 to the Harvard Digestive Diseases Center. The Kraehenbuhl laboratory is supported by Swiss National Science Foundation Grant 31.37155.93 and Swiss League against Cancer Grant 373.89.2.

## References

Amerongen, H. M., Weltzin, R. A., Farnet, C. M., Michetti, P., Haseltine, W. A., and Neutra, M. R. (1991). Transepithelial transport of HIV-1 by intestinal M cells: A mechanism for transmission of AIDS. *J. Acquired Immune Defic. Syndr.* **4**, 760–765.
Amerongen, H. M., Wilson, G. A. R., Fields, B. N., and Neutra, M. R. (1994). Proteolytic processing of reovirus is required for adherence to intestinal M cells. *J. Virol.* **68**, 8428–8432.

Apter, F. M., Michetti, P., Winner III, L. S., Mack, J. A., Mekalanos, J. J., and Neutra, M. R. (1993). Analysis of the roles of anti-lipopolysaccharide and anti-cholera toxin IgA antibodies in protection against *Vibrio cholerae* and cholera toxin using monoclonal IgA antibodies *in vivo*. *Infect. Immun.* **61,** 5279–5285.

Bliska, J. B., Galan, J. E., and Falkow, S. (1993). Signal transduction in the mammalian cell during bacterial attachment and entry. *Cell (Cambridge, Mass.)* **73,** 903–920.

Bye, W. A., Allan, C. H., and Trier, J. S. (1984). Structure, distribution and origin of M cells in Peyer's patches of mouse ileum. *Gastroenterology* **86,** 789–801.

Clark, M. A., Jepson, M. A., Simmons, N. L., Booth, T. A., and Hirst, B. H. (1993). Differential expression of lectin-binding sites defines mouse intestinal M-cells. *J. Histochem. Cytochem.* **41,** 1679–1687.

Dertzbaugh, M. T., and Elson, C. O. (1991). Cholera toxin as a mucosal adjuvant. *In* "Topics in Vaccine Adjuvant Research" (D. R. Spriggs and W. C. Koff, eds.), pp. 119–132. CRC Press, Boca Raton, Florida.

Ermak, T. H., and Owen, R. L. (1986). Differential distribution of lymphocytes and accessory cells in mouse Peyer's patches. *Anat. Rec.* **215,** 144–152.

Ermak, T. H., Steger, H. J., and Pappo, J. (1990). Phenotypically distinct subpopulations of T cells in domes and M-cell pockets of rabbit gut-associated lymphoid tissues. *Immunology* **71,** 530–537.

Falk, P., Roth, K. A., and Gordon, J. I. (1994). Lectins are sensitive tools for defining the differentiation programs of epithelial cell lineages in the developing and adult mouse gastrointestinal tract. *Am. J. Physiol.* **266,** G987–G1003.

Farstad, I. N., Halstensen, T. S., Fausa, O., and Brandtzaeg, P. (1994). Heterogeneity of M cell-associated B and T cells in human Peyer's patches. *Immunology* **83,** 457–464.

Fujimura, Y., Kihara, T., and Mine, H. (1992). Membranous cells as a portal of *Yersinia pseudotuberculosis* entry into rabbit ileum. *J. Clin. Electron Microsc.* **25,** 35–45.

Giannasca, P. J., Giannasca, K. T., Falk, P., Gordon, J. I., and Neutra, M. R. (1994). Regional differences in glycoconjugates of intestinal M cells in mice: Potential targets for mucosal vaccines. *Am. J. Physiol.* **267,** G1108–G1121.

Grutzkau, A., Hanski, C., Hahn, H., and Riecken, E. O. (1990). Involvement of M cells in the bacterial invasion of Peyer's patches: A common mechanism shared by *Yersinia enterocolitica* and other enteroinvasive bacteria. *Gut* **3,** 1011–1015.

Haneberg, B., Kendall, D., Amerongen, H. M., Apter, F. M., Kraehenbuhl, J. P., and Neutra, M. R. (1994). Induction of secretory immune responses in small intestine, colon-rectum, and vagina measured with a new method for collection of specific IgA from local mucosal surfaces. *Infect. Immun.* **62,** 15–23.

Hopkins, S., Kraehenbuhl, J. P., Schoedel, F., Potts, A., Peterson, D., De Grandi, P., and Nardelli-Haefliger, D. (1995). A recombinant *Salmonella typhimurium* vaccine induces local immunity by four different routes of immunization. *Infect. Immun.* **63,** 3279–3286.

Inman, L. R., and Cantey, J. R. (1983). Specific adherence of *Escherichia coli* (strain RDEC-1) to membranous (M) cells of the Peyer's patch in *Escherichia coli* diarrhea in the rabbit. *J. Clin. Invest.* **71,** 1–8.

Ito, S. (1974). Form and function of the glycocalyx on free cell surfaces. *Philos. Trans. R. Soc. London (Biol.)* **268,** 55–66.

Jarry, A., Robaszkiewicz, M., Brousse, N., and Potet, F. (1989). Immune cells associated with M cells in the follicle-associated epithelium of Peyer's patches in the rat. *Cell Tissue Res.* **225,** 293–298.

Jones, B. D., Ghori, N., and Falkow, S. (1994). *Salmonella typhimurium* initiates murine infection by penetrating and destroying the specialized epithelial M cells of the Peyer's patches. *J. Exp. Med.* **180,** 15–23.

Kohbata, S., Yokobata, H., and Yabuuchi, E. (1986). Cytopathogenic effect of *Salmonella typhi* GIFU 10007 on M cells of murine ileal Peyer's patches in ligated ileal loops: An ultrastructural study. *Microbiol. Immunol.* **30,** 1225–1237.

Langman, J. M., and Rowland, R. (1986). The number and distribution of lymphoid follicles in the human large intestine. *J. Anat.* **194,** 189–194.

Madara, J. L., Nash, S., Moore, R., and Atisook, K. (1990). Structure and function of the intestinal epithelial barrier in health and disease. *Monogr. Pathol.* **31,** 306–324.

Maury, J., Nicoletti, C., Guzzo-Chambraud, L., and Maroux, S. (1995). The filamentous brush border glycocalyx, a mucin-like marker of enterocyte hyper-polarization. *Eur. J. Biochem.* **228,** 323–331.

Mestecky, J., Abraham, R., and Ogra, P. L. (1994). Common mucosal immune system and strategies for the development of vaccines effective at mucosal surfaces. *In* "Handbook of Mucosal Immunology" (P. L. Ogra, J. Mestecky, and M. E. Lamm, eds.), pp. 357–372. Academic Press, New York.

Mooseker, M. (1985). Organization, chemistry and assembly of the cytoskeletal apparatus of the intestinal brush border. *Ann. Rev. Cell Biol.* **1,** 209–241.

Nedrud, J. G., and Lamm, M. E. (1991). Adjuvants and the mucosal immune system. *In* "Topics in Vaccine Adjuvant Research" (D. R. Spriggs and W. C. Koff, eds.), pp. 54–67. CRC Press, Boca Raton, Florida.

Nedrud, J. G., Liang, X. P., Hague, N., and Lamm, M. E. (1987). Combined oral/nasal immunization protects mice from Sendai virus infection. *J. Immunol.* **139,** 3484–3492.

Neutra, M. R., and Kraehenbuhl, J. P. (1992). Transepithelial transport and mucosal defence. The role of M cells. *Trends Cell Biol.* **2,** 134–138.

Neutra, M. R., Phillips, T. L., Mayer, E. L., and Fishkind, D. J. (1987). Transport of membrane-bound macromolecules by M cells in follicle-associated epithelium of rabbit Peyer's patch. *Cell Tissue Res.* **247,** 537–546.

Neutra, M. R., Wilson, J. M., Weltzin, R. A., and Kraehenbuhl, J. P. (1988). Membrane domains and macromolecular transport in intestinal epithelial cells. *Am. Rev. Respir. Dis.* **138,** S10–S16.

Neutra, M. R., Michetti, P., and Kraehenbuhl, J. P. (1994a). Secretory immunoglobulin A: structure, synthesis, and function. *In* "Physiology of the Gastrointestinal Tract" (L. R. Johnson, ed.), pp. 975–1009. 3rd Ed. Raven, New York.

Neutra, M. R., Giannasca, P. J., Giannasca, K. T., and Kraehenbuhl, J. P. (1994b). M cells and microbial pathogens. *In* "Infections of the GI Tract" (M. J. Blaser, P. D. Smith, J. I. Ravdin, H. B. Greenberg, and R. L. Guerrant, eds.), pp. 163–178. Raven, New York.

Neutra, M. R., Pringault, E., and Kraehenbuhl, J. P. (1996). Antigen sampling across epithelial barriers and induction of mucosal immune responses. *Annu. Rev. Immunol.* **14,** 275–300.

Nibert, M. L., Furlong, D. B., and Fields, B. N. (1991). Mechanisms of viral pathogenesis. *J. Clin. Invest.* **88,** 727–734.

Ogra, P. L., and Karzon, D. T. (1969). Distribution of poliovirus antibody in serum, nasopharynx and alimentary tract following segmental immunization of lower alimentary tract with poliovaccine. *J. Immunol.* **102,** 1423–1430.

O'Leary, A. D., and Sweeney, E. C. (1986). Lymphoglandular complexes of the colon: Structure and distribution. *Histopathology* **10,** 267–283.

Owen, R. L., Pierce, N. F., Apple, R. T., and Cray, W. C. J. (1986). M cell transport of *Vibrio cholerae* from the intestinal lumen into Peyer's patches: A mechanism for antigen sampling and for microbial transepithelial migration. *J. Infect. Dis.* **153,** 1108–1118.

Pace, J., Hayman, M. J., and Galan, J. E. (1993). Signal transduction and invasion of epithelial cells by *S. typhimurium. Cell (Cambridge, Mass.)* **72,** 505–514.

Pappo, J., and Ermak, T. H. (1989). Uptake and translocation of fluorescent latex particles by rabbit Peyer's patch follicle epithelium: A quantitative model for M cell uptake. *Clin. Exp. Immunol.* **76,** 144–148.

Pierce, F. N., and Cray, W. C. J. (1982). Determinants of the localization, magnitude, and duration of a specific mucosal IgA plasma cell response in enterically immunized rats. *J. Immunol.* **128,** 1311–1315.

Sansonetti, P. J. (1991). Genetic and molecular basis of epithelial cell invasion by *Shigella* species. *Rev. Infect. Dis.* **13,** 285–292.

Semenza, G. (1986). Anchoring and biosynthesis of stalked brush border membrane glycoproteins. *Annu. Rev. Cell Biol.* **2,** 255–314.

Sicinski, P., Rowinski, J., Warchol, J. B., Jarzcabek, Z., Gut, W., Szczygiel, B., Bielecki, K., and Koch, G. (1990). Poliovirus type 1 enters the human host through intestinal M cells. *Gastroenterology* **98,** 56–58.

Uchida, J. (1987). An ultrastructural study on active uptake and transport of bacteria by microfold cells (M cells) to the lymphoid follicles in the rabbit appendix. *J. Clin. Electron Microsc.* **20,** 379–394.

Walker, R. I., Schauder-Chock, E. A., and Parker, J. L. (1988). Selective association and transport of *Campylobacter jejuni* through M cells of rabbit Peyer's patches. *Can. J. Microbiol.* **34,** 1142–1147.

Wassef, J. S., Keren, D. F., and Mailloux, J. L. (1989). Role of M cells in initial antigen uptake and in ulcer formation in the rabbit intestinal loop model of Shigellosis. *Infect. Immun.* **57,** 858–863.

Winner III, L. S., Mack, J., Weltzin, R. A., Mekalanos, J. J., Kraehenbuhl, J. P., and Neutra, M. R. (1991). New model for analysis of mucosal immunity: Intestinal secretion of specific monoclonal immunoglobulin A from hybridoma tumors protects against *Vibrio cholerae* infection. *Infect. Immun.* **59,** 977–982.

Wolf, J. L., Rubin, D. H., Finberg, R. S., Kauffman, R. S., Sharpe, A. H., Trier, J. S., and Fields, B. N. (1981). Intestinal M cells: A pathway for entry of reovirus into the host. *Science* **212,** 471–472.

# Chapter 3

# Toward an *in Vitro* Model for Microorganism Transport and Antigen Sampling through the Epithelial Digestive Barrier

Eric Pringault

*Swiss Institute for Experimental Cancer Research and Institute of Biochemistry, University of Lausanne, Switzerland, and Pasteur Institute, 75015 Paris, France*

## I. INTRODUCTION

Differentiation of specific epithelial cell lineages during development, as well as epithelial plasticity in response to hetelogous cell-to-cell cross-talk during adult life, accounts for the large variety of functions which are performed by the several hundred square meters of mucosal surfaces found in the human body. Among their functions, mucosa should sample antigens and microorganisms from the outside world, in order to trigger the development of either tolerance or immune responses (Neutra *et al.*, 1995).

In simple epithelia, this sampling and transport of antigens is restricted to sites where the mucosal surface contacts organized lymphoid tissue, which is overlaid by a special epithelium, i.e., the follicle-associated epithelium (FAE). Such structures are found in the nasal cavity, the bronchi (Sminia *et al.*, 1989), and the gut.

In the gut, this structure is called Peyer's patch, and forms a distinct functional unit specialized to trigger a local immune response. Nutritional functions and antibacterial defenses are lost at these sites (Neutra and Kraehenbuhl, 1992). The M cells, a specialized cell type found scattered in the follicle-associated epithelium, play a key role in mucosal immunity by their capacity to sample and transport macromolecules (Owen, 1977; Neutra *et al.*, 1987), microorganisms (Wolf *et al.*, 1981; Owen *et al.*, 1986; Kohbata *et al.*, 1986), and inert particles (Lefevre *et al.*, 1978; Pappo and Ermak, 1989) from the lumen into the underlying lymphoid tissue. M cells can be distinguished by electron microscopy from neighboring enterocytes by the absence of a brush border and a huge invagination of the basoleral membrane, forming a pocket which contains lymphocytes and/or macrophages. The lack of a typical brush border and its associated glycocalix could facilitate access and adherence of particles and microorganisms, while the basolateral membrane of M cells interacts with cells of the mucosal immune system (Bhalla and Owen, 1983).

Most studies on M cells have been restricted to morphological analyses. Since M cells are a minority cell population, the obtainment of substantial amounts of enriched or purified M-cell preparation cannot be achieved, thus precluding biochemical studies. Furthermore, attempts to identify specific markers (monclonal antibodies or specific cDNAs) have failed. Whether M cells are of epithelial, intestinal, or mesenchymal origin has been controversial.

## II. EPITHELIAL ORIGIN OF M CELLS

As a first attempt to study the ontogeny and mechanism of M-cell formation, we have investigated the expression of three tissue-specific cytoskeletal proteins (cytokeratins, vimentin, and villin) that are reliable markers of cell origin. These proteins also play crucial roles in the specific shape of epithelial cells and assembly of the highly specialized apical cell surface of enterocytes.

### A. Mouse M Cells Do Not Express the Mesenchymal Marker Vimentin

Expression of vimentin, an intermediate filament protein absent in epithelial cells but present in mesenchymal cells, has been reported in M cells from rabbit FAE, together with epithelial-specific cytokeratins (Gebert et al., 1992; Gebert and Hach, 1992). This observation has greatly contributed to the controversy about M-cell origin (epithelial vs mesenchymal). However, these data do not rule out phenotypic plasticity of M cells under certain conditions, which would allow the coexpression of these two types of intermediate filaments, as observed in epithelial cells when grown in vitro.

The localization of cytokeratins and vimentin was analyzed on mouse FAE by immunocytochemistry. Epithelial-specific cytokeratins were expressed in both absorptive enterocytes and M cells, while vimentin was not detected in mouse FAE. To further confirm the absence of vimentin expression in mouse FAE cells, we took advantage of transgenic mice in which the nls-lacZ gene was introduced into one allele of the vim locus by homologuous recombination (Colucci-Guyon et al., 1994). In such mice, the vimentin promotor drives the expression of the nuclear β-galactosidase in all vimentin-expressing cells. No nuclear β-galactosidase activity was detected in M cells of Peyer's patch FAE from these mice, while endothelial cells and macrophages were strongly positive (Kerneis et al., 1996).

### B. Cytosolic Distribution of Villin in M Cells Correlates with the Absence of Brush Border

In intestinal cells, assembly of the F-actin network in the brush border occurs as a stepwise process (Coluccio and Bretscher, 1989; Shibayama et al., 1987) that requires the expression and the recruitment of specific actin binding proteins (Matsudaira and Burgess, 1979), including villin (Bretscher and Weber, 1980; Pringault *et al.*, 1991) and fimbrin (Matsudaira and Burgess, 1979). Villin was demonstrated to be a key component of brush-border assembly (Friederich *et al.*, 1989, 1990; Costa de Beauregard *et al.*, 1995) and displays a tissue-specific pattern of expression, mainly in epithelial cells developing a brush border (Robine *et al.*, 1985; Pringault *et al.*, 1986). In addition, this protein was shown to be expressed early in the differentiation of endodermic and committed intestinal cells, and has been used as a marker to identify their derivatives (Maunoury *et al.*, 1988, 1992). In adult small and large intestine, villin is already expressed in the proliferative cell compartment located in the crypts, in addition to the differentiated enterocytes lining the villi (Robine *et al.*, 1985; Boller *et al.*, 1988). Villin was not detected in nonepithelial cells at any stage of development or in adults.

Therefore, whether or not villin expression is found in M cells could have important implications for the understanding of their origin, their differentiation, and the molecular mechanisms underlying their specialized functions.

We have shown that villin was expressed in both enterocytes and M cells from the FAE (Kernéis *et al.*, 1996). This protein had an unusual cytoplasmic distribution in FAE cells lacking a brush border and in cells displaying an intraepithelial pocket filled with lymphocytes. Thus, the cytoplasmic distribution of villin provides a new identification criteria for M cells and reflects the reorganization of the F-actin network, which correlates with the inability of M cells to assemble a brush border.

Villin expression in M cells is consistent with their epithelial intestinal origin and confirms that M cells and adjacent absorptive enterocytes both derive from the same stem cells anchored in the crypts.

It has been established that villin plays a key role in the organization and plasticity of the F-actin network. First, spontaneous brush-border assembly, *in vivo* and in intestinal cultured cells, occurs with increased expression of villin and concomitant recruitment of the protein to the apex of the cell (Robine *et al.*, 1985). Second, when villin is overexpressed in fibroblast-like CV1 cells following cDNA transfection, villin induces the formation of microvilli containing F-actin bundles (Friederich *et al.*, 1989). Third, suppression of villin expression by antisense RNAs in cultured enterocytes prevents the brush-border assembly and the localization of intestine-specific hydrolases in the apical membrane (Costa de Beauregard *et al.*, 1995). F-actin disappears from the cell apex while stress fibers develop at the base of the cells, without altering the epithelial polarity. This redistribution of the F-actin network and the loss of brush-border assembly can be reversed by blocking the effect of antisense RNAs.

In M cells, villin accumulates at high levels in the cytoplasm but seems to be unable to exert its morphogenic effect, reflected by the absence of induction of microvillus growth and brush-border assembly. The molecular mechanism blocking brush-border assembly has not yet been elucidated. *In vitro* studies have demonstrated that villin controls the gelation/solation of F-actin in a calcium-dependent manner (Glenney *et al.,* 1981), by inducing bundling of preformed F-actin filaments in the absence of calcium, whereas increasing the calcium concentration induces severing of F-actin filaments by villin. The unusual distribution of villin in M cells could reflect a bias in favor of the severing activity, due to an increase in local calcium concentration. Alternatively, M cells could express another actin-binding protein which competes with villin and blocks brush-border assembly.

### C. Mouse FAE Displays Intermediate Phenotypes between Absorptive Enterocytes and M Cells

Intermediate phenotypes with moderate levels of cytoplasmic villin and hypomorphic brush borders were also observed. Such heterogeneity suggests that there is a continuum between well-differentiated enterocytes with a well-developed brush border and cells lacking a brush border and unable to recruit cytoplasmic villin to the apex. A similar heterogeneity has been reported for apical alkaline phosphatase, which is absent in M cells but is associated with the brush border of fully differentiated enterocytes (Owen and Bhalla, 1983). This observation raises again (Smith and Peacock, 1992) the question of whether M cells arise from the conversion of fully differentiated enterocytes.

### III. EXPERIMENTAL APPROACHES TO INDUCE FAE PROPERTIES AND M CELL FORMATION

As demonstrated for the villus-associated epithelium (Gordon and Hermiston, 1994), FAE renewal is dependent on the proliferation of crypt cells surrounding the follicle. Stem cells of these follicle-associated crypts are unusual in that they are the outset of two distinct axes of migration/differentiation. Cells on one wall of the crypt differentiate into absorptive enterocytes, enteroendocrine, or goblet cells that migrate onto villi. On the opposite wall of the same crypt, cells differentiate into absorptive enterocytes displaying several distinct features and M cells.

It has been demonstrated that differentiation of villus-associated enterocytes require interactions with fibroblasts from the lamina propria and components from the extracellular matrix (Kedinger, 1994). In the follicle-associated epithelium, M cells establish intimate contact with underlying B and T cells, as well as antigen-presenting cells. However, these transmission electron microscopy studies give only a "snapshot" of a section of a Peyer's patch, and do not provide evidence that lymphoid cells are permanent or transient residents of this pocket or that FAE and M cell formation require a paracrine or cell contact-mediated cross-talk with the lymphoid compartment of the Peyer's patch.

New experimental approaches have thus been developed to investigate the role of immune cells in the mechanism of FAE and M-cell formation, and to address the following question: can enterocytes be converted into cells sharing properties with M cells?

### A. Transfer of Peyer's Patch Lymphocytes into Intestinal Ectopic Sites Converts the Villus-Associated Epithelium into a Follicle-Associated Epithelium Containing M Cells

Injection of freshly isolated lymphoid follicle cells under the duodenal mucosa of a recipient mouse, in a location devoided of endogenous follicle or Peyer's patch (Fig. 1), induces after several days the formation of structures similar to Peyer's patches. These Peyer's patch-like structures display a normal composition of immune cells compared to the endogenous Peyer's patches (i.e., a majority of CD4$^+$ T cells, a very small number of CD8$^+$ T cells, B cells expressing IgM, and a germinative center with IgA-positive cells). The epithelium covering these induced patches displays the characteristics of FAE (loss of polymeric immunoglobulin receptor expression, apparition of binding sites for the lectin *Ulex Europaus Agglutinin 1* on the membrane of a subpopulation of cells) and contains typical M cells. In contrast, the injection of thymocytes of 3-month-old mice did not induce these structures.

This indicates that the normal distribution of Peyer's patches in the mouse intestine depends on sites of lymphocyte homing through high endothelial venules, and that the vascularization system can by-passed by direct injection. Furthermore, FAE and M-cell differentiation can be specifically induced from any intestinal crypt from which a villus-type differentiation normally originates.

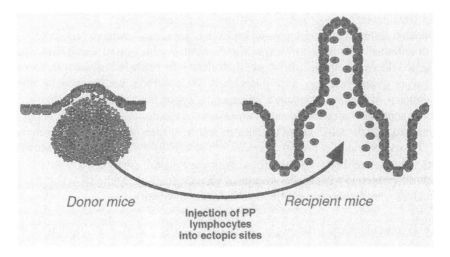

**FIGURE 1.** Ectopic transfer of Peyer's patch follicle cells under the duodenal mucosa of a recipient mouse. Peyer's patch follicle cells are freshly isolated from the intestine of a donor Balb/c mouse, and injected under the duodenal mucosa of a recipient mouse, in a place devoided of Peyer's patches. After 8 to 9 days, the injected segment is resected and immunomorphorlogic analyses are performed.

## B. Peyer's Patch Lymphocytes Induce Brush-Border Effacement, Membrane Ruffling, and Latex Bead Translocation in a Cultured Human Intestinal Cell Line

M cells could arise either from fully differentiated enterocytes present in the induced FAE (conversion) or directly from immature crypt cells (independent differentiation program). In the first case, the M-cell phenotype corresponds to the aspect of an enterocyte having acquired a new specialized function of lumen-to-follicle transcytosis, concommitant to interaction with one of several lymphocytes. To perform this function, the enterocyte disassembles its brush border, reorganizes its cytoskeleton network, and changes its columnar shape. Whether or not these modifications are reversible has to be considered. In the first hypothesis, M cell as a specific entity is unlikely. In the second case, cross-talk with lymphoid cells triggers an M-cell differentiation program in immature crypt cells in a process close to that postulated for other mucosal cell types, such as goblet cells or enteroendocrine cells. Committed M cells never acquire absorptive enterocyte characteristics (for instance, they never assemble a brush border) but instead acquire their specific functions.

Thus, we tried to induce FAE properties, starting from already well-differentiated intestinal cell lines, and establish coculture conditions with immune and epithelial cells which mimic the *in situ* situation.

A coculture system composed of intestinal cells and follicle cells has been developed. Caco-2 clone1 cells, selected for a well-developed homogenous brush border and a widespread sucrase–isomaltase expression (Costa de Beauregard *et al.*, 1995), were grown upside down on 3-$\mu$m porous filters. After confluency, lymphoid follicle cells were introduced in the basolateral chamber and cocultured with intestinal cells for 1 to 7 days (Fig. 2). Follicle cells passed through the filter, digested the extracellular matrix, and homed into the epithelial monolayer. Epithelial polarity and tightness were maintained. We observed that decrease of apical expression of sucrase isomaltase, disorganization of the brush border, and occasional apparition of apical membrane ruffles were correlated with the homing of lymphoid follicle cells. These changes in apical surface properties were followed by the acquisition of a vectorial (apical to basolateral) translocation of inert particles (fluorescent latex beads). Thus, lymphoepithelial contacts have converted well-differentiated villus-type absorptive enterocytes into epithelial cells sharing structural and functional properties with FAE and M cells.

## IV. CONCLUSIONS

The phenomenology described in the experimental induction of FAE properties and M-cell formation, *in vivo* and *in vitro,* emphasizes the critical role of the immune system in the differentiation of epithelial inductive sites for mucosal immunity.

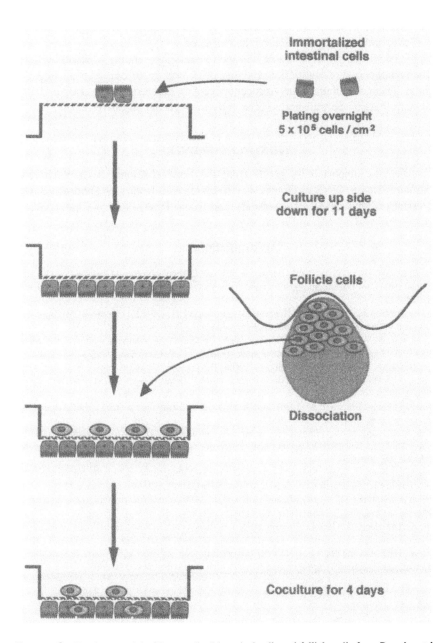

*FIGURE 2.* Coculture model of immortalized intestinal cells and follicle cells from Peyer's patches. Intestinal cells (CaCO2 clone 1 cells) are plated in a reverse orientation on 3-$\mu$m porous filters. Cells are grown several days after confluency and freshly isolated follicle cells from Peyer's patches of a donor Balb/c mouse are then introduced in the basolateral chamber. The effect of lymphoepithelial cross-talk is analyzed after 1 to 7 days of coculture.

The coculture model allows the study of lymphoepithelial cross-talk at the molecular level and the identification of the mediators.

Such a coculture model will also be used to study the genetics, the cell biology, and the pathogenesis of enteric invasive bacterial pathogens (Salmonella, Shigella, Yersinia). This could help to develop genetically modified strains as antigen delivery vectors that can be transported efficiently through the digestive barrier.

## ACKNOWLEDGMENTS

This study was supported by grants from the Fonds National de la Recherche Scientifique Suisse (FNRS, Grant 31-37612.93), and from the Sandoz, (Basel, Switzerland), Zyma (Nyon, Switzerland), and Ipsen (Paris, France) Fundations.

## REFERENCES

Bhalla, D. K., and Owen, R. L. (1983). Migration of B and T lymphocytes to M cells in Peyer's patch follicle epithelium: An autoradiographic and immunocytochemical study in mice. *Cell. Immunol.* **81,** 105–117.

Boller, K., Arpin, M., Pringault, E., Mangeat, P., and Reggio, H. (1988). Differential distribution of villin and villin mRNA in mouse intestinal epithelial cells. *Differentiation* **39,** 51–57.

Bretscher, A., and Weber, K. (1980). Villin is a major protein of the microvillus cytoskeleton which binds both G and F-actin in a calcium dependant manner. *Cell (Cambridge, Mass.)* **20,** 839–847.

Colucci-Guyon, E., Portier, M. M., Dunia, I., Paulin, D., Pournin, S., and Babinet, C. (1994). Mice lacking vimentin develop and reproduce without an obvious phenotype. *Cell (Cambridge, Mass.)* **79,** 678–694.

Coluccio, L. M., and Bretscher, A. (1989). Reassociation of microvilli core proteins making a microvillar core *in vitro. J. Cell Biol.* **108,** 495–502.

Costa de Beauregard, M. A., Pringault, E., Robine, S., and Louvard, D. (1995). Suppression of villin expression by antisense RNA impairs brush border assembly in polarized epithelial intestinal cells. *EMBO J.* **14,** 409–421.

Friederich, E., Huet, C., Arpin, M., and Louvard, D. (1989). Villin induces microvilli growth and actin redistribution in transfected fibroblasts. *Cell (Cambridge, Mass.)* **59,** 461–475.

Friederich, E., Pringault, E., Arpin, M., and Louvard, D. (1990). From the structure to the function of villin, an actin-binding protein of the brush border. *BioEssays* **12,** 403–408.

Gebert, A., and Hach, G. (1992). Vimentin antibodies stain membranous epithelial cells in the rabbit bronchus-associated lymohoid tissue (BALT). *Histochemistry* **98,** 271–273.

Gebert, A., Hach, G., and Bartels, H. (1992). Co-localization of vimentin and cytokeratins in M-cells of rabbit gut-associated lymphoid tissue (GALT). *Cell Tissue Res.* **269,** 331–340.

Glenney, J., Jr., Geisler, N., Kaulfus, P., and Weber, K. (1981). Demonstration of at least two different actin binding sites in villin, a calcium-regulated modulator of F-actin organization. *J. Biol. Chem.* **256,** 8156–8161.

Gordon, J. I., and Hermiston M. L. (1994). Differentiation and self-renewal in the mouse gastrointestinal epithelium. *Curr. Opin. Cell Biol.* **6,** 795–803.

Kedinger, M. (1994). What triggers intestinal cells to move or stay and to proliferate and differentiate? *Gastroenterology* **107,** 885–888.

Kernéis, S., Bogdanova, A., Colucci-Guyon, E., Kraehenbuhl, J. P., and Pringault, E. (1996). Cytosolic distribution of villin in M cells from mouse Peyer's patches with the absence of a brush-border. *Gastroenterology* **110,** 515–521.

Kohbata, S., Yokobata, H., and Yabuuchi, E. (1986). Cytopathogenic effect of *Salmonella typhi* GIFU 10007 on M cells of murine ileal Peyer's patches in ligated ileal loops: An ultrastructural study. *Microbiol. Immunol.* **30**, 1225–1237.

Lefevre, M. E., Olivo, R., and Joel, D. D. (1978). Accumulation of latex particles in Peyer's patches and their subsequent appearance in villi and mesenteric lymph nodes. *Proc. Soc. Exp. Biol. Med.* **59**, 298–302.

Matsudaira, P. T., and Burgess, D. R. (1979). Identification and organization of the components in the isolated microvillus cytoskeleton. *J. Cell Biol.* **83**, 667–673.

Maunoury, R., Robine, S., Pringault, E., Huet, C., Guenet, J. L., Gaillard, J. A., and Louvard, D. (1988). Villin expression in the visceral endoderm and in the gut anlage during early mouse embryogenesis. *EMBO J.* **7**, 3321–3329.

Maunoury, R., Robine, S., Pringault, E., Leonard, N., Gaillard, J. A., and Louvard, D. (1992). Developmental regulation of villin gene expression in the epithelial cell lineages of mouse digestive and urogenital tracts. *Development (Cambridge, UK)* **115**, 717–728.

Neutra, M. R., and Kraehenbuhl, J. P. (1992). Transepithelial transport and mucosal defence: The role of M cells. *Trends Cell Biol.* **2**, 134–138.

Neutra, M. R., Phillips, T. L., Mayer, E. L., and Fishkind, D. J. (1987). Transport of membrane-bound macromolecules by M cells in follicle-associated epithelium of rabbit Peyer's patch. *Cell Tissue Res.* **247**, 537–546.

Neutra, M. R., Pringault, E., and Kraehenbuhl, J. P. (1995). Epithelial cells and mucosal immunity. *Annu. Rev. Immunol.* **14**, 275–300.

Owen, R. L. (1977). Sequential uptake of horseradish peroxidase by lymphoid follicle epithelium of Peyer's patches in the normal unobstructed mouse intestine: An ultrastructural study. *Gastroenterology* **72**, 440–451.

Owen, R. L., and Bhalla, D. K. (1983). Cytochemical analysis of alkaline phosphatase and esterase activities and of lectin-binding and anionic sites in rat and mouse Peyer's patch M cells. *Am. J. Anat.* **168**, 199–212.

Owen, R. L., Pierce, N. F., Apple, R. T., and Cray, W. C., Jr. (1986). M cell transport of *Vibrio cholerae* from the intestinal lumen into Peyer's patches: A mechanism for antigen sampling and for microbial transepithelial migration. *J. Infect. Dis.* **153**, 1108–1118.

Pappo, J., and Ermak, T. H. (1989). Uptake and translocation of fluorescent latex particles by rabbit Peyer's patch follicle epithelium: A quantitative model for M cell uptake. *Clin. Exp. Immunol.* **76**, 144–148.

Pringault, E., Arpin, M., Garcia, A., Findori, J., and Louvard, D. (1986). A human cDNA villin clone to investigate the differentiationof intestinal and kidney cells *in vivo* and in culture. *EMBO J.* **5**, 3119–3124.

Pringault, E. Robine, S., and Louvard, D. (1991). Structure of the human villin gene. *Proc. Natl. Acad. Sci. U.S.A.* **88**, 10811–10815.

Robine, S., Huet, C., Moll, R., Sahuquillo-Merino, C., Coudrier, E., Zweibaum, A., and Louvard, D. (1985). Can villin be used to identify malignant and undifferentiated normal digestive epithelial cells? *Proc. Natl. Acad. Sci. U.S.A.* **82**, 8488–8492.

Shibayama, T., Carboni, J. M., and Mooseker, M. S. (1987). Assembly of the intestinal brush border: Appearance and distribution of microvillar core proteins in developing chick enterocytes. *J. Cell Biol.* **105**, 335–344.

Sminia, T., van der Brugge-Gamelkoorn, G. J., and Jeurissen, S. H. M. (1989). Structure and function of bronchus-associated lymphoid tissue (BALT). *Crit. Rev. Immunol.* **9**, 119–151.

Smith, M. W., and Peacock, M. A. (1992). Microvillus growth and M-cell formation in mouse Peyer's patch follicle-associated epithelial tissue. *Exp. Physiol.* **77**, 389–392.

Wolf, J. L., Rubin, D. H., Finberg, R., Kauffman, R. S., Sharpe, A. H., Trier, J. S., and Fields, B. N. (1981). Intestinal M cells: A pathway for entry of reovirus into the host. *Science* **212**, 471–472.

# Chapter 4

# Role of Dendritic Cells, Macrophages, and $\gamma\delta$ T Cells in Antigen Processing and Presentation in the Respiratory Mucosa

P. G. Holt, D. J. Nelson, A. S. McWilliam, D. Cooper, D. Strickland, and J. W. Upham

*TVW Telethon Institute for Child Health Research,*
*West Perth, Western Australia 6872,*
*Australia*

## I. Introduction

Immune responses to inhaled antigens are regulated to a large extent by interactions between three cell populations: dendritic cells, resident tissue macrophages, and CD8$^+$ T cells. Recent studies in our lab on the characterization of these cell populations are reviewed below.

## II. Dendritic Cells

### A. Distribution and Surface Phenotype

Two distinct populations of dendritic cells (DC) exist within the respiratory tract (Holt *et al.*, 1988, 1989, 1990, Schon-Hegrad *et al.*, 1991), within the epithelium of the conducting airways and in the parenchyma of the peripheral lung, respectively. An additional population is found within the nasal mucosa, particularly in the region of the nasal turbinates (Nelson *et al.*, 1994) The majority of these cells constitutively express class II MHC antigen (Ia), but recent studies have identified the presence of a significant Ia $-$ subset in the airway epithelium (Nelson *et al.*, 1994).

### B. Function

The primary role of these DC is in surveillance for inhaled antigen, which they sequester and store in immunogenic form for subsequent presentation to T cells (Holt *et al.*, 1988, 1992, 1993). Analogous to epidermal Langerhans cells, their capacity for antigen presentation is limited during the epithelial phase of their life cycle, and this function develops only after exposure to GM-CSF (Holt *et al.*,

*Essentials of Mucosal Immunology*  Copyright © 1996 by Academic Press, Inc. All rights of reproduction in any form reserved.

1992, 1993), which is not envisaged to occur normally until their migration to regional lymph nodes [RLN (Holt *et al.*, 1993)]. In addition, the capacity of these DC to respond to GM-CSF is inhibited *in situ* by soluble signals (notably TNFα and NO) from resident tissue macrophages (Holt *et al.*, 1993).

### C. Population Dynamics

In the steady state, the half-life of the airway DC population is around 2 days, in contrast to ≥7 days and ≥15 days for similar populations in the deep lung and epidermis, respectively (Holt *et al.*, 1994). This rapid turnover is matched only by DC populations in the gut wall, reflecting the importance of these cells in antigen surveillance at the major "front-line" mucosal sites in the body.

### D. Response to Inflammation

Following inhalation of aerosols containing bacterial LPS (Schon-Hegrad *et al.*, 1991), or, in particular whole killed bacteria (McWilliam *et al.*, 1994), large numbers of DC are rapidly recruited into the airway epithelium with kinetics identical to those of PMN. Over the ensuing 48 hr, the majority of immigrants migrate further to RLN, presumably displaying the antigens encountered at the inflammatory site (McWilliam *et al.*, 1994).

The airway epithelial DC network also upregulates in chronic inflammation, increasing in both number and intensity of Ia expression (McWilliam *et al.*, 1994).

### E. Steroid Regulation of Airway DCs

Exposure to topical (inhaled) steroids lowers DC density in the airways of normal rats by 40–50% within 2–3 days, and rapid rebound ensues after withdrawal of drug, within the same time frame (Nelson *et al.*, 1995). High-dose systemic dexamethasone is considerably more potent, and reduces their density by ≥80% within 2–3 days (Nelson *et al.*, 1995).

Topical and systemic steroids are highly effective in prevention of DC recruitment during inflammation (Nelson *et al.*, 1995), but are ineffective in inhibition of the *in vitro* DC response to GM-CSF (Holt *et al.*, 1996).

### F. Ontogeny

In rats, the airway and lung DC networks mature postnatally from Ia- precursors that commence seeding into fetal respiratory tract tissues during late intrauterine development (Nelson *et al.*, 1994). Between birth and weaning, DC increase in both number and Ia expression, this process occurring most rapidly at sites of maximum inflammatory stimulation from the outside environment (especially the nasal turbinates; Nelson *et al.*, 1994).

During the early postnatal period, cells of the networks are relatively refractory to both GM-CSF and IFNγ stimulation, and moreover the capacity of the network to upregulate in response to local inflammatory challenge (e.g., by bacteria) is severely limited, relative to adults (Nelson and Holt, in press).

The overall rate of postnatal maturation of the airway DC network in rats parallels the development of their capacity to mount IgG responses to the inhaled antigens (McMenamin *et al.*, 1995). and accordingly we have postulated that the DC are "rate limiting" in the postnatal development of local immune competence in the respiratory tract.

## III. ENDOGENOUS TISSUE MACROPHAGES IN REGULATION OF THE LOCAL EXPRESSION OF T-CELL IMMUNITY

### A. Suppression of T-Cell Proliferation

Previous studies have established that endogenous macrophages in respiratory tract tissues, including those in the lung interstitum (Holt *et al.*, 1985), the airway mucosa (Holt *et al.*, 1988), and in particular the pulmonary alveolar macrophage (PAM) population present on the lumenal surface of the lung and airways (Holt, 1993), are capable of directly inhibiting the capacity of T cells to respond to DC-mediated activation (or to other stimuli such as mitogens) via proliferation.

### B. Cytokine Secretion in the Absence of Proliferation

Our recent work, however, indicates that this process is considerably more complex than hitherto recognized. It is now evident that despite their inability to proliferate in the presence of PAM, T cells undergo the full gamut of functional changes associated with activation. These include $Ca^{2+}$ flux, TCR downmodulation, CD28 upregulation, cytokine (including IL-2) secretion, and IL-2R $\alpha\beta$ expression; however, they appear unable to transduce signals downstream of IL-2R engagement, and remain locked in the $G_0/G_1$ phase of the cell cycle (Strickland *et al.*, 1994; Strickland, Kees and Holt, submitted for publication. Strickland, Upham *et al.*, 1995).

### C. Reversibility of PAM Effects

An important finding relative to interpretation of the biological significance of this phenomenon is that of its reversibility. Thus, following separation of antigen-stimulated T cells from PAM, even after 3 days in coculture, the hitherto "suppressed" T cells rapidly commence proliferation (Strickland *et al.*, 1994).

### D. The *in Vivo* Role of PAM-Mediated T-Cell Suppression

We interpret these findings as follows. Rather than suppression of T-cell functions, this mechanism provides the means to fine-tune the local expression of T-cell immunity by limiting the T-effector response at the individual cell level to a "single hit." Thus, incoming T cells can respond locally to antigen and secrete their full repertoire of cytokines, but are unable to expand clonally. However, the latter can occur following the subsequent migration of the T cells to RLN, thus contributing to the maintenance of immunological memory relating to antigens encountered in the lung.

### E. Cytokine-Mediated Alterations in the Functional Phenotype of PAM

Culture of PAM in GM-CSF, particularly in the presence of TNF$\alpha$, transiently downmodulates the T-cell suppressive properties of PAM, rendering them permissive for T-cell proliferation (Bilyk and Holt, 1993). However, if culture in the presence of GM-CSF is prolonged beyond 24–48 hr, the PAM spontaneously revert to their original phenotype (Bilyk and Holt, 1995), possibly as a result of tachyphylaxis of GM-CSF receptors. TGF$\beta$ exerts similar effects, and the effects of these cytokines appear to be mediated via inhibition of NO production (Bilyk and Holt, 1995). This provides a potential mechanism for bypassing PAM suppression and facilitating the transient local expression of T-cell immunity, in the face of immunoinflammatory challenge (Bilyk and Holt, 1993, 1995).

### F. Mechanism(s) of PAM-Mediated T-Cell Suppression

In the rat and the mouse, it is clear that NO production plays a central role in this process (Bilyk and Holt, 1995; Strickland et al., 1994, and submitted; Upham et al., 1995), with smaller contributions from TGF$\beta$, IL-1R antagonist, and PGE$_2$; in humans, despite similar overall effects of PAM on T cells (Upham et al., 1995; Upham, Strickland, Robinson, and Holt, submitted), we have been unable to ascribe a role to NO or any of the aforementioned mediators.

## IV. CD8$^+$ T-Cell Regulation of Primary Immune Responses to Inhaled Antigen

Our laboratory has been involved in the study of regulation of primary IgE responses to inhaled antigen for several years (reviewed in Holt and McMenamin, 1989), and has described an important role for CD8$^+$ T cells.

Thus, exposure of animals to aerosolized antigen triggers a transient, self-limiting IgE/IgG$_1$ response, often with concomitant preservation of IgG$_{2a/2b}$ and IgA responses; subsequent parenteral challenge of animals reveals "tolerance" with respect to IgE/IgG$_1$ and DTH responses to the antigen, a phenomenon which can be adoptively transferred by purified CD8$^+$ (but not CD4$^+$) T cells. This process represents the respiratory tract equivalent of oral tolerance, achieved by feeding low doses of antigen.

## A. Cytokine Responses during "Tolerance" Induction

Recent studies indicate that during the early phase of this process, during which low-level IgE is being produced (specific to the challenge antigen), the immune response in the lymph nodes draining the airway mucosa is dominated by CD4[+] T cells which secrete both IL-2 and IL-4 (McMenamin and Holt, 1993). As IgE production wanes, the cytokine response progressively changes to IFN$\gamma$ production by MHC class I-restricted antigen-specific CD8[1] T cells, the initial *in vitro* activation of which is dependent on IL-2 released by MHC class II-restricted antigen-specific CD4[+] T cells (McMenamin and Holt, 1993).

Evidence for the latter is provided by *in vitro* experiments demonstrating that IFN$\gamma$ production was blocked by MoAbs against MHC class II or CD4, and the blocking was reversible by rec IL-2. Additionally, IFN$\gamma$ production was blockable by anti-MHC-class I MoAb, and this was not reversible by rec IL-2, identifying the ultimate effector cell as a MHC class I-restricted CD8[+] T cell responding to nominal (in this case OVA) antigen (McMenamin and Holt, 1993). This process accordingly appears analogous to classical "immune deviation."

## B. The Role of $\gamma\delta$ T Cells

In adoptive transfer experiments, the CD8[+] T cell was identified initially as CD3[+] but $\alpha\beta$ TCR, suggesting a role for either CD8[+] $\gamma\delta$T or CD8[+] $\alpha\beta$T cells with temporarily downmodulated TCR (McMenamin *et al.*, 1991).

Direct evidence in support of the former was provided in follow-up studies involving positive selection of mouse $\gamma\delta$ T cells employing the GL-3 MoAb (McMenamin *et al.*, 1994) and selection of rat $\gamma\delta$ T cells via the V6-5 MoAb from Dr T. Hunig (McMenamin *et al.*, 1995). In both studies, immune deviation was transferable by as few as 50–500 positively selected $\gamma\delta$ T, cells, and additionally appeared antigen-specific as shown by crossover experiments with a second antigen (McMenamin *et al.*, 1994, 1995).

Immunohistochemical studies (unpublished) indicate that unlike skin and gut mucosa, which contain large numbers of $\gamma\delta$ T cells, the normal airway mucosa contain very few of these cells; given the initial site at which they appear in this system [viz. the regional lymph node, as inferred by earlier adoptive transfer experiments (Sedgwick and Holt, 1985)], we surmise that they are part of the central $\gamma\delta$ T pool, as opposed to the mucosal dwelling population.

Studies are in progress to identify the antigen-presenting cells responsible for their initial activation, and in particular the role of migrating airway intraepithelial DC.

## ACKNOWLEDGMENTS

This work is supported by the NH&MRC of Australia, and GLAXO.

# REFERENCES

Bilyk, N., and Holt, P. G. (1993). Inhibition of the immunosuppressive activity of resident pulmonary alveolar macrophages by granulocyte/macrophage colony-stimulating factor. *J. Exp. Med.* **177**, 1773–1777.

Bilyk, N., and Holt, P. G. (1995). Cytokine modulation of the immunosuppressive phenotype of pulmonary alveolar macrophages via regulation of nitric oxide production. *Immunology* **86**, 231–237.

Holt, P. G. (1993). Regulation of antigen-presenting cell function(s) in lung and airway tissues. *Eur. Respir. J.* **6**, 120–129.

Holt, P. G., and McMenamin, C. (1989). Defence against allergic sensitization in the healthy lung: The role of inhalation tolerance. *Clin. Exp. Allergy* **19**, 255–262.

Holt, P. G., Degebrodt, A., Venaille, T., O'Leary, C., Krska, K., Flexman, J., Farrell, H., Shellam, G., Young, P., Penhale, J., Robertson, T., and Papadimitriou, J. M. (1985). Preparation of interstitial lung cells by enzymatic digestion of tissue slices: Preliminary characterization by morphology and performance in functional assays. *Immunology* **54**, 139–147.

Holt, P. G., Schon-Hegrad, M. A., and Oliver, J. (1988). MHC class II antigen-bearing dendritic cells in pulmonary tissues of the rat. Regulation of antigen presentation activity by endogenous macrophage populations. *J. Exp. Med.* **167**, 262–274.

Holt, P. G., Schon-Hegrad, M. A., Phillips, M. J., and McMenamin, P. G. (1989). Ia-positive dendritic cells form a tightly meshed network within the human airway epithelium. *Clin. Exp. Allergy* **19**, 597–601.

Holt, P. G., Schon-Hegrad, M. A., Oliver, J., Holt, B. J., and McMenamin, P. G. (1990). A contiguous network of dendritic antigen-presenting cells within the respiratory epithelium. *Int. Arch. Allergy Appl. Immunol.* **91**, 155–159.

Holt, P. G., Oliver, J., McMenamin, C., and Schon-Hegrad, M. A. (1992). Studies on the surface phenotype and functions of dendritic cells in parenchymal lung tissue of the rat. *Immunology* **75**, 582–587.

Holt, P. G., Oliver, J., Bilyk, N., McMenamin, C., McMenamin, P. G., Kraal, G., and Thepen, T. (1993). Downregulation of the antigen presenting cell function(s) of pulmonary dendritic cells *in vivo* by resident alveolar macrophages. *J. Exp. Med.* **177**, 397–407.

Holt, P. G., Haining, S., Nelson, D. J., and Sedgwick, J. D. (1994). Origin and steady-state turnover of class II MHC-bearing Dendritic Cells in the epithelium of the conducting airways. *J. Immunol.* **153**, 256–261.

Holt, P. G., Thomas, J. A., McWilliam, A. S., and Nelson, D. J. (1996). Steroids inhibit recruitment of Dendritic Cells into the airway epithelium, but do not prevent their functional activation by GM-CSF. Submitted.

McMenamin, C., and Holt, P. G. (1993). The natural immune response to inhaled soluble protein antigens involves major histocompatibility complex (MHC) class I-restricted CD8+ T cell-mediated but MHC class II-restricted CD4+ T cell-dependent immune deviation resulting in selective suppression of IgE production. *J. Exp. Med.* **178**, 889–899.

McMenamin, C., Oliver, J., Girn, B., Holt, B. J., Kees, U. R., Thomas, W. R., and Holt, P. G. (1991). Regulation of T-cell sensitization at epithelial surfaces in the respiratory tract: Suppression of IgE responses to inhaled antigens by CD3+ TcR α-/β-lymphocytes (putative γ/δ T cells). *Immunology* **74**, 234–239.

McMenamin, C., Pimm, C., McKersey, M., and Holt, P. G. (1994). Regulation of CD4+-TH-2-dependent IgE responses to inhaled antigen in mice by antigen-specific γ/δ T-cells. *Science* **265**, 1859–1861.

McMenamin, C., McKersey, M., Kuhnlein, P., Hunig, T., and Holt, P. G. (1995). γ/δ T-cells downregulate primary IgE responses in rats to inhaled soluble protein antigens. *J. Immunol.* **154**, 4390–4394.

McWilliam, A. S., Nelson, D., Thomas, J. A., and Holt, P. G. (1994). Rapid Dendritic Cell recruitment is a hallmark of the acute inflammatory response at mucosal surfaces. *J. Exp. Med.* **179,** 1331–1336.

Nelson, D. J., and Holt, P. G. Defective regional immunity in the respiratory tract of neonates is attributable to hyporesponsiveness of local Dendritic Cells to activation signals. *J. Immunol.* in press.

Nelson, D. J., McMenamin, C., McWilliam, A. S., Brenan, M., and Holt, P. G. (1994). Development of the airway intraepithelial Dendritic Cell network in the rat from class II MHC (Ia) negative precursors: Differential regulation of Ia expression at different levels of the respiratory tract. *J. Exp. Med.* **179,** 203–212.

Nelson, D. J., McWilliam, A. S., Haining, S., and Holt, P. G. (1995). Modulation of airway intraepithelial Dendritic Cells following exposure to steroids. *Am. J. Respir. Crit. Care Med.* **151,** 475–481.

Schon-Hegrad, M. A., Oliver, J., McMenamin, P. G., and Holt, P. G. (1991). Studies on the density, distribution, and surface phenotype of intraepithelial class II major histocompatibility complex antigen (Ia)-bearing dendritic cells (DC) in the conducting airways. *J. Exp. Med.* **173,** 1345–1356.

Sedgwick, J. D., and Holt, P. G. (1985). Induction of IgE-secreting cells and IgE isotype-specific suppressor T cells in the respiratory lymph nodes of rats in response to antigen inhalation. *Cell. Immunol.* **94,** 182–194.

Strickland, D. H., Kees, U. R., and Holt, P. G. (1994). Suppression of T-cell activation by Pulmonary Alveolar Macrophages: dissociation of effects on TcR, IL-2R expression, and proliferation. *Eur. Resp. J.* in press.

Strickland, D. H., Kees, U. R., and Holt, P. G. Regulation of T-cell activation in the lung: Alveolar macrophages induce reversible T-cell anergy *in vivo* associated with inhibition of IL-2R signal transduction. Submitted.

Strickland, D. H., Kees, U. R., and Holt, P. G. Regulation of T-cell activation in the lung: Isolated lung T-cells exhibit surface phenotypic characteristics of recent activation including downmodulated TcR, but are locked into $G_0/G_1$ phase of the cell cycle. Submitted.

Upham, J. W., Strickland, D. H., Bilyk, N., Robinson, B. W. S., and Holt, P. G. (1995). Alveolar macrophages from humans and rodents selectively inhibit T-cell proliferation but permit T-cell activation and cytokine secretion. *Immunology* **84,** 142–147.

Upham, J. W., Strickland, D. H., Robinson, B. W. S., and Holt, P. G. (1996). Alveolar macrophages selectively inhibit T-cell proliferation but not expression of effector function. Submitted.

## Chapter 5

# Nonprofessional Antigen Presentation: New Rules and Regulations

L. Mayer, X. Y. Yio, A. Panja, and N. Campbell

*Division of Clinical Immunology,
The Mount Sinai Medical Center,
New York, New York 10029*

Recent studies from a number of laboratories have supported the existence of nonprofessional antigen-presenting cells (1). By definition this means that such cells are not macrophages, dendritic cells, or B cells; more concretely, this means that cells do not constitutively express class II molecules, do not express conventional costimulatory molecules for T-cell activation, or are poorly phagocytic. The emerging concept is that interaction of T cells with such antigen-presenting cells results in the induction of anergy or no activation at all (2). This may be one of the bases for the prevention of autoimmune responses. In the systemic immune system it is advantageous for the host to block autoantigen recognition early on. Such inhibition may be easy to regulate in the antigen-pristine environment of the spleen, lymph nodes, etc.

In the gastrointestinal tract the demands upon the immune system are different. There is a marked difference in antigen load, with the intestine constantly exposed to dietary, viral, and bacterial products, antigens that would evoke active immune responses if administered systemically. However, there are differences here too. Antigens that pass through the gastrointestinal (GI) tract are affected by multiple factors that alter their form, including salivary secretions, gastric acid, pancreatic proteases, and bile acids. Thus, by the time Ags reach the mucosal immune system they may be nonantigenic (di- and tripeptides) or processed to a form that is distinct from that which would result from processing by systemic antigen presenting cells (APC)s. This luminal preprocessing is coupled with a battery of unique sites where antigen can gain access to the mucosal immune system, the M cell, and the absorptive epithelium. It has become quite clear that the intestinal epithetial cells (IEC) can no longer viewed as a passive player in the immune responses seen in the gut. Several laboratories have documented that IEC can process and present antigen to primed T cells *in vitro* (3–6).

*Essentials of Mucosal Immunology* Copyright © 1996 by Academic Press, Inc. All rights of reproduction in any form reserved.

In addition, IEC produce a number of immunoregulatory cytokines and in turn possess receptors for cytokines which can alter APC function (7–10). However, there are several features of the IEC that place it in a unique position, acting as an APC. First, these cells are poorly phagocytic and fail to process large macromolecules in a manner similar to that of monocytes/macrophages (11). Thus, Ags sampled by IEC may be incapable of "normal" antigen presentation by conventional restriction elements. This processing defect may be less critical given the preprocessing of Ag that occurs in the lumen. However, the wide array of peptides which can be presented is lost in this process. Second, and potentially related to this, is the finding that IEC can express nonclassical restriction elements CD1 and Tl in mouse and CD1d in man (12–14). These class Ib molecules are nonpolymorphic but are capable of binding peptides and interestingly nonpeptide antigens. One important recent finding is the fact that they bind larger peptides than class I and class II molecules can, allow for overhang of peptides beyond the antigen binding groove, and, as is the case for CD1, have endosomal localization motifs (15). Thus these are class I-like molecules that can travel in a class II compartment and potentially bind to exogenous Ags that have been subjected to limited processing. The fact that CD1d can function in such a system has been supported by experiments documenting that antibodies to CD1d can inhibit T-cell proliferation induced by normal IEC (15) and the cytolysis of IEC by intraepithelial lymphocytes (IEL) (16). These antibodies have no effect on T-cell activation induced by monocytes or dendritic cells. Conversely, mAbs directed against conventional restriction elements (class Ia and class II) are incapable of inhibiting T-cell proliferation in T-cell:IEC cocultures (17). Thus IEC appear to be unconventional in many ways.

However, probably the most intriguing finding has been the preferential activation of CD8$^+$ suppressor T cells by normal IEC. Similar results have been obtained in rat and man (3,5). This is not to say that CD4$^+$ T cells cannot be activated in these cocultures. Purified populations of CD4$^+$ T cells proliferate quite well in response to class II antigen-expressing IEC (6,18). In fact, under these conditions proliferation can be inhibited by antibodies to class II. However when bulk populations of T cells are stimulated, CD8$^+$ T-cell proliferation predominates. Functionally these cells are noncytolytic and suppress broadly in an antigen-unrestricted fashion in man (5). Phenotypically these cells are CD8$\alpha_\beta$$^+$, CD28$^-$, IL-2R$^+$. To date we have been unable to reproducibly demonstrate suppressor factor production (e.g., IL-10, TGF$\beta$) by these activated cells.

The obvious question is how these cells get activated. mAb inhibition experiments have shown that CD8 itself is important and the activation of a CD8-associated src-like tyrosine kinase, p56lck, is a necessary but not sufficient event (17). It appears then that a molecule expressed by IEC is capable of binding to and crosslinking CD8. The obvious candidate, class Ia molecules, neither activates p56lck nor restricts T cell:IEC interactions.

Given the data reported above it would seem that CD1d might be a candidate

## Possible roles of gp180

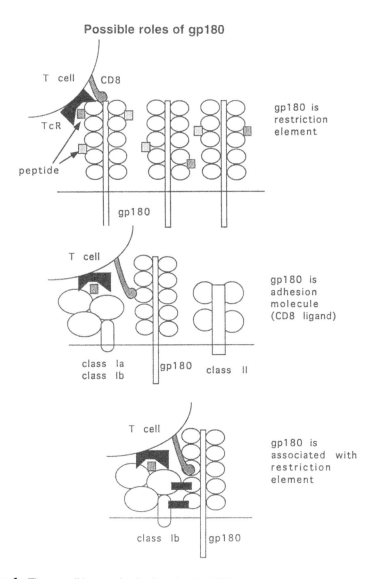

**FIGURE 1.** Three possible scenarios for the role of gp180 in regulating mucosal immune responses. In the first scenario gp180 is a novel restriction element capable of binding peptides and associating with both the T-cell receptor (TCR) and CD8. In this capacity gp180 would be class I-like. The second scenario suggests that gp180 does not associate with the T-cell receptor but is capable of binding to CD8 as described in the text. In this context gp180 is functioning as an adhesion molecule. The third scenario is where gp180 cannot associate with the TCR itself but does associate with either a conventional or nonclassical restriction element on the epithelial cell. Here the TCR is engaged by the restriction element and CD8 is brought in to the coreceptor complex by gp180 ligation.

for such a regulatory molecule. However, thus far there are no data which support that CD1d can bind to CD8. Furthermore, antibodies to CD1d which block IEC-induced T-cell proliferation fail to block p56lck activation. Furthermore, CD1d transfectants (kind gift of Dr. Richard Blumberg—Brigham & Women's Hospital, Boston, MA) fail to activate p56lck in murine T-cell hybridomas transfected with full-length CD8$\alpha$ cDNA. Finally, mAbs to CD1d also appear to inhibit CD4$^+$ T-cell proliferation induced by some IEC preparations, suggesting that the effects of this class Ib molecule are not CD8-restricted.

In order to define a novel CD8 ligand on IEC, we generated a series of mAbs against normal IEC. The criteria for selection were: first, that the mAbs be epithelial cell specific; second, that they inhibit CD8$^+$ T-cell proliferation induced by normal IEC; and third, that they inhibit activation of CD8$\alpha$-associated p56lck. Two mAbs recognizing a 180-kDa glycoprotein (gp180) were identified, B9 and L12. Both mAbs recognize distinct carbohydrate epitopes on the gp180 molecule. This molecule was purified by mAb B9 affinity chromatography and was shown to bind to CD8$^+$ T cells and activate CD8 associated p56lck. Further characterization awaits its cloning, but gp180, from its structure, appears to be more of an adhesion molecule. One would then have to speculate that gp180 associates with a surface molecule that is capable of binding to the T-cell antigen receptor either alone or when complexed to gp180. The predicted scenarios for gp180 function are depicted in Fig. 1. The currently favored model is one where gp180 associates with a class Ib molecule. This would explain the presentation of exogenous antigen to CD8$^+$ T cells by IEC, the presence of predominantly CD8$^+$ T cells in the IEC compartment, and the poor activation of mucosal lymphocytes by conventional APCs. Intrinsically this makes sense as the cost of immunodysregulation in the gut is clear: inflammation and the loss of functional integrity of the GI tract. A distinct set of rules and regulations are in order for an immune system with such inflammatory potential.

## ACKNOWLEDGMENTS

Supported by PHS Grants AI 23504, AI 24671, and DK 44156.

## REFERENCES

1. Wiman, K., Curman, B., Forsum, U., Klareskug, L., Malmnas-Tjernlund, U., Rask, L., Tragardh, L., and P. A. Peterson, (1978). Occurrence of a Ia antigens on tissues of nonlymphoid origin. *Nature (London)* **276,** 711.
2. Lenschow, D. J., and Bluestone, J. A. (1993). T cell co-stimulation and *in vivo* tolerance. *Curr. Opin. Immunol.* **5**(5), 747–752.
3. Bland, P. W., and Warren, L. G. (1986). Antigen presentation by epithelial cells of rat small intestine. I. Selective induction of suppressor T cells. *Immunology* **58,** 9.
4. Bland, P. W., and Warren, L. G. (1986). Antigen presentation by epithelial cells of rat small intestine. I. Kinetics. Antigen specificity and blocking by anti Ia antisera. *Immunology* **58,** 1.

5. Mayer, L., and Shlien, R. (1987). Evidence for function of a Ia molecule on gut epithelial cells in man. *J. Exp. Med.* **166,** 1471.
6. Kaiserlian, D., Vidal, K., and Revillard, J. P. (1989) Murine enterocytes can present soluble antigen to specific class II restricted . CD4+ T cells. *Eur. J. Immunol.* **19,** 1513.
7. Deem, R. L., Shanahan, F., and Targan, S. R. (1990). Triggered mucosal T cells release TNFa and IFN g which kill human colonic epithelial cells. *Gastro* **98,** A444 (1990).
8. Madara, J. C., and Staffork, J. (1989). Interferon g directly affects barrier function of cultured intestinal epithelial monolayers. *J. Clin. Invest.* **83,** 724–727.
9. Chang, F. B., Musch, M. and Mayer, L. (1990). IL-1 and IL-3 regulation short circuit current in the chicken enterocyte. *Gastroenterology* **98,** 1518.
10. Ciacci, C. Mahida, Y. R., Dignass, A., Koizumi, M., Podolsky, D. K. (1993). Functional interleukin-2 receptors on intestinal epithelial cells. *J. Clin. Invest.* **92**(1), 527–532.
11. Bland, P. W., and Whiting, C. V. (1989). Antigen processing by isolated rat intestinal villus enterocytes. *Immunology* **68,** 497.
12. Bleicher, P. A., Balk, S. P., Hagen, S. J., Blumberg, R. S., Flotte, T. J., and Terhorst, C. (1990). Expression of murine CD1 on gastrointestinal epithelium. *Science* **250,** 679.
13. Blumberg, R. S., Terhorst, C., Bleicher, P. McDermott, F. V., et al. (1991). Expression of a non-polymorphic MHC class I-like molecule. CD1d, by human intestinal epithelial cells. *J. Immunol.* **147,** 2518.
14. Hershberg, R., Eghtesady, P., Sydora, B., Brorson, K., *et al.* (1990). Expression of the thymus leukemia antigen in mouse intestinal epithelium. *Proc. Natl. Acad. Sci. U.S.A.* **87,** 9727–9731.
15. Panja, A., Blumberg, R. S., Balk, S. P., Mayer, L. (1993). CD1d is involved in T cell: Epithelial cell interactions. *J. Exp. Med.* **178,** 1115.
16. Sydora, B. C., Mixter, P. F., Holcombe, H. R., Eghtesady, P., *et al.* (1993). Intestinal intraepithelial lymphocytes are activated and cytolytic but do not proliferate as well as other T cells in response to mitogenic signals. J *Immunol.* **150,** 2179–2191.
17. Li, Y., Yio, X. Y., and Mayer, L. (1995). Human intestinal epithelial cell induced CD8+ T cell activation is mediated through CD8 and the activation of CD8-associated p56[lck] *J. Exp. Med.* in press.
18. Mayer, L., Siden, E., Becker, S., and Eisenhardt, D. (1990). Antigen handling in the intestine mediated by normal enterocytes. *In* "Advances in Mucosal Immunology" (T. MacDonald, S. Challacombe, P. W. Bland, C. R. Stokes, R. V. Heatly, A. N. Mowat, eds.), pp. 23–28. Kluwer, Dordrecht, The Netherlands.

*part*

# II

# ROLE OF EPITHELIAL CELLS IN MUCOSAL IMMUNITY

## Chapter 6

# Intestinal Epithelial Cells: An Integral Component of the Mucosal Immune System

Martin F. Kagnoff, Lars Eckmann, Suk-Kyun Yang, George Huang, Hyun C. Jung, Sharon L. Reed, and Joshua Fierer

*Department of Medicine, University of California, San Diego, La Jolla, California 92093*

## I. INTRODUCTION

Intestinal epithelial cells compose a barrier that separates the host's internal milieu from the external environment. These cells have been studied extensively in the past because of their essential role in secretory and absorptive processes. More recent studies show that intestinal epithelial cells can be regarded also as an integral and essential component of the host's innate and acquired immune system. Thus, intestinal epithelial cells constitutively express, or can be induced to express, HLA class II molecules (Mayer *et al.,* 1991) known to be important in antigen presentation, classical class I as well as nonclassical HLA class Ib molecules such as CD1d (Blumberg *et al.,* 1991) and the neonatal Fc receptor for IgG, receptors for the cytokines IL-1, IL-2, IL-4, IL-6, IFN$\gamma$, and TGF$\beta$1 (Ciacci *et al.,* 1993; Mulder *et al.,* 1990; Fantini *et al.,* 1992; Ullmann *et al.,* 1992; Raitano and Korc, 1993; Reinecker and Podolsky, 1995), complement components (C3, C4, factor B) (Andoh *et al.,* 1993), eicosanoids (Eckmann *et al.,* 1995a), and, as will be discussed in this chapter, an array of proinflammatory cytokines and the adhesion molecule ICAM-1 (Jung *et al.,* 1995; Eckmann *et al.,* 1993a; Yang *et al.,* 1995; Huang *et al.,* 1995a). In this contemporary view, intestinal epithelial cells communicate with other mucosal cells via a spectrum of mediators that have both autocrine and paracrine activities (Fig. 1). These mediators act on the intestinal epithelial cells themselves, as well as on intraepithelial lymphocytes (IEL) in the paracellular space, and on lymphoid cells, mononuclear phagocytes, neutrophils, mast cells, and eosinophils in the adjacent lamina propria. These latter cells also act as important components of the host's cytokine cascade and, as such, release additional mediators which have further autocrine and paracrine effects on epithelial cells, as well as lymphoid and mononuclear cells in the lamina propria. These cascades of mediator release and mediator activity are finely regulated both to

*Essentials of Mucosal Immunology* Copyright © 1996 by Academic Press, Inc. All rights of reproduction in any form reserved.

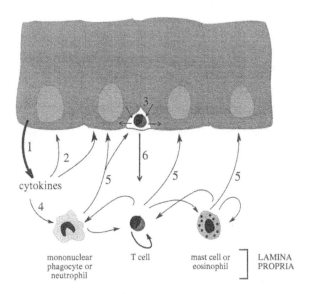

**FIGURE 1.** Intestinal epithelial cells are an integral component of a communications network. Cytokines produced by intestinal epithelial cells (1) can have autocrine or paracrine effects on other epithelial cells (2) as well as stimulate IEL (3) and cells within the lamina propria (4). Lamina propria cells activated by epithelial cell cytokines in turn release mediators (5) which act on epithelial cells as well as other cell populations within the lamina propria. Intraepithelial lymphocytes also release cytokines that influence epithelial cell growth and differentiation as well as the function of underlying cells in the lamina propria (6).

induce and to downregulate appropriate host immune and inflammatory responses at mucosal surfaces.

## II. REGULATED PRODUCTION OF PROINFLAMMATORY CYTOKINES BY HUMAN COLON EPITHELIAL CELLS

### A. Constitutive and Regulated Production of Proinflammatory Cytokines in Response to Agonist Stimulation

We have characterized the constitutive and regulated production of proinflammatory cytokines in response to agonists using human colon cancer cell lines (Eckmann *et al.*, 1993a; Jung *et al.*, 1995; Yang *et al.*, 1995). In undertaking these studies, we reasoned that, despite their transformed nature, if an identical array of proinflammatory cytokines was expressed and upregulated in several cell lines of different origin, the regulated expression of those cytokines would likely prove to be a general property of normal colon epithelial cells as well, unless the expression, or lack of expression, of a specific cytokine was causally related to the transformation process.

Human colon epithelial cell lines can constitutively express a broad array of cytokines including C–X–C and C–C chemokines, as well as GM-CSF and TNFα (Table I). Each of these cytokines promotes the inflammatory response and can be upregulated in the cell lines by TNFα and/or IL-1. Human colon epithelial cells also express TGFβ1, a cytokine with potent activity with respect to downregulating inflammatory and immune responses (Eckmann et al., 1993a; Jung et al., 1995; Yang et al., 1995) and stimulating isotype switching to the IgA class (Kim and Kagnoff, 1990; van Vlasselaer et al., 1992). Unlike the proinflammatory cytokines, expression of TGF$_{\beta 1}$ was not significantly altered following TNFα or IL-1 stimulation. Importantly, none of the human intestinal colon cell lines express immunoregulatory cytokines such as IL-2, IL-4, IL-5, IL-12p40, or IFNγ (Eckmann et al., 1993a), constitutively or following agonist stimulation.

Studies to address the mechanisms by which proinflammatory cytokines are upregulated in colon epithelial cells in response to agonist stimulation have focused on agonist-induced expression of the prototypic C–X–C chemokine IL-8, a cytokine important for neutrophil chemotaxis and activation (Eckmann et al., 1993a; Jung et al., 1995). Stimulation of several human colon cancer cell lines (e.g., T84, Caco-2, HT29, SW620) with TNFα or IL-1 upregulated IL-8 gene transcription, IL-8 mRNA levels, and IL-8 secretion in TNFα or IL-1-responsive colon cell lines (Eckmann et al., 1993a). IL-8 gene transcription, mRNA levels, and protein secretion increased rapidly in the first 2–4 hr following agonist stimulation and declined over the ensuing several hours, despite continued agonist stimulation (Fig. 2). The cytokines IFNγ, EGF, and IL-6 by themselves had little, if any, stimulatory effect on IL-8 production by the cell lines. However, in combination with TNFα, there was marked potentiation of the upregulation of the IL-8 response (Eckmann et al., 1993a).

## B. Bacterial Invasion Is a Potent Stimulus for the Production of Proinflammatory Cytokines by Colon Epithelial Cells

Invasion of the intestinal mucosal surfaces by pathogenic bacteria is accompanied by an acute inflammatory response typically characterized by a marked infiltration

TABLE I

HUMAN COLON EPITHELIAL CELL LINES CAN EXPRESS A
BROAD ARRAY OF PROINFLAMMATORY CYTOKINES

| C–X–C chemokines | C–C chemokines | Other proinflammatory cytokines |
| --- | --- | --- |
| IL-8 | MCP-1 | GM-CSF |
| GROα | MIP-1α | TNFα |
| GROβ | MIP-1β | |
| GROγ | RANTES | |
| ENA-78 | | |

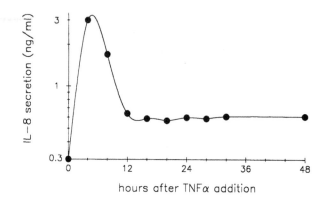

**FIGURE 2.** Time course of TNFα-stimulated IL-8 secretion by the human T84 colon cancer cell line. Confluent T84 cell monolayers were stimulated with TNFα for up to 48 hr. IL-8 secretion was determined for each time point by removing the medium and, subsequently, incubating the cells in freshly added medium containing TNFα for a 4-hr period. (From Eckmann *et al.*, 1993a, with permission of the authors.)

of neutrophils. To understand the mechanisms that underlie this acute inflammatory response, it is important to define the proinflammatory signals involved and to identify the crucial cells that produce these signals. We asked whether intestinal epithelial cells, which are the first host cells to come into contact with an invading pathogen, serve as an early signaling system to adjacent and underlying inflammatory cells following invasion by bacteria. We demonstrated that IL-8 secretion by human colon epithelial cell lines was rapidly upregulated in response to coculture with several different gram-negative and gram-positive bacteria (Table II), but not in response to coculture with similar inocula of noninvasive bacteria (Eckmann *et al.*, 1993b). Consistent with the interpretation that cellular invasion was required for induction of the epithelial cytokine response, cytochalasin D, which blocks actin polymerization and bacterial entry in epithelial cells, abrogated the ability of highly invasive *Salmonella* strains to induce an IL-8 response in colon epithelial cell monolayers (Eckmann *et al.*, 1993b). The IL-8 response is not entirely dependent on the specific mechanism that is used by the bacteria to enter the host cells, or the intracellular bacterial location, since entry mechanisms and intracellular "lifestyle" differ among the invasive bacteria studied. Moreover, IL-8 mRNA expression by cultured colon epithelial cells increases within 2–3 hr of infection and declines rapidly thereafter. This suggests that intestinal epithelial cells play an important role by providing early signals for the initiation of an acute mucosal inflammatory response. Later during the course of infection, it is likely that inflammatory cells themselves become the dominant producers of IL-8 as long as the bacteria and their products remain within the mucosa. Finally, we note that IL-8 secretion was observed predominantly from the basolateral surface of polarized monolayers of T84 cells in response to TNFα stimulation or bacterial invasion

TABLE II

INVASIVE BACTERIA THAT HAVE BEEN
DEMONSTRATED TO STIMULATE IL-8 SECRETION
BY HUMAN COLON EPITHELIAL CELL LINES

*Salmonella dublin* Lane
Enteroinvasive *Escherichia coli*
*Shigella dysenteriae*
*Yersinia enterocolitica*
*Listeria monocytogenes*

(Eckmann *et al.,* 1993a,b). This vectorial secretion may be important for establishing a chemotactic gradient for the migration of neutrophils to the epithelial layer following invasion of the epithelium by pathogenic bacteria.

Further studies assessed the levels of constitutive and regulated expression of members of the GRO family of C–X–C chemokines that act as potent neutrophil chemoattractants and activators, and of MCP-1 and MIP-1$\beta$, which are prototypic members of the C–C family of chemokines that function as chemoattractants and activators of cells of the monocyte/macrophage lineage and T cells. Like IL-8, mRNA levels for the GRO family of chemokines (i.e., GRO$\alpha$, $\beta$, $\gamma$) were markedly upregulated following infection of epithelial monolayers with invasive bacteria (Yang *et al.,* 1995). This was also the case, although to a lesser extent, for MCP-1 and MIP-1$\beta$ (Jung *et al.,* 1995; Yang *et al.,* 1995). In addition to chemokines, the proinflammatory cytokines GM-CSF and TNF$\alpha$ also are upregulated following microbial invasion of colon epithelial cells (Jung *et al.,* 1995). These latter cytokines are of particular relevance given their known potential for autocrine effects on epithelial cells (e.g., increased HLA class II expression) and paracrine effects on monocytes/macrophages and dendritic cells in the mucosa. Our *in vitro* studies were confirmed *in vivo* using freshly isolated colon epithelial cells that were infected with bacteria *in vitro* or stimulated with various agonists (Jung *et al.,* 1995). In addition to the cytokines mentioned above, freshly isolated human colon epithelial cells, but not the cell lines, produced IL-6 (Jung *et al.,* 1995). In summary, invasion of epithelial cells by bacteria or, alternatively, stimulation of epithelial cells with proinflammatory agonists such as TNF$\alpha$ or IL-1 defines two paradigms for upregulating the expression and secretion of proinflammatory cytokines by epithelial cells.

## III. CYTOLYTIC PATHOGENS: A FURTHER PARADIGM FOR UPREGULATION OF PROINFLAMMATORY CYTOKINES BY INTESTINAL EPITHELIAL AND STROMAL CELLS

Cytolytic pathogens, such as *Entamoeba histolytica* trophozoites, damage the human colonic epithelium in focal areas resulting in extensive cell lysis and the development of mucosal ulcerations. The acute response of the host likely determines whether or not the infection will spread systemically. We have focused on the mechanism by which the host signals the stimulation of an acute inflammatory response following infection with cytolytic pathogens using *E. histolytica* trophozoites as a model system. For these studies, human colon epithelial cell lines and intestinal stromal cells, such as colonic fibroblasts and intestinal smooth muscle cells as well as human liver cells, were cocultured with *E. histolytica* trophozoites. Coculture of these cells with *E. histolytica* trophozoites resulted in increased secretion of an array of chemoattractant and proinflammatory cytokines that included IL-8, GROα, GM-CSF, and, in some cases, IL-6 (Eckmann *et al.*, 1995b). Each of these cytokines has an important role in the initiation and perpetuation of the inflammatory response. Since IL-8 released in this system is a potent chemoattractant and activator for neutrophils, we again focused on the IL-8 response to examine the specific mechanisms that are responsible for upregulation of proinflammatory cytokines in response to *E. histolytica*.

### A. Increased IL-8 Production Is Associated with Host Cell Lysis

We found that the mechanisms responsible for initiating the proinflammatory cytokine cascade in response to cytolytic *E. histolytica* trophozoites differ from those of bacterial invasion. Maximal IL-8 secretion in the *E. histolytica*-infected cocultures was confined to a relatively narrow range of trophozoite inoculum with maximal IL-8 secretion being obtained when approximately 50% of the monolayers were lysed (Eckmann *et al.*, 1995b). Upregulation of IL-8 in the cocultures was accompanied by increased transcription from the IL-8 promoter, and time course studies revealed increased levels of IL-8 mRNA and increased IL-8 secretion as early as 2 hr after addition of *E. histolytica* trophozoites (Eckmann *et al.*, 1995b).

### B. IL-1$_\alpha$ in Host Cell Lysates Activates IL-8 Secretion

IL-8 secretion by the cocultures required the presence of viable trophozoites, and was not induced by *E. histolytica* membrane molecules or secreted *E. histolytica* products. Moreover, maximal IL-8 secretion was seen under conditions which resulted in substantial cell lysis. We therefore investigated the possibility that components of damaged host cells that are released during lysis may stimulate the remaining viable cells in the monolayers to secrete IL-8. This, in fact, was the case since cell lysates induced IL-8 secretion when added to freshly cultured cells.

Several cytokines, including TNFα and IL-1, are known to be produced by the cells used in these studies (Eckmann *et al.*, 1995b) and were considered as candidate agonists for the upregulation of IL-8. In the case of colon fibroblasts and human intestinal smooth muscle cells, and in the case of some but not all of the colon epithelial cell lines, the majority of the IL-8 stimulating activity was shown to be due to the cellular release of preformed IL-1α, but not due to TNFα or IL-

$1\beta$ in the cell lysates (Fig. 3). Moreover, blocking the activity of IL-1$\alpha$ that was released during the course of *E. histolytica* coculture abrogated the upregulation of IL-8 as well as the other cytokines (Eckmann *et al.*, 1995b).

In contrast to the colon fibroblast and smooth muscle cells, induction of IL-8 responses by some of the colon epithelial cell lines was shown to be due to a different mechanism. Colon epithelial cells such as HT29 lack preformed IL-1$\alpha$ and increased IL-8 production was not due to target cell lysis. In those cells, increased IL-8 production was shown to be mediated by adherence of viable *E. histolytica* to the target cells by a galactose-inhibitable amoebic adherence protein (Eckmann *et al.*, 1995b; Petri *et al.*, 1987). The intracellular mechanisms involved in inducing the IL-8 response in that case appeared to require, at least in part, an increase in intracellular calcium levels (Eckmann *et al.*, 1995b).

## IV. EXPRESSION OF ADHESION MOLECULES ON COLON EPITHELIAL CELLS FOLLOWING MICROBIAL INVASION

Adhesion molecules on epithelial cells and counterligands on neutrophils may play a key role in the interaction between neutrophils and epithelial cells that are relevant early in the course of bacterial invasion. Our studies focused on ICAM-1 which is an important ligand for $\beta 2$ integrins on neutrophils. ICAM-1 is constitutively expressed at low, but detectable, levels on several human colon epithelial cell lines. Following coculture of these lines with invasive gram-positive or gram-

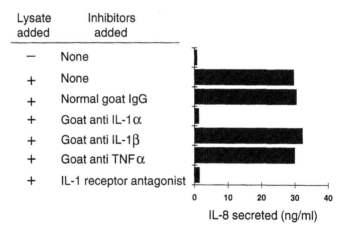

**FIGURE 3.** IL-1$\alpha$ released from cells lysed by *E. histolytica* trophozoites can stimulate IL-8 secretion by healthy cells. Anti-cytokine antibodies or IL-1 receptor antagonist were added to lysates from *E. histolytica*-damaged cells, after which the ability of the lysates to stimulate IL-8 secretion by viable test cells was assessed. As shown, anti-IL-1$\alpha$ antibodies or IL-1 receptor antagonist blocked greater than 90% of the lysate-induced IL-8 response, whereas antibodies against IL-1$\beta$ or TNF$\alpha$ had no affect on the IL-8 response.

negative bacteria, but not noninvasive bacteria, ICAM-1 mRNA expression and surface ICAM-1 levels were markedly increased (Huang *et al.,* 1995b). Moreover, ICAM-1 upregulation, to a sufficient extent, was independent of the autocrine release of TNFα, a known stimulant of ICAM-1 expression, by the cells. Using a neutrophil adhesion assay, we further demonstrated that increased expression of ICAM-1 is paralleled by increased neutrophil adhesion to the epithelial monolayers. Such adhesion could be blocked largely by antibodies to ICAM-1 on intestinal epithelial cells and completely by antibodies to CD18 on neutrophils. These *in vitro* data suggest that bacterial invasion of colon epithelial cells can upregulate the expression of adhesion molecules on epithelial cells and promote neutrophil adherence to bacterially infected cells. If paralleled *in vivo,* this may aid in the destruction of bacteria as they pass through the epithelial mucosal barrier. Moreover, increased ICAM-1 expressed on the epithelial cells may function as a putative costimulatory molecule for the activation of adjacent and underlying T cells in the mucosa.

## V. Summary

Colon epithelial cells coordinately express an array of proinflammatory cytokines and other key signaling molecules following bacterial invasion. Each of these signals has a well-recognized role in activation of the host inflammatory response. In this respect, colon epithelial cells appear to be programmed to act as sensors and to provide signals for the activation of the mucosal inflammatory response in the early phases following microbial invasion.

## Acknowledgments

This work was supported by NIH Grant DK35108. L.E. was supported by a Senior Research Fellowship Award from the Crohn's & Colitis Foundation, and G.H. was supported by NIH Training Grants DK07202 and CA09174.

## References

Andoh, A., Fujiyama, Y., Bamba, T., and Hosoda, S. (1993). Differential cytokine regulation of complement C3, C4, and factor B synthesis in human intestinal epithelial cell line, Caco-2. *J. Immunol.* **151,** 4239–4247.

Blumberg, R. S., Terhorst, C., Bleicher, P., McDermott, F. V., Allan, C. H., La, J. S., and Balk, S. P. (1991). Expression of a nonpolymorphic MHC class I-like molecule, CD1 intestinal epithelial cells. *J. Immunol.* **147,** 2518–2524.

Ciacci, C., Mahida, Y. R., Dignass, A., Koizumi, M., and Podolsky, D. K. (1993). Functional interleukin-2 receptors on intestinal epithelial cells. *J. Clin. Invest.* **92,** 527–532.

Eckmann, L., Jung, H. C., Schuerer-Maly, C. C., Panja, A., Morzycka-Wroblewska, E., and Kagnoff, M. F. (1993a). Differential cytokine expression by human intestinal epithelial cell lines: Regulation expression of interleukin-8. *Gastroenterology* **105,** 1689–1697.

Eckmann, L., Kagnoff, M. F., and Fierer, J. (1993b). Epithelial cells secrete the chemokine interleukin-8 in response to bacterial entry. *Infect. Immun.* **61,** 4569–4574.

Eckmann, L., Kagnoff, M. F., and Stenson, W. F. (1995a). *Salmonella* invasion upregulates cyclooxygenase expression and PGE2 production by intestinal epithelial cells. *Clin. Exp. Immunol.* **76,** S86 (Abstract).

Eckmann, L., Reed, S. L., Smith, J. R., and Kagnoff, M. F. (1995b). *Entamoeba histolytica* trophozoites induce an inflammatory cytokine response by cultured human cells through the paracrine action of cytolytically released interleukin-1$\alpha$. *J. Clin. Invest.* **96,** 1269–1279.

Fantini, J., Bolmont, C., and Yahi, N. (1992). Tumor necrosis factor-alpha stimulates both apical and basal production of HIV in polarized human intestinal HT29 cells. *Immunol. Lett.* **34,** 85–90.

Huang, G. T.-J., Eckmann, L., Fierer, J., and Kagnoff, M. F. (1995a). Human colon epithelial cells upregulate ICAM-1 expression following bacterial invasion. *Clin. Exp. Immunol.* **76,** S86 (Abstract).

Huang, G. T.-J., Eckmann, L., Fierer, J., and Kagnoff, M. F. (1995b). Increased ICAM-1 expression on human colon epithelial cells in response to bacterial invasion. *Gastroenterology* **108,** A839 (Abstract).

Jung, H. C., Eckmann, L., Yang, S.-K., Panja, A., Fierer, J., Morzycka-Wroblewska, E., and Kagnoff, M. F. (1995). A distinct array of proinflammatory cytokines is expressed in human colon epithelial cells in response to bacterial invasion. *J. Clin. Invest.* **95,** 55–65.

Kim, P.-H., and Kagnoff, M. F. (1990). Transforming growth factor $\beta$1 increases IgA isotype switching at the clonal level. *J. Immunol.* **145,** 3773–3778.

Mayer, L., Eisenhardt, D., Salomon, P., Bauer, W., Plous, R., and Piccinini, L. (1991). Expression of class II molecules on intestinal epithelial cells in humans. Differences between normal and inflammatory bowel disease. *Gastroenterology* **100,** 3–12.

Mulder, K. M., Zhong, Q., Choi, H. G., Humphrey, L. E., and Brattain, M. G. (1990). Inhibitory effects of transforming growth factor beta 1 on mitogenic response, transforming growth factor alpha, and c-myc in quiescent, well-differentiated colon carcinoma cells. *Cancer Res.* **50,** 7581–7586.

Petri, W. A., Smith, R. D., Schlesiner, P. H., Murphy, C. F., and Ravdin, J. I. (1987). Isolation of the galactose-binding lectin that mediates the *in vitro* adherence of *Entamoeba histolytica. J. Clin. Invest.* **80,** 1238–1244.

Raitano, A. B., and Korc, M. (1993). Growth inhibition of a human colorectal carcinoma cell line by interleukin 1 is associated with enhanced expression of gamma-interferon receptors. *Cancer Res.* **53,** 636–640.

Reinecker, H.-C., and Podolsky, D. K. (1995). Human intestinal epithelial cells express functional cytokine receptors sharing the yc chain of the interleukin-2 receptor. *Clin. Exp. Immunol.* **76,** S4 (Abstract).

Ullmann, C. D., Schlom, J., and Greiner, J. W. (1992). Interleukin-6 increases carcino-embryonic antigen and histocompatibility leukocyte antigen expression on the surface of human colorectal carcinoma cells. *J. Immunother.* **12,** 231–241.

van Vlasselaer, P., Punnonen, J., and de Vries, J. E. (1992). Transforming growth factor-beta directs IgA switching in human B cells. *J. Immunol.* **148,** 2062–2067.

Yang, S.-K., Eckmann, L., and Kagnoff, M. F. (1995). Colon epithelial cells express a broad array of chemokines. *Clin. Immunol. Immunopathol.* **76,** S4 (Abstract).

# Chapter 7

# Bacterial Activation of Mucosal Cytokine Production

Catharina Svanborg, William Agace, Spencer Hedges, Maria Hedlund, and Majlis Svensson

*Department of Medical Microbiology, Division of Clinical Immunology, Lund University, 22362 Lund, Sweden*

## I. INTRODUCTION

Mucosal surfaces form barriers that prevent microbes from the external environment from reaching internal organs. Epithelial cells have traditionally been regarded as rather passive cellular elements, responsible for keeping the mucosal barrier together. Due to their important role in transport of s-IgA, they have been included in the mucosal immune system (5, 6). It is becoming increasingly clear that epithelial cells act as "arbitrators" between the outside world and the mucosal immune system, and that they possess intricate means of sensing external stimuli, and of emitting signals that alter the function of adjacent or distant cells. They are, at once, the target of attaching microorganisms in the lumen and of mediators from cells in the mucosal environment, and as such are essential for the outcome of the cross-talk between bacteria and their hosts.

Pathogens express virulence factors that enable them to overcome mucosal defenses and tilt the balance in the cross-talk in their favor. The pathogens use specific adherence factors to localize to the site of infection; they secrete toxins that trigger changes in the mucosal barrier and cross the mucosa with the help of invasion factors. Recent studies have shown that inflammation is a key to the very early steps in the pathogenesis of mucosal infections, and that the virulence factors can act by directly triggering inflammatory processes in the mucosa.

We became interested in mucosal inflammation—one outcome of the cross-talk—because of observations made in urinary tract infections (UTI). The symptoms and signs of acute UTI are, to a great extent, attributable to the inflammatory response that the bacteria induce when they enter the urinary tract. There is elevated temperature, an acute-phase response in serum (C-reactive protein, CRP; erythrocyte sedimentation rate, ESR), a local inflammatory response in the urine (excretion of neutrophils and tubular proteins), and a mucosal immune response dominated by s-IgA antibodies. These host response parameters suggested to us that the mucosa produced cytokines in response to infection, and that these cytokines were involved as mediators of disease. This review summarizes some aspects of our studies on mucosal cytokine responses to bacterial infection that were discussed during the 8th International Congress on Mucosal Immunology in San Diego, July 1995 (Abstracts P-152, O-240, O-502, O-503, O-506, P-597).

## II. INFECTION AND EPITHELIAL CYTOKINE RESPONSES

A mucosal cytokine response to infection was first shown to occur in mice and in patients colonized with *Escherichia coli* in the urinary tract (7–9). Interleukin 6 (IL-6) and IL-8 were shown to be secreted into the urine within minutes of local challenge with *E. coli.* Cytokine responses were also detected in adults and children with different forms of UTI (10, 11). Subsequent studies have shown that cytokine production occurs during a variety of mucosal infections in humans (for review see 12).

The rapid local cytokine response to UTI suggested to us that resident mucosal cells were the primary responders in this process. The urinary tract mucosa differs from that of other mucosal sites in that it lacks organized lymphoid tissue, goblet cells, etc. Epithelial cells are the dominating cellular elements. Furthermore, the epithelial cells are the target of uropathogenic *E. coli* that attach to these cells with a high degree of specificity. We therefore decided to focus on the epithelial cells, as a probable source of the mucosal cytokine response (13). *E. coli* was first shown to trigger cytokine secretion by kidney and bladder cell lines (13, 14). Bacteria stimulated *de novo* synthesis of cytokine-specific mRNAs for IL-1$\alpha$, IL-1$\beta$, IL-6, and IL-8, and the accumulation of intracellular protein (15, 16). The cytokine repertoir was, however, restricted as compared to nonepithelial cells like macrophages (16). Subsequent studies have shown that epithelial cells from other mucosal sites also secrete cytokines when exposed to pathogens (for review see 12). This ability of microbes to trigger epithelial cytokine responses thus appears to be a general feature of host–parasite interactions at mucosal sites.

## III. ROLE OF THE CERAMIDE SIGNALING PATHWAY IN THE CYTOKINE RESPONSES TO P-FIMBRIATED *ESCHERICHIA COLI*

Uropathogenic *E. coli* attach to human urinary tract epithelial cells through fimbriae-associated adhesins that bind to receptor epitopes on host glycoconjugates (17). Adherence to human urinary tract epithelial cells is a virulence factor for uropathogenic *E. coli;* adhering strains cause up to 90% of uncomplicated acute pyelonephritis episodes, but are rare among *E. coli* not causing UTI (20). P fimbriae show a more clear-cut association to the inflammatory response and to disease than other fimbrial types expressed by uropathogens (21). P fimbriae carry lectin domains that bind specifically to Galα1-4Galβ-containing oligosaccharides, the carbohydrate portion of the globoseries of glycolipids (22–24). Attachment has been shown to increase both the cytokine response in the mouse urinary tract and the cytokine response of uroepithelial cells exposed to bacteria *in vitro* (14, 18, 19).

There are several indications that the P fimbriae contribute to the induction of cytokine responses. P-fimbriated *E. coli* elicited a higher IL-6 response than isogenic strains lacking the fimbriae. Isolated P fimbriae with an intact lectin domain were shown to trigger an IL-6 response, while lectin-deficient fimbriae failed to do so (14). Cytokine activation by P fimbriae was dependent on glycolipid receptor expression, in that treatment of the cells with PDMP, an inhibitor of ceramide glycosylation, reduced receptor expression, attachment, and cytokine activation (18).

The oligosaccharide receptor epitopes recognized by P fimbriae are bound to ceramide in the outer leaflet of the lipid bilayer (22, 24). Ceramide has recently become recognized a second messenger in the sphingomyelin signal transduction pathway. Ceramide is released from sphingomyelin following the action of sphingomyelinase (25). The hydrolysis of sphingomyelin can also occur upon exposure of cells to exogenous agonists that activate endogenous sphingomyelinases. Such agonists include TNFα, IL-1$_\beta$, NGF, and FAS (25–29). We have demonstrated that P-fimbriated *E. coli* activate the ceramide signalling pathway, and we propose that this activation contributes to the epithelial cytokine response induced by the P-fimbriated *E. coli* in uroepithelial cells (Hedlund *et al.*, submitted for publication).

Two approaches were used to study *E. coli* activation of the ceramide pathway in A498 cells (a human kidney cell line). The release of ceramide was studied in unlabeled cells and was quantitated by *in vitro* phosphorylation with diacylglycerol kinase. With this assay P-fimbriated *E. coli* and sphingomyelinase were shown to stimulate the release of ceramide. Isogenic strains expressing a different lectin, type 1 fimbriae, did not cause the release of ceramide in the cells despite the fact that these bacteria activated IL-6.

Released ceramide is phosphorylated to ceramide-1-phosphate through the action of ceramide-activated protein kinases. We quantitated the phosphorylation of ceramide to ceramide-1-phosphate in cells prelabeled with $^{32}$P. P-fimbriated *E. coli* and sphingomyelinase were shown to induce the formation of ceramide-1-phosphate. In contrast, type 1-fimbriated *E. coli* or nonfimbriated controls did not cause ceramide phosphorylation.

The ceramide-activated protein kinase CAPK is a serine–threonine kinase (29). We therefore examined the effect of serine–threonine protein kinase inhibitors on the *E. coli*-induced cytokine response. PMA, a known activator of these kinases, was used as a control. Staurosporin and K252a were found to reduce the IL-6 response of the cells to PMA. These agents also inhibited the IL-6 response to P-fimbriated *E. coli*. Tyrosine-kinase inhibitors (genistein and tyrphostin) had no effect. The involvement of serine–threonine kinases in the P fimbriae-induced cytokine response is consistent with the involvement of the ceramide pathway in the bacterially induced IL-6 response.

Further evidence for specificity was obtained by comparing type 1-fimbriated and P-fimbriated *E. coli*. Both types of fimbriae mediated attachment to the A498 cells and enhanced the cytokine response in those cells. The IL-6 response to type 1 fimbriae differed, however, in sensitivity to protein kinase inhibitors from that of P fimbriae. The response to type 1 fimbriae was insensitive to serine–threonine protein kinase inhibitors, but partially affected by tyrosine kinase inhibitors. This suggested that type 1-fimbriated *E. coli* activated the epithelial cytokine response via a different pathway than the P-fimbriated strains.

The mechanism of P-fimbriae-induced ceramide release needs to be defined. *Staphylococcus aureus* and other bacteria are known to secrete sphingomyelinase. The *E. coli* strains produced low levels of acid and neutral sphingomyelinases, but there was no evidence for a difference in sphingomyelinase activity related to fimbrial type or evidence of activation upon contact with the cells. Low levels of sphingomyelinase activity were also detected in the cells, but no activation upon contact with the bacteria was observed.

LPS is known to be a poor activator of epithelial cell cytokine responses. Recently, Joseph *et al.* showed that ceramide and LPS have sufficient structural homology that LPS can replace ceramide as an activator of serine–threonine protein kinases in cells that express CD-14 (30). Since the A498 cells used in our experiments do not express CD-14, we exposed the A498 cells to LPS in the presence of human serum known to contain soluble CD-14 that might reconstitute this deficiency. There was no enhancement of the IL-6 response. Furthermore, if LPS were the principal activator of ceramide release and IL-6 production, P- and type 1-fimbriated *E. coli* would be expected to generate a similar response. These strains attach in similar numbers to the A498 cells and would therefore be expected to deliver LPS to the cell surface with similarly efficiency. The difference in ceramide release and insensitivity to serine–threonine kinase inhibitors between strains differing in fimbrial expression suggested that the fimbrial receptor specificity influenced the transmembran signalling pathway.

*Pseudomonas aeruginosa* fimbriae have been shown to enhance the cytokine responses of respiratory tract epithelial cells (31). A low-molecular-mass product of *P. aeruginosa*, the autoregulator was suggested to further activate epithelial cell cytokine production. The transmembrane signalling events involved in these processes remain to be defined.

## IV. Do P-Fimbriated *Escherichia coli* Invade Uroepithelial Cells?

Studies on intestinal epithelial cells have suggested that bacterial invasion is essential for the induction of cytokine responses. Invasive *Salmonella, Yersinia, Shi-*

*gella, Listeria,* and *E. coli* induced IL-8 secretion in colonic epithelial cells, but LPS and a noninvasive *E. coli* strain did not (32). More recently, invasive strains were shown to activate a wide range of cytokines (Monocyte Chemotactic Protein-1 (MCP-1), Granulocyte Macrophage-Colony Stimulating Factor, IL-8, and TNF) in colon epithelial cell lines, and MCP-1, IL-8, and IL-6 in primary cell cultures (see Chapter 6).

Several observations have suggested that invasion may occur during the pathogenesis of urinary tract infection. *E. coli* spread from the local site of infection in the urinary tract to the blood stream in about 30% of patients with acute pyelonephritis (33). The blood isolates express P fimbriae even more frequently than *E. coli* strains that cause acute pyelonephritis in patients without urosepsis (34, 35). Consequently, P-fimbriated *E. coli* appear to have enhanced ability to cross the epithelial barrier. This may involve attachment followed by invasion through epithelial cells or the destruction of the epithelial barrier via other mechanisms.

We examined the interaction of P-fimbriated *E. coli* with human uroepithelial cell layers using a human kidney cell line grown in Transwell units. Four aspects of the bacterial interactions with the cells were studied.

1. Bacterial transmigration across confluent cell layers, determined by viable counts.

2. Changes in the morphology of the cell layer, determined by scanning and transmission EM.

3. Bacterial cytotoxicity fo the cells, detected by cell viability assay.

4. Invasion into the cell studied with the gentamicin assay.

Urosepsis isolates, recombinant strains differing in P fimbrial expression, and nonfimbriated controls were used. The urosepsis strains were found to pass the cell layers and to multiply in the lower well. Passage was associated with attachment of bacteria to the upper surface of the cells, detachment of the cells, and induction of cell death. There was no evidence that invasion through epithelial cells occurred frequently or contributed to bacterial passage in a significant way. The P-fimbriated strains showed enhanced passage across the cell layer and enhanced survival compared to the nonfimbriated vector control strains. The nonfimbriated bacteria did not attach to the cell monolayer, cause detachment, or pass across the cell layer in significant numbers. These results suggest that the early cytokine response of epithelial cells does not require invasion by P-fimbriated *E. coli.* Furthermore, the results demonstrate that bacteria cause major changes to the cell layer. These changes are likely to facilitate the passage of bacteria across the mucosal lining. The molecular mechanisms need to be defined.

## V. Epithelial Cells in Mucosal Cytokine Networks

The ability of epithelial cells to secrete cytokines and to respond to exogenous cytokines provides a basis for cytokine networking. Epithelial cell involvement in mucosal cytokine networks was first postulated when IL-1 and TNF were shown to stimulate epithelial IL-8 secretion (36). It was suggested at the time that stimulated macrophages could serve as a source of inflammatory cytokines during mucosal infections: these cytokines would stimulate epithelial cell IL-8 responses. Subsequent studies have shown that proinflammatory cytokines (IL-1, TNF) can stimulate IL-6 and IL-8 secretion in a variety of epithelial cells (12).

T cells and intraepithetial lymphocytes (IELs) regulate mucosal immune responses. These cells are localized near epithelial cells, and some of their regulatory effects may be achieved through interactions with those cells. T cells, and immunoregulatory cytokines produced mainly by T cells, have been shown to influence epithelial cell functions including the expression of class II antigens, secretory component, and ICAM-1 (37–40). We have shown that immunoregulatory cytokines stimulate epithelial cell cytokine production and modify the epithelial cell cytokine responses to bacteria (41).

Cells of the Th1 subtype are commonly defined by their ability to secrete IL-2 and IFNγ. We found no effect of IL-2 on epithelial cell IL-6 or IL-8 production. IFNγ had a stimulatory effect on IL-6, but no effect on the IL-8 production. Cells of the Th2 subtype are commonly defined by their ability to secrete IL-4, IL-5, IL-10, and IL-13. These cytokines were found to activate IL-6 (IL-4, IL-5, IL-10, and IL-13) and IL-8 responses (IL-4 and IL-13). Other immunoregulatory cytokines (TGFβ1 and IL-12) induced IL-6 but not IL-8 production.

IFNγ and IL-4 had strong and partially opposite effects on the epithelial cell cytokine responses to E. coli. IL-4 was identified as a positive regulator of IL-6 responses, and acted in synergy with E. coli on the IL-6 response. This implies that IL-4 can enhance mucosal IL-6 responses to infection, and thereby promote IL-6-mediated effects such as acute-phase responses and IgA-committed B cell maturation. It should be emphasized that IL-4 is not only a T-cell product. IL-4 can be produced by mucosal mast cells in response to inflammatory stimuli.

IFNγ was a less effective stimulant of IL-6 and IL-8 production at both the protein and mRNA levels than IL-4, and it did not induce IL-6 production in synergy with E. coli. The epithelial cell cytokine response to IFNγ was more complex than that observed with IL-4 since it both inhibited and enhanced the levels of secreted cytokines. IFNγ decreased the IL-8 levels when added as a costimulant with the bacteria, and decreased both the IL-6 and IL-8 levels when added to E. coli-primed cells. In contrast, the IL-6 and IL-8 responses to E. coli stimulation were enhanced by IFNγ priming of the epithelial cells.

These observations have several interesting implications for the regulation of mucosal responses to microbial challenge. Immune responses that favor the expansion of Th2 cell populations, or that induce IL-4 secretion, would strongly enhance epithelial IL-6 production in response to gram-negative bacteria. Thus, as a consequence of the activation of mucosal Th2 or mast cells there would be increases in IL-6-dependent B cell and inflammatory responses. Conversely, immune responses that favor the expansion of Th1 cell populations, or that induce IFNγ secretion, would either inhibit or enhance the cytokine response to bacteria depending on the sequence of activation. In the naive mucosa, where epithelial cells are first stimulated by bacteria, the subsequent exposure to IFNγ would lower IL-6 and IL-8 levels and lower the inflammatory response. This situation might occur in the newborn intestine, or at normally sterile mucosal sites that become exposed to bacteria. In the event of *de novo* bacterial exposure of an IFNγ-primed site, there would be an enhanced IL-6 response and no inhibition of IL-8 levels. These phenomena need to be addressed in *in vivo* models; however, the novel effects of IL-4 and IFNγ presented in this study provide a mechanism whereby activated T cells can regulate epithelial cell cytokine responses to bacteria.

## VI. NEUTROPHIL RECRUITMENT TO THE MUCOSA

Mucosal infections cause a rapid neutrophil influx to the site of infection (42). The molecular mechanisms that explain the increase in urinary neutrophil numbers are gradually becoming understood. We have recently shown that urinary tract epithelial cells participate in transepithelial neutrophil migration in two ways: (a) by secreting neutrophil chemoattractants and (b) by the expression of cell adhesion molecules (12, 43–46).

### A. Neutrophil Chemoattactants

Mucosal infections of the urinary and respiratory tract are accompanied by a local IL-8 response. IL-8 is a member of the α-chemokine family (C–X–C) of cytokines with chemotactic activity for neutrophils (43). In patients with UTI and in patients deliberately colonized with *E. coli* in the urinary tract, levels of urinary IL-8 correlate strongly with urinary neutrophil numbers (9). The neutrophil chemotactic activity of infected urine was reduced by 50% *in vitro* by monoclonal antibodies to IL-8 (46). Taken together these observations suggest that IL-8 is an important neutrophil chemoattractant in UTI. The role of IL-8 for neutrophil migration accross uroepithelial cell layers was further analyzed in an *in vitro* model. *E. coli* and IL-1 were shown to induce neutrophil migration across kidney and bladder epithelial layers in the Transwell model system (44, 45). Anti-IL-8 antibody completely blocked the IL-1- and *E. coli*-induced transepithelial migration (45).

### B. Bacteria Upregulate Epithelial of ICAM-1 Expression

We examined the role of cell adhesion molecules in transuroepithelial neutrophil migration. Epithelial cell lines and normal urinary tract epithelial cells were found to express ICAM-1, but not ICAM-2 or E-selectin. *E. coli* and IL-1 upregulated the expression of ICAM-1 on the epithelial cell surface and antibodies to ICAM-1 blocked from 60–80% of *E. coli*-induced transepithelial neutrophil migration. The neutrophil receptor for ICAM-1 was tentatively identified as the β2-integrin

CD11b/CD18 (Mac-1) since antibodies to CD11b and CD18 but not to CD11a blocked the *E. coli*-induced transepithelial neutrophil migration (44).

## VII. ROLE OF MUCOSAL INFLAMMATION AND NEUTROPHIL INFLUX IN THE CLEARANCE OF UTI

Earlier studies on antibacterial mucosal defenses emphasized how mucosal immune mechanisms cooperate to prevent inflammation. In contrast, we have proposed that mucosal inflammation plays an essential role for the resistance to infection, at least in the urinary tract. This was first indicated by studies in a murine UTI model. C3H/HeJ mice, which have a defective response to LPS, were found to be highly susceptible to intravesical infection with *E. coli* compared to C3H/HeN normal mice (42, 47). Analysis of their mucosal inflammatory responses showed that the urinary neutrophil and IL-6 levels were significantly lower in C3H/HeJ mice (7, 42, 48). LPS hyporesponder mice of the C57BL/10ScCr background are also more susceptible to experimental UTI, and have a reduced inflammatory response compared to normal C57BL/6J mice (48). The presence of neutrophils in the urine in both mouse backgrounds corresponded with clearance of infection. Further studies showed that pharmacological inhibitors of inflammation severely inhibited the ability of C3H/HeN mice to clear acute UTI (49). A role for neutrophils in the clearance of UTI was confirmed by Miller and co-workers (50), who showed that treatment of rats with anti-neutrophil serum led to a 1000-fold increase in bacterial numbers in infected kidneys.

So why do the bacteria trigger a cytokine response that causes inflammation and activates antibacterial defenses at mucosal sites? It is likely that continued investigations will identify benefits gained by the pathogens in the process. The cross-talk between microbes and host mucosae is exquisitely regulated by mechanisms that will continue to puzzle and fascinate, as will the paradox of human health in a microbe-rich environment.

### ACKNOWLEDGMENTS

This study was supported by grants from the Swedish Medical Research Council, the Medical Faculty, Lund University, the Österlund and Crawford foundations, and the Royal Physiographic Society.

### REFERENCES

1. Freter, R. (1969). Studies on the mechanism of action of intestinal antibody in experimental cholera. *Texas Rep. Biol. Med.* **22,** 299–316.
2. Williams, R. C., and Gibbons, R. J. (1972). Inhibition of bacterial adherence by secretory immunoglobulin A: A mechanism of antigen disposal. *Science* **177,** 697–699.
3. Svanborg-Edén, C. and Svennerholm, A.-M. (1978). Secretory immunoglobulin A and G antibodies prevent adhesion of *Escherichia coli* to human urinary tract epithelial cells. *Infect. Immun.* **22,** 790–797.

4. Svanborg-Edén, C., Freter, R., Hagberg, L., Hull, R., Hull, S., Leffler, H., and Schoolnik, G. (1982). Inhibition of experimental ascending urinary tract infection by a receptor analogue. *Nature* **298,** 560–562.

5. Brandtzaeg, P. (1973). Structure, synthesis and external transfer of mucosal immunoglobulins. *Ann. Inst. Pasteur/Immunol.* **124C,** 417–438.

6. Brandtzaeg, P., Krajci, P., Lamm, M., Kaetzel, C. S. (1994). Epithelial and hepatobiliary transport of polymeric immunoglobulins. *In* "Handbook of Mucosal Immunology" (P. L. Ogra, M. E. Lamm, J. R. McGhee, J. Mestecky, W. Strober, and J. Bienenstock, Eds), pp. 113–123. Academic Press, San Diego.

7. de Man, P., van Kooten, C., Aarden, L., Engberg, I., Linder, H., and Svanborg-Edén, C. (1989). Interleukin-6 induced at mucosal surfaces by gram-negative bacterial infection. *Infect. Immun.* **57,** 3383–3388.

8. Hedges, S., Anderson, P., Lidin-Janson, G., de Man, P., and Svanborg, C. (1991). Interleukin-6 response to deliberate colonization of the human urinary tract with gram-negative bacteria. *Infect. Immun.* **59,** 421–427.

9. Agace W., Hedges S., Ceska M., and Svanborg, C. (1993). Interleukin-8 and the neutrophil response to mucosal gram-negative infection. *J. Clin. Invest.* **92,** 780–785.

10. Hedges, S., Stenquist, K., Lidin-Janson, G., Martinell, J., Sandberg, T., and Svanborg, C. (1992). Comparison of urine and serum concentrations of Interleukin-6 in women with acute pyelonephritis or asymptomatic bacteriuria. *J. Infect. Dis.* **166,** 653–656.

11. Benson, M., Andreasson, A., Jodal, U., Karlsson, Å., Rydberg, J., and Svanborg, C. (1994). Interleukin-6 in childhood urinary tract infection. *Pediatr. Infect. Dis. J.* **13,** 612–616.

12. Hedges, S., Agace, W., and Svanborg, C. (1995). Epithelial cytokine responses and mucosal cytokine networks. *Trends in Microbiol.* **3,** 266–270.

13. Hedges, S., de Man, P., Linder, H., van Kooten, C., and Svanborg-Edén, C. (1990). Interleukin-6 is secreted by epithelial cells in response to gram-negative bacterial challenge. *In* "Advances in Mucosal Immunology. Intrenational Conference of Mucosal Immunity" (T. MacDonald, Ed.), pp. 144–148, Kluwer, London.

14. Hedges, S., Svensson, M., and Svanborg, C. (1992). Interleukin-6 response of epithelial cell lines to bacterial stimulation *in vitro*. *Infect. Immun.* **60,** 1295–1301.

15. Hedges, S., Agace, W., Svensson, M., Sjögren, A-C., Ceska, M., and Svanborg, C. (1994). Uropithelial cells are a part of a mucosal cytokine network. *Infect. Immun.* **62,** 2315–2321.

16. Agace, W., Hedges, S., Andersson, U., Andersson, J., Ceska, M., and Svanborg, C. (1993). Selective cytokine production by epithelial cells following exposure to *Escherichia coli*. *Infect. Immun.* **61,** 602–609.

17. Leffler, H., and Svanborg-Edén, C. (1986). *In* "Microbial lectines and agglutinins" (D. Mirelman, Ed.), pp. 84–110. John Wiley & Sons, Inc., New York.

18. Svensson, M., Lindstedt, R., Radin, N., and Svanborg, C. (1994). Epithelial glucosphingolipid expression as a determinant of bacterial adherence and cytokine production. *Infect. Immun.* **62,** 4404–4410.

19. Linder, H., Engberg, I., Mattsby-Baltzer, I., Jann, K., and Svanborg-Edén, C. (1988). Induction of inflammation by *Escherichia coli* on the mucosal level: Requirement of adherence and endotoxin. *Infect. Immun.* **56,** 1309–1313.

20. Svanborg-Edén, C., Hanson, L. Å., Jodal, U., Lindberg, U., and Sohl-Åkerlund, A. (1976). Variable adherence to normal urinary tract epithelial cells of *Escherichia coli* strains associated with various forms of urinary tract infection. *Lancet* **II,** 490–492.

21. Leffler, H., and Svanborg-Edén, C. (1981). Glycolipid receptors for uropathogenic *Escherichia coli* on human erythrocytes and uroepithelial cells. *Infect. Immun.* **34,** 920.

22. Leffler, H., and Svanborg-Edén, C. (1980). Chemical identification of a glycosphingolipid receptor for *Escherichia coli* attaching to human urinary tract epithelial cells and agglutinating human erythrocytes. *FEMS Microbiol. Lett.* **8,** 127–134.

23. Källenius, G., Möllby, R., Svensson, S. B., Winberg, J., Lundblad, S., Svensson, S., and Cedergren, B. (1980). The Pk antigen as a receptor for the hemagglutination of pyelonephritogenic *E.coli*. *FEMS Microbiol. Lett.* **7**, 297–302.

24. Bock, K., Breimer, M. E., Brignole, A., Hansson, G. C., Karlsson, K.-A., Larsson, G., Leffler, H., Samuelsson, B., Strömberg, N., Svanborg-Edén, C., and Thurin, J. (1985). Specificity of binding of a strain of uropathogenic *Escherichia coli* to Gal$\alpha$-14Gal$\beta$ containing glycosphingolipids. *J. Biol. Chem.* **260**, 8545–8551.

25. Weigmann, K., Schütze, S., Muchleidt, T., Witte, D., and Krönke, M. (1994). Functional dichotomy of neutral and acidic sphingomyelinases in tumor necrosis factor signalling. *Cell* **78**, 1005–1015.

26. Mathias, S., Younes, A., Kan, C. C., Orlow, I., Joseph, C., and Kolesnick, R. N. (1993). Activation of the sphingolmyelin signalling pathway in intact EL4 cells and in cell-free system by IL-1$_\beta$. *Science* **259**, 519–522.

27. Okazaka, T., Bell, R. M., and Hannun, Y. A. (1989). Sphingomyelin turn-over induced by vitamin D$_3$ in HL-60 cells. Role in cell differentiation. *J. Biol. Chem.* **264**, 19076–19080.

28. Mathias, S., Dressler, K. A., and Kolesnick, R. N. (1991). Characterization of a ceramide-activated protein kinase: Stimulation by tumor necrosis factor $\alpha$. *Proc. Natl. Acad. Sci. USA* **88**, 10009–10013.

29. Ballour, L. F., Chao, C. P., Holness, M. A., Barker, S. C., and Raghow, R. (1992). Interleukin-1 mediated PGE$_2$ production and sphingomyelin metabolism. Evidence for the regulation of cyclooxygenase gene expression by sphingosine and ceramide. *J. Biol. Chem.* **267**, 20044–20050.

30. Joseph, C. K., Wright, S. D., Bornmann, W. G., Randolph, J. T., Kumar, E. R., Bittman, R., Liu, J., and Kolesnick, R. N. (1994). Bacterial lipopolysaccharide has structural similarity to ceramide and stimulates ceramide-activated protein kinase in myeloid cells. *J. Biol. Chem.* **269**, 17606–17610.

31. di Mango, E., Zar, H. J., Bryan, R., Prince, and Diverse, A. *P. aeruginosa* gene products stimulate respiratory epithelial cells to produce IL-8. (In preparation).

32. Eckman, L., Kagnoff, M. F., and Fierer, J. (1993). Epithelial cells secrete the chemokine Interleukin-8 in response to bacterial entry. *Infect. Immun.* **61**, 4569–4574.

33. Johnson, J. R., Roberts, P. L., and Stamm, W. E. (1987). P fimbriae and other virulence factors in *Escherichia coli* urosepsis: Association with patients' characteristics. *J. Infect. Dis.* **156**, 225–229.

34. Johnson, J. (1991). Virulence factors in *Escherichia coli* urinary tract infection. *Clin. Microbiol. Rev.* **4**, 80–128.

35. Otto, G., Sandberg, T., Marklund, B.-I., Ulleryd, P., and Svanborg, C. (1993). Virulence factors and pap genotype in *E. coli* isolates from women with acute pyelonephritis with or without bacteremia. *Clin. Infect. Dis.* **17**, 448–456.

36. Standiford, T. J., Kunkel, S. L., Basha, M. A., Chensue, S. W., Lynch III, J. P., Toews, G. B., Westwick, J., and Strieter, R. M. (1990). Interleukin-8 gene expression by a pulmonary epithelial cell line. A model for cytokine networks in the lung. *J. Clin. Invest.* **86**, 1945–1953.

37. Cerf-Bensussan, N., Quaroni, A., Kurnick, J., and Bhan, A. (1984). Intraepithelial lymphocytes modulate Ia expression by intestinal epithelial cells. *J. Immunol.* **132**, 2244–2252.

38. Kvale, D., Brandtzaeg, P., and Lövhaug, D. (1988). Up-regulation of the expression of secretory component and HLA molecules in a human colonic cell line by tumour necrosis factor-$\alpha$ and gamma interferon. *Scand. J. Immunol.* **28**, 351–357.

39. Kvale, D., Krajci, P., and Brandtzaeg, P. (1992). Expression and regulation of adhesion molecules ICAM-1 (CD54) and LFA-3 (CD58) in human intestinal epithelial cell lines. *Scand. J. Immunol.* **35**, 669–676.

40. Sollid, L. M., Kvale, D., Brandtzaeg, P., Markussen, G., and Thorsby, E. (1987). Interferon-$\gamma$ enhances expression of secretory component, the epithelial receptor for polymeric immunoglobulins. *J. Immunol.* **138**, 4303.

41. Hedges, S., Bjarnadottir, M., Agace, W., Hang, L., and Svanborg, C. Immunoregulatory cytokines

modify *Escherichia coli* induced epithelial cell IL-6 and IL-8 responses. *Infect. Immun.* Submitted for publication.

42. Shahin, R., Engberg, I., Hagberg, I., and Svanborg-Edén, C. (1987). Neutrophil recruitment and bacterial clearance correlated with LPS nonresponsiveness in local gram-negative infection. *J. Immunol.* **10**, 3475–3480.

43. Baggiolini, M., Dewald, B., and Moser, B. (1994). Interleukin-8 and related chemotactic cytokines-CXC and CC chemokines. *Adv. Immunol.* **55**, 97–179.

44. Agace, W., Patarroyo, M., Svensson, M., Carlemalm, E., and Svanborg, C. (1995). *Escherichia coli* induce trans-uroepithelial neutrophil migration by an ICAM-1 dependant mechanism. *Infect. Immun.*, in press.

45. Agace, W., Godaly, G., Ceska, S., and Svanborg, C. (1995). *Escherichia coli* induced trans-uroepithelial migration is IL-8 dependent. In preparation.

46. Ko, Y. C., Mukaida, N., Ishiyama, S., Tokue, A., Kawai, T., Matsushima, K., and Kasahara, T. (1993). Elevated Interleukin-8 levels in the urine of patients with urinary tract infections. *Infect. Immun.* **61**, 1307–1314.

47. Hagberg, L., Hull, R., Hull, S., McGhee, J. R., Michalek, S. M., and Svanborg-Edén, C. (1984). Difference in susceptibility to gram-negative urinary tract infection between C3H/HeJ and C3H/HeN mice. *Infect. Immun.* **46**, 839–844.

48. Agace, W., Hedges, S., and Svanborg, C. (1992). Lps genotype in the C57 black mouse background and its influence on the Interleukin-6 response to *E.coli* urinary tract infection. *Scand. J. Immun.* **35**, 531–538.

49. Linder, H., Engberg, I., van, K. C., deMan, P., and Svanborg,-Edén, C. (1990). Effects of anti-inflammatory agents on mucosal inflammation induced by infection with gram-negative bacteria. *Infect. Immun.* **58**, 2056–2060.

50. Miller, T., Findon, G., and Cawley, S. (1987). Cellular basis of host defence in pyelonephritis. III. Deletion of individual components. *Br. J. Exp. Pathol.* **68**, 377–388.

# Chapter 8

# MHC-like Molecules on Mucosal Epithelial Cells

Richard S. Blumberg,* Neil Simister,† Andreas D. Christ,* Esther J. Israel,‡
Sean P. Colgan,§ and Steven P. Balk‖

*Gastroenterology Division, Brigham and Women's Hospital, Harvard Medical School, Boston,
Massachusetts 02115; †Rosensteil Center for Basic Biomedical Research, Brandeis University,
Waltham, Massachusetts 02254; ‡Division of Pediatric Gastroenterology and Nutrition,
Massachusetts General Hospital, Harvard Medical School, Boston, Massachusetts 02115;
§Department of Anesthesia, Brigham and Women's Hospital, Harvard Medical School,
Boston, Massachusetts 02115; and ‖Hematology–Oncology Division, Beth Israel Hospital,
Harvard Medical School, Boston, Massachusetts 02115

## I. Summary

MHC class Ib molecules are nonpolymorphic MHC class I-like molecules which fulfill functions divergent from the classisal, MHC class Ia molecules. The human intestine is a unique immunologic compartment, which expresses two of these molecules: the neonatal Fc receptor for IgG (FcRn) and CD1. The FcRn is expressed by adult enterocytes in that mRNA, protein, and Fc binding of IgG characteristic of this molecule can be detected. This suggests that the FcRn is functional beyond the neonatal period which has important implications for mucosal immune regulation. Whereas CD1d is expressed by intestinal epithelial cells (IEC) and upregulated here by IFN$\gamma$, CD1a, b, and c are expressed primarily on mononuclear cells of the lamina propria. CD1d can be recognized in its native form on IECs by peripheral CD8$^+$ T cells. CD8$^+$ intestinal intraepithelial lymphocyte (IEL) T-cell clones can recognize several members of the CD1 gene family in a transfected HLA-A,B negative, B-cell line. The IEC appears to express at least two forms of CD1d, a cell surface and intracellular form. The cell surface form that is likely recognized by peripheral CD8$^+$ T cells is distinct from all previously described class 1 MHC molecules, suggesting that it is transported to the cell surface by a distinct pathway and does not function as a conventional antigen-presenting molecule. This form is expressed independently of $\beta_2$M, without N-linked carbohydrate side-chain modification. Complex transcriptional processing of CD1d also occurs. Thus, distinct structural isoforms of CD1d are detectable which may function in IEL–mucosal T cell interactions.

*Essentials of Mucosal Immunology*   Copyright © 1996 by Academic Press, Inc. All rights of reproduction in any form reserved.

## II. STRUCTURE AND FUNCTION OF MHC CLASS Ia MOLECULES

The classical MHC class I or class Ia genes consist of a few highly polymorphic loci on mouse chromosome 17 (H-2 K, D, and L) and human chromosome 6 (HLA A, B, and C) (Yewdell and Bennick, 1992). The MHC class Ia molecule is expressed on the cell surface as a 43- to 45-kDa glycosylated, transmembrane heavy chain that is noncovalently associated with $\beta$2-microglobulin ($\beta_2$M), a 12-kDa nonglycosylated protein that is encoded outside the MHC genetic locus. The class Ia molecules bind short (approximately nine amino acids) peptides in their $\alpha$1 and $\alpha$2 domains that are derived from the degradation of cytoplasmic proteins and are delivered to the class Ia molecule by transporter associated proteins *(Tap)* of the endoplasmic reticulum (Monaco, 1992). The $\alpha$1 and $\alpha$2 domains, which comprise the peptide binding pocket or groove, contain the majority of the allelic polymorphism (Bjorkman *et al.*, 1987).

These molecules thus display on the cell surface a composite of the internal antigenic experience of the cell for presentation to CD8$^+$ T cells in contradistinction to class II MHC which display a composite array of external antigenic events for presentation to CD4$^+$ T cells (Neefjes and Pleogh, 1992). The three ingredients of this tripartite complex (classical class I heavy chain, $\beta_2$M, and nominal peptide) are prerequisite for the functional expression of the MHC class Ia molecule (Yewdell and Bennick, 1992). Binding of the CD8 coreceptor to conserved amino acid sequences contained within the $\alpha$3 domain of the class I heavy chain provides signals to the T cell through a CD8 associated kinase, *lck,* and a stabilizing environment for the sampling of peptide components contained within the MHC class I groove by the T cell receptor (TCR), most commonly an $\alpha\beta$ heterodimer (Rudd, 1990; Weiss, 1990). When the appropriate conformation is presented for TCR binding, a signal is delivered to the T cell via the CD3 complex which leads, appropriately, to cytolysis of the cell expressing the internal deleterious event as reflected in the abnormal MHC class Ia display. Thus the MHC class Ia proteins are ubiquitously expressed, polymorphic molecules that bind a large variety of peptide antigens for presentation to CD8$^+$ T cells whose primary function is likely cytolysis.

## III. STRUCTURE AND FUNCTION OF MHC CLASS Ib MOLECULES

The host also maintains a quantitatively larger number of nonclassical, or MHC class Ib, molecules whose function is less clear but may be targeted to specific tasks of immunologic recognition (Stroynowski, 1990; Shawar *et al.*, 1994). These molecules do not fall into a specific gene family and their designation as distinct molecules is partly historical. The genes for the known class Ib molecules are either linked or unlinked to the MHC locus on chromosome 6 and 17 of the human and mouse, respectively. In general, the MHC-unlinked class Ib genes possess significantly less homology and conservation of function with the class Ia gene members than the MHC-linked class Ib molecules. The MHC-linked class Ib molecules of the mouse are encoded within three genetic regions: Q, T, and M. The number of class Ib genes is strain-specific with some mouse strains such as BALB/ C possessing almost 35 of these genes. The human MHC locus is less well studied but contains at least 18 class I-related genes, 4 of which likely encode functional MHC class Ib proteins (HLA-E, F, G, and the MHC class I chain-related gene A which is closely linked to the HLA-B locus) (Houlihan *et al.*, 1995; Bahranm *et al.*, 1994). The non-MHC-linked class Ib genes are represented by the CD1 locus in human and mouse (Yu and Milstein, 1989), an Fc receptor for IgG in rat, mouse, and humans (Simister and Mostov, 1989; Ahouse *et al.*, 1993; Story *et al.*, 1994), and a zinc-associated $\alpha$2-glycoprotein in humans (Araki *et al.*, 1988). Cytomegalovirus also expresses a class I-like molecule which binds $\beta_2$M and likely plays a role in viral pathogenicity (Grundy *et al.*, 1987). An activated protein C receptor on endothelium also exhibits homology to the $\alpha$1 and $\alpha$2 domains of CD1 (Fukudome and Esmon, 1994), indicating that the MHC class I-related structure may serve diverse functional purposes.

The characteristics of the MHC class Ib molecules would appear to fall on a continuum in comparison to the products of the class Ia locus with several similarities (Stroynowski, 1990; Shawar *et al.*, 1994). First, the MHC class Ia and Ib molecules have a similar exon organization which generally consists of eight exons encoding a 5' untranslated and leader peptide, the coding regions for the N-terminal, membrane distal, or extracellular, immunoglobulin-like $\alpha$1–3 domains, each approximately 90 amino acids in length, a transmembrane domain, a cytoplasmic tail, and a 3' untranslated region. Second, many of the contact sites for $\beta_2$M that have been previously defined for the class Ia proteins are likely conserved in the MHC-linked class Ib molecules (Tyson-Calnon *et al.*, 1991). The MHC-unlinked, class Ib molecules exhibit less conservation of these sites which may correlate with a less stringent requirement for $\beta_2$M in assembly. This includes CD1 (Balk *et al.*, 1994) and the Zn-$\alpha$2-glycoprotein (Araki *et al.*, 1988). Third, many of the consensus residues for binding CD8, which have been identified in the $\alpha$3 domain of human and mouse class Ia molecules, may be conserved in the class Ib molecules. In addition, at least two class Ib molecules, mouse thymus leukemia antigen (TL) and CD1, have been shown to bind CD8 (Teitell *et al.*, 1991; Castaño *et al.*, 1995). Finally, many of the class Ib molecules have been shown to function as TCR ligands, or restriction elements, for T cells in either antigen specific or alloantigen *in vitro* model systems for $\alpha\beta$ and $\gamma\delta$ T cells expressing either the CD8 or double-negative (CD4$^-$CD8$^-$) phenotype (Porcelli *et al.*, 1992). Of interest, double-negative T cells represent a minor subset of oligoclonal T cells in the peripheral blood that may be expanded in autoimmunity (Porcelli *et al.*, 1993).

There are, however, several major differences which represent distinguishing features that demarcate these molecules from the class Ia molecules (Stroynowski, 1990; Shawar *et al.*, 1994). First, there is a notable absence of allelic polymorphism. In contrast to the dozens of alleles described for the class Ia genes which may vary by as much as 25% at the amino acid level in the $\alpha 1$ and $\alpha 2$ domains, the class Ib genes display limited allelism that is usually limited to a few amino acid substitutions. Thus, they are considered to be nonpolymorphic. Second, the tissue distribution of many of the class Ib molecules is limited to certain tissues and/or cell types, in contrast to the almost ubiquitous expression of the class Ia molecules. These include: preferential expression of mouse TL (T-locus), mouse and human CD1d, and the mouse, rat, and human neonatal FcR for IgG on IEC; expression of mouse Q10 by the liver; restriction of human HLA-G and zinc-$\alpha 2$-glycoprotein to the syncytiotrophoblast and serum, respectively; and the restriction of human CD1a, b, and c expression to thymocytes in thymus and Langerhans cells, B cells, and activated monocytes in the periphery. Third, there is marked plasticity in the protein products of the class Ib genes via the use of alternate transcripts generating proteins that are transmembrane, glycolipid-anchored, or secreted. Finally, in those examples in which bound antigens have been identified, there is a tendency to display a specialization for the presentation of particular, perhaps nonpeptide, antigen or for particular nonantigen presentation functions. For example, the M3 gene of the mouse H2-M locus binds a single class of peptides that are N-formylated, a characteristic of prokaryotic proteins, for presentation to cytotoxic T lymphocytes (Kurlander *et al.*, 1992). Notably, the class Ia groove is incompetent to bind N-formylated peptides. Other examples include: Qa-1, which may bind heat-shock protein peptides; Qa-2, which binds a variety of nonpeptides similar to class Ia molecules that fall into a consensus for epithelial pathogens (Rötzschke *et al.*, 1993); the neonatal FcR, which binds immunoglobulin of the $\gamma$ class on the apical surface of the enterocyte for transcytosis to the basolateral surface (Simister and Rees, 1985); and CD1b, which binds mycobacterial lipids (Beckman *et al.*, 1994). Finally, although these bound antigens may be loaded in a *Tap*-dependent mechanism, similar to class Ia, it is becoming increasingly evident that several class Ib molecules may be processed for transport to the cell surface for function via an alternative pathway. This notably includes the mouse TL and mouse and human CD1 antigens which localize to the IEC and can be stably expressed on the cell surface of the *Tap*-negative cells (de la Salle *et al.*, 1994; M. Kronenberg, personal communication). FcRn binds no peptide but rather IgG (Burmeister *et al.*, 1994a,b). This indicates that many of the class Ib molecules may employ novel pathways of biosynthesis distinct from the class Ia molecules.

Taken together, these characteristics suggest that the class Ib molecules are nonpolymorphic, class I-like molecules which may function as ligands for discrete subpopulations of T cells, especially cytolytic CD8$^+$ T cells and double-negative (CD4$^-$CD8$^-$) T cells, in discrete topological tissue niches and/or, in many cases, may be specialized to present a distinct, often unique, class of peptide or non-peptide antigen. They thus complement the ubiquitous polymorphic class Ia molecules which may be viewed as protection of the species from unforeseen pathogenic events whose tight control is important in preventing or avoiding auto-immunity.

## IV. THE HUMAN INTESTINAL EPITHELIAL COMPARTMENT

The human gut-associated lymphoid tissue (GALT) is a specialized organ compartment which likely utilizes class Ib molecules for specific purposes. The epithelium of the intestine, in particular, is a unique immunological compartment that is predominantly composed of essentially two cell types, CD8$^+$ T cells and the IEC, the latter of which are increasingly being recognized as unique antigen-presenting cells (Mayer, 1991; Blumberg and Balk, 1994). The IEC is likely involved in monitoring luminal antigenic events. This may occur via IEC regulation of paracellular uptake of antigen, direct uptake and processing of antigen by the IEC, or the transcellular transport of antigen by the IEC to subepithelial immune cells (Mayer, 1991). The class Ib molecule described for transport of IgG may be involved in this process (see below).

The majority of the CD8$^+$ T cells, or intestinal IEL, express the $\alpha\beta$ TCR and the minority express the $\gamma\delta$ TCR. These iIELs almost uniformly express CD45RO, a marker for antigen education or memory, and the unique mucosal integrin, $\alpha^E\beta_7$ (or HML-1), which likely marks iIELs for homing to the basolateral surface of intestinal epithelium (Jarry et al., 1990). iIELs exhibit marked cytolytic activity in several in vitro model systems including redirected lysis, the lysis of epithelial tumor cell lines, and the presence of cytolytic granules (Taunk et al., 1992; Guy-Grand et al., 1991; Sydora et al., 1993). Given their low proliferative potential in a variety of systems, this suggests that their primary end-stage function is cytolysis (Ebert, 1989). In addition, despite the contiguity to the intestinal lumen and the potential exposure to a variety of dietary and microbial antigens with the expectation that the TCR repertoire of the iIEL will be markedly polyclonal, as each T cell recognizes a distinct antigen via its TCR, an examination of the TCR repertoire by a variety of PCR-based techniques shows that the TCR repertoire of both $\alpha\beta$ and $\gamma\delta$ iIELs is surprisingly oligoclonal (Balk et al., 1991; Blumberg et al., 1993; VanKerckhove et al., 1992; Gross et al., 1994; Chowers et al., 1994). This indicates that the intestinal epithelium is colonized by a large mass of limited number of T-cell clones which likely recognize a limited range of antigens in the context of a class I-related ligand on the IEC. This, in turn, implicates class Ib molecules due to their qualities as nonpolymorphic ligands for unique classes of CD8$^+$ T cells.

The remainder of this chapter will thus focus on two class Ib molecules which are expressed on human IECs: the neonatal FcR for IgG (FcRn) and CD1.

## V. The FcRn in Human Intestine

The FcRn, which has been cloned from rat (Simister and Mostov, 1989), mouse (Ahouse *et al.*, 1993), and human (Story *et al.*, 1994), consists of a 40- to 50-kDa heavy chain, which has significant structural similarities to major histocompatibility complex (MHC) class I molecules. FcRn is responsible for the passive acquisition of maternal IgG across epithelial cells of the placenta antenatally in humans and postnatally across the epithelial cells of the intestine in rats, mouse, and humans. This process is specific for the Fc portion of IgG, but not IgA and IgM. Binding of IgG occurs preferentially at acidic pH (pH < 6), the pH of endosomes and the neonatal intestinal lumen, but not at neutral pH, the pH of the interstitium. Cocrystallographic analysis of FcRn with IgG shows that the putative groove for peptide formed by the $\alpha$1 and $\alpha$2 is lost due to a Pro[162] residue (Burmeister *et al.*, 1994a,b). IgG is bound primarily on the outer face of the $\alpha$ helix formed by the $\alpha$2 domain with contact sites at the junction of the CH2–CH3 domains of IgG (Kim *et al.*, 1994). This region of IgG is histidine-rich, which likely accounts for the pH dependence of binding. Thus, receptor-bound IgG on the apical surface of the polarized epithelium is transferred to the basolateral surface of the epithelial cell by this molecule within a transcytotic pathway wherein discharge of IgG occurs. The FcRn-associated pathway is also capable of transporting IgG/immune complexes (Rodewald *et al.*, 1979), suggesting that the FcRn may function in both passive acquisition of IgG and specific luminal sampling of antigen. This suggests that the FcRn pathway may shape the immature mucosal and systemic immune system.

We have recently observed that functional expression of the FcRn may also occur beyond the neonatal period and in tissues other than intestine and placenta, where most passive acquisition of IgG has been shown to occur. Expression of the FcRn has been observed on the cell surface of adult rat hepatocytes (Blumberg *et al.*, 1995). This expression is preferentially enriched on apical membrane domains supporting a potential interaction with IgG in the biliary lumen. These findings suggest that the MHC class I-related FcR may be expressed in a variety of developmental and anatomic contexts.

We have recently cloned a human homolog of the rat and mouse MHC class I-related neonatal FcR from human placenta (Story *et al.*, 1994). This cDNA has significant homology with the previously cloned rat and mouse isoforms. Using this cDNA as a probe, significant amounts of message could also be demonstrated in adult human intestine (Story *et al.*, 1994). This message can be localized to IECs (data not shown). We have also recently cloned by PCR full-length transcripts from neonatal and adult human intestine. Sequencing of these PCR amplification products has revealed nearly identical sequences from human placenta (Story *et al.*, 1994), fetal intestine, and adult intestine (data not shown). Thus, a gene product similar to fetal intestine is found to be transcribed beyond the neonatal period in normal adult human IECs.

The detection of specific transcripts for the FcRn suggests that FcRn might be functional in adult human intestine. Western blotting of normal adult human small and large intestine with an anti-peptide antiserum raised in rabbits against peptides contained within the $\alpha 2$ domain of FcRn has revealed evidence of specific bands consistent with the MHC class I-related FcRn in both tissues (data not shown). This protein is likely functional since T84 cells, an IEC line, and normal adult enterocytes specifically bind Fc fragments of IgG at pH 6 but not pH 8 (data not shown). This indicates that functional FcR binding activity, distinctive of this receptor, is observed *in vivo* in adult humans.

Thus, the human homolog of the mouse and rat FcRn that was recently cloned from human placenta is functionally expressed in adult IECs. This indicates that FcRn is present in the intestine through a wide range of ages in the host, indicating that the FcRn may subserve specific age-related functions. The implications of these observations for the adult mucosal immune system need to be established. There are two functional possibilities which, in turn, reflect the possible vectoral direction of FcRn bulk flow: either basolateral to apical or apical to basolateral. In the former model, the adult FcRn might be responsible for transporting IgG and/or IgG immune complexes into the lumen for immune exclusion and/or immune complex elimination. This, in turn, might provide an explanation for the IgG which is normally observed within the intestinal lumen. In the latter model, the adult FcRn might be responsible for the transport of IgG and/or IgG immune complexes from the lumen to the interstitium. Parenthetically, clinical studies in humans suggest that macromolecular absorption of antigens likely continues at low levels normally throughout life (Walker and Isselbacher, 1974). Model system studies in whole animals, such as the hamster, further suggest that this process is transcellular across the enterocyte and involves immunoglobulin (Bockman and Winborn, 1968). This supports the supposition that an FcRn for immunoglobulin may reside on the luminal surface of the enterocyte and remain functional in adult life for the purposes of immune complex sampling which may be delivered to subepithelial immune cell elements which are competent to process, present, and respond to macromolecular antigens. Thus, when expressed in adult tissues, the FcRn may fulfill an important luminal immunosurveillance function through the immunoregulation of subepithelial mucosal immune cells.

## VI. CD1 IN THE HUMAN INTESTINE

As described above, the intestinal epithelium contains a limited number of cytolytic $CD8^+$ $CD45RO^+$ $HML-1^+$ $\alpha\beta$ T cell clones that likely recognize a limited range of class I-related antigenic events on an IEC and are unlikely to recognize luminal events. These observations strongly suggest a role of iIELs in local microenvironment immunosurveillance and functionally implicate class Ib molecules as potential ligands for human iIELs in view of their nonpolymorphic structure, function as T-cell ligands for CD8$^+$ T cells, and localized expression on IECs in mouse systems.

In the human, the best candidate ligands are members of the CD1 gene family in view of the known tissue distributions of the mouse class Ib molecules (Bleicher et al., 1990). The CD1 gene family contains five members, CD1A–E,[1] which map to chromosome 1. A gene product for CD1E has not been identified (Calabi and Bradbury, 1991). CD1A–D fall into two groups based on nucleotide and deduced amino acid sequence: CD1A–C and CD1D, the latter of which is most homologous to mouse CD1 (Balk et al., 1989), and likely a rat homolog (Ichimiya et al., 1994). Human CD1D shares 60% amino acid homology in the $\alpha$1 and $\alpha$2 domains with mouse CD1 in comparison to 30–40% homology with CD1A–C. CD1A–C, on the other hand, share 50–60% amino acid sequence homology with each other in these domains. CD1a–c and CD1d likely also differ in tissue distribution, antigens presented, and responsive T-cell populations. CD1a–c are primarily thymic antigens which are expressed on thymocytes and in a restricted fashion on certain professional antigen-presenting cells such as B cells, Langerhans cells, and activated monocytes (Calabi and Bradbury, 1991; Kasinrerk et al., 1993). The data to date support the notion that CD1a–c fulfill a function in the presentation of bacterial and mycobacterial antigens to double-negative T cells (Dellabona et al., 1993; Porcelli et al., 1992). CD1d is expressed at lower levels in the thymus than CD1a–c and is expressed in a wide variety of tissues (Canchis et al., 1993). Within these tissues, a predilection is observed for epithelial cell expression (Blumberg et al., 1991; Canchis et al., 1993). This cellular specificity is reminiscent of previous observations with the MHC class I chain-related gene product (Bahranm et al., 1994). Although not yet observed for human CD1d, the mouse homolog of CD1d, CD1.1, has been shown to bind 22-amino-acid peptides with a distinctive hydrophobic motif for presentation to CD8$^+$ T cells (Castaño et al., 1995).

Using two monoclonal antibodies (mAb) originally raised against mouse CD1.1, the homolog of human CD1d, we have previously shown that, similar to mouse CD1, human CD1d is constitutively expressed by normal IECs (Blumberg et al., 1991; Canchis et al., 1993). Although CD1a, b, and c are regularly observed to be expressed by lamina propria mononuclear cells, especially in inflammation, there is little if any CD1a–c expression by IECs (T. Halstensen, personal communication). Occasionally, small numbers of CD1a$^+$ IECs are observed under inflammatory conditions such as celiac sprue and inflammatory bowel disease (data not shown). Thus, CD1d is the dominant CD1 family member expressed by IECs.

Although constitutively expressed on the IEC, CD1d expression appears to be regulated by cytokines found in the local intestinal milieu. Using a cell surface ELISA and mAbs 1H1 and 3C11, we have recently shown that CD1d expression

---

[1] By convention, CD1 genes are designated by capital letters (CD1A–E) and CD1 proteins by lower case letters (CD1a–d).

is upregulated by epithelial exposure to IFNγ. This appears to be specific for IFNγ since IEC exposure to IL-2, GM-CSF, IL-4, IL-5, IL-6, and TNFα resulted in no observable change in CD1d expression (data not shown). However, this effect is modest, increasing expression only 1.5- to 2.0-fold. Thus, similar to class I and II MHC proteins and ICAM-1, IFNγ regulates the cell surface expression of CD1d on IECs (Kaiserlian et al., 1991). This is different from CD1a, b, and c, which are induced by GM-CSF and IL-4 on monocytes, suggesting differences in regulation in comparison to CD1d (Porcelli et al., 1992; Kasinrerk et al., 1993).

CD1d is likely a ligand for CD8⁺ T cells. Previous studies by Mayer et al. have shown that IECs stimulate the proliferation of peripheral blood CD8⁺ T cells (Mayer and Eisenhardt, 1990). T-cell proliferation increases with increasing numbers of stimulating IECs. This proliferation can be abrogated nearly completely by the 3C11 monoclonal antibody, suggesting a functional role for the epitope recognized by this mAb (Panja et al., 1993). As a corollary, iIEL T-cell clones can recognize CD1 expressed on B-cell transfectants in a cytolytic assay, a likely major function of these cells. As can be seen in Table I, the dominant CD8⁺ T-cell clones from three donors were analyzed for cytolytic activity at an effector:target ratio of 10:1 using a $^{51}$Cr-labeled HLA-A,B-negative B-cell line transfected with either CD1a, b, c, d or the transfection vector alone (mock). Table I shows percentage killing. Note the consistent lysis of the CD1d transfectant and, to a somewhat lesser extent, the CD1a and c transfectants. Note that the three clones, I5.R5–7, express the dominant TCR in donor one of a recent publication (Blumberg et al., 1993). Thus, CD1d expressed on the cell surface of human IECs is a ligand for CD8⁺ T cells and human CD8⁺ iIEL T-cell clones expressing dominant TCRs specifically recognize CD1, especially the CD1d gene product, on B-cell transfectants in vitro.

TABLE I

CYTOTOXIC CELL ACTIVITY OF NORMAL HUMAN iIELs

| Target cells | iIEL T cell clones | | | | | |
|---|---|---|---|---|---|---|
| | 11.A1 | 11.A2 | 10.A1 | 5.R5 | 5.R6 | 5.R7 |
| C1R-mock | 5.6 | 0.7 | 3.4 | 11.0 | 2.8 | 2.6 |
| C1R-CD1a | 10.4 | 16.6 | 2.9 | 22.0 | 8.3 | 10.8 |
| C1R-CD1b | 3.0 | 4.7 | 0.4 | 7.5 | 6.9 | 9.4 |
| C1R-CD1c | 19.0 | 47.9 | 14.2 | 32.0 | 15.3 | 40.0 |
| C1R-CD1d | 23.5 | 55.1 | 14.2 | 31.2 | 21.0 | 39.0 |

Note. The HLA-A,B-negative cell lines transfected with either the CD1a, b, c, or d cDNAs or the vector alone (mock) (Balk et al., 1991), were labeled with $^{51}$Cr and used as targets in a 4-hr chromium release assay. The effector cells are normal human iIEL T cell clones obtained by limiting dilution of iIEL cell lines from the fresh iIELs of three donors described in Blumberg et al. (1993). The percentage cytotoxicity at an effector:target ratio of 10:1 is shown.

The CD1d on the cell surface of the targets used in the cytotoxicity assay is different from the CD1d on the cell surface of IECs. The CD1d target used in the cytolytic assay was transfected with the CD1d cDNA originally cloned from a thymus library (Balk *et al.*, 1989). Analysis of the cell surface protein on this transfectant by immunoprecipitation of iodinated proteins with an antipeptide antiserum raised in rabbits against the $\alpha1$ and $\alpha2$ domains of CD1d shows a 44- to 48-kDa smear consistent with the predicted amino acid sequence derived from this cDNA (Blumberg *et al.*, 1991). Immunoprecipitation of iodinated cell surface proteins from human IECs reveals, however, a 37-kDa protein without N-linked carbohydrate side chains, which is expressed on the cell surface independently of $\beta_2M$ (Balk *et al.*, 1994). Proof of identity was provided by a peptide map of the eluted IEC 37-kDa band in comparison to a V8 protease digestion of bacterially synthesized CD1d (Balk *et al.*, 1994). Thus, the structure of CD1d expressed on the surface of IECs is characterized by the absence of N-linked carbohydrate side chains and independence from $\beta_2M$. This form is different from that expressed on CD1d B cell transfectants which are targets for cytolytic iIEL T-cell clones. Although the function of this form of CD1d is presently unknown, the results by Panja *et al.* (1993) suggest a role in proliferation of CD8$^+$ T cells which implicates this molecular form in the expansion of specific CD8$^+$ iIELs.

The derivation of this 37-kDa form of CD1d is unclear but could represent either alternate transcription or post-translational modification mechanisms. Presently, the latter is favored. As can be seen in Fig. 1, the IEC cell surface form of CD1d coresolves with deglycosylated CD1d from a CD1d-transfected $\beta_2M$-negative melanoma cell line. This suggests that biosynthesis of CD1d is novel.

Equally intriguing have been preliminary observations on a potential intracellular IEC form of CD1d. In Fig. 2, plasma membranes (representing both internal and external, or cell surface, membrane-associated proteins) of the T84 cell line or normal human IECs from colon were solubilized in NP40 and immunoprecipitated with the 3C11 monoclonal antibody, and the immunoprecipitates resolved by SDS–PAGE under nonreducing conditions. Western blotting with an anti-peptide antiserum raised against the $\alpha1$ and $\alpha2$ domains of CD1d identified two bands: the monomeric 37-kDa band, originally identified on the cell surface (Balk *et al.*, 1994), and a monomeric 55-kDa band. This latter form is also notable for resistance to N-glycanase digestion and a weak or absent association with $\beta_2M$ (data not shown).

The ability to detect multiple structural isoforms in human IECs is reminiscent of studies with other class Ib molecules including other CD1 family members and HLA-G, for example. Woolfson and Milstein (1994) have analyzed CD1a and CD1c transcripts by PCR and have detected multiple structural variants that are generated by different splicing patterns. In the case of CD1a, three distinct protein isoforms were defined: a secreted form, a *bone fide* $\beta_2M$-associated transmembrane form, and an intracellular form which was retained with the endoplasmic reticulum. At least five alternate splicing products of HLA-G have also been de-

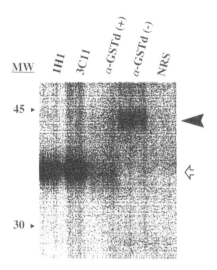

**FIGURE 1.** Immunoprecipitation of cell surface CD1d. Cell surface proteins of normal human IECs and the $\beta_2$M negative cell line, FO-1, transfected with the full-length CD1d cDNA (Balk *et al.,* 1989) were radiolabeled with [125]I and a lysate of proteins was prepared in NP40 as a detergent. Immunoprecipitates were prepared with either the IH1 and 3C11 mAbs or a polyclonal antiserum raised in rabbits against a GST–CD1d fusion protein ($\alpha$-GSTd). The $\alpha$-GSTd immunoprecipitates were either treated (+) or not treated (−) with N-glycanase. NRS represents normal rabbit serum as a control. The immunoprecipitates were resolved under reducing conditons and exposed on a Phosphorimager (Molecular Dynamics). The closed arrow indicates the glycosylated CD1d and the open arrow the deglycosylated (or nonglycosylated) CD1d.

fined, three of which have been shown to encode distinct proteins (Fujii *et al.,* 1994). Two of these are soluble molecules, one of which is likely unassociated with $\beta_2$M.

Given these observations with other class Ib molecules and our ability to detect distinct protein species in IECs by Western blotting, we analyzed CD1D transcription in human IECs by 3'-RACE. This has also revealed a series of alternatively spliced products. One transcript terminates in a cryptic polyadenylation site in the intron between the $\alpha2$ and $\alpha3$ domain exons. A second transcript deletes the transmembrane region exon while a third deletes the $\alpha3$ domain exon (data not shown). Whether these alternatively spliced CD1D transcripts encode functional protein needs to be established.

Nonetheless, the detection of these different structural forms within IECs by analysis of CD1d protein and CD1D transcripts raises the possibility of a role for these forms within the intestinal epithelial compartment, especially with respect to iIEL expansion and function. The dramatic colonization of the epithelium with a limited number of CD8[+] T-cell clones seems unlikely to be a stochastic or random event, suggesting that an IEC ligand, or ligands, exists for a limited number of

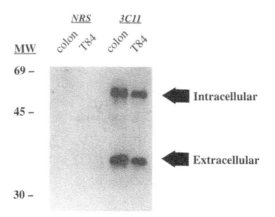

**FIGURE 2.** Western blotting of IEC CD1d. Plasma membranes from normal human colonic IECs or the T84 cell line were solubilized in immunoprecipitation buffer containing NP40 as a detergent and immunoprecipitated with either normal rat serum (NRS) or the 3C11 monoclonal antibody (mAb). The immunoprecipitates were resolved by SDS–PAGE under nonreducing conditions, transferred to nitrocellulose by Western blotting and immunoblotted with an anti-CD1d antipeptide antiserum. The resultant bands were detected with a horseradish peroxidase-conjugated secondary antibody and enhanced chemiluminescence (Amersham).

cytolytic $\alpha\beta$ TCR$^+$ (and likely $\gamma\delta$ TCR$^+$) CD8$^+$ T cell clones, which results in the TCR-specific recruitment and/or expansion in the basal state. Our studies raise the possibility that alternative isoforms of CD1d on IECs, perhaps presenting a limited array of nonconventional antigens, may perform these functions. Cytokines such as IFN$\gamma$ could upregulate this form of CD1d, resulting in the further recruitment and/or expansion of appropriate iIEL clones. It could further be speculated that IEC alterations during injury may lead to limited antigenic differences, which may trigger the cytolytic activity of these clonally expanded iIELs. This cytolytic signal may be another isoform of CD1d, such as the intracellular form described here, other members of the CD1 gene family, or other cell surface proteins yet to be defined, such as gp180 (Yio *et al.*, 1995). Given the observations of dendritic epidermal cells in mouse skin which utilize an invariant $\gamma\delta$ TCR that appears to be specific for an antigen expressed on stressed keratinocytes, these putative events may be a general property of the mucosal/epithelial surfaces (Havran *et al.*, 1991).

## REFERENCES

Ahouse, J. J., Hagerman, C. L., Mittal, P., Gilberg, D. J., Copeland, N. G., Jenkins, N. A., and Simister, N. E. (1993). Mouse MHC class I-like Fc receptor encoded outside the MHC. *J. Immunol.* **151,** 6076–6088.

Araki, T., Gejyo, F., Takagaki, K., Haupt, H., Schwick, H. G., Burgi, W., Marti, T., Schaller, J., Rickli, E., Brossmer, R., Atkinson, P. H., Putnam, F. W., and Schmid, K. (1988). Complete amino acid sequence of human plasma Zn-$\alpha_2$-glycoprotein and its homology to histocompatibility antigens. *Proc. Natl. Acad. Sci. U.S.A.* **85**, 679–683.

Bahranm, S., Bresnahan, M., Geraghty, D. E., and Spies, T. (1994). A second lineage of mammalian major histocompatibility complex class I genes. *Proc. Natl. Acad. Sci. U.S.A.* **91**, 6259, 6263.

Balk, S. P., Bleicher, P. A., and Terhorst, C. (1989). Isolation and characterization of a cDNA and gene coding for a fourth CD1 molecule. *Proc. Natl. Acad. Sci. U.S.A.* **86**, 252–256.

Balk, S. P., Ebert, E. C., Blumenthal, R. V., Landau, S. B., Wucherpfennig, K. W., McDermott, F. V., and Blumberg, R. S. (1991). Oligoclonality and recognition of CD1 by human intestinal intraepithelial lymphocytes. *Science* **253**, 1411–1415.

Balk, S. P., Burke, S., Polischuk, J. E., Frantz, M. E., Yang, L., Porcelli, S., Colgan, S. P., and Blumberg, R. S. (1994). $\beta_2$-microglobulin—independent MHC class Ib molecule expressed by human intestinal epithelium. *Science* **265**, 259–62.

Beckman, E. M., Porcelli, S. A., Morita, C. T., Behar, S. M., Furlong, S. T., and Brenner, M. B. (1994). Recognition of a lipid antigen by CD1-restricted $\alpha\beta^+$ T cells. *Nature (London)* **372**, 691–694.

Bjorkman, P. J., Saper, M. A., Samraoui, B., Bennett, W. S., Strominger, J. L., and Wiley, D. C. (1987). The foreign antigen binding site and T cell recognition regions of class I histocompatibility antigens. *Nature (London)* **329**, 512–518.

Bleicher, P. A., Balk, S. P., Hagen, S. J., Blumberg, R. S., Flotte, T. J., and Terhorst, C. (1990). Expression of murine CD1 on gastrointestinal epithelium. *Science* **250**, 679–682.

Blumberg, R. S., and Balk, S. P. (1994). Intraepithelial lymphocytes and their recognition of nonclassical MHC molecules. *Int. Rev. Immunol.* **11**, 15–30.

Blumberg, R. S., Terhorst, C., Bleicher, P., Allan C., McDermott, F. V., Landau, S. B., Trier, J., and Balk, S. P. (1991). Expression of nonpolymorphic MHC class I-like molecule, CD1d, by human intestinal epithelial cells. *J. Immunol.* **147**, 2518–2524.

Blumberg, R. S., Yockey, C. E., Gross, G. G., Ebert, E. C., and Balk, S. P. (1993). Human intestinal intraepithelial lymphocytes are derived from a limited number of T cell clones that utilize multiple V$\beta$ T cell receptor genes. *J. Immunol.* **150**, 5144–5153.

Blumberg, R. S., Koss, T., Story, C. M., Barisani, D., Polischuk, J., Lipin, A., Pablo, L., Green, R., and Simister, N.E. (1995). A major histocompatibility complex class I-related Fc receptor for IgG in rat hepatocytes. *J. Clin. Invest.* **95**, 2397–2402.

Bockman, D. E., and Winborn, W. B. (1968). Light and electron microscopy of intestinal ferritin absorption: Observations in sensitized and non-sensitized hamsters *(Mesocricetus auratus)*. *Anat. Rec.* **155**, 603–622.

Burmeister, W. P., Gastinel, L. N., Simister, N. E., Blum, M. L., and Bjorkman, P. J. (1994a). Crystal structure at 2.2 Å resolution of the MHC-related neonatal Fc receptor. *Nature (London)* **372**, 336–343.

Burmeister, W. P., Huber, A. H., and Bjorkman, P. J. (1994b). Crystal structure of the complex of rat neonatal Fc receptor with Fc. *Nature (London)* **372**, 379–383.

Calabi, F., and Bradbury, A. (1991). The CD1 system. A review. *Tissue Antigens* **137**, 1–9.

Canchis, P. W., Bhan, A. K., Landau, S. B., Yang, L., Balk, S. P., and Blumberg, R. S. (1993). Tissue distribution of the non-polymorphic major histocompatibility complex class I-like molecule, CD1d. *Immunology* **80**, 561–565.

Castaño, A. R., Tangri, S., Miller, J. E. W., Holcombe, H. R., Jackson, M. R., Huse, W. D., Kronenberg, M., and Peterson, P. A. (1995). Peptide binding and presentation bymouse CD1. *Science* **269**, 223–226.

Chowers, Y., Holtmeier, W., Harwood, J., Morzycka-Wroblewska, E., and Kagnoff, M. (1994). The V$\delta$ T cell receptor repertoire in human small intestine and colon. *J. Exp. Med.* **180**, 183–190.

de la Salle, H., Hanau, D., Fricker, D., Urlacher, A., Kelly, A., Salamero, J., Powis, S. H., Donato, L., Bausinger, H., Laforet, M., Jeras, M., Spehner, D., Bieber, T., Falkenrodt, A., Cazenave, J.-P., Trowsdale, J., and Tongio, M.-M. (1994). Homozygous human TAP peptide transporter mutation in HLA class I deficiency. *Science* **265**, 237–240.

Dellabona, P., Casorati, G., Friedli, B., Angman, L., Sallusto, F., Tunnacliffe, A., Roosneek, E., and Lanzavecchia, A. (1993). *In vivo* persistence of expanded clones specific for bacterial antigens within the human T cell receptor $\alpha/\beta$ CD4$^-$8$^-$ subset. *J. Exp. Med.* 1763–1771.

Ebert, E. C. (1989). Proliferative responses of human intraepithelial lymphocytes to various T-cell stimuli. *Gastroenterology* **97,** 1372–1381.

Fujii, T., Ishitani, A., and Geraghty, D. E. (1994). A soluble form of the HLA-G antigen is encoded by a messenger ribonucleic acid containing intron 4. *J. Immunol.* **153,** 5516–5524.

Fukudome, K., and Esmon, C. T. (1994). Identification, cloning, and regulation of a novel endothelial cell protein C/activated protein C receptor. *J. Biol. Chem.* **263,** 26486–26491.

Gross, G. G., Schwartz, V. L., Stevens, C., Ebert, E. C., Blumberg, R. S., and Balk, S. P. (1994). Distribution of dominant T cell receptor $\beta$ chains in human intestinal mucosa. *J. Exp. Med.* **180,** 1337–1344.

Grundy, J. E., McKeating, J. A., Ward, P. J., Sanderson, A. R., and Griffiths, P. D. (1987). $\beta_2$ microglobulin enhances the infectivity of cytomegalovirus and when bound to the virus enables class I HLA molecules to be used as a virus receptor. *J. Gen. Virol.* **68,** 793–803.

Guy-Grand, D., Malassis-Seris, M.., Briottet, C., and Vassalli, P. (1991). Cytotoxic differentiation of mouse gut thymodependent and independent intraepithelial T lymphocytes is induced locally. Correlation between functional assays, presence of perforin and granzyme transcripts, and cytoplasmic granules. *J. Exp. Med.* **173,** 1549–1552.

Havran, W. L., Chien, Y.-H., and Allison, J. P. (1991). Recognition of self antigens by skin-derived T cells with invariant $\gamma\delta$ antigen receptors. *Science* **252,** 1430–1432.

Houlihan, J. M., Biro, P. A., Harper, H. M., Jenkinson, H. J., and Holmes, C. H. (1995). The human amnion is a site of MHC class Ib expression: Evidence for the expression of HLA-E and HLA-G. *J. Immunol.* **154,** 5665–5674.

Ichimiya, S., Kikuchi, K., and Matsuura, A. (1994). Structural analysis of the rat homologue of CD1. Evidence for evolutionary conservation of he CD1D class and widespread transcription by rat cells. *J. Immunol.* **153,** 1112–1123.

Jarry, A., Cerf-Bensussan, N., Brousse, N., Selz, F., and Guy-Grand, D. (1990). Subsets of CD3$^+$ (T cell receptor $\alpha/\beta$ or $\gamma/\delta$) and CD3 lymphocytes isolated from normal human gut epithelium display phenotypical features different from their counterparts in peripheral blood. *Eur. J. Immunol.* **20,** 1097–1103.

Kaiserlian, D., Rigal, D., Abello, J., and Revillard, J. P. (1991). Expression, function and regulation of the intercellular adhesion molecule-1 (ICAM-1) on human intestinal epithelial cell lines. *Eur. J. Immunol.* **21,** 2415–21.

Kasinrerk, W., Baumruker, T., Majdic, O., Knapp, W., and Stockinger, H. (1993). CC1 molecule expression on human monocytes induced by granulocyte-macrophage colony-stimulating factor. *J. Immunol.* **150,** 579–584.

Kim, J.-K., Tsen, M.-F., Ghetie, V., and Ward, E. S. (1994). Localization of the site of the murine IgG1 molecule that is involved in binding to the murine intestinal Fc receptor. *Eur. J. Immunol.* **24,** 2429–2434.

Kurlander, R. J., Shawar, S. M., Brown, M. L., and Rich, R. R. (1992). Specialized role for a murine class I-b MHC molecule in prokaryotic host defenses. *Science* **257,** 678–679.

Mayer, L. (1991). Antigen presentation in the intestine. *Curr. Opin. Gastroenterol.* **7,** 446–449.

Mayer, L., and Eisenhardt, D. (1990). Lack of induction of suppressor T cells by intestinal epithelial cells from patients with inflammatory bowel disease. *J. Clin. Invest.* **86,** 1255–1260.

Monaco, J. J. (1992). A molecular model of MHC class-I-restricted antigen processing. *Immunol. Today* **13,** 173–179.

Neefjes, J. J., and Pleogh, H. L. (1992). Intracellular transport of MHC class II molecules. *Immunol. Today* **13,** 179–184.

Panja, A., Blumberg, R. S., Balk, S. P., and Mayer, L. (1993). CD1d is involved in T cell–intestinal epithelial cell interactions. *J. Exp. Med.* **178,** 1115–1119.

Porcelli, S., Morita, C. T., and Brenner, M. B. (1992). CD1b restricts the response of human CD4⁻8⁻ T lymphocytes to a microbial antigen. *Nature (London)* **360**, 593–596.

Porcelli, S., Yockey, C. E., Brenner, M. D., and Balk, S. P. (1993). Analysis of T cell antigen receptor (TCR) expression by human peripheral blood CD8αβ T cells demonstrates preferential use of several Vβ genes and an invariant TCRα chain. *J. Exp. Med.* **178**, 1–16.

Rodewald, R., Abrahamson, D. R., and Powers, A. (1979). Intestinal absorption of immune complexes by neonatal rats: A route of antigen transfer from mother to young. *Science* **206**, 567–569.

Rötzschke, O., Falk, K., Stevanović, Grahovac, B., Soloski, M. J., Jung, G., and Rammensee, H.-G. (1993). Qa-2 molecules are peptide receptors of higher stringency than ordinary class I molecules. *Nature (London)* **361**, 642–644.

Rudd, C. E. (1990). CD4, CD8 and the TCR–CD3 complex: A novel class of protein–tyrosine kinase receptor. *Immunol. Today* **11**, 400–406.

Shawar, S. M., Vyas, J. M., Rodgers, J. R., and Rich, R. R. (1994). Antigen presentation by major histocompatibility complex class I-ʙ molecules. *Annu. Rev. Immunol.* **12**, 839–880.

Simister, N. E., and Mostov, K. E. (1989). An Fc receptor structurally related to MHC class I antigens. *Nature (London)* **337**, 184–187.

Simister, N. E., and Rees, A. R. (1985). Isolation and characterization of an Fc receptor from neonatal rat small intestine. *Eur. J. Immunol.* **15**, 733–738.

Story, C. M., Mikulska, J. E., and Simister, N. E. (1994). A major histocompatibility complex class I-like Fc receptor cloned from human placenta: Possible role in transfer of immunoglobulin G from mother to fetus. *J. Exp. Med.* **180**, 2377–2381.

Stroynowski, I. (1990). Molecules related to class-I major histocompatibility complex antigens. *Annu. Rev. Immunol.* **8**, 501–530.

Sydora, B. C., Mixter, P. F., Holcombe, H. R., Eghtesady, P., Williams, K., Amaral, M. C., Nel, A., and Kronenberg, M. (1993). Intestinal intraepithelial lymphocytes are activated and cytolytic but do not proliferate as well as other T cells in response to mitogenic signals. *J. Immunol.* **150**, 2179–2191.

Taunk, J., Roberts, A. I., and Ebert, E. C. (1992). Spontaneous cytotoxicity of human intraepithelial lymphocytes against epithelial cell tumors. *Gastroenterology* **102**, 69–75.

Teitell, M., Mescher, M. F., Olson, C. A., Littman, D. R., and Kronenberg, M. (1991). The thymus leukemia antigen binds human and mouse CD8. *J. Exp. Med.* **174**, 1131–1138.

Tyson-Calnon, A., Grundy, J. E., and Perkins, S. J. (1991). Molecular comparisons of the β₂-microglobulin-binding site in class I major-histocompatibility-complex α-chains and proteins of related sequences. *Biochem. J.* **277**, 259–369.

Van Kerckhove, C., Russell, G. J., Deusch, K., Reich, K., Bhan, A. K., DerSimonian, H., and Brenner, M. B. (1992). Oligoclonality of human intestinal intraepithelial T cells. *J. Exp. Med.* **175**, 57–63.

Walker, W. A., and Isselbacher, K. J. (1974). Uptake and transport of macromolceules by the intestine: Possible role in clinical disorders. *Gastroenterology* **78**, 531–550.

Weiss, A. (1990). Structure and function of the T cell antigen receptor. *J. Clin. Invest.* **86**, 1015–1022.

Woolfson, A., and Milstein, C. (1994). Alternative splicing generates secretory isoforms of human CD1. *Proc. Natl. Acad. Sci. U.S.A.* **91**, 6683–6687.

Yewdell, J. W., and Bennink, J. R. (1992). Cell biology of antigen processing and presentation to major histocompatibility complex class I molecule-restricted T lymphocytes. *Adv. Immunol.* **52**, 1–123.

Yio, X. Y., Toy, L. S., Lin, A. Y., Honig, S., and Mayer, L. (1995). Expression of the CD8 ligand, gp180, by epithelial cells from patients with IBD. *Gastroenterology* **108**, A947.

Yu, C. Y., and Milstein, C. (1989). A physical map linking the five CD1 human thymocyte differentiation antigen genes. *EMBO J.* **8**, 3727–3732.

# Chapter 9

# Regulatory Peptides and Integration of the Intestinal Epithelium in Mucosal Responses

Daniel K. Podolsky

*Department of Medicine, Gastrointestinal Unit and Center for the Study of Inflammatory Bowel Disease, Department of Medicine, Massachusetts General Hospital at Harvard Medical School, Boston, Massachusetts 02114*

In recent years, it has become increasingly clear that the intestinal epithelial cells have key functions in addition to digestion and nutrient absorption. The epithelium is poised to serve as both the key physical barrier to the complex mixture of microorganisms and potentially toxic compounds present in the lumen and the frontier of the mucosal immune system. Intestinal epithelial cells are capable of producing a variety of cytokines and other regulatory factors which can affect functional regulation of the epithelium itself through autocrine and paracrine mechanisms as well as functional integration with lamina propria populations. The bidirectional nature of this cytokine network is now apparent with the demonstration that both rat and human intestinal epithelial-derived cell lines possess a much greater array of cytokine receptors than previously anticipated.

Regulatory peptides encompass structurally diverse peptides identified variously as peptide growth factors, interleukins, interferons, neuropeptides, hormones, and colony-stimulating factors (Nathan and Sporn, 1991). Several cytokines have been found to be expressed by constituents of the intestinal mucosa and to modulate intestinal epithelial cell populations. They include transforming growth factor $\beta$ (TGF$\beta$), transforming growth factor $\alpha$ (TGF$\alpha$), interleukin-1 (IL-1), tumor necrosis factor $\alpha$ (TNF$\alpha$), and interferon-$\gamma$ (IFN$\gamma$) (Shirota 1990; Madara and Strafford, 1989; Takacs *et al.,* 1988; Wu and Miyamoto, 1990; Chang *et al.,* 1990). These cytokines also exert potent effects on constituents of the mucosal immune system.

A high degree of redundancy is present within the "network" of cytokines found in the intestinal mucosa: a single cytokine can be produced by a wide variety of cells, and conversely each may act on a variety of distinct cell populations with diverse bioactivities. Both epithelial and immune cell populations may produce many or all of these cytokines in addition to serving as target cells. These observations lend support to the notion that a complex network of cytokines may have an important role in the regulation of a range of biological processes within the intestinal mucosa, e.g., regulation of epithelial cell proliferation and differentiation.

## I. REGULATORY PEPTIDES MODULATE EPITHELIAL PROLIFERATION AND FUNCTION

The intestinal mucosa is distinguished by a dynamic population of epithelial cells at its surface which undergoes nearly complete turnover every few days (Lipkin 1963). Despite continued loss of mature epithelial cells from villus tips and their replacement from the crypts, the integrity of the mucosal barrier and other functions are preserved. It is evident that these processes require precise regulation of proliferation and differentiation. In addition to peptide factors, components of the extracellular matrix and mesenchyme are also likely to be important.

Nontransformed cell lines from rat small intestinal epithelium, designated IEC-6, IEC-17, and IEC-18, have provided useful models to study the contribution of extracellular matrix and peptide factors in intestinal epithelial cell proliferation and differentiation. These cell lines retain many of the characteristics of crypt cells (Quaroni *et al.,* 1979). It has been reported that the cells can be induced to differentiate into mature epithelial cell types (enterocytes, goblet, endocrine, and Paneth cells) by association with fetal rat gut mesenchyme (Hahn *et al.,* 1990). In addition, enterocyte differentiation has been reported when IEC-6 cells were grown on a complex extracellular matrix without additional cellular elements (Carroll *et al.,* 1988).

Epidermal growth factor (EGF), a homolog of transforming growth factor (TGF$\alpha$), stimulates proliferation of IEC cell lines. In contrast, TGF$\beta$ is a very potent inhibitor of proliferation (Kurokawa and Podolsky, 1987). In addition to inhibition of proliferation, TGF$\beta_1$ also induces some features of the differentiated phenotype in IEC cells. Both TGF$\alpha$ and TGF$\beta$ are produced by the IEC cell lines and their expression appears to be controlled by autocrine mechanisms (Suemori *et al.,* 1991a). Addition of EGF (as a surrogate for TGF$\alpha$) to subconfluent cells resulted in enhanced expression of TGF$\alpha$ mRNA which peaked at 3–6 hr. Subsequently TGF$\alpha$ expression declined in parallel with increasing expression of TGF$\beta_1$ in the IEC cells. In contrast, addition of TGF$\beta$ to subconfluent IEC cells resulted in both autocrine induction of its own expression and suppression of TGF$\alpha$ expression. These observations suggest that an initial proliferative stimulus is reinforced by autocrine induction of TGF$\alpha$ but is ultimately downregulated through parallel induction of TGF$\beta$ expression.

The physiological relevance of these studies (on the IEC cells) is underscored by the observed expression of TGF$\alpha$ and TGF$\beta$ mRNA and protein in primary rat intestinal epithelial cells (Koyama and Podolsky, 1989; Barnard *et al.,* 1989). Expression of EGF could not be demonstrated, suggesting that TGF$\alpha$ and other members of the EGF family (e.g., amphiregulin) may be the physiological ligands for previously described EGF receptors on the basolateral surface of normal intestinal epithelial cells. Interestingly, a gradient of TGFα expression was observed among isolated primary intestinal epithelial cells. Paradoxically, preferential expression was seen in villus cells with progressively lower amounts in the crypts. In contrast, highest levels of TGFβ mRNA expression were found in the crypts with progressively lower levels in villus cell populations, although TGFβ peptides may be more widely distributed. The predominance of TGFβ in crypt populations may imply the need for a constitutive restraint on proliferation. These gradients of expression may suggest mechanisms for regulation of proliferation but other functions of the peptides cannot be excluded. EGF, and by implication TGFα, can modulate nutrient and electrolyte transport as well as disaccharidase expression in enterocytes.

Following recognition of the role of the growth factors TGFα and TGFβ in modulating proliferation of intestinal epithelial cells, studies from this laboratory demonstrated the presence of functional IL-2 receptors in the IEC-6 cell line derived from normal rat crypt epithelium as well as primary rat enterocytes (Ciacci *et al.,* 1993a). IL-2 was found to enhance production of TGFβ and promote cell migration in *in vitro* wounding models *(vide infra)*. In subsequent studies, these studies have been extended with the demonstration of functional IL-2 receptors on human colonic epithelial-derived cell lines (Reinecker and Podolsky, 1995).

These studies have led to the recognition that intestinal epithelial cells may respond to an even broader range of cytokines whose receptors share a component of the IL-2 receptor complex (Reinecker and Podolsky, 1995). IL-2 signalling requires the dimerization of the IL-2 receptor β (IL-2Rβ) and common γ (γc) chains. The γc is also a component of the receptors for IL-4, IL-7, and IL-9. To assess the extent and role of the receptor signal transducing system utilizing the γc chain on human intestinal epithelial cells, the expression of γc, IL-2Rβ, and receptor chains specific for IL-4, IL-7, and IL-9 was assessed by reverse transcription-coupled PCR on human intestinal epithelial cell lines and on isolated primary human intestinal epithelial cells. CaCO2, HT-29, and T-84 cells were found to express transcripts for the γc and IL-4R chains constitutively. IL-2Rβ chain expression was demonstrated in CaCO2 and HT-29 but not in T-84 cells. None of the cell lines expressed mRNA for the IL-2Rα chain. After stimulation with epidermal growth factor for 24 hr CaCO2, HT-29, and T-84 cells expressed transcripts for IL-7R. In addition, CaCO2 and HT-29 cells expressed mRNA for the IL-9R. Receptors for IL-2, IL-4, IL-7, and IL-9 on intestinal epithelial cell lines appeared to be functional; stimulation with these cytokines caused rapid tyrosine phosphorylation of several cellular proteins. Of note, the pattern of proteins undergoing tyrosine phosphorylation in the intestinal epithelial lines in response to these cytokines was distinct from that observed in lymphocytes exposed to these same ligands. These findings suggest that the pathways of response to cytokines in epithelial cells may be distinguished from those delineated in lymphocytes and macrophages. The relevance of the observations in intestinal epithelial cell lines for intestinal epithelial function *in vivo* was supported by the demonstration of transcripts for γc, IL-2Rβ, IL-4R, IL-7R, and IL-9R in primary human intestinal epithelial cells.

## II. Cytokines and Response to Mucosal Injury

The mucosal epithelium of the alimentary tract forms a barrier to the broad spectrum of noxious substances present within the lumen. Rapid resealing of this barrier following injury is essential to preservation of normal homeostasis. Observations made over the past several years have demonstrated the capability of the gastrointestinal tract to rapidly reestablish continuity of the surface epithelium after extensive destruction. This process, which occurs following various forms of injury both *in vitro* and *in vivo*, has been called epithelial restitution (Waller *et al.,* 1988; Silen, 1987; Lacy 1988; Feil *et al.,* 1987). Restitution occurs by migration of viable epithelial cells from areas adjacent to or just beneath the injured surface to cover the denuded area; restitution *in vivo* has been observed to occur within minutes to hours. The rapidity of this process suggests that cellular proliferation is not essential to restitution. Regeneration through epithelial cell proliferation and differentiation of surface mucosal cells occurs subsequent to this initial response to reestablish the continuity of the epithelial surface (Rutten and Ito, 1983; Moore *et al.,* 1989; Nusrat *et al.,* 1992).

Initial studies in this laboratory using an *in vitro* model of epithelial restitution demonstrated that TGFβ promotes intestinal epithelial restitution (Ciacci *et al.,* 1993b). However, as noted above, the broad spectrum of regulatory peptides generally known as cytokines has been demonstrated to be present within the intestinal mucosa and may serve as important modulators of epithelial cell function.

The effects of various cytokines and peptide growth factors were studied in an *in vitro* model of intestinal epithelial restitution (Dignass *et al.,* 1993a). Standard "wounds" were established in confluent monolayers of the intestinal cell line IEC-6, and migration was quantitated in the presence or absence of the physiologically relevant cytokines EGF, IL-1β, IL-6, TNFα, IFNγ, and PDGF. TGFα, EGF, IL-1β, and IFNγ enhanced epithelial cell restitution by 2.3- to 5.5-fold. Basic FGF (fibroblast growth factor), KGF (keratinocyte growth factor), and HGF (hepatocyte growth factor) had similar effects (Dignass *et al.,* 1994a,b,c). In contrast, IL-6, TNFα, and PDGF had no effect on cell migration, suggesting that the enhancing activity of the other cytokines was not a nonspecific effect. Enhancement of restitution was independent of proliferation. The restitution-promoting cytokines TGFα, EGF, IL-1β, and IFNγ increase the production of bioactive TGFβ1 peptide in wounded IEC-6 cell monolayers. The promotion of IEC-6 restitution by various cytokines could be completely blocked by addition of immunoneutralizing anti-TGFβ1, suggesting that various cytokines that are expressed in intestinal mucosa promote epithelial restitution after mucosal injury through increased production of bioactive TGFβ1 in epithelial cells.

## III. TREFOIL PEPTIDES AND EPITHELIAL INTEGRITY

Although the epithelium represents the cellular frontier of the mucosa, it has long been recognized that the apical surface of this population is covered by a viscoelastic coat secreted by the goblet cells (or mucous cells in the stomach), which occupies the interface between the lumen and the mucosa. This coat has been presumed to contribute to mucosal protection in conjunction with other potential functions. However, there has been little insight into its biochemical and functional properties in direct support of this concept.

The viscoelastic gel overlying the mucosa is formed largely by the secreted products of the goblet cell population. Among these, the high-molecular-weight mucin glycoproteins have been the best recognized. Although these highly heterogeneous and extensively glycosylated glycoproteins presumably contribute to gel formation, their functional importance remains incompletely understood. More recently, mucus-producing cells have been recognized to secrete large amounts of trefoil peptides in conjunction with mucin glycoproteins. The mammalian trefoil peptide family is composed of at least three small peptides sharing a distinctive motif of six cysteine residues in a module (designated a trefoil or a "P" domain), which leads to the formation of three intrachain loops through disulfide bond formation (Thim et al., 1988, 1989, 1994). These peptides are expressed in a complementary organ-specific pattern throughout the gastrointestinal tract, which seems to have been highly conserved through evolution. pS2 expression is found in the proximal stomach, human spasmolytic polypeptide (HSP) in the distal stomach and biliary tree (and pancreas in some animals), and intestinal trefoil factor (ITF) throughout the small and large intestine (Podolsky et al., 1993; Suemori et al., 1991a; Rio et al., 1988; Jeffrey et al., 1994; Hanby et al., 1993a,b; Lefebvre et al., 1993; Rio et al., 1991; Tomasetto et al., 1990; Chinery et al., 1992). These peptides are secreted onto the luminal surface, where they are present in the viscoelastic mucus gel.

In order to define the biochemical properties which enable these peptides to exert protective effects at the lumenal surface, human and rat intestinal trefoil factors (HITF and RITF) have been purified from colonic and intestinal mucosa, respectively, by ammonium sulfate precipitation of soluble proteins from mucosal scrapings, followed by sequential chromatography on DEAE-cellulose and reverse-phase HPLC to yield homogenous proteins on SDS–PAGE recognized by anti-ITF antisera. Native ITF was found to exist as monomer and dimer species of apparent molecular weight 6.8 and 14 kDa. Recombinant ITFs produced using the baculovirus expression cloning system were found to occur as spontaneously formed dimers which comigrated with native ITFs and were recognized by anti-ITF antisera. Recombinant RITF and HITF were resistant to digestion by pancreatic and gastrointestinal tract digestive proteases as assessed by electrophoretic migration and immunoreactivity with anti-ITF antisera. Addition of either RITF or HITF to a solution of purified human colonic mucin glycoproteins resulted in macromolecular complex formation. Comparable aggregation was observed with the addition of another trefoil peptide, HSP (human spasmolysin). Aggregation appeared to depend on ITF dimer formation; monomeric ITF had no effect on light scattering but could competitively inhibit HSP-induced aggregation of mucin glycoproteins. Thus, trefoil peptides are structurally suited to retain biological function in the hostile environment of the mucosal surface and may facilitate protection through direct complex formation with mucin glycoproteins, the other dominant product of goblet cell populations.

Although the trefoil peptides and mucin glycoproteins are among the most abundant products of the gastrointestinal tract mucosa and in aggregate seem to form the mucus gel that composes the interface between mucosa and lumen throughout the gastrointestinal tract, their full functional role has not yet been defined. Ectopic expression of trefoil peptides adjacent to areas of ulceration provides circumstantial evidence for a role in wound healing (Hanby et al., 1993a; Rio et al., 1991; Wright et al., 1990, 1993). While expression of a protein in metaplastic tissue does not necessarily reflect an important physiologic function, it should be noted that expression of trefoil peptides is highly induced in animal models of gastrointestinal ulceration. In a rat model of gastric ulceration induced by glacial acetic acid, a 1000-fold increase in immunoreactive ITF in the surrounding tissue was observed, compared to only 4-fold induction of rSP by Day 40 when healing was nearly complete (Taupin et al., 1994). As assessed by immunohistochemistry, highest levels of expression of these trefoil peptides was present in proximity to the ulcer with diminishing levels at greater distances from the lesion. In contrast, a similar model of ulceration induced by application of acetic acid to rat intestinal serosa demonstrated greater increases in rSP expression than that observed for ITF (Cook et al., 1994). While some groups have reported alterations in trefoil peptides immediately after injury (Stettler et al., 1995), others note that increased expression occurs in a substantially delayed time frame (Cook et al., 1995) that would seem to preclude a primary role in healing.

The presence of high concentrations of trefoil peptides and mucin glycoproteins on the luminal surface of the normal gastrointestinal tract due to constitutive production suggests that these factors play an important role in sustaining normal mucosal function. In recent studies, cooperative interaction between trefoil peptides and mucin glycoproteins was observed to protect the integrity of model intestinal epithelial monolayers against a variety of injurious agents (Dignass et al., 1994c). Addition of recombinant trefoil peptides human spasmolytic polypeptide, rat and human intestinal trefoil factor to subconfluent nontransformed rat intestinal epithelial cell lines (IEC-6 and IEC-17), human colon cancer-derived cell lines (HT-29 and CaCO2), or nontransformed fibroblasts (NRK and BHK) had no significant effect on proliferation. However, addition of the trefoil peptides to wounded monolayers of confluent IEC-6 cells in the in vitro model of epithelial restitution described above resulted in a 3- to 6-fold increase in the rate of epithelial migration into the wound. Stimulation of restitution by the trefoil peptide HSP was enhanced in a cooperative fashion by the addition of mucin glycoproteins purified from the colon or small intestine of either rat or man, achieving up to a 15-fold enhancement in restitution. No synergistic effect was observed following the addition of nonmucin glycoproteins. In contrast to cytokine stimulation of intestinal epithelial cell restitution, which is mediated through enhanced TGFβ bioactivity, trefoil peptide and trefoil peptide–mucin glycoprotein stimulation of restitution was not associated with alteration in concentrations of bioactive TGFβ and was not affected by the presence of immunoneutralizing anti-TGFβ antiserum. Collectively, these findings suggest that the trefoil peptides which are secreted onto the lumenal surface of the gastrointestinal tract may act in conjunction with the mucin glycoprotein products of goblet cells to promote reestablishment of mucosal integrity after injury through mechanisms distinct from those which may act at the basolateral pole of the epithelium.

In addition to promoting healing of epithelial monolayers after injury, recent studies demonstrate that trefoil peptides and mucin glycoproteins act in a cooperative fashion to protect monolayers of intestinal epithelial cells against a variety of injurious agents (Kindon et al., 1995). Intestinal epithelial cell lines form a relatively impermeable barrier to the inert marker mannitol when grown on a supporting membrane. Injurious agents, including C. difficile toxin A and bile salts (taurocholic acid and oleic acid), damage the integrity of the monolayer barrier, with penetration of the marker mannitol. Both native and recombinant rITF or hITF, or HSP in combination with gastrointestinal tract-derived mucin glycoproteins when applied to the monolayer prior to adding the agent, markedly diminished the injury. Although the addition of either a trefoil peptide or a mucin glycoprotein individually conferred protection, combinations of a trefoil peptide and a mucin glycoprotein provided increased protection in an additive and perhaps synergistic fashion. These effects too appear to be generic to trefoil peptides and gastrointestinal tract mucin glycoproteins. Thus, protection conferred by combinations of gastric mucin glycoproteins with either native or recombinant ITF, or colonic mucin glycoprotein with recombinant hSP, was similar to that observed with combinations of colonic mucin glycoproteins and ITF, or gastric mucin glycoprotein with hSP. Similarly, the source species (human or rat) did not appear to alter the additive nature of the effect, with combinations of rat and human proteins conferring protection similar to combinations of trefoil peptides and mucin glycoprotein from the same species. Non-mucin glycoproteins alone or in combination with trefoil peptides were ineffective in protecting against injury. These studies provide further evidence of a generalized interaction between trefoil peptides and mucin glycoproteins within the gastrointestinal tract, and for a role in the prevention of injury to the mucosal epithelium. Further studies are needed to define whether the protective effects of trefoil peptide and mucin glycoprotein combinations result from stabilization of the physical structure of mucin, or a more direct effect on the epithelium via specific receptors, or both.

Recent studies have supported the inference that the effects observed in vitro parallel properties of trefoil peptides exerted *in vitro* (Babyatsky *et al.*, 1996). Oral rHSP and ITF markedly protected against both ethanol- and indomethacin-induced gastric injury in rats when given up to 6 hr prior to injury. No protection against ethanol injury was noted after intraperitoneal administration of rHSP. Intraperitoneal rHSP protected against indomethacin-induced injury only at the maximal dose given (15 mg). Neither rHSP or ITF altered gastric pH. Protection was not associated with systemic absorption of trefoil peptides. These findings support the conclusion that the viscoelastic gel formed by these constituents *in vivo* provides an important defense mechanism protecting the mucosa from injury as well as facilitating repair after injury has occurred.

## ACKNOWLEDGMENTS

The author thanks the many colleagues who contributed to studies mentioned in this report: Drs. M. Babyatsky, C. Ciacci, A. Dignass, Y. Mahida, H-C. Reinecker, S. Suemori, K. Devaney, and H. Kindon. These studies were suggested by NIH Grants DK 46906, DK 41557, and P30 DK 43351.

## REFERENCES

Babyatsky, M. N., DeBeaumont, M. Thim, L., and Podolsky, D. K. (1996). Oral trefoil peptides protect against ethanol and indomethacin-induced gastric injury in bats. *Gastroenterology,* **110,** 489–497.

Barnard, J. A., Beauchamp, R. D., Coffey, R. J., and Moses, H. L. (1989). Regulation of intestinal epithelial cell growth by transforming growth factor type $\beta$. *Proc. Natl. Acad. Sci. U.S.A.* **86,** 1578–1582.

Carroll, K. M., Wong, T. T., Drabik, D. L., and Chang, E. B. (1988). Differentiation of rat small intestine epithelial cells by extracellular matrix. *Am. J. Physiol.* **254,** G355–G360.

Chang, E. B., Musch, M. V., and Mayer, L. (1990). Interleukinss 1 and 3 stimulate anion secretion in chicken intestine. *Gastroenterology* **98,** 1518–1524.

Chinery, R., Poulson, R., Rogers, L. A., Jeffery, R. E., Longcroft, J. M., Hanby, A. M., and Wright, N. A. (1992). Localization of intestinal trefoil-factor mRNA in rat stomach and intestine by hybridization *in situ*. *Biochem. J.* **285,** 5–8.

Ciacci, C., Mahida, Y. R., Dignass, A., Koizumi, M., and Podolsky, D. K. (1993a). Functional interleukin-2 receptors on intestinal epithelial cells. *J. Clin. Invest.* **92,** 527–532.

Ciacci, C., Lind, S. E., and Podolsky, D. K. (1993b). Transforming growth factor $\beta$ regulation of migration in wounded rat intestinal epithelial monolayers. *Gastroenterology* **105,** 93–101.

Cook, G. A., Skultety, K. J., Yeomans, N. D., and Giraud, A. S. (1994). Increased trefoil peptide expression in a rat model of intestinal repair. *Gastroenterology* **106,** A195 (Abstract).

Cook, G. A., *et al.* (1995). Trefoil peptide expression falls following gastric mucosal injury but is induced in a TGF$\alpha$-dependent manner late in repair. *Gastroenterology* **108,** A75 (Abstract).

Dignass, A. U., and Podolsky, D. K. (1993). Cytokine modulation of intestinal epithelial cell restitution: Central role of transforming growth factor $\beta$. *Gastroenterology* **105,** 1323–1332.

Dignass, A. U., Tsunekawa, S., and Podolsky, D. K. (1994a). Fibroblast growth factors modulate intestinal epithelial cell growth and migration. *Gastroenterology* **106,** 1254–1262.

Dignass, A. U., Lynch-Devaney, and Podolsky, D. K. (1994b). Hepatocyte growth factor/scatter factor modulates intestinal epithelial cell proliferation and migration. *Biochem. Biophys. Res. Commun.* **202,** 701–709.

Dignass, A. K., Kindon, H., Thim, L., and Podolsky, D. K. (1994c). Trefoil peptides promote epithelial migration through a transforming growth factor β-independent pathway. *J. Clin. Invest.* **94,** 376–383.

Feil, W., Lacy, E. R., Wong, Y. M., Burger, D., Wenzl, E., Starlinger, M., and Schiessel, R. (1989). Rapid epithelial restitution of human and rabbit colonic mucosa. *Gastroenterology* **97,** 685–701.

Feil, W., Wenzl, E., Vattay, P., Starlinger, M., Sogukoglu, T., and Schiessel, R. (1987). Repair of rabbit duodenal mucosa after acid injury *in vivo* and *in vitro*. *Gastroenterology* **92,** 1973–1986.

Hahn, U., Stallmach, A., Hahn, E. G., and Riecken, E. O. (1990). Basement membrane components are potent promoters of rat intestinal epithelial cell differentiation *In Vitro*. Gastroenterology **98,** 322–335.

Hanby, A. M., Poulsom, P., Singh, S., Jankowski, J., Hopwood, D., Elia, G., Rogers, L., Patel, K., and Wright, N. A. (1993a). Hyperplastic polyps: A cell lineage with both synthesizes and secretes trefoil-peptides and has phenotypic similarity with the ulcer-associated cell lineage. *Am. J. Pathol.* **142,** 663–68.

Hanby, A. M., Poulsom, R., Singh, S., Elia, G., Jeffery, R. E., and Wright, N. A. (1993b). Spasmolytic polypeptide is a major antral peptide: Distribution of the trefoil peptides human spasmolytic polypeptide and pS2 in the stomach. *Gastroenterology* **105,** 1110–1116.

Jeffrey, G. P., Oates, P. S., Wang, T. C., Babyatsky, M. V., and Brand, S. J. (1994). Spasmolytic polypeptide: A trefoil peptide secreted by rat gastric mucous cells. *Gastroenterology* **106,** 336–345.

Kindon, H., Pothoulakis, C., Thim, L., Lynch-Devany, K., and Podolsky, D. K. (1995). Trefoil peptide protection of intestinal epithelial barrier function: Cooperative interaction with mucin glycoprotein. *Gastroenterology* **109,** 516–523.

Koyama, S., and Podolsky, D. K. (1989). Differential expression of transforming growth factors α and β in rat intestinal epithelial cells. *J. Clin. Invest.* **83,** 1768–1773.

Kurokawa, M. (1987). Effects of growth factors on an intestinal epithelial cell line: Transforming growth factor β inhibits proliferation and stimulates differentiation. *Biochem. Biophys. Res. Commun.* **142,** 775–782.

Lacy, E. R. (1988). Epithelial restitution in the gastrointestinal tract. *J. Clin. Gastroenterol.* **10**(Suppl. 1), 72–77.

Lefebvre, O., Wolf, C., Kedinger, M., Chenard, M. P., Tomasetto, C., Chambon, P., and Rio, M. C. (1993). The mouse one P-domain (pS2) and two P-domain (mSP) genes exhibit distinct patterns of expression. *J. Cell Biol.* **122,** 191–98.

Lipkin, M. (1963). Cell proliferation kinetics in the gastrointestinal tract of man. II. Cell renewal in stomach, ileum, colon, and rectum. *Gastroenterology* **45,** 721–729.

Madara, J. L., and Stafford, J. (1989). Interferon-gamma directly affects barrier function of cultured intestinal epithelial monolayers. *J. Clin. Invest.* **83,** 724–727.

Moore, R., Carlson, S., and Madera, J. L. (1989). Rapid barrier restitution in an *in vitro* model of intestinal epithelial injury. *Lab. Invest.* **60,** 237–244.

Nathan, C., and Sporn, M. (1991). Cytokines in context. *J. Cell Biol.* **113,** 981–986.

Nusrat, A., Delp, C., and Madar, J. L. (1992). Intestinal epithelial restitution. *J. Clin. Invest.* **89,** 1501–1511.

Podolsky, D. K., Lynch-Devaney, K., Stow, J. L., Oates, P., Murgue, B., De-Beaumont, M., Sands, B. E., and Mahida, Y. R. (1993). Identification of human intestinal trefoil factor: Goblet cell-specific expression of a peptide targeted for apical secretion. *J. Biol. Chem.* **268,** 6694–6702.

Quaroni, A., Wands, J., Trelstad, R. L., and Isselbacher, K. J. (1979). Epitheloid cell cultures from rat small intestine. *J. Cell Biol.* **80,** 245–265.

Reinecker, H.-C., and Podolsky, D. K. (1995). Human intestinal epithelial cells express functional cytokine receptors sharing the common γc chain of the interleukin 2 receptor. *Proc. Natl. Acad. Sci. U.S.A.* **92,** 8353–8357.

Rio, M. C., Bellocq, J. P., Daniel, J. Y., Tomasetto, C., Lathe, R., Chenard, M. P., Batzenschlager, A., and Chambon, P. (1988). Breast cancer-associated pS2 protein: Synthesis and secretion by normal stomach mucosa. *Science* **241,** 705–708.

Rio, M.-C., Chenard, M. P., Wolf, C., Marcellin, L., Tomasetto, C., Lathe, R., Bellocq, J. P., and Chambon, P. (1991). Induction of pS2 and hSP genes as markers of mucosal ulceration of the digestive tract. *Gastroenterology* **100,** 375–379.

Rutten, M. J., and Ito, S. (1983). Morphology and electrophysiology of guinea pig gastric mucosal repair *in vitro. Am J. Physiol.* **244G,** 171–182.

Shirota, J. (1990). Interleukin 6 and its receptor are expressed in human intestinal epithelial cells. *Virchows Arch. B. Cell Pathol.* **58,** 303–308.

Silen, W. (1987). Gastric mucosal defense and repair. *In* "Physiology of the Gastrointestinal Tract" (L. R. Johnson, ed.), 2nd Ed., pp. 1044–1069. Raven, New York.

Stettler, C., Schmassmann, A., Poulsom, R., Hirschi, C., Flogerzi, B., Matsumoto, K., Nakamura, T., and Halter, F. (1995). Effect of hepatocyte growth factor on expression of trefoil peptides in injured gastric mucosa. *Gastroenterology* **108,** A226 (Abstract).

Suemori, S., Ciacci, C., and Podolsky, D. K. (1991a). Regulation of transforming growth factor expression in rat intestinal epithelial cell lines. *J. Clin. Invest.* **87,** 2216–2221.

Suemori, S., Lynch-Devaney, K., and Podolsky, D. K. (1991b). Identification and characterization of rat intestinal trefoil factor: Tissue- and cell-specific member of the trefoil protein family. *Proc. Natl. Acad. Sci. U.S.A.* **88,** 11017–11021.

Takacs, L., Kovacs, E. J., Smith, M. R., Young, H. A., and Durum, S. K. (1988). Detection of IL-1 alpha and IL-1 beta gene expression by *in situ* hybridization. Tissue localization of IL-2 mRNA in the normal C57BL/6 mouse. *J. Immunol.* **141,** 3081–3095.

Taupin, D. R., Cook, G. A., Yeomans, N. D., and Giraud, A. S. (1994). Increased trefoil peptide expression occurs late in the healing phase in a model of gastric ulceration in the rat. *Gastroenterology* **106,** A195 (Abstract).

Thim, L. (1989). A new family of growth factor-like peptides: 'Trefoil' disulfide loop structures as a common feature in breast cancer associated peptide (pS2), pancreatic spasmolytic polypeptide (PSP), and frog skin peptides (spasmolysins). *FEBS Lett.* **250,** 85–90.

Thim, L. (1988). A surprising sequence homology. *B. J. Lett.* **253,** 309.

Thim, L. (1994). Trefoil peptides: A new family of gastrointestinal molecules. *Digestion* **55,** 353–360.

Tomasetto, C., Rio, M. C., Gautier, C., Wolf, C., Hareuveni, M., Chambon, P., and Lathe, R. (1990) "hSP, the domain-duplicated homolog of pS2, is co-expressed with pS2 in stomach but not in breast carcinoma. *EMBO J.* **9,** 407–414.

Waller, D. A., Thomas, N. W., and Self, T. J. (1988). Epithelial restitution in the large intestine of the rat following insult with bile salts. *Virchows Arch. A, Pathol. Anat. Histopathol.* **414,** 77–81.

Wright, N. A., Poulson, R., Stamp, G. W., Hall, P. A., Jeffery, R. E., Longcroft, J. M., Rio, M. C., Tomasetto, C., and Chambon, P. (1990). Epidermal growth factor (EGF/URO) induce expression of regulatory peptides in damaged human gastrointestinal tissues. *J. Pathol.* **162,** 279–284.

Wright, N. A., Poulson, R., Stamp, G. W., Van Noorden, S., Sarraf, C., Elia, G., Ahnen, D., Jeffery, R., Longcroft, J., Pike, C., *et al.* (1993). Trefoil peptide gene expression in gastrointestinal epithelial cells in inflammatory bowel disease. *Gastroenterology* **104,** 12–20.

Wu, S. G., and Miyamoto, T. (1990). Radioprotection of the intestinal crypts of mice by recombinant human interleukin-1α. *Radiat. Res.* **123,** 112–115.

# Chapter 10

# Role of Stromal–Epithelial Cell Interactions and of Basement Membrane Molecules in the Onset and Maintenance of Epithelial Integrity

M. Kedinger,* C. Fritsch,* G. S. Evans,† A. De Arcangelis,* V. Orian-Rousseau,* and P. Simon-Assmann*

*INSERM Research Unit 381, Ontogenesis and Pathology of the Digestive Tract, 67200 Strasbourg, France; and † University of Sheffield, Department of Pediatrics, The Sheffield Children's Hospital, Sheffield S10 2TH, England*

## I. Introduction

The intestinal mucosa is routinely exposed to an enormous number of macromolecules and potential pathogens; therefore the maintenance of the integrity of the epithelial barrier is of particular importance in the physiopathology of this organ. The morphological and functional steady state of the mucosa depends primarily on an appropriate ratio of epithelial cell proliferation and maturation.

In the mature organ, the single-layered small intestinal epithelium is compartmentalized: deep crypts contain the stem cells and proliferative cells, and villi protruding in the lumen are composed of highly polarized and tightly linked absorptive cells. The onset and maintenance of this morphological and functional organization result from various intrinsic properties of the cells, hormonal regulations, and intercellular signaling. The cell types involved in this signaling network are present in the epithelium itself (like endocrine, goblet, Paneth cells, and intraepithelial lymphocytes) and in the underlying connective tissue (the lamina propria) that comprise various immunocompetent cells, endothelial and muscle cells, neurons, and fibroblasts. Interestingly, a fibroblastic cell layer is closely apposed to the epithelial layer.

The intestinal anlagen are formed early in development and consist of a poorly differentiated stratified epithelium derived from the endoderm, which is surrounded by undifferentiated intestinal mesenchymal cells. During morphogenesis, a single-layered epithelium is formed in parallel to the outgrowth of villi; the mesenchyme differentiates into the outer muscle layers and the cellular elements of the submucosal and mucosal connective tissue. Among these latter cells are the

111

subepithelial juxta-parenchymal cells. A complex network of extracellular matrix molecules which forms the basement membrane is present between the epithelial and fibroblastic cell layers from the earliest stages of intestinal development and from the crypts to the villi.

This article will focus on the role of heterologous cell interactions between epithelial and mesenchymal cells, and of basement membrane molecules in the morphological and functional integrity of the gut epithelium. The potential involvement of these cellular and molecular components in the process of inflammation will be discussed.

## II. Epithelial–Mesenchymal Cell Interactions

### A. Morphological Observations of the Intestinal Epithelial–Mesenchymal Interface

At fetal stages corresponding to 7–8 weeks in human, at 12 or 14 days in mouse or rat, the intestinal epithelial–mesenchymal interface is characterized by the fact that the basal surface of the deepest layer of endodermal cells is delineated by a regular basement membrane underlined by elongated mesenchymal cells. Later on, when villus morphogenesis takes place, the basement membrane is interrupted, allowing direct contact between both cell compartments through cytoplasmic processes which extend either from the base of the epithelial cells (Mathan *et al.*, 1972) or from the mesenchymal cells (Colony and Conforti, 1993). In the mature intestine, small fenestrations in the basement membrane are observed in the upper two-thirds of the villi where basal protrusions of the epithelial cells can be seen (Komuro and Hashimoto, 1990). These scanning and transmission electron microscopy observations, e.g., direct cell–cell contact as well as heterologous cells separated by a basement membrane, suggest that cell communications could occur via local paracrine factors (see The Mesenchymal Cell Compartment) and/or via cell–matrix molecules (see Experimental Observations . . .) signaling.

### B. Experimental Observations of Reciprocal Permissive and Inductive Cell Interactions

The comparison of monocultures of isolated intestinal endodermal or epithelial cells and of mesenchymal-derived cells with cocultures of endodermal–mesenchymal cells stressed the importance of heterologous cell contacts for epithelial cell cytodifferentiation (Kedinger *et al.,* 1987). A similar conclusion was drawn from gastric anlagen cocultured on both sides of Nucleopore filters, in which epithelial differentiation occurred only when the diameter of the pores allowed migration of mesenchymal cells to the epithelial side of the filter (Takiguchi-Hayashi and Yasugi, 1990). The morphological and biochemical follow-up of grafted hybrid intestines—composed of epithelial/mesenchymal anlagen taken either from different species (chick/rodent) or from different levels of the gastrointestinal tract—allowed us to demonstrate that the mesenchyme plays most often a permissive role in the morphogenesis and cytodifferentiation of the endoderm. As an example, cross-associations comprising rat proximal (jejunal) endoderm and distal (ileal) mesenchyme, or vice versa, develop hybrid structures in which epithelial cells express an enzymatic pattern characteristic of the original level of the endoderm. This has been illustrated clearly for the peculiar maintenance in the proximal epithelium, and shut down in the distal epithelium of lactase mRNA and protein at stages corresponding to the postweaning period (Duluc et al., 1994). However, the involvement of additional inductive interactions has been emphasized by the "intestinalization" of chick gizzard and of rodent colon endoderm by the small intestinal mesenchyme. This latter aspect, illustrated by the induction by the small intestinal mesenchyme of sucrase in epithelial cells deriving from the colon endoderm (Duluc et al., 1994), is of particular interest since colonic cancer cells express small intestinal-like phenotypes. Reciprocal instructive interactions have also been demonstrated in associations developed from gut endoderm surrounded by skin fibroblasts. In this case, intestinal epithelial cells induce skin fibroblasts to form subnormal lamina propria and muscle layers (Kedinger et al., 1990). Finally, recombination experiments showed that mature tissular components—crypt epithelial cells as well as fibroblasts from the lamina propria—retain properties similar to those of their embryonic counterpart (Haffen et al., 1983; Kedinger et al., 1986).

### C. The Mesenchymal Cell Compartment

As described in the two preceding paragraphs, there are compelling reasons to argue that intestinal mesenchymal cells have significant roles in intestinal mucosal development and physiology. Because of their localization at the epithelium–lamina propria interface, the subepithelial (myo)-fibroblastic cells may be involved in signal transmission between these compartments. The current knowledge about the subepithelial mesenchymal cells has been summarized in a recent review (Valentich and Powell, 1994). Among the various putative effectors described in various tissues, the two following examples illustrate partially the molecular nature of signals given by the intestinal mesenchyme and received by epithelium allowing morphogenesis, differentiation, or growth.

*In situ* hydridization of the developing gut revealed a mesenchymal expression of epimorphin, a component shown to be involved in epithelial morphogenesis such as lung tubular formation and hair follicle growth (Hirai et al., 1992). More precisely, epimorphin mRNA was detected at early development stages in clusters of mesenchymal cells surrounding the gut endoderm, and later on in cells underlying the intervillus epithelium (Goyal et al., 1995). A similar localization has been reported for scatter factor/hepatocyte growth factor (SF/HGF) mRNA (Sonnenberg *et al.*, 1993). SF/HGF is a secreted glycoprotein which acts in a paracrine fashion on epithelial cell growth and movements, and thus on morphogenesis. Interestingly, transcripts of the SF/HGF receptor, the C-met tyrosine kinase, are detected in the intestinal epithelial cells (Sonnenberg *et al.*, 1993). The receptors have been shown to be distributed on the basolateral surface of the epithelial cells in the colon (Crepaldi *et al.*, 1994). The complementary expression of SF/HGF and its receptors in the two-cell compartments suggests one possible molecular mechanism for mesenchymal–epithelial interactions.

In an attempt to characterize more precisely the properties of individual intestinal stromal cells in terms of (1) their production of—or response to—local paracrine factors (cytokines) and extracellular matrix (ECM) molecules, and (2) their effect on epithelial cells, we raised permanently growing fibroblast lines derived from postnatal rat intestinal lamina propria (G. Evans, personal communication). A first set of experiments shows that the conditioned culture medium collected from these lines contains some factors implicated in epithelial–mesenchymal cell interactions. In particular SF/HGF and also basic fibroblast growth factor (bFGF) which also interacts with basement membrane heparan sulfate proteoglycan to form a complex that binds to and activates the cell surface FGF receptors. In a second series of experiments, we have selected two morphologically different stable clones, F1G9 and A1F1, from one pleiomorphic fibroblast line. These two clones exhibit characteristic growth responses to cytokines. The proliferation of the former line is inhibited by TGF$\beta$1, that of the latter by IL-2. In addition, TGF$\beta$ induces a large proportion of F1G9 cells to express smooth muscle $\alpha$-actin, but this factor does not promote increased expression of this molecule in the A1F1 clone. As for the effects of these mesenchymal cell lines on epithelial cells, different effects on promoting growth and differentiation have also been observed.

Experimental approaches, including cocultures of fetal intestinal endodermal cells and of the fibroblast cell lines and grafts of associations comprising intact endoderms wrapped in fibroblastic cell sheets, were used to analyze the response of the epithelial cells. We observed that A1F1 cells stimulated growth of the endodermal cells, while F1G9 cells rather induced their differentiation. In addition, the morphology of the developed hybrid associations was different; they form, respectively, deep glands and villus–crypt structures (Fritsch *et al.*, manuscript in preparation).

Taken together, these observations and experiments strongly suggest that specific mesenchymal cell populations can direct intestinal development and differentiation; furthermore, their nature and properties can be influenced by various cytokines produced by the epithelium or the immunocompetent cells present in the lamina propria. Dysfunction of signal transmission emanating from the mesenchymal cells may be a crucial determinant in the pathogenesis of intestinal inflammatory disease (see Valentich and Powell, 1994).

## III. Extracellular Matrix Molecules and Cell Interactions: An Integrated Interplay Controlling the Physiological Steady State of the Intestinal Tissue

### A. ECM Components in the Developing and Mature Gut

Because of its strategic location between the epithelial cells and the adjacent mesenchymal cells, the basement membrane (BM) may play a crucial role in regulating the communication between these two cell compartments. BMs are specialized sheet-like ECM that separate the parenchymal cells from the connective tissue in most tissues. ECM molecules are considered as dynamic effectors in morphogenesis and in generation and maintenance of epithelial cell polarity. This exoskeleton interacts with cell surface receptors such as integrins which transduce information from the cell environment to the intracellular compartment.

The current knowledge on the location, nature, and developmental or spatial variations of the ECM molecules expressed in the intestinal tissue has been reviewed recently (Simon-Assmann *et al.*, 1995). The ubiquitous BM molecules, laminin, type IV collagen, nidogen, and perlecan are found in the subepithelial intestinal BM. To illustrate the diversity in the expression, molecular composition, and localization of the intestinal BM, laminin represents an interesting example. At least three isoforms of the laminin (LN) family are expressed in the gut subepithelial BM: LN-1, LN-2, and LN-5. Laminins are trimeric cross-shaped molecules characterized by one long arm comprising the helicoidal association of the C-terminal end of the three peptides and by three short arms corresponding to the single N-terminal ends of each constituent chain. Laminin-1 ($\alpha 1$, $\beta 1$, $\gamma 1$ chains) is expressed at the intestinal epithelial–mesenchymal interface in intestinal anlagen (11/12 days in the mouse/rat embryos, 7 weeks in human fetuses). From a biosynthetic point of view, large amounts of LN-1 with the highest $\alpha 1$ versus $\beta 1/\gamma 1$ chains ratio are produced during intestinal morphogenesis/differentiation (Simo *et al.*, 1991). In contrast to LN-1, the first expression of LN-2 ($\alpha 2$, $\beta 1$, $\gamma 1$ chains) is delayed and corresponds to the stage of crypt formation (after birth in rodents, $\approx 15$ weeks in human) where these molecules are confined. In the human mature organ, LN-1 and LN-2 have a complementary localization (Fig. 1), with LN-1 underlying the villus epithelial cells and LN-2 the crypt cells (Simon-Assmann *et al.*, 1994; Beaulieu and Vachon, 1994). Finally, LN-5 ($\alpha 3$, $\beta 3$, $\gamma 2$ chains), which is found like LN-1 at the level of the villus, is characterized in the mouse intestine by a dissociation in chain expression due to a late appearance of $\alpha 3$ chains (Orian-Rousseau *et al.*, 1996). Such a distinct distribution of each LN molecule together with their specific binding to various integrins strongly suggests their participation in different cellular behavior such as proliferation, migration, and differentiation.

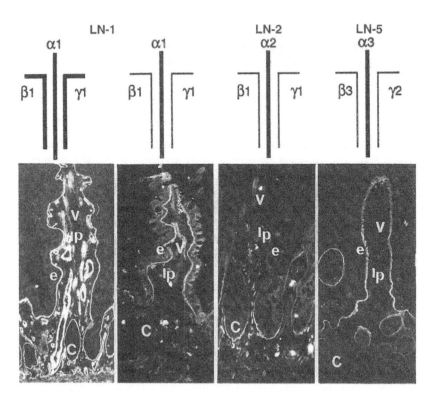

*FIGURE 1.* Differential expression of laminin isoforms in human adult intestine. The molecule or individual chains immunodetected with the corresponding antibodies are indicated on top of the micrographs. (e) Epithelial cells, (lp) lamina propria, (V) villus, (C) crypt.

## B. Involvement and Role of BM Molecules in Cell Interaction-Dependent Differentiation

A variety of experimental observations performed in various cell systems including intestinal cells point to the fact that the organization of a true BM requires the intimate contact between epithelial and mesenchymal cells. Experimentally, although each cell compartment cultured independently is able to synthesize some BM molecules, no authentic BM—visualized with specific antibodies or as an electron-dense material—can be elaborated unless heterologous cocultures are employed. In this case, laminin, type IV collagen, nidogen, and perlecan are deposited at the epithelial/mesenchymal interface (Simon-Assmann *et al.,* 1988).

The absolute requirement of close cell contacts for BM formation can be explained by the data obtained from the analysis of chick–rodent epithelial–mesenchymal hybrid associations developed as grafts in chick embryos or in nude mice (Fig. 2A). In these hybrid intestines, the deposition of BM components is traced

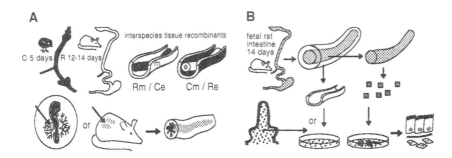

**FIGURE 2.** Schematic representation of interspecies recombination experiments (A) and of cocultures (B). (A) Intestinal anlagen taken from 5-day-chick (C) embryos or 12/14-day-rodent (R) fetuses (12 days in mouse, 14 days in rat) are dissociated enzymatically by collagenase and then mechanically to separate the endoderm from the mesenchyme. Interspecies recombinants comprising rodent mesenchyme (m) and chick endoderm (e) (Rm/Ce) or vice versa (Cm/Re) are grafted in the coelom of 3-day-chick embryos or under the skin (or kidney capsule) in nude mice. (B) 14-day fetal rat intestinal endodermal microexplants are seeded on top of confluent fetal mesenchymal cells or lamina propria fibroblasts or other nonintestinal fibroblasts as controls. The hybrid intestines/or cocultures are recovered after various time periods and processed for immunocytochemistry and biochemical analysis.

with species-specific antibodies. From these observations we conclude that the subepithelial BM is composed of molecules deposited either by the epithelial or mesenchymal compartment alone, or by both compartments for some BM constituents. In addition, variations in the cellular origin can be observed as a function of the development of the hybrids. The detailed conclusions drawn from this study are summarized in Table I (for references see Simon-Assmann *et al.*, 1995). These data stress the importance not only of the heterologous cell contacts but also of

*TABLE I*

SUMMARY OF THE EPITHELIAL OR MESENCHYMAL ORIGIN OF THE DIFFERENT BM
MOLECULES IN CHICK/RODENT HYBRID INTESTINES DEVELOPED FOR, RESPECTIVELY,
3, 6–8, AND 13 DAYS IN CHICK EMBRYOS

| Stages of development of the hybrid intestine | BM molecules | Perlecan | Type IV collagen | Nidogen | LN-1 $\beta1\gamma1$ chains | LN-1 $\alpha1$ chain | LN-5 $\gamma2$ chain |
|---|---|---|---|---|---|---|---|
| Early stages | Epithelium | + | + | − | + | + | + |
|  | Mesenchyme | − | + | + | + | − | − |
| Villus formation | Epithelium | + | − | − | + | + | + |
|  | Mesenchyme | − | + | + | + | − | + |
| Final maturation | Epithelium | + | − | − | + | + | − |
|  | Mesenchyme | − | + | + | + | + | + |

the maturation state of each tissue compartment. This also underlies the reciprocal, permissive, or instructive cell interactions that lead to the elaboration of the appropriate exoskeleton.

Experimental evidence supporting a role for BM molecules in cell differentiation is given by the chronological steps in the formation of cell–cell contacts, BM, and expression of epithelial differentiation markers which occur in cocultures of early embryonic intestinal endodermal cells and mesenchymal cells (Fig. 2B). Furthermore, in this model, the expression of apical hydrolases can be blocked by anti-laminin antibodies added in the coculture medium (Simo *et al.*, 1992). A similar inhibition of the epithelial cell polarization or of tissular morphogenesis was obtained using antibodies directed against various laminin domains in the kidney and lung (for references see Simon-Assmann *et al.*, 1995). In more recent experiments, LN-1 $\alpha$1 chain expression in the colonic cancer cell line Caco-2 was inhibited by stably transfecting the cells with an antisense cDNA to this molecule. This led to particularly interesting and informative data on the role of this molecule (De Arcangelis *et al.*, 1996). Caco-2 cells were chosen because, in contrast to most other colonic cancer cell lines, (1) they are highly polarized and differentiated in culture, (2) they express the constituent $\alpha$1 chain of LN-1, and (3) they form a BM when cocultured on top of mesenchymal cells (Bouziges *et al.*, 1991a). The absence of $\alpha$1 chain expression in the transfected clones altered the secretion of the complementary $\beta$1/$\gamma$1 chains of laminin. As a consequence (Fig. 3), no BM

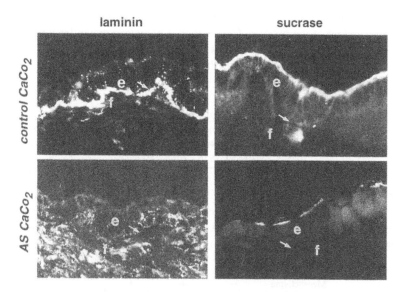

**FIGURE 3.** Immunocytochemical detection of laminin-1 and sucrase on cryosections of cocultures. Control Caco2 cells or LN1$\alpha$1 chain antisense-transfected cells are cultured on top of fetal skin fibroblasts. Arrows indicate the Caco2-fibroblast interface. (e) Caco2 cells, (f) fibroblasts.

was formed in cocultures despite the production of type IV collagen and nidogen by the mesenchymal cell compartment. Finally, the polarization and differentiation characteristics of the cells were strikingly disturbed. These experiments clearly demonstrate the requirement for laminin-1 for epithelial cell differentiation, which is also indicated by the villus localization of this laminin isoform.

The potential role of the $\alpha2$ chain in the maintenance of an extracellular microenvironment specific to the crypt cell compartment was analyzed in a mutant $\alpha2$-deficient mouse (*dy/dy* mouse). The major phenotype of these mice, which die prematuraly, is a severe muscular dystrophy (see in Simon-Assmann *et al.*, 1994). Neither the overall gross morphology of the intestine, including the formation of crypts, nor the cytodifferentiation from the stem cells, including that of Paneth cells at the bottom of the crypts, was modified (Simon-Assmann *et al.*, 1994). This observation either means that LN-2 $\alpha2$ chain does not act on the maintenance of the crypt steady state, or that replacement pathways can occur. This might be the case in the *dy/dy* mouse since in contrast to the human intestine, LN-1 $\alpha1$ is also found in the crypt BM.

### C. ECM Remodeling in Inflammatory Bowel Disease

It is well documented that matrix molecules play an essential role in wound healing and fibrosis. The chronology of the events which occur in both cases are: (1) an inflammatory phase with inflammatory cell recruitement and function, resulting in an important release of cytokines; (2) a proliferative phase characterized by the expansion of the fibroblast population responding to locally produced cytokines and peptide growth factors; and (3) a remodeling phase characterized by the production of extracellular matrix molecules (mainly connective tissue components, e.g., collagens I and III, fibronectin, chondronectin, and proteoglycans; Postlethwaite and Kang, 1992). The role of the lamina propria fibroblasts in this increased ECM synthesis has been shown by Stallmach and colleagues (1992). These matrix molecules are involved in the restoration of the wound which is normally followed by resorption of the inflammatory site and suppression of further matrix formation. However, regulatory imbalances may result in pathological consequences, characterized by the inappropriate deposition of fibrotic tissue and/or unresolved inflammatory responses. Such a situation is well documented in Crohn's disease where fibrosis may lead to intestinal strictures (Matthes *et al.*, 1992).

It is now recognized that changes in ECM synthesis, accumulation, and catabolism may account for the initiation and progression of many acquired diseases. Thus, by analogy with the wound repair model, one can speculate that an enhanced or abnormal release of cytokines—by immunocompetent, epithelial, or mesenchymal cells—may modulate the synthesis and/or degradation of ECM molecules including those at the epithelium/mesenchyme interface. This could alter cell interactions and finally lead to an imbalance between epithelial cell proliferation and differentiation. The three following examples reported for inflammatory bowel disease (IBD) illustrate how changes of the extracellular microenvironment may lead to morphological disruption of the tissue. First, in intestinal biopsies taken from patients with active Crohn's disease, an increased immunostaining of hyaluronan (HA) in the distended lamina propria was observed together with an increased luminal release. This was interpreted by the authors as an indication of increased villus permeability (Ahrenstedt *et al.*, 1992). HA is a large polyanionic molecule which could favor cell movements and tissue remodeling by preventing the accessibility to the cell receptors of ECM molecules involved in cell polarization and differentiation. It is tempting to correlate these observations made in Crohn's biopsies to the high synthesis of HA by the fetal intestine (Bouziges *et al.*, 1991b) when morphogenetic remodeling occurs. Interestingly, IL1 has been shown to increase HA synthesis (Postlethwaite and Kang, 1992). Second, a substantial loss of sulfated glycosaminoglycans from the subepithelial basement membrane is described in IBD and in particular for Crohn's disease, and was associated with areas of TNFα-producing macrophages (Murch *et al.*, 1993). TNFα could inhibit the synthesis of sulfated GAGs and thus disrupt the continuity of the basement membrane. Besides, TNFα is known to induce apoptosis in target cells. The third example illustrating changes in the ECM patterning concerns tenascin. Although tenascin is not considered a BM molecule, it is concentrated just beneath the epithelial cells. In normal gut it is expressed with an increasing gradient from base to the tip of the villi in the small intestine and restricted to the mucosal surface in the colon. This peculiar localization together with the fact that tenascin disturbs epithelial cell adhesion to the ECM substrate *in vitro* suggests that this molecule exerts a physiological role in the shedding of the intestinal epithelial cells (Probstmeier *et al.*, 1990). Riedl and collaborators (1992) describe that tenascin content at the basement membrane level is heavily increased in the inflamed mucosa and extends toward the bottom of the crypts. The overexpression of this molecule in areas outside the normal desquamation compartment might cause an overall decreased adherence of the epithelium in inflamed mucosa. This may also indicate a role for TGF$_\beta$ in these diseases since this molecule has been reported to increase tenascin synthesis (Postlethwaite and Kang, 1992).

## IV. Conclusion and Perspectives

The biology of the epithelial–mesenchymal cell interactions has been studied extensively in morphogenesis and differentiation in various organs, and we start now to understand part of the molecular signaling that controls cell communications. The lesson drawn from the observations and experimental works in this domain is that each developmental—injured or healing—stage may depend on appropriate local concentrations of ECM proteins, autocrine factors (like SF/HGF), or other cytokines and growth factors at the epithelial–mesenchymal junction. There are complex and intricated interactions between the various effectors: ECM molecules, integrins, and ECM degradation enzymes are either up- or downregulated by cytokines; similarly some cytokines upregulate and others downregulate the expression of growth factors, which in turn controls the expression of enzymes involved in matrix degradation. The production of all these components and of their receptors by the epithelial or mesenchymal cells depend on cell interactions; this partially corresponds to an autocrine loop of control additionnally modulated by the other cell present locally, like the immunocompetent cells and neurons. Any stage of dysregulation in their expression may result in morphological and functional alterations.

Much remains to be done to highlight the nature of the cells and to identify the factors involved in the cell interactions allowing the maintenance of an appropriate adult morphology and function. Although the concept of the epithelial stem cell has been well documented and the crypt cellular and molecular microenvironment has been described, the mechanisms involved in the regulation of this peculiar epithelial–mesenchymal unit remain obscure. In addition, little is known about the biology of the mesenchymal cell compartment: is there a persistent stem cell population or do phenotypic changes recorded in pathological stages result from cell plasticity? A better understanding of individual mesenchymal cell populations requires the characterization of specific markers and the definition of the basic production of the different molecules quoted above as well as of their response to cytokines, hormones, regulatory peptides. This information will undoubtly help our understanding of normal and pathological cell interactions. Furthermore, the use of techniques allowing a tissue- and time-specific knock-out of the potential effectors will bring more focused insight into these mechanisms.

## REFERENCES

Ahrenstedt, O., Knutson, L., Hallgren, R., and Gerdin, B. (1992). Increased luminal release of hyaluronan in uninvolved jejunum in active Crohn's disease but not in inactive disease or in relatives. *Digestion* **52,** 6–12.

Beaulieu, J. F., and Vachon, P. H. (1994). Reciprocal expression of laminin A-chain isoforms along the crypt-villus axis in the human small intestine. *Gastroenterology* **106,** 829–839.

Bouziges, F., Simo, P., Simon-Assmann, P., Haffen, K., and Kedinger, M. (1991a). Altered deposition of basement-membrane molecules in co-cultures of colonic cancer cells and fibroblasts. *Int. J. Cancer* **48,** 101–108.

Bouziges, F., Simon-Assmann, P., Simo, P., and Kedinger, M. (1991b). Changes in glycosaminoglycan expression in the rat developing intestine. *Cell Biol. Int. Rep.* **15,** 97–106.

Colony, P. C., and Conforti, J. C. (1993). Morphogenesis in the fetal rat proximal colon. Effects of cytochalasin-D. *Anat. Rec.* **235,** 241- 252.

Crepaldi, T., Pollack, A. L., Prat, M., Zborek, A., Mostov, K., and Comoglio, P. M. (1994). Targeting of the SF/HGF receptor to the basolateral domain of polarized epithelial cells. *J. Cell Biol.* **125,** 313–320.

De Arcangelis, A., Neuville, P., Boukamel, R., Lefebvre, O., Kedinger, M., and Simon-Assmann, P. (1996). Inhibition of laminin $\alpha$1-chain expression leads to alteration of basement membrane assembly and cell differentiation. *J. Cell Biol.* **133,** in press.

Duluc, I., Freund, J.-N., Leberquier, C., and Kedinger, M. (1994). Fetal endoderm primarily holds the temporal and positional information required for mammalian intestinal development. *J. Cell Biol.* **126,** 211–221.

Goyal, A., Grapperhaus, K.J., Swietlicki, E., and Rubin, D.C. (1995). Characterization of rat intestinal epimorphin expression suggests a role in crypt-villus morphogenesis. *Gastroenterology* **108(Suppl.),** A727.

Haffen, K., Lacroix, B., Kedinger, M., and Simon-Assmann, P. (1983). Inductive properties of fibroblastic cell cultures derived from rat intestinal mucosa on epithelial differentiation. *Differentiation* **23,** 226–233.

Hirai, Y., Takebe, K., Takashina, M., Kobayashi, S., and Takeichi, M. (1992). Epimorphin. A mesenchymal protein essential for epithelial morphogenesis. *Cell (Cambridge, Mass.)* **69,** 471–481.

Kedinger, M., Simon-Assmann, P. M., Lacroix, B., Marxer, A., Hauri, H. P., and Haffen, K. (1986). Fetal gut mesenchyme induces differentiation of cultured intestinal endoderm and crypt cells. *Dev. Biol.* **113,** 474–483.

Kedinger, M., Simon-Assmann, P., Alexandre, E., and Haffen, K. (1987). Importance of a fibroblastic support for *in vitro* differentiation of intestinal endodermal cells and for their response to glucocorticoids. *Cell Differ.* **20,** 171–182.

Kedinger, M., Simon-Assmann, P., Bouziges, F., Arnold, C., Alexandre, E., and Haffen, K. (1990). Smooth muscle actin expression during rat gut development and induction in fetal skin fibroblastic cells associated with intestinal embryonic epithelium. *Differentiation* **43,** 87–97.

Komuro, T., and Hashimoto, Y. (1990). 3-Dimensional structure of the rat intestinal wall mucosa and submucosa. *Arch. Hist. C.* **53,** 1–21.

Mathan, M., Hermos, J. A., and Trier, J. S. (1972). Structural features of the epithelio–mesenchymal interface of rat duodenal mucosa during development. *J. Cell Biol.* **52,** 577–588.

Matthes, H., Herbst, H., Schuppan, D., Stallmach, A., Milani, S., Stein, H., and Riecken, E. O. (1992). Cellular localization of procollagen gene transcripts in inflammatory bowel diseases. *Gastroenterology* **102,** 431–442.

Murch, S. H., MacDonald, T. T., Walker-Smith, J. A., Levin, M., Lionetti, P., and Klein, N. J. (1993). Disruption of sulphated glycosaminoglycans in intestinal inflammation. *Lancet* **341,** 711–714.

Orian-Rousseau, V., Aberdam, D., Fontao, L., Chevalier, L., Meneguzzi, G., Kedinger, M., and Simon-Assmann, P. (1996). Developmental expression of laminin-5 and HD1 in the intestine: epithelial to mesenchymal shift for the laminin γ2 chain subunit deposition. *Dev. Dynamics* **205,** in press.

Postlethwaite, A. E., and Kang, A. H. (1992). Fibroblasts and matrix proteins. *In* "Inflammation: Basic Principles and Clinical Correlates" (J. I. Gallin *et al.,* eds.), 2nd Ed., pp. 747–773. Raven, New York.

Probstmeier, R., Martini, R., and Schachner, M. (1990). Expression of J1/tenascin in the crypt-villus unit of adult mouse small intestine. Implications for its role in epithelial cell shedding. *Development (Cambridge, U.K.)* **109,** 313–321.

Riedl, S. E., Faissner, A., Schlag, P., von Herbay, A., Koretz, K., and Moller, P. (1992). Altered content and distribution of tenascin in colitis, colon adenoma, and colorectal carcinoma. *Gastroenterology* **103,** 400–406.

Simo, P., Simon-Assmann, P., Bouziges, F., Leberquier, C., Kedinger, M., Ekblom, P., and Sorokin, L. (1991). Changes in the expression of laminin during intestinal development. *Development (Cambridge, U.K.)* **112,** 477–487.

Simo, P., Simon-Assmann, P., Arnold, C., and Kedinger, M. (1992). Mesenchyme-mediated effect of dexamethasone on laminin in cocultures of embryonic gut epithelial cells and mesenchyme-derived cells. *J. Cell Sci.* **101,** 161–171.

Simon-Assmann, P., Bouziges, F., Arnold, C., Haffen, K., and Kedinger, M. (1988). Epithelial–mesenchymal interactions in the production of basement membrane components in the gut. *Development (Cambridge, U.K.)* **102,** 339–347.

Simon-Assmann, P., Duclos, B., Orian-Rousseau, V., Arnold, C., Mathelin, C., Engvall, E., and Kedinger, M. (1994). Differential expression of laminin isoforms and α6-β4 integrin subunits in the developing human and mouse intestine. *Dev. Dynamics* **201,** 71–85.

Simon-Assmann, P., Kedinger, M., De Arcangelis, A., Orian-Rousseau, V., and Simo, P. (1995). Extracellular matrix components in intestinal development. *Experientia (Basel)* **51,** 883–900.

Sonnenberg, E., Meyer, D., Weidner, K. M., and Birchmeier, C. (1993). Scatter factor/hepatocyte growth factor and its receptor, the c-met tyrosine kinase, can mediate a signal exchange between mesenchyme and epithelia during mouse development. *J. Cell Biol.* **123,** 223–235.

Stallmach, A., Schuppan, D., Riese, H. H., Matthes, H., and Riecken, E. O. (1992). Increased collagen type III synthesis by fibroblasts isolated from strictures of patients with Crohn's disease. *Gastroenterology* **102,** 1920–1929.

Takiguchi-Hayashi, K., and Yasugi, S. (1990). Transfilter analysis of the inductive influence of proventricular mesenchyme on stomach epithelial differentiation of chick embryos. *Roux Arch. Dev. Biol.* **198,** 460–466.

Valentich, J. D., and Powell, D. W. (1994). Intestinal subepithelial myofibroblasts and mucosal immunophysiology. *Curr. Opin. Gastroenterol.* **10,** 645–651.

# Chapter 11

# Neuroendocrine Regulation of Mucosal Immune Responses

Hiroshi Nagura, Mitsuru Kubota, and Noriko Kimura

*Department of Pathology, Tohoku University School of Medicine,
Sendai 980–77, Japan*

The primary function of intestine is to digest and absorb various essential nutrients into the circulation. The course of this activity has the consequence that the mucosal surface extends to the largest area of the body in contact with the external environment, and that the intestinal mucosa is exposed to a wide variety of antigens derived from resident and invading microorganisms as well as foods. The absorption of these antigens must be limited by a mucosal surface barrier, which allows absorption of nutrient molecules. This mucosal barrier is created and maintained by the mucosal immune defense system, in addition to nonimmunological physiological barrier including motility, mucus, and cell turnover (Russell and Walker, 1990; Nagura, 1992; Sanderson and Walker, 1994). Through such mechanisms the mucosal immune system contributes to the maintenance of the intestinal mucosal milieu and functions, and to the maintenance of overall body metabolic integrity. Thus the mucosal immune system, like all other homeostatic systems, is necessary to be under neuroendocrine regulation.

The interaction between the neuroendocrine system and the immune system has been recognized for many years, and it has recently become apparent that the neuroendocrine system can influence the immune responses, particularly in the mucosal immune system (e.g., Roszman *et al.,* 1985; Stead *et al.,* 1987; Croitoru *et al.,* 1990; Befus, 1993; Nagura *et al.,* 1994). Thus, abnormalities of the neuroendocrine–immune interactions may be important in disease pathogenesis of immune-inflammatory disorders in the intestine, including inflammatory bowel disease (IBD) and food allergy (Koch *et al.,* 1987; Kubota *et al.,* 1992; Kimura *et al.,* 1992; Nagura *et al,* 1994). The study of the morphologic, pathophysiologic, and molecular bases of this interaction has become the subject of intensive research. In this article we will briefly review the information available to date on the advance in this field concerning neuroendocrine–mucosal immune interaction and intestinal immuno-inflammatory disorders.

## I. The Intestinal Neuroendocrine and Immune Systems

The intestinal neuroendocrine system consists of an extensive network of the enteric nervous system and specialized epithelial endocrine cells, which constitute a "diffuse neuroendocrine system" (Gabella, 1970; Ferri et al., 1983; Polak and Bloom 1983; Kimura et al., 1994). Although initially only three gastrointestinal neuropeptides were recognized, during the past few years a number of new peptides have been discovered and each ascribed to a specific nerve fiber and/or endocrine cells (Jaffe, 1979; Croitoru et al., 1990; Pascual et al., 1994).

### A. Mucosal Nerve Networks

The enteric nervous system is a specialized component of the autonomic nervous system with a number of tissue-specific features. The majority of the neurons of the mucosal and submucosal plexus contain neuropeptide transmitters, including vasoactive intestinal peptide (VIP), substance P (SP), and somatostatin (SOM), which are also found in the central nervous system (Table I) (Croitoru et al., 1990; Pascual et al., 1994). The density of nerves in the intestinal mucosa is quite enormous. Their distribution is divided into three patterns, i.e., (1) dense networks around crypts, (2) along capillaries, and (3) networks without relation to crypts and capillaries, but with occasional relation to immune effector cells in the lamina propria (Kimura et al., 1994; Nagura et al., 1994) (Fig. 1). According to Ferri et al. (1983), it has been calculated that the linear density of VIP-containing nerve fibers (VIP nerves) in the human intestinal lamina propria is on the order of 30 m/cm$^3$. The lamina propria is also richly populated with a diffuse collection of

*TABLE I*

DISTRIBUTION OF GUT HORMONES IN THE GASTROINTESTINAL MUCOSA

| Gut hormones | Endocrine cells | Localization of endocrine cells | | | | | Gut nerves | Central nerve system |
| | | Gastric body | Gastric antrum | Upper small intestine | Lower small intestine | Large intestine | | |
|---|---|---|---|---|---|---|---|---|
| VIP | − | − | − | − | − | − | + | + |
| Somatostatin | D | + | + | + | + | + | + | + |
| Substance P | EC | − | + | + | + | − | + | + |
| Enkephaline | ND | + | + | + | + | − | + | + |
| Neurotensine | N | + | − | + | + | − | − | + |
| Gastrin | G | − | + | + | − | − | − | − |
| Serotonin | EC | − | + | + | + | + | − | − |

*Note.* +, positive, −, negative, ND, not determined.

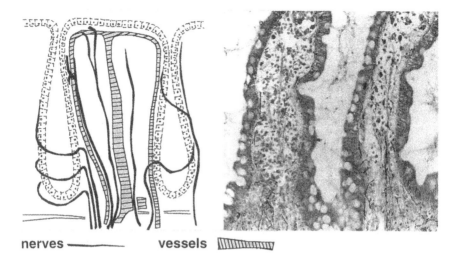

**nerves ————    vessels** [illustration]

*FIGURE 1.* The distribution of VIP nerves in the intestinal mucosa. They are distributed (1) around crypts, (2) along capillaries, and (3) without relation to crypts and capillaries, but with occasional relation to immune effector cells in the lamina propria.

lymphocytes, plasma cells, and cells of a monocyte-macrophage lineage (Brandt-zaeg *et al.,* 1989; Nagura, 1992), and consequently these immunocytes are within one cell distance of nerve fibers in the lamina propria and can reach close proximity to nerves by chance alone. Further, their inherent mobility enhances the opportunity of neural–immune interactions, suggesting they are innervated transiently. The close approximation between immunocytes and peptidergic nerves suggests their intimate cross-communication, and the mucosal localization of neuropeptides indicates that their release locally can directly affect the function of epithelial cells, vascular endothelial cells, and immunocytes.

## B. Mucosal Endocrine Cells

Endocrine cells are widely distributed throughout the gastrointestinal mucosa, and the gastrointestinal tract has recently been recognized as a major endocrine system. Neuropeptides found in the enteric nerves are simultaneously localized in these mucosal endocrine cells and central nervous system (Jaffe, 1979; Polak and Bloom, 1982) (Table I), that is, neuropeptides in the intestinal mucosa are produced by nerves and cells belonging to the amine precursor uptake and decarboxylation (APUD) system (Pearse and Polak, 1971). Intestinal endocrine cells are usually pyramidal and frequently have long apical processes extending toward the lumen of glands (Fujita and Kobayashi, 1977). Ultrastructurally characteristic intracytoplasmic dense-core granules allow for their classification, and some of these

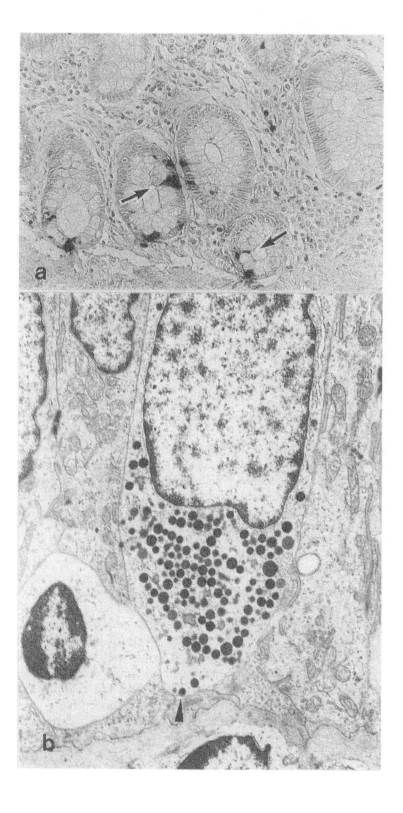

granules attach to the basal plasma membrane faced to the basement membrane, suggesting a paracrine function (Fig. 2).

VIP, first identified for its potent vasodilatory properties (Said and Mutt, 1970), is not found in the endocrine cells of adult human intestine, but VIP mRNA is still localized (Kubota et al., 1994a). Other possible sources of neuropeptides in the intestinal mucosa include cells not normally considered as a part of the nervous or APUD systems. Immunocytes have been also shown to synthesize VIP, SP, and SOM (O'Dorisio et al., 1980; O'Dorisio, 1986; Pascaul and Bost, 1990). These mucosal localizations of neuropeptides suggest that their release locally could directly affect both epithelial cell and lymphocyte functions, and these findings lead us to speculate that the neurohormonal–immune network is functionally bidirectional.

## II. NEUROPEPTIDE RECEPTORS ON IMMUNOCYTES IN THE INTESTINAL MUCOSA

When considering the above-mentioned neuroendocrine–immune communication, we must examine the distribution of neuropeptide receptors in the intestine. To date over 20 neuropeptides and neuroendocrine hormone receptors have been identified on immunocytes, such as mononuclear and polymorphonuclear leukocytes (Bost, 1988; Croitoru et al., 1990; Pascaul et al., 1994; Kubota et al., 1994b). Conversely, several examples of immune modification of neurohormonal elements of the central nervous system have been reported. Cells of the mucosal immune system must be continuously exposed to locally and systemically derived neuropeptides in the microenvironment of the intestinal mucosa. The demonstration of neuropeptide receptors on mucosal immunocytes supports the notion of the neuroendocrine–immune communication in the intestine.

### A. VIP Receptor on Macrophages and Follicular Dendritic Cells

According to our recent observations, VIP receptor was expressed on follicular dendritic cells (FDC) in the germinal center of Peyer's patches and macrophages in the intestinal lamina propria (Kubota et al., 1994a; Nagura et al., 1994) (Fig. 3). In normal adult human colon, macrophages are distributed in the lamina propria along the surface epithelial layer, and approximately 60% of these macrophases express VIP receptor. Immunoelectron microscopically, VIP receptor was linearly expressed on the plasma membrane of labryrinth-like cytoplasmic processes, which are characteristic to FDC. In fetus and neonates, however, VIP re-

---

FIGURE 2. The distribution (a) and the ultrastructure (b) of intestinal endocrine cells. Intestinal endocrine cells are usually pyramidal and frequently have long apical processes extending toward the lumen of gland (→). They have dense-core granules in the basal cytoplasm, and some of these granules attach to the basement membrane (▶).

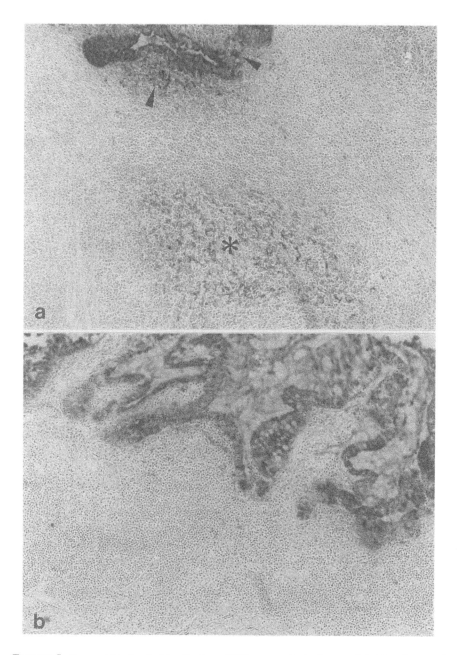

***FIGURE 3.*** Immunohistochemical localization of VIP receptor in the human adult (a) and neonatal
(b) small intestines. In the adult intestine, VIP receptor is expressed on follicular dendrictic cells in the
germinal center of Peyer's patches (∗) and macrophages in the lamina propria (▶). In the neonatal
intestine, however, VIP receptor is absent in these cells.

ceptor was absent in these cells despite the presence of VIP nerves and VIP endocrine cells in the intestinal mucosa, and became positive following the appearance of IgA plasma cells in the lamina propria when the mucosal immune system matured.

It has been well documented that neuropeptides modulate a variety of macrophage functions (Morley *et al.*, 1987; Zwilling, 1994), as shown in Table II. VIP and opioids, for example, mainly suppress, and substance P and neurotensin upregulate or activate these functions (Foris *et al.*, 1984; Hartung, 1988; Lotz *et al.*, 1988; Segura *et al.*, 1992). Thus, VIP participates in the regulation of mucosal immune responses through macrophages and FDC under physiological conditions; that is, it is obvious that VIP must modulate T- or B-cell functions via macrophages and FDC, where VIP receptor is expressed.

### B. Neuropeptide Receptors on Lymphocytes and Epithelial Cells

Direct neuropeptide modulation of T- and B-lymphocyte functions has been also reported. According to Stanisz *et al.* (1986), VIP inhibited the level of IgA in the culture supernatant of Peyer's patch cells. By contrast, SP enhanced the level of IgA in similar cultures. Furthermore, receptors for VIP and SP have been found on both T and B lymphocytes (Croitoru *et al.*, 1990; Pascaul *et al.*, 1994). Although the role of neuropeptide receptors on T lymphocytes has been less well studied than that of B lymphocytes, Ottaway (1984) reported that preincubation of the T lymphocytes with VIP decreased the rate of entry of cells into Peyer's

TABLE II

EFFECT OF NEUROPEPTIDE ON MACROPHAGE FUNCTION

| Neuropeptide | Effect on macrophage |
|---|---|
| VIP | Suppresses macrophage function |
| | Stimulates increase in cAMP |
| | Inhibits respiratory burst |
| | Stimulates phagocytic function through PKC activation |
| Substance P | Is a macrophage activator |
| | Stimulates phagocytosis and respiratory burst |
| | Enhances IL-1 and TNF$\alpha$ production |
| Neurotensin | Stimulates macrophage activity |
| | Stimulates phagocytosis and cytokin production |
| | Augments tumor cell killing |
| Opioids | Suppresses macrophage function |
| | Decreases phagocytosis and respiratory burst |
| | Reduces HLA-DR expression |
| Growth hormone | Is a macrophage activator |
| | Augments $O_2$ production |
| | Activates phagocytosis and microbial killing |

patches and mesenteric lymph nodes *in vivo*. This suggests that VIP has an important regulatory effect on the traffic of lymphocytes into tissues (Ottaway, 1984), and the potential regulation of lymphoid cell migration by the neuropeptide could provide an important mechanism by which immune function may be cordinated with other neurophysiological controls. In addition, Croitoru *et al.* (1990) reported the SP-stimulation of natural killer activity by murine intraepithelial lymphocytes, a T-cell population with diverse cytotoxic ability (London, 1994).

Limited papers are also available on the effect of neuropeptide receptors on intestinal epithelial cells. One study assessed the contribution of neuropeptides to secretory component (SC) secretion by epithelial cells, and proved that VIP was effective in stimulating SC release (Kelleher *et al.*, 1991). VIP was also shown to be a potent stimulant of intestinal secretion (Jaffe, 1979). These findings suggest the presence of VIP receptor on enterocytes.

## III. MUCOSAL IMMUNE RESPONSES AND THE HYPOTHALAMIC–PITUITARY–ADRENAL AXIS

The physiologic responses to psychological stressors are known to be mediated by either the autonomic nerve system, including neuropeptide-containing nerves, or the hypothalamic–pituitary–adrenal (HPA) axis. There is growing evidence that a cascade of hormones in response to a variety of stimuli to the hypothalamus have immune effects as well (Berczi, 1991; Gaillard, 1994). Glucocorticoids, for example, exert a negative control over the secretion of peptides from both the HPA axis and the immune system. Inflammatory cytokines have also been shown to modulate HPA axis acting at all three levels, hypothalamus, pituitary gland, and adrenal gland. IL-1 and IL-6 stimulate hormone secretion of the PHA axis at all three levels, whereas tumor necrosis factor (TNF) inhibits adrenocorticotropic hormone (ACTH) release, aldosteron synthesis, and ACTH-induced corticosteron secretion (Gaillard, 1994; Zwilling, 1994).

### A. HPA Axis and Intestinal Leukocytes

The profound influence of steroid hormones on lymphoid tissues was first shown by Selye in 1936, and ACTH and corticosteron were the first therapeutic agents capable of relieving the symptoms of immunoinflammatory diseases. ACTH has an anti-inflammatory and immunosuppressive effect, which can be reproduced by the administration of glucocorticoid. Such an ACTH effect is found to be infective in adrenolectomized animals (Berczi, 1991). Glucocorticoid, however, influences leukocyte recirculation by causing neutrophilia, with concomitant decrease of lymphocytes and monocytes by acting on the vascular endothelium (Chung *et al.*, 1986).

The HPA axis regulates macrophage function by producing a cascade of hormones in response to a variety of stimule (Zwilling, 1994), and activation of the HPA axis suppresses the major histocompatibility complex (MHC) class II antigen expression by macrophages by preventing MHC class II transcription, and also inhibits phagocytosis and antitumor activity. The suppression coincides with peak levels of plasma corticosteron.

### B. HPA Axis and Intestinal Epithelial Cells

Villous epithelial cells of the small intestine are always positive for MHC class II antigens as shown in macrophages (Nagura *et al.*, 1991). Under physiological conditions, however, crypt epithelial cells of the small intestine and those of the colonic gland do not express MHC class II antigens. In actively inflamed lesions of ulcerative colitis, MHC class II antigen is induced to express on the colonic epithelial cells (Matsumoto *et al.*, 1989), and this expression is reported to be induced by cytokines such as interferon-$\gamma$ secreted by activated macrophages. The activation of the HPA axis suppresses such activated macrophage function, and results in suppressing inflammation (Zwilling *et al.*, 1990; Zwilling, 1994).

Aldosterone, of which secretion is influenced by TNF from activated macrophages, plays a role in the regulation of aldosterone-sensitive sodium transport and water absorption by the human proximal, colon and these epithelial cells constitutively express receptor for aldosterone (Fukushima *et al.*, 1991).

Figure 4 is a schematic illustration of the neuroendocrine–immune network. Psychological stresses activate the HPA axis followed by the modulation of immuno-inflammatory responses.

### IV. INTESTINAL INFLAMMATION AND ABNORMAL NEUROHORMONAL REGULATION OF MUCOSAL IMMUNE RESPONSES

In the normal intestinal mucosa, significant numbers of VIP and SP nerves are intimately associated with glands, blood vessels, and immune effector cells (Kimura *et al.*, 1994; Nagura *et al.*, 1994), on which receptors for these neuropeptides have been found (Bost, 1988; Croitoru *et al.*, 1990; Pascaul *et al.*, 1994; Kubota *et al.*, 1994a). Degenerative and proliferative changes in neuropeptide-containing enteric nerves are consistent features of the pathology of the inflammatory bowel disease (IBD), ulcerative colitis, and Crohn's disease (Koch *et al.*, 1987; Kubota *et al.*, 1992; Kimura *et al.*, 1994), and delayed expression of these receptors on mucosal immune effector cells of infants influence the responsiveness of macrophages to food and microbial antigens and to develop influenced allergic disorders in the intestinal mucosa.

### A. Inflammatory Bowel Disease

Ulcerative colitis, for example, is known as an idiopathic chronic inflammatory disease of the intestinal mucosa, and characterized by prolonged clinical course and inflammation (MacDermott and Stenson, 1988). Degeneration and subsequent

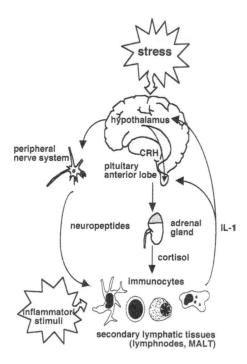

**FIGURE 4.** Schematic illustration of neuroendocrine–immune network. Psychological stresses activate the HPA axis. This activation suppresses immune/inflammatory reaction mediated by a cascade of hormones produced by endocrine organs in the HPA axis. Stresses on the hypothalamus also modulate the function of immunocytes by neuropeptides such as VIP. In the opposite direction, immuno/inflammatory responses stimulate the HPA axis via stimulation of a cascade of inflammatory cytokines.

absence or proliferation of nerves in the inflammatory mucosal lesions have been demonstrated by the immunohistochemical technique (Koch *et al.*, 1987; Kubota *et al.*, 1992; Kimura *et al.*, 1994). In the hypervascular areas of inflamed mucosa of ulcerative colitis patients, increasing VIP and SP innervations are observed along the proliferating, dilated, venule-like blood vessels, and in severe inflammatory lesions, both nerves decrease, and are almost absent around crypt abscess.

These findings show that enteric nerves degenerate in the severely inflamed mucosa, and subsequently regenerate or proliferate simultaneously with the regeneration of structural components of the intestinal mucosa, such as blood vessels and glands. In contrast, increased concentration of immunoreactive SP and also β-endorphin, a neuropeptide found in the colonic mucosa, have been described in the colonic mucosa with chronic persistent states of ulcerative colitis (Goldin *et al.*, 1989). This may cause the persistence of inflammation in the colonic mucosa.

We postulate that the loss and/or abnormality of neuropeptide innervation is a result of inflammatory damage to enteric nerves and that it may contribute to the disorder of mucosal immunoregulation (Kimura *et al.,* 1994; Nagura *et al.,* 1994). Following this loss of neuroimmune regulation, inflammation may become more pronounced, resulting in further neuronal and other tissue damages.

## B. Infantile Enteropathy

The appearance of VIP receptor on macrophages and FDC and the disappearance of VIP endocrine cells are closely related to the maturity of the mucosal immune system, similar to IgA plasma cell appearance in the intestinal lamina propria (Kubota *et al.,* 1994a,b; Nagura *et al.,* 1994) and disappearance of secretory IgA binding to the jejunal villous epithelium and Fc-mediated IgG uptake, which are characteristic features of neonate before the mucosal immune system matures (Nagura *et al.,* 1978) (Table III).

Delayed-type hypersensitivity in the infantile intestinal mucosa is characterized by a infantile enteropathy, and immaturity or certain regulation abnormalities of the mucosal immune system are shown to be important in the pathogenesis (Jackson *et al.,* 1983). As mentioned previously, VIP is involved in the regulation of mucosal immune responses, and their regulation abnormalities cause various intestinal disorders. In infants of atopic dermatitis with food allergy (Sampson, 1989), although macrophages and FDC in the intestinal lamina propria have already appeared, VIP receptor is not expressed on these immunocytes, and VIP does not bind on them (H. Nagura, M. Kubota, and N. Kimura, unpublished data). In the

*TABLE III*

DEVELOPMENTAL ASPECTS OF NEUROHORMONAL REGULATION ON
THE IMMUNOLOGIC FUNCTION OF THE HUMAN INTESTINE

|  | Neonates | Children/adults |
|---|---|---|
| Lamina propria |  |  |
| IgA plasma cell | − | +[a] |
| Macrophage, FDC | + | + |
| VIP receptor (macrophage, FDC) | − | + |
| VIP nerve | + | + |
|  |  |  |
| Epithelium |  |  |
| SC synthesis (crypts, villi) | − ~ ± | +[a] |
| HLA-DR expression (villi) | − | + |
| S-IgA binding (villi, jejunum) | + | − |
| IgG uptaking (villi, jejunum) | + | −[b] |
| (Fc receptor-mediated) |  |  |
| VIP edocrine cell | + | −(mRNA+) |

*Note.* +, positive; ±, weakly positive; −, negative.
[a] SC-mediated S-IgA transport.
[b] Closure.

TABLE *IV*

EXPRESSION OF VIP RECEPTOR AND FOOD ALLERGY

|  | VIP nerve | VIP receptor | |
|---|---|---|---|
|  |  | Mφ | FDC |
| Benign rectal bleeding | + | − | − |
| Atopic dermatitis (rectal biopsy) | + | −(↑) | − |
| Ulcerative colitis (children) | +(↓) | +(↑) | + |
| Age-matched healthy controls | + | + | + |

*Note.* ↑, increased number; ↓, decreased number.

same aged infants, VIP receptor is demonstrated on macrophages and FDC simultaneously with the occurrence of IgA plasma cells in the lamina propria.

The correlation between the expression of VIP and VIP receptor and the intestinal inflammatory disorders is summarized in Table IV. This shows that the distribution abnormalities of VIP receptor and/or its ligand may cause and maintain the immunoregulatory disorder of the mucosal immune system.

## V. CONCLUSION

We have provided here evidence for the existence of a communication network between the neuroendocrine and mucosal immune systems. Neuropeptides and cytokines are regarded as rapid modulators of neuroendocrine and immunoinflammatory mechanisms, and the shared expression of their receptors by elements of both systems supports the existence of neuroendocrine–mucosal immune interactions (Fig. 5). Abnormalities of such interactions are important in the disease

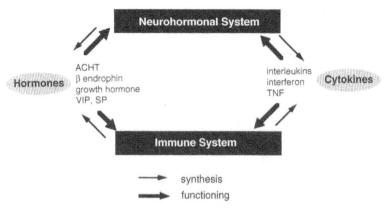

FIGURE 5. Schematic illustration of the cross-talk between neurohormonal and immune systems. The communication network between two systems is mediated by hormones and cytokines.

pathogenesis of immuno-inflammatory disorders in the intestine, including IBD and food allergy.

## REFERENCES

Befus, A. D. (1993). Neuromodulation of gastrointestinal immune and inflammatory responses. In "Immuno-Pharmacology of the Gastrointestinal System" (J. L. Wallace, ed.), pp. 1–14. Academic Press, New York.

Berczi, I. (1991). Neurohormonal–immune interaction. In "Functional Endocrine Pathology" (K. Kovacs and S. L. Assa, eds.), Vol. 2, pp 990–1004. Blackwell, Oxford.

Bost, K. L. (1988). Hormone and neuropeptide receptors on mononuclear leukocytes. Prog. Allergy **43**, 68–63.

Brandtzaeg, P., Halstensen, T. S., Kett, K., Krajci, P., Kvale, D., Rogunum, T. O., Scott, H., and Sollid, L. M. (1989). Immunobiology and immunopathology of human gut mucosa: Humoral immunity and intraepithelial lymphocytes. Gastroenterology **97**, 1562–1584.

Chung, H.-T., Samlowshi, W. E., and Daynes, R. A. (1986). Modification of the murine immune system by glucocorticoids: Alteration of the tissue localization properties of circulating lymphocytes. Cell. Immunol. **101**, 571–585.

Croitoru, K., Ernst, P. B., Stanisz, A. M., Stead, A. M., Stead, R. H., and Bienenstock, J. (1990). Neuroendocrine regulation of the mucosal immune system. In "Immunology and Immunopathology of the Liver and Gastrointestinal Tract" (S. R. Targan and F. Shanahan, eds.), pp. 183–201. Igaku-Shoin, New York.

Ferri, G.-L., Adrian, T. E., Ghatel, M. A., O'Shaughnessy, D. J., Plobert, L., Lee, Y. C., Buchan, A. M. J., Polak, J. M., and Bloom, S. R. (1983). Tissue localization and relative distribution of regulatory peptides in separated layer from the human bowel. Gastroenterology **84**, 777–786.

Foris, G., Medgyesi, G. A., Gyimesi, E., and Hawck, M. (1984). Metenkephalin induced alterations of macrophage functions. Mol. Immunol. **21**, 747–750.

Fujita, T., and Kobayashi, S. (1977). Structure and function of gut endocrine cells. Int. Rev. Cytol. **6**(Suppl.), 187–233.

Fukushima, K., Sasano, H., Nagura, H., Sasaki, I., Matsuno, S., and Krozowski, Z. S. (1991). Immunohistochemical localization of mineralocorticoid receptor in human gut. Tohoku J. Exp. Ed. **65**, 155–163.

Gabella, G. (1979). Innervation of the gastrointestinal tract. Int. Rev. Cytol. **59**, 129–193.

Gaillard, R. C. (1994). Effects of cytokines on the hypothalamo-pituiary-adrenal axis. In "Advances in Psychoneuroimmunology" (I. Berczi and J. Szelenyi, eds.), pp. 137–148. Plenum, New York.

Goldin, E., Karmeli, F., Selinger, Z., and Rachmilewitz, D. (1989). Colonic substance P levels are increased in ulcerative colitis and decreased in chronic severe constipation. Dig. Dis. Sci. **34**, 1193–1198.

Hartung, H.-P. (1988). Activation of macrophages by neuropeptides. Brain, Behav. Immun. **2**, 275–281.

Jackson, D., Walker-Smith, J. A., and Phillps, A. D. (1983). Macromolecular absorption by histologically normal and abnormal small intestinal mucosa in childhood: An in viro study using organ cutture. J. Pediatr. Gastroenterol. Nutr. **2**, 235–242.

Jaffe, B. M. (1979). Hormones of the gastrointestinal tract. In "Endocrinology" (L. J. DeGroot, G. F. Cahill, Jr., W. D. Odell, L. Martini, J. T. Potts, Jr., D. H. Nelson, E. Steinberger, and A. L. Winegrad, eds.). Vol. 3, pp. 1669–1678. Grune & Stratton, New York.

Kelleher, R. S., Hann, L. E., Edward, J. A., and Sullivan, D. A. (1991). Endocrine, neural, and immune control of secretory component output by lacrimal gland acinar cells. J. Immunol. **146**, 3405–3412.

Kimura, M., Hiwatashi, N., Masuda, T., Nagura, H., and Toyota, T. (1992). Immunohistochemical distribution of VIP-containing nerve fibers in colonic mucosa from patients with ulcerative colitis. Biomed. Res. **13**(Suppl. 2), 81–84.

Kimura, M., Masuda, T., Hiwatashi, N., Toyota, T., and Nagura, H. (1994). Changes in neuropeptide-containing nerves in human colonic mucosa with inflammatory bowel disease. *Pathol. Int.* **44,** 624–634.

Koch, T. R., Carney, J. A., and Go, V. L. W. (1987). Distribution and quantitation of gut neuropeptides in normal intestine and inflammatory bowel disease. *Dig. Dis. Sci.* **32,** 360–376.

Kubota, Y., Petras, R. E., Ottaway, C. A., Tubbs, R. R., Farmer, R. G., and Fiocchi, S. (1992). Colonic vasoactive intestinal peptide nerves in inflammatory bowel disease. *Gastroenterology* **102,** 1242–1251.

Kubota, M., Ohtani, H., Kimura, N., and Nagura, H. (1994a). VIP-receptor on follicular dendritic cells in Peyer's patches of human neonates. *In* "Current Topics in Mucosal Immunology 1993" (M. Tsuchiya, J. Yodoi, T. Hibi, and S. Miura, eds.), pp. 267–270. Excepta Medica, Amsterdam.

Kubota, M., Ohtani, H., Kimura, N., Matsumoto, S., and Nagura, H. (1994b). Localization and binding of neuropeptides on the lymphoid apparatus of the infantile intestine. *Dig. Organ Immunol.* **29,** 67–72.

London, S. D. (1994). Cytotoxic lymphocytes in mucosal effector sites. *In* "Handbook of Mucosal Immunology" (P. L. Ogra, J. Mesteckey, M. E. Lamm, W. Strober, J. R. McGhee, and J. Bienenstock, eds.), pp. 325–332. Academic Press, San Diego.

Lotz, M., Vaughan, J. H., and Carson, D. A. (1988). Effects of neuropeptides on production of inflammatory cytokines by human monocytes. *Science* **241,** 1218–1221.

MacDermott, R. P., and Stenson, W. F. (1988). Alteration of the immune system in ulcerative colitis and Crohn's disease. *Adv. Immunol.* **42,** 285–323.

Matsumoto, T., Kitano, A., Nakamura, S., Kobayashi, K., and Nagura, H. (1989). Possible role of vascular endothelial cells in immune responses in colonic mucosa examined immunocytochemically in subject with and without ulcerative colitis. *Clin. Exp. Immunol.* **78,** 424–430.

Morley, J. E., Kay, N. E., Solomon, G. F., and Plotnikoff, N. P. (1987). Neuropeptides: Conductors of the immune orchestra. *Life Sci.* **41,** 527–544.

Nagura, H. (1992). Mucosal defense mechanism in health and disease; Role of the mucosal immune system. *Acta Pathol. Jpn.* **42,** 387–400.

Nagura, H., Nakane, P. K., and Brown, W. R. (1978). Breast milk IgA binds to jejunal epithelium in suckling rats. *J. Immunol.* **128,** 1333–1339.

Nagura, H., Ohtani, H., Masuda, T., Kimura, M., and Nakamura, S. (1991). HLA-DR expression on M cells overlying Peyer's patches is a common feature of human small intestine. *Acta Pathol. Jpn.* **441,** 818–823.

Nagura, H., Kimura, M., Kubota, M., and Kimura, N. (1994). Nuroendocrine-immune interaction in the gastrointestinal tract. *In* "Advances in Psychoneuroimmunology" (I. Berczi and J. Szelenyi, eds.), pp. 253–261. Plenum, New York.

O'Dorisio, M. S. (1986). Neuropeptides and gastrointestinal immunity. *Am. J. Med.* **81**(Suppl. 6B), 74–82.

O'Dorisio, M. S., O'Dorisio, T. M., Cataland, S., and Balcerzak, S. P. (1980). VIP as a biochemical marker for polymorphonuclear leucocytes. *J. Lab. Clin. Med.* **96,** 666–672.

Ottaway, C. A. (1984). *In Vivo* alteration of receptors for vasoactive intestinal peptide changes in the *in vivo* localization of mouse T cells. *J. Exp. Med.* **160,** 1054–1069.

Pascual, D. W., and Bost, K. L. (1990). Substance P production by macrophage cell lines: A possible autocrine function for this neuropeptides. *Immunology* **71,** 52–56.

Pascual, D. W., Stanisz, A. M., and Bost, K. L. (1994). Functional aspects of the peptidergic circuit in mucosal immunity. *In* "Handbook of Mucosal Immunology" (O. P. L. Ogra, J. Mestecky, M. E. Lamm, W. Strober, J. R. McGhee and J. Bienenstock, eds.), pp. 203–216, Academic Press, San Diego.

Pearse, A. G. E., and Polak, J. M. (1971). Neural crest origin of the endocrine polypeptide (APUD) cells of the gastrointestinal tract and pancreas. *Gut* **12,** 783–788.

Polak, J. M., and Bloom, S. R. (1982). Distribution and tissue localization of VIP in the central nervous system and seven peripheral organs. In "Vasoactive Intestinal Peptide" (S. I. Said, ed.), pp. 107–112, Raven, New York.

Roszman, T. L., Jackson, J. C., Cross, R. J., Titus, M. J., Markesbery, W. R., and Brooks, W. H. (1985). Neuroanatomic and neurotransmitter influences on immune function. *J. Immunol.* **135,** 769s–772s.

Russell, G. J., and Walker, W. A. (1990). Role of the intestinal barrier and antigen uptake. In "Immunology and Immunopathology of the Liver and Gastrointestinal Tract" (S. R. Targan and F. Shanahan, eds.), pp. 15–31. Igaku-Shoin, New York.

Said, S. I., and Mutt, V. (1970). Polypeptide with broad biological activity: Isolation from small intestine. *Science* **169,** 1217–1218.

Sampson, H. A. (1989). Role of food allergy and mediator release in atopic dermatitis. *J. Allergy Clin. Immunol.* **81,** 635–645.

Sanderson, I. R., and Walker, W. A. (1994). Mucosal barrier. In "Handbook of Mucosal Immunology" (P. L. Ogra, J. Mestecky, M. E. Lamm, W. Strober, J. R. McGhee, and J. Bienenstock, eds.), pp. 263–274. Academic Press, San Diego.

Segura, J. J., Guerrero, J. M., Goberna, R., and Calvo, J. R. (1992). Stimulatory effect of vasoactive intestinal peptide (VIP) on cyclic AMP production in rat peritoneal macrophages. *Reg. Pept.* **37,** 195–203.

Selye, H. (1936). Thymus and adrenals in response of the organism to injuries and intoxications. *Br. J. Exp. Pathol.* **17,** 234–248.

Stanisz, A. M., Befus, D., and Bienenstock, J. (1986). Differential effects of vasoactive intestinal peptide, substance P, and somatostatin on immunoglobulin synthesis and proliferation by lymphocytes from Peyer's patches, mesenteric lymphodes, and spleen. *J. Immunol.* **136,** 152–156.

Stead, R., Bienenstock, J., and Stanisz, A. M. (1987). Neuropeptide regulation of mucosal immunity. *Immunol. Rev.* **100,** 333–359.

Zwilling, B. S. (1994). Neuroimmunonodulation of macrophage function. In "Handbook of Human Stress and Immunity" (R. Graser and J. K. Glaser, eds.), pp. 53–76. Academic Press, San Diego.

Zwilling, B. S., Dinkins, M., Christner, R., Faris, M., Griffin, A., Hilburger, M., McPeek, M., and Pearl, D. (1990). Restraint stress induced suppression of major histcompatibility class expression by murine peritoneal macrophages. *J. Neuroimmunol.* **29,** 125–130.

# Chapter 12

# New Insights into Epithelial Cell Function in Mucosal Immunity: Neutralization of Intracellular Pathogens and Excretion of Antigens by IgA

Michael E. Lamm,* John G. Nedrud,* Charlotte S. Kaetzel,† and Mary B. Mazanec‡

*Departments of *Pathology and ‡Medicine, Case Western Reserve University, Cleveland, Ohio 44106; and †Department of Pathology and Laboratory Medicine, Markey Cancer Center, University of Kentucky, Lexington, Kentucky 40536*

## I. INTRODUCTION AND BARRIER FUNCTION OF IgA

The epithelial cells lining a mucous membrane form a barrier that separates the interior of the body from the external environment. Therefore, antibodies in the mucosal secretions, principally IgA, have an opportunity to interact with antigens of microbes, food, and inhaled substances while they are external to the body proper and in this way keep foreign matter from entering tissues. This immune exclusion or barrier function of secretory IgA has been appreciated for some time and forms much of the rationale behind the expanding efforts to develop vaccines that are geared to stimulating secretory rather than serum antibodies.

Although the immune exclusion function of secretory IgA has long been accepted, it is only recently that experimental systems became available to prove it. Under natural conditions of infection or following deliberate immunization, the immune response is always heterogeneous and includes multiple isotypes of antibody as well as cellular immunity. Immune responses limited to the production of IgA antibodies are never observed. Thus, assignment of an immune barrier function to IgA antibodies in the mucosal secretions was based largely on correlations between resistance to infection and the time course and quantitative dominance of antibodies of the IgA isotype (Lamm, 1976; Mestecky and McGhee, 1987) and on studies *in vitro* showing that IgA antibodies can inhibit bacterial adherence to epithelial cells (Svanborg-Eden and Svennerholm, 1978; Williams and Gibbons, 1972). The possibility of proving that lumenal IgA antibodies are truly capable of mediating immune exclusion arose when methods were developed for producing

141

IgA monoclonal antibodies, e.g., by emphasizing the lymphoid tissue associated with the gut to enhance the frequency of B cells making IgA antibodies when immunizing mice prior to preparing hybridomas. With IgA monoclonal antibodies having specificity for microbial pathogens in hand, it then became possible to test experimentally by means of passive immunization whether lumenal IgA antibody as the only immunological effector was indeed capable of preventing infection when given to mice that were subsequently challenged with the pathogen.

Our own studies to address this question used Sendai virus, a parainfluenza virus that is a natural respiratory pathogen of rodents. We showed that IgA monoclonal antibodies with specificity for the viral hemagglutinin, an envelope protein, were capable of inhibiting infection if placed in the respiratory tract (Mazanec *et al.*, 1987). Work by others (Renegar and Small, 1991; Weltzin *et al.*, 1994) in the respiratory tract with influenza and respiratory syncytial virus and in the intestinal tract with several bacterial pathogens (Apter *et al.*, 1993; Czinn *et al.*, 1993; Michetti *et al.*, 1992) also demonstrated that IgA antibodies can inhibit mucosal infection. The inference from these experiments is that a small, preexisting quantity of specific IgA antibody in the mucosal secretions should be capable under natural conditions of preventing or mitigating infection by a microbial pathogen since the quantities of infectious agents to which individuals tend to be exposed are relatively small. Effective amounts of such preexisting secretory IgA antibodies could be present as a result of prior infection or deliberate immunization with the same or a related agent.

The cited studies of passive immunization with IgA monoclonal antibodies emphasize the point that preexisting IgA antibodies in the mucosal secretions can indeed prevent infection. If, however, there is insufficient secretory IgA antibody to prevent infection, does this imply that IgA has little further to offer in the way of host defense? In this regard, our recent studies suggest to the contrary that as mucosal IgA antibodies begin to be formed during the course of an infection, they may be able to contribute to recovery in two ways. First, we shall consider the possibility that IgA antibodies can neutralize intracellular pathogens inside epithelial cells. Then we shall discuss an excretory function for IgA. These possibilities arise from the natural route by which newly synthesized mucosal IgA reaches the secretions.

IgA is the main isotype of antibody in the external secretions for two reasons: the overwhelming majority of the abundant plasma cells in the lamina propria of mucous membranes make IgA and the epithelial cells lining mucous membranes express on their basolateral surface a receptor, the polymeric Ig receptor, that is specific for oligomeric IgA, and also IgM, a pentameric Ig (Lamm, 1976; Mestecky and McGhee, 1987). IgA secreted from local plasma cells can bind to the polymeric Ig receptor. The complex is then endocytosed into the epithelial cells and passes via vesicles to the apical surface, where proteolytic cleavage splits the polymeric Ig receptor at the junction of its extracellular and transmembrane domains such that the former domain, together with its bound IgA, is released into the secretions as secretory IgA (Mostov, 1994; Solari and Kraehenbuhl, 1985). Thus, secretory IgA consists of a molecule of oligomeric IgA coupled to the extracellular domain of its receptor.

## II. INTRAEPITHELIAL NEUTRALIZATION OF VIRUSES

It occurred to us that IgA antibodies, during their transport across epithelial cells, might be able to neutralize viruses that were infecting the cells by an intracellular action. We decided to test this possibility experimentally. Our initial studies were carried out *in vitro* with polarized monolayers of epithelial cells that synthesize and express the polymeric Ig receptor. When grown on permeable membranes the cells retain their apical to basal polarity, and diffusion of molecules between adjacent cells is prevented by their tight junctions. Such polarized cell monolayers model a mucosal epithelium and offer a good system for testing whether IgA antibodies and viral components can meet intracellularly and whether this can lead to neutralization of virus.

In this system we have worked with two viruses, Sendai and influenza (Mazanec *et al.,* 1992, 1995a). If the cells are infected from above and monoclonal IgA antibodies against envelope protein are introduced below the monolayer, two-color immunofluorescence demonstrates that antibody and viral protein colocalize (Table I). Moreover, if virus is quantified in the fluid above the monolayer and in cell lysates, it can be demonstrated that specific oligomeric IgA antibody inhibits the production of virus. The specificity of the virus neutralization is demonstrated by controls in which specific oligomeric IgA monoclonal antibody is compared with irrelevant oligomeric IgA antibody (which can be taken up by the epithelial cells but fails to neutralize virus and is not held by viral antigen so as to be visible by

*TABLE I*

SUMMARY OF INTRACELLULAR VIRUS NEUTRALIZATION EXPERIMENTS[a]

| Virus | Antibody | Neutralization of virus | Ig visualized |
|-------|----------|-------------------------|---------------|
| Yes | Specific oligomeric IgA | Yes | Yes |
| Yes | Irrelevant oligomeric IgA | No | No |
| No | Specific oligomeric IgA | No | No |
| Yes | Specific IgG | No | No |

[a] Epithelial monolayers were infected with Sendai or influenza virus from above and exposed to monoclonal antibodies from below. Specific antibodies are to envelope protein. Subsequently, virus was quantified and Ig was examined by immunofluorescence. Only specific oligomeric IgA antibody neutralizes virus, and only this antibody in infected cells is sufficiently retained intracellularly to be observed by immunofluorescence. Although irrelevant oligomeric IgA is transcytosed under these conditions, it is not held up by the viral antigen in infected cells so as to be demonstrable by immunofluorescence.

immunofluorescence) and with anti-viral monomeric IgA or IgG (which, although specific, cannot neutralize virus because they have no affinity for the polymeric Ig receptor and are therefore incapable of being endocytosed).

In addition to *in vitro* evidence of the sort just described, we also have evidence that IgA antibodies can neutralize virus inside mucosal epithelial cells *in vivo*. For example, we have compared the efficacy of intravenously injected IgA and IgG monoclonal antibodies to the same envelope protein of Sendai virus in conferring resistance to mice challenged with virus in the respiratory tract. Even though the serum antibody levels of the IgA and IgG antibodies were comparable and IgG, being smaller than oligomeric IgA, should diffuse more easily out of the blood-stream into respiratory tissue, the IgA antibodies were more effective in fighting infection (M. B. Mazanec, M. E. Lamm, J. G. Nedrud, and C. S. Kaetzel, unpublished results). We believe that these preliminary results support the idea that the IgA antibodies were more effective because those that did get into respiratory tissues were, unlike the IgG antibodies, capable of being taken up by receptor-mediated endocytosis into the epithelial cells lining the upper respiratory tract where they could inhibit virus.

Although, as discussed above, we believe we have good evidence that IgA antibodies can inhibit virus production in epithelial cells by acting intracellularly, we do not know exactly where the antibody is acting. The concept of intracellular neutralization of virus by IgA antibody obviously requires that at some point in transcytosis of IgA across the epithelial cell following its internalization via the polymeric Ig receptor, some of the antibody has access to its particular antigen at a locus in the cell that is involved in the virus life cycle. In theory, endocytosed IgA antibody specific for a viral component could meet its antigen at a number of cellular sites depending on the particular virus and its life cycle and on the specificity of the antibody. For example, replication of virus could be inhibited: at the stage of virus entry at the plasma membrane of the epithelial cell; at the time of uncoating; at the sites of synthesis, processing, or export of envelope protein; during the synthesis of components of the nucleocapsid; or at the time of assembly or release from the cell. If the antibody is specific for an envelope protein, then a likely site is the secretory pathway for export of newly synthesized cellular glyco-proteins or final assembly of the virus at the cell membrane. If the antibody is specific for an internal component of the virus, it could potentially act at the cytoplasmic site of synthesis of the viral core or at final assembly. Preliminary studies suggest that IgA antibodies against viral nucleoproteins may be able to inhibit virus production but are less efficient than antibodies against envelope proteins (Mazanec *et al.*, 1995b).

Although the details of the life cycles of many viruses are well understood, the same is not yet true for the epithelial transcytosis of IgA. It is accepted that after its internalization at the basolateral surface of the cell, IgA is transported inside vesicles. A simple model is that the original endocytotic vesicle moves to the apex of the cell, fuses with the apical plasma membrane, and releases its IgA after cleavage of the polymeric Ig receptor. However, recent data indicate that the process is more complicated and that vesicular exchange takes place between a system of basolateral early endosomes and apical recycling endosomes, which may be a particularly important locus for protein sorting (Apodaca et al., 1994). Such interactions might well allow at least some of the vesicles transporting IgA to have an opportunity to fuse with other vesicles that are involved in the production, transport, or assembly of viral components. This kind of interaction is especially likely in the case of viral envelope glycoproteins, which pass through the Golgi and trans-Golgi network and may well intersect endosomes (Volz et al., 1995). Moreover, it is consistent with the immunofluorescence data showing colocalization of envelope protein and IgA antibody (Mazanec et al., 1992, 1995a). If fusion of vesicles in the secretory pathway with vesicles transcytosing IgA is indeed a mechanism of virus neutralization, such vesicular fusion could be typical of transcytotic vesicles in general, an offshoot of the main transcytotic pathway, or characteristic of particular proteins or cells such that some of the IgA being transcytosed meets components of a virus that happens to be infecting the cell.

Regardless of the true site(s) and mechanism(s) of intracellular neutralization of viruses by IgA antibody within epithelial cells, if the phenomenon should prove to be a mechanism of host resistance to infection in vivo, it would be a notable exception to the long-established rule that immune-mediated resistance to intracellular pathogens depends on cell-mediated immunity (T cells, NK cells) and that humoral antibodies are ineffective once pathogens are inside cells. Instead, by inhibiting intracellular pathogens within cells (at least in the special case of epithelial cells that express polymeric Ig receptor), IgA antibodies as well as cell-mediated immune mechanisms could play a role in recovery from infection.

## III. Excretory Function of IgA

Thus far we have considered IgA's function in host defense in two contexts, within the mucosal secretions and within the epithelial lining of mucous membranes. There is yet a third locus where we believe IgA can serve in protection of the host, namely the extracellular space of the mucosal lamina propria, which comprises the layer of loose connective tissue underlying the epithelial basement membrane. Here the extracellular fluid has a high content of IgA secreted by the abundant local plasma cells. This is the source of the IgA that eventually reaches the secretions. However, we believe this IgA can begin to function in host defense even before it reaches the epithelium and the secretions by combining with antigens in the lamina propria. This possibility arises because intact or partially degraded antigens that are inhaled or ingested or are derived from the intestinal microflora can to some extent cross the mucosal lining (Husby et al., 1985; Paganelli et al., 1981), as can microorganisms during inapparent or clinically apparent infections (Jones et al., 1994; Takeuchi, 1967; Wolf et al., 1981). Locally produced specific IgA antibodies can then be expected to bind to these antigens. We believe that IgA immune complexes formed in this way in the lamina propria are an ongoing occurrence, which is magnified during mucosal infections.

The question of the fate of such locally formed immune complexes then arises. Although some of them could be absorbed into the systemic circulation, we believe the majority are instead efficiently transported directly through the mucosal epithelium by the identical mechanism utilized by free oligomeric IgA. The IgA portion of the complex binds to the polymeric Ig receptor and the transport process across the epithelium works the same regardless of whether or not the Fab portions of the IgA are occupied by antigen. Functioning in this way, mucosal IgA is in effect serving as an excretory antibody to eliminate antigens from the body. In a sense, IgA antibodies in the lamina propria can provide a second layer of immune exclusion to back up the primary immune exclusion barrier in the lumen. This second barrier can reduce the body's burden of immune complexes by preventing their access to the systemic circulation. A particular advantage for having the IgA isotype play this excretory role is that it is relatively noninflammatory (Pfaffenbach et al., 1982). Thus, abundant immune complexes can be formed within mucosal tissues as a regular event without instigating an adverse inflammatory reaction, as would be the case if the complexes were formed with IgG, IgM, or IgE antibodies.

The ability of IgA antibodies to transport antigens across epithelial cells from basal to apical can be readily demonstrated experimentally in the same two-chamber polarized epithelial monolayer system that was used to study intracellular neutralization of viruses by IgA (Kaetzel et al., 1991, 1994). If soluble immune complexes containing specific oligomeric IgA antibody are placed below the monolayer, the immune complexes are soon detectable within the epithelial cells and subsequently in the fluid bathing the apical epithelial surface (Table II). If, on the other hand, the antibody in the immune complexes is monomeric and hence

*TABLE II*

TRANSPORT OF IMMUNE COMPLEXES ACROSS
EPITHELIAL MONOLAYERS[a]

| Immune complex | Transport |
| --- | --- |
| Ag + oligomeric IgA | Yes |
| Ag + monomeric IgA | No |
| Ag + IgG | No |

[a] Soluble, radioactive immune complexes placed below polarized epithelial monolayers were tested for transport into the fluid above the cells. Transport occurs when the antibody is oligomeric IgA, which can bind to the polymeric Ig receptor.

unable to bind to the polymeric Ig receptor, the complexes are not transported. However, mixed complexes in which monomeric and oligomeric antibody are bound to the same molecule of multivalent antigen are transported (Kaetzel *et al.*, 1994). The determining factor for transport of an immune complex is thus the presence of an oligomeric antibody molecule; other molecules bound to it will also be transported regardless of whether the binding is direct, as with a molecule of antigen, or indirect, as with a molecule of monomeric antibody also bound to the same molecule of antigen. The transported immune complexes remain intact, with little evidence of degradation during passage through the cells.

In addition to this *in vitro* evidence, we also have preliminary evidence from studies *in vivo* in mice that IgA immune complexes in the intestinal lamina propria can be transported through the epithelium. In these experiments mice are immunized to a foreign protein via the gastrointestinal tract to induce a mucosal IgA antibody response. Subsequently a bolus of antigen is given intestinally or systemically, after which antigen can be visualized immunohistochemically in small intestinal crypt cells, which transport IgA, but not in small intestinal villus cells, which do not transport IgA as well. The interpretation is that immune complexes formed in the intestinal mucosa and containing IgA antibody are being excreted through the crypt cells.

## IV. CONCLUSIONS

For IgA's role in mucosal defense we envision a three-tiered system (Fig. 1). First, IgA antibodies in the lumenal secretions act as an initial immune exclusion barrier to help keep antigens from attaching to and penetrating the mucosal epithelium. Such antibodies in the lumen would be particularly adept at preventing infection. When protective mechanisms are insufficient, however, a mucosal infection can be established, in which case one would expect an antibody response to ensue. If the pathogen is still present as IgA antibodies begin to be formed locally, then the second and third levels of IgA defense function can begin to operate. In the case of intracellular pathogens like viruses or invading bacteria, intraepithelial cell neutralization could take place. If microbial pathogens have penetrated all the way into the lamina propria, they or their antigens can form immune complexes with IgA antibodies. Such complexes can then be excreted through the mucosal epithelium into the lumen. IgA antibodies functioning in these ways at the second and third levels of mucosal defense can thus help in recovery from infection. In this light the significance of IgA in host defense extends well beyond the traditional view of a lumenal barrier for helping to prevent infection. We believe that the expanded view of IgA's potential functions in mucosal defense presented here lends further support to the importance of developing vaccines that are capable of stimulating potent, long-lasting IgA antibody responses to microbial pathogens that enter through or infect mucous membranes.

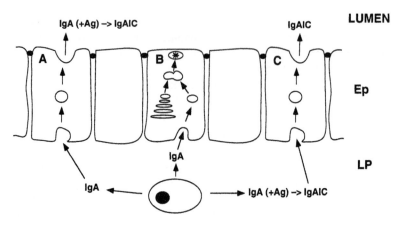

**FIGURE 1.** The three levels where mucosal IgA is proposed to function in host defense are illustrated in this diagram of a lining epithelium. IgA is secreted from plasma cells in the lamina propria. In cell A, after entry by receptor-mediated endocytosis, IgA is transported in vesicles through the cell into the lumenal secretions, where it has an opportunity to complex antigens. In cell B, which is infected by a virus, it is suggested that vesicles transcytosing IgA can fuse with vesicles leaving the Golgi and containing newly synthesized virus protein (indicated by the *), allowing intracellular neutralization of the virus by specific antibody. In cell C, IgA antibody–antigen complexes that were formed in the lamina propria are internalized and transported to the lumen in similar fashion to free IgA in cell A.

## ACKNOWLEDGMENTS

This research was supported by NIH Grants AI-26449, AI-32588, CA-51998, and HL-37117.

## REFERENCES

Apodaca, G., Katz, L., and Mostov, K. E. (1994). Receptor-mediated transcytosis of IgA in MDCK cells is via apical recycling endosomes. *J. Cell Biol.* **125,** 67–86.

Apter, F. M., Michetti, P., Winner III, L. S., Mack, J. A., Mekalanos, J. J., and Neutra, M. R. (1993). Analysis of the roles of antipolysaccharide and anti-cholera toxin immunoglobulin A (IgA) antibodies in protection against *Vibrio cholerae* and cholera toxin by use of monoclonal IgA antibodies *in vivo. Infect. Immun.* **61,** 5279–5285.

Czinn, S. J., Cai, A., and Nedrud, J. G. (1993). Protection of germ-free mice from infection by *Helicobacter felis* after active oral or passive IgA immunization. *Vaccine* **11,** 637–642.

Husby, S., Jensenius, J. C., and Svehag, S. E. (1985). Passage of undegraded dietary antigen into the blood of healthy adults: Quantitation, estimation of size distribution, and relation of uptake to levels of specific antibodies. *Scand. J. Immunol.* **22,** 83–92.

Jones, B. D., Ghori, N., and Falkow, S. (1994). *Salmonella typhimurium* initiates murine infection by penetrating and destroying the specialized epithelial M cells of the Peyer's patches. *J. Exp. Med.* **180,** 15–23.

Kaetzel, C. S., Robinson, J. K., Chintalacharuvu, K. R., Vaerman, J.-P., and Lamm, M. E. (1991). The polymeric immunoglobulin receptor (secretory component) mediates transport of immune complexes across epithelial cells: A local defense function for IgA. *Proc. Natl. Acad. Sci. U.S.A.* **88,** 8796–8800.

Kaetzel, C. S., Robinson, J. K., and Lamm, M. E. (1994). Epithelial transcytosis of monomeric IgA and IgG cross-linked through antigen to polymeric IgA. A role for monomeric antibodies in the mucosal immune system. *J. Immunol.* **152,** 72–76.

Lamm, M. E. (1976). Cellular aspects of immunoglobulin A. *Adv. Immunol.* **22,** 223–290.

Mazanec, M. B., Nedrud, J. G., and Lamm, M. E. (1987). Immunoglobulin A monoclonal antibodies protect against Sendai virus. *J. Virol.* **61,** 2624–2626.

Mazanec, M. B., Kaetzel, C. S., Lamm, M. E., Fletcher, D., and Nedrud, J. G. (1992). Intracellular neutralization of virus by immunoglobulin A antibodies. *Proc. Natl. Acad. Sci. U.S.A.* **89,** 6901–6905.

Mazanec, M. B., Coudret, C. L., and Fletcher, D. R. (1995a). Intracellular neutralization of influenza virus by IgA anti-HA monoclonal antibodies. *J. Virol.* **69,** 1339–1343.

Mazanec, M. B., Coudret, C. L., McCool, T., Baldwin, P., and Fletcher, D. R. (1995b). Intracellular interaction between IgA antibody and viral nucleoprotein. *Clin. Immunol. Immunopathol.* **76,** S115.

Mestecky, J., and McGhee, J. R. (1987). Immunoglobulin A (IgA): Molecular and cellular interactions involved in IgA biosynthesis and immune response. *Adv. Immunol.* **40,** 153–245.

Michetti, P., Mahan, M. J., Slauch, J. M., Mekalanos, J. J., and Neutra, M. R. (1992). Monoclonal secretory immunoglobulin A protects mice against oral challenge with the invasive pathogen *Salmonella typhimurium. Infect. Immun.* **60,** 1786–1792.

Mostov, K. E. (1994). Transepithelial transport of immunoglobulins. *Annu. Rev. Immunol.* **12,** 63–84.

Paganelli, R., Lennsky, R. J., and Atherton, D. S. (1981). Detection of specific antigen within circulating immune complexes. Validation of the assay and its application to food antigen-antibody complexes found in healthy and food-allergic subjects. *Clin. Exp. Immunol.* **46,** 44–53.

Pfaffenbach, G., Lamm, M. E., and Gigli, I. (1982). Activation of the guinea pig alternative complement pathway by mouse IgA immune complexes. *J. Exp. Med.* **155,** 231–247.

Renegar, K. B., and Small, Jr., P. A. (1991). Passive transfer of local immunity to influenza virus infection by IgA antibody. *J. Immunol.* **146,** 1972–1978.

Solari, R., and Kraehenbuhl, J.-P. (1985). The biosynthesis of secretory component and its role in the transepithelial transport of IgA dimer. *Immunol. Today* **6,** 17–20.

Svanborg-Eden, C., and Svennerholm, A.-M. (1978). Secretory immunoglobulin A and G antibodies prevent adhesion of *Escherichia coli* to human urinary tract epithelial cells. *Infect. Immun.* **22,** 790–797.

Takeuchi, A. (1967). Electron microscopic studies of experimental Salmonella infection. I. Penetration into the intestinal epithelium by *Salmonella typhimurium. Am. J. Pathol.* **50,** 109–136.

Volz, B., Orberger, G., Parwall, S., Hauri, H.-P., and Tauber, R. (1995). Selective re-entry of recycling cell surface glycoproteins to the biosynthetic pathway in human hepatocarcinoma HepG2 cells. *J. Cell Biol.* **130,** 537–551.

Weltzin, R., Hsu, S. A., Mittler, E. S., Georgakopoulos, K., and Monath, T. P. (1994). Intranasal monoclonal immunoglobulin A against respiratory syncytial virus protects against upper and lower respiratory tract infections in mice. *Antimicrob. Agents Chemother.* **38,** 2785–2791.

Williams, R. C., and Gibbons, R. J. (1972). Inhibition of bacterial adherence by secretory immunoglobulin A: A mechanism of antigen disposal. *Science* **177,** 697–699.

Wolf, J. L., Rubin, D. H., Finberg, R., Kauffman, R. S., Sharpe, A. H., Trier, J. S., and Fields, B. N. (1981). Intestinal M cells: A pathway for entry of reovirus into the host. *Science* **212,** 471–472.

# Chapter 13

# Structure and Function of the Polymeric Immunoglobulin Receptor in Epithelial Cells

James E. Casanova

*Pediatric Gastroenterology,*
*Massachusetts General Hospital East,*
*Charlestown, Massachusetts 02129*

## I. Introduction

More than 30 years ago, antigenic differences between serum IgA and secretory IgA (S-IgA) led to the discovery that S-IgA contained an additional polypeptide chain of approximately 70 kDa, which has come to be called secretory component (SC) (Hanson, 1961; Tomasi *et al.,* 1965). It was subsequently found that IgM was also associated with SC in mucosal secretions (Thompson, 1970; Brandtzaeg, 1975; Arnold *et al.,* 1977). In 1974, Brandtzaeg demonstrated that antisera raised against SC stained the basolateral plasma membranes of epithelial cells in mucosal tissues, leading to the hypothesis that SC served as a receptor for polymeric immunoglobulins (Brandtzaeg, 1974). This hypothesis at first seemed paradoxical. How could a soluble protein function as a receptor? And why was SC membrane-bound in epithelial cells but freely soluble in secretions? These questions were resolved when Mostov and co-workers used anti-SC antisera to immunoprecipitate *in vitro* translation products of rabbit liver mRNA, demonstrating that SC was synthesized as a larger precursor form (Mostov *et al.,* 1980). Furthermore, translation in the presence of microsomal membranes revealed that this precursor was indeed an integral membrane protein with a protease-accessible cytoplasmic domain of approximately 15 kDa and was capable of binding dimeric IgA *in vitro*. The precursor–product relationship between this larger transmembrane form and soluble SC was directly demonstrated by pulse–chase analysis in metabolically labeled HT-29 cells (Mostov and Blobel, 1982), rabbit mammary lobules (Kuhn and Kraehenbuhl, 1982), and rat liver (Sztul *et al.,* 1985). This transmembrane protein has been variously referred to as membrane secretory component (mSC), transmembrane SC (tmSC), and the more descriptive polymeric immunoglobulin receptor (pIgR).

151

The complex cellular itinerary of the pIgR was first elucidated by Sztul and co-workers in rat liver, and has since been found to be similar in other tissues and cultured cells (Fig. 1). Newly synthesized receptors are transported to the basolateral cell surface (sinusoidal membrane in hepatocytes) where ligand is bound. It should be noted that all subsequent transport processes occur independently of receptor occupancy. Receptor/ligand complexes (or unoccupied receptors) are then rapidly internalized in clathrin-coated pits and enter an acidic endosomal compartment, along with other receptors and their respective ligands. In the relatively low pH of this compartment (pH 6.0–6.5) many ligands dissociate from their receptors; however, IgA remains tightly bound under these conditions. Ultrastructural studies have revealed that the pIgR becomes sequestered in a subcompartment of the endosome, where it is packaged into transcytotic carrier vesicles (Geuze et al., 1984). Transport of these vesicles to the apical cell surface (bile canaliculus in hepatocytes) appears to be facilitated by microtubules, as treatment of cells with nocodazole or other microtubule-depolymerizing agents substantially inhibits transport (Breitfeld et al., 1990; Hunziker et al., 1990). At some point during the transport process, a disulfide bond forms between the receptor and one of the IgA monomers, linking them covalently. Upon arrival at the apical plasma membrane, the extracellular domain of the receptor is proteolytically cleaved, producing SC which, along with bound IgA, is released into secretions.

## II. STRUCTURE OF THE pIgR

### A. Ectodomain

The primary structure of the pIgR has been determined by cDNA cloning and/or direct protein sequencing from rabbit (Mostov et al., 1984), rat (Banting et al., 1989), human (Eiffert et al., 1984; Krajci et al., 1989), bovine (Kulseth et al., 1995), and murine (Piskurich et al., 1995) sources. The receptors from all five species are approximately 65% homologous, although higher degrees of homology are observed in regions with conserved function (Piskurich et al., 1995, see below). As predicted by the biochemical data, the receptor consists of a single transmembrane protein of 750–755 amino acids, with a single transmembrane domain (Fig. 2). A member of the immunoglobulin superfamily, the extracellular, ligand-binding domain consists of five Ig-like subdomains, the first four of which are similar to Ig variable regions and the fifth to Ig constant regions (Mostov et al., 1984). Interestingly, in the species for which genomic sequence has been determined, each of the Ig domains is encoded by a single exon, except for domains 2 and 3, which are contained within a single large exon (Deitcher and Mostov, 1986; Krajci et al., 1992). In rabbits, this large exon can be removed by alternative splicing, giving rise to a small form of the receptor that retains a high affinity for IgA (Deitcher and Mostov, 1986).

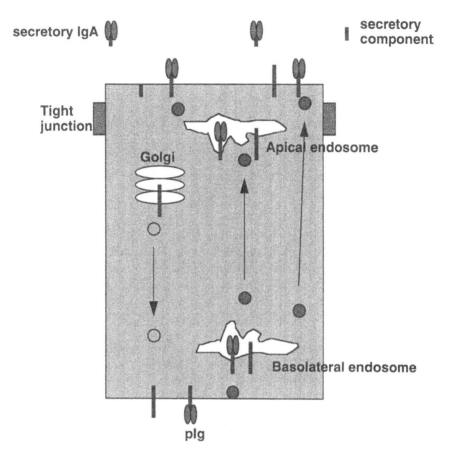

**FIGURE 1.**  Intracellular transport of the pIgR in epithelial cells. The receptor is designated by a thick black line, exocytic vesicles by open circles, transcytotic vesicles by shaded ones. Two pathways to the apical surface are shown, one direct and one via apical endosomes. Experimental evidence exists for both hypotheses.

Ig domains are characteristically composed of two antiparallel $\beta$ sheets, connected and stabilized by a disulfide bond (Williams and Barclay, 1988). This characteristic "long" disulfide bond links cysteine residues that are 62–70 amino acids apart in the linear sequence, but brought into close proximity by protein folding. In addition, computer modeling has suggested that many of the Ig-like domains contain "short" disulfide bonds, where the participating cysteines are separated by 6–9 residues (Eiffert *et al.*, 1984). These shorter bonds are conserved in domains 1 and 5 in all species but their presence in domains 2, 3, and 4 is more variable (Piskurich *et al.*, 1995). Moreover, domain 5 contains a conserved "extra" disulfide

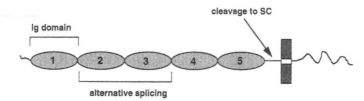

**FIGURE 2.** Domain organization of the pIgR. The extracellular domain contains five immunoglobu-lin-like domains (shaded ovals). Each Ig domain is contained on a separate exon, except domains 2 and 3 which are on a single large exon, which can be excised by alternative splicing in rabbits. Cleavage to SC occurs in the stalk domain connecting the SC portion to the membrane. The plasma membrane is represented by a shaded rectangle, the transmembrane helix as a white box.

bond of intermediate length (34 residues) that undergoes rearrangement during the covalent linkage with IgA. In this process, $Cys^{467}$ of the human pIgR has been found to link with $Cys^{311}$ of one $\alpha$ chain of the IgA dimer (Fallgreen-Gebauer *et al.,* 1993).

## B. Ligand Binding

As described above, the pIgR is specific for the polymeric immunoglobulins IgA and IgM (pIgs) and does not bind monomers. Numerous investigators have examined the binding of these ligands to SC *in vitro,* and in most species, IgM binds with a higher affinity than does polymeric IgA (summarized by Brandtzaeg, 1985). Although a subject of some controversy, the bulk of evidence suggests that binding of pIgs to SC appears to require the presence of J chain. Brandtzaeg and Prydz found that the binding of IgA polymers to HT29 cells expressing the pIgR correlated directly with J chain content (Brandtzaeg and Prydz, 1984). More recently Hendrickson and co-workers (1995) have shown that IgA from J-chain deficient mice, although polymeric, is transported neither from blood to bile *in vivo,* nor across monolayers of pIgR-expressing Madin-Darby Canine Kidney (MDCK) cells *in vitro.*

The binding of pIgs to the receptor is thought to be a two-stage process, involving an initial, noncovalent interaction between the ligand and elements of the first Ig-like domain, followed by formation of a disulfide bridge between a cysteine residue in domain 5 ($Cys^{467}$ in human) and one of the IgA heavy chains ($Cys^{311}$) as described above. Disulfide bond formation is thought to occur following internalization of receptor–ligand complexes and, at least in liver, has been shown to be a late event in the transcytotic process (Chintalacharuvu *et al.,* 1994). It has been hypothesized that disulfide bond formation is catalyzed by the presence of protein disulfide isomerase in endosomes, transcytotic carrier vesicles, or both. However covalent linkage of dIgA with free SC has been observed *in vitro,* suggesting that a catalyzing agent is unnecessary.

What are the structural determinants on the pIgR that specify ligand binding? Several lines of evidence suggest that the first Ig-like domain contains the primary site(s) of noncovalent interaction. First, only proteolytic or recombinant fragments of the receptor that contain domain 1 retain the capacity to bind ligand (Frutiger *et al.,* 1986; Bakos *et al.,* 1991a; Bakos *et al.,* 1994). Second, monoclonal antibodies specific for epitopes in domain 1 can compete with IgA for binding to the receptor (Bakos *et al.,* 1991). Third, synthetic peptides corresponding to sequences within domain 1 can bind IgA in an ELISA-based assay (Bakos *et al.,* 1991a). However, in this last case, peptides bound both monomeric and polymeric IgA, with an equivalent affinity that was two orders of magnitude less than that of native SC. This finding suggested that either structural constraints imposed by protein folding or additional binding determinants were required for optimal affinity and specificity.

The structural homology between the pIgR and other members of the Ig superfamily makes it possible to construct reasonably accurate computer models of the individual Ig-like domains, using the crystallographic coordinates of related molecules as a framework (Eiffert *et al.,* 1984; Beale and Coadwell, 1987; Bakos *et al.,* 1993; Coyne *et al.,* 1994). Based on such models, the synthetic peptide encompassing residues 15–37 of human pIgR which binds with highest affinity to IgA is predicted to span the loop connecting $\beta$ strands B and C of domain 1. This loop corresponds to the CDR1 loop of true immunoglobulins (Bakos *et al.,* 1993). The CDRs (Complementarity Determining Regions) of Igs are the hypervariable regions whose sequences determine antigen specificity. Each antigen binding site consists of three CDRs from the light chain and three from the heavy chain, which are brought into close proximity by lateral associations between the two chains. CDR-like loops in the T-cell coreceptors CD4 and CD8 have also been shown to be required for interaction with MHC class II and class I, respectively (Salter *et al.,* 1990; Fleury *et al.,* 1991; Sanders *et al.,* 1991).

Examination of the sequence spanning CDR1 in domain 1 of the pIgR reveals that it is almost identical among human, rabbit, rat, mouse, and bovine receptors (Fig. 3), suggesting a conserved function. Moreover, there is no discernible homology between CDR1 in domain 1 and the corresponding CDR1 loops in domains 2–5, which, combined with the data described above, further implies a functional role for domain 1.

Mutagenesis of individual amino acids in CDR1 demonstrated that a subset of these residues are indeed critical for binding of dimeric IgA to the native pIgR (Coyne *et al.,* 1994). The key residues are clustered toward the C terminus of the loop and are notable for the fact that they are either charged (Arg[37], His[38], Arg[40]) or polar (Ser[34], Asn[36], Ser[39]).[1] They may therefore participate in either electrostatic interactions or hydrogen bonding with adjacent residues in the IgA dimer.

Mutagenesis of either CDR2 or CDR3 in domain 1, by replacement with their

---

[1] Amino acid assignments are from the sequence of Mostov *et al.* (1984).

```
            1< leader peptide ><Domain 1-->                              CDR1            70
    Mouse   MRLYLFTLLV TVFSGVSTK. .....SPIFG PQEVSSIEGD SVSITCYYPD TSVNRHTRKY WCRQGASGMC
     Rat    MRLSLFALLV TVFSGVSTQ. .....SPIFG PQDVSSIEGN SVSITCYYPD TSVNRHTRKY WCRQGANGYC
   Bovine   MSRLFLACLL AIFPVVSMK. .....SPIFG PEEVTSVEGR SVSIKCYYPP TSVNRHTRKY WCRQGAQGRC
    Human   MLLFVLTCLL AVFPAISTK. .....SPIFG PEEVNSVEGN SVSITCYYPP TSVNRHTRKY WCRQGARGGC
   Rabbit   MALFLLTCLL AVFSAATAQS SLLGPSSIFG PGEVNVLEGD SVSITCYYPT TSVNRHSRKF WCREEESGRC
 Consensus  M-LFLL--L- -VF--VS--- -----SPIFG P-EV-S-EG- SVSITCYYP- TSVNRHTRKY WCRQGA-G-C

            71  CDR2                                            CDR3            >< 140
    Mouse   TTLISSNGYL SKEYSGRANL INFPENNTFV INIEQLTQDD TGSYKCGLGT SNRGLSFDVS LEVSQVPELP
     Rat    ATLISSNGYL SKEYSGRASL INFPENSTFV INIAHLTQED TGSYKCGLGT TNRGLFFDVS LEVSQVPEFP
   Bovine   TTLISSEGYV SDDYVGRANL TNFPESGTFV VDISHLTHKD SGRYKCGLGI SSRGLNFDVS LEVSQDPAQA
    Human   ITLISSEGYV SSKYAGRANL TNFPENGTFV VNIAQLSQDD SGRYKCGLGI NSRGLSFDVS LEVSQGPGLL
   Rabbit   VTL.ASTGYT SQEYSGRGKL TDFPDKGEFV VTVDQLTQND SGSYKCGVGV NGRGLDFGVN VLVSQKPE..
 Consensus  -TLISS-GY- S-EY-GRA-L -NFPE--TFV V-I--LTQ-D -G-YKCGLG- --RGL-FDVS LEVSQ-P---

            141 Domain 2-->                                                    210
    Mouse   SDTHVYTKDI GRNVTIECPF KRENVPSKKS LCKKTNQSCE LVIDST..EK VNPSYIGRAK LFMKGTDLTV
     Rat    NDTHVYTKDI GRTVTIECRF KEGNAHSKKS LCKKRGEACE VVIDST..EY VDPSYKDRAI LFMKGTSRDI
   Bovine   SHAHVYTVDL GRTVTINCPF TNFPESGTFV LCKKTIQDCF QVVDST..GY VSNSYKDRAH ISILGTNTLV
    Human   NDTKVYTVDL GRTVTINCPF KTENAQKRKS LYKQIGLYPV LVIDSS..GY VNPNYTGRIR LDIQGTGQLL
   Rabbit   PDDVVYKQYE SYTVTITCPF TYATRQLKKS FYKVEDGELV LIIDSSSKEA KDPRYKGRIT LQIQSTTAKE
 Consensus  -D--VYT-D- GRTVTI-CPF ---N----KS LCK------- -VIDS----- V-P-Y--R-- L---GT----

            211                        ><Domain 3-->                           280
    Mouse   FYVNISHLTH NDAGLYICQA GEGPSADKKN VDLQVLAPEP ELLYKDLRSS VTFECDLGRE VANEAKYLCR
     Rat    FYVNISHLIP SDAGLYVCQA GEGPSADKNN ADLQVLEPEP ELLYKDLRSS VTFECDLGRE VANDAKYLCR
   Bovine   FSVVINRVKL SDAGMYVCQA GDDAKADKIN IDLQVLEPEP ELVYGDLRSS VTFDCSLGPE VANVPKFLCQ
    Human   FSVVINQLRL SDAGQYLCQA GDDSNSNKKN ADLQVLKPEP ELVYEDLRGS VTFHCALGPE VANVAKFLCR
   Rabbit   FTVTIKHLQL NDAGQYVCQS GSDPTAEEQN VDLRLLT..P GLLYGNLGGS VTFECALDSE DANAVASLRQ
 Consensus  F-V-I--L-- -DAG-YVCQA G----ADK-N -DLQVL-PEP EL-Y-DLR-S VTFEC-LG-E VAN--K-LC-

            281                                                               350
    Mouse   M.NKETCDVI INTLGKRDPD FEGRILITPK DDNGRFSVLI TGLRKEDAGH YQCGAHSSGL PQEGWPIQTW
     Rat    K.NKETCDVI INTLGKRDPA FEGRILLTPR DDNGRFSVLI TGLRKEDAGH YQCGAHSSGL PQEGWPVQAW
   Bovine   KKNGGACNVV INTLGKKAQD FQGRIVSVPK D.NGVFSVHI TSLRKEDAGR YVCGAQPEGE PQDGWPVQAW
    Human   QSSGENCDVV VNTLGKKRAPA FEGRILLNPQ DKDGSFSVVI TGLRKEDAGR YLCGAHSDGQ LQEGSPIQAW
   Rabbit   VRGG...NVV IDSQGTIDPA FEGRILFT.K AENGHFSVVI AGLRKEDTGN YLCGVQSNGQ SGDG.PTQLR
 Consensus  ------C-VV INTLGK--P- FEGRIL--P- D-NG-FSV-I TGLRKEDAG- Y-CGA-S-G- -QEG-P-Q-W
```

***FIGURE 3.*** Alignment of receptor sequences from mouse (Piskurich *et al.,* 1995), rat (Banting *et al.,* 1989), human (Krajci *et al.,* 1989), bovine (Kulseth *et al.,* 1995), and rabbit (Mostov *et al.,* 1984) sources. The rabbit sequence has been updated to correct two errors in the reported sequence (replacement of $Thr^{36}$ with Asn, and replacement of the sequence from $Arg^{570}$ to $Glu^{592}$ in the stalk region with $Ala^{570}$–$Lys^{594}$, caused by three missing nucleotides in the original sequence). Alignment was performed using the GCG programs PILEUP and PRETTY. Locations of the cleaved leader peptide, Ig domains, and stalk region are indicated above the sequence. The transmembrane domain is in italics. Regions important to receptor function are in bold type. CDR1, CDR2, and CDR3 are thought to constitute the primary site of noncovalent interaction with plg. The predicted site of SC cleavage is marked by an X. Cytoplasmic residues involved in basolateral sorting are proximal to the transmembrane domain. Tyrosines involved in clathrin-mediated endocytosis are marked with an asterisk, phosphorylation sites with a P.

domain 2 counterparts, was also found to completely abrogate ligand binding (Coyne *et al.,* 1994), suggesting that all three CDRs participate in the interaction with dIgA. In CD4, CDR1 and CDR3 have been shown to interact with determinants on MHC class II complexes (Fleury *et al.,* 1991), while in CD8, CDR 1 and CDR2 interact with the heavy chain of MHC class I (Salter *et al.,* 1990; Sanders *et al.,* 1991). This, however, is the first indication that all three CDRs can be utilized in a nonantigen interaction.

```
         351      ><Domain 4-->                                                      420
   Mouse  QLFVNEESTI PNRRSVVKGV TGGSVAIACP YNPKESSSLK YWCRWEGDGN GHCPALVGTQ AQVQEEYEGR
     Rat  QLFVNEESTI PNSRSVVKGV TGGSVAIVCP YNPKESSSLK YWCHWEADEN GRCPVLVGTQ ALVQEGYEGR
  Bovine  QLFVNEETAI PASPSVVKGV RGGSVTVSCP YNPKDANSAK YWCHWEEAQN GRCPRLVESR GLIKEQYEGR
   Human  QLFVNEESTI PRSPTVVKGV AGSSVAVLCP YNRKESKSIK YWCLWEGAQN GRCPLLVDSE GWVKAQYEGR
  Rabbit  QLFVNEEIDV SRSPPVLKGF PGGSVTIRCP YNPKRSDSHL QLYLWEGSQ. TRHLLVDSGE GLVQKDYTGR
Consensus  QLFVNEE--I P-S--VVKGV -GGSV-I-CP YNPKES-S-K YWC-WE---N GRCP-LV--- --V---YEGR

         421                                              ><Domain 5--> 490
   Mouse  LALFDQPGNG TYTVILNQLT TEDAGFYWCL TNGDSRWRTT IELQVAEATR EPNLEVTPQN ATAVLGETFT
     Rat  LALFDQPGSG AYTVILNQLT TQDSGFYWCL TDGDSRWRTT IELQVAEATK KPDLEVTPQN ATAVIGETFT
  Bovine  LALLTEPGNG TYTVILNQLT DQDTGFYWCV TDGDTRWIST VELKVVQG.. EPSLKV.PKN VTAWLGEPLK
   Human  LSLLEEPGNG TFTVILNQLT SRDAGFYWCL TNGDTLWRTT VEIKIIEG.  EPNLKV.TGN VTAVLGETLK
  Rabbit  LALFEEPGNG TFSVVLNQLT AEDEGFYWCV SDDDESLTTS VKLQIVDGEP SPTID....K FTAVQGEPVE
Consensus  LALF--PGNG TYTVILNQLT --D-GFYWC- T-GD--W-TT VEL-V-E--- -P-L-V-P-N -TAV-GE---

         491                                                                       560
   Mouse  VSCHYPCKFY SQEKYWCKWS NKGCHILPSH DEGARQSSVS CDQSSQLVSM TLNPVSKEDE GWYWCGVKQG
     Rat  ISCHYPCKFY SQEKYWCKWS NDGCHILPSH DEGARQSSVS CDQSSQIVSM TLNPVKKEDE GWYWCGVKEG
  Bovine  LSCHFPCKFY SFEKYWCKWS NRGCSALPTQ NDGPSQAFVS CDQNSQVVSL NLDTVTKEDE GWYWCGVKEG
   Human  VPCHFPCKFS SYEKYWCKWN NTGCQALPSQ DEGPSKAFVN CDENSRLVSL TLNLVTRADE GWYWCGVKQG
  Rabbit  ITCHFPCKYF SSEKYWCKWN DHGCEDLPT. KLSSSGDLVK CNNN.LVLTL TLDSVSEDDE GWYWCGAKDG
Consensus  --CHFPCKFY S-EKYWCKW- N-GC--LP-- -EG-----V- CD--S--VSL TL--V--EDE GWYWCGVK-G

         561                            ><Stalk domain            630
   Mouse  QTYGETTAIY IAVEERTR.. ........GS SHVNPTDANA RAKVAL...E EEVVDSSISE KENKAIPNPG
     Rat  QVYGETTAIY VAVEERTR.. ........GS PHINPTDANA RAKDAP...E EEAMESSVRE DENKANLDPR
  Bovine  PRYGETAAVY VAVESRVK.. ·........GS QGAKQVKA.A PAGAA..... ...IQSRAGE IQNKALLDPS
   Human  HFYGETAAVY VAVEER.... ........KA AGSRDVSL.A KADAAP...D EKVLDSGFRE IENKAIQDPR
  Rabbit  HEFEEVAAVR VELTEPAKVA VEPAKVPVDP AKAAPAPAEE KAKAAVPSAQ EKAVVPIVKE AENKVVQKPR
Consensus  --YGET-AVY VAVEER---- ---------- -------A-A -A--A----- E----S---E -ENKA---P-

         631 X                                < transmembrane domain  > 700
   Mouse  PFANEREIQN VRDQAQENRA SGDAGSADGQ SRSSSSKVLF STLVPLGLVL AVGAIAVWVA RVRERKNVDR
     Rat  LFADEREIQN AGDQAQENRA SGNAGSAGGQ ..SGSSKVLF STLVPLGLVL AVGAVAVWVA RVRERKNVDR
  Bovine  FFAKE....S VKDAAGGPGA PADPGRPTGY ..SGSSKALV STLVPLALVL VAGVVAIGVV RARHRKNVDR
   Human  LFAEKKAVAD TRDQADGSRA SVDSGSSEEQ ..SGSSRALV STLVPLGLVL AVGAVAVGVA RARHRKNVDR
  Rabbit  LLAEEVAVQS AEDPASGSRA SVDASSASGQ ..SGSAKVLI STLVPLGLVL AAGAMAVAIA RARHRNVDR
Consensus  LFA-E----- --D-A---RA S-D-GS--GQ --SGSSK-L- STLVPLGLVL A-GAVAV-VA R-RHRKNVDR

         P  *                                                             P   770
   Mouse  MSISSYRTDI SMADFKNSRD LGGNDNMGAS PDTQQTVIEG KDEIVTTTEC TAEPEESKKA KRSSKEEADM
     Rat  MSISSYRTDI SMGDFRNSRD LGGNDNMGAT PDTQQETVLEG KDEIETTTEC TTEPEESKKA KRSSKEEADM
  Bovine  ISIRSYRTDI SMSDFENSRD FEGRDNMGAS PEAQETSLGG KDEFATTTED TVESKEPKKA KRSSKEEADE
   Human  VSIRSYRTDI SMSDFENSRD FGANDNMGAS SITQETSLGG KEEFVATTES TTETKEPKKA KRSSKEEADM
  Rabbit  VSIGSYRTDI SMSDLENSRE FGAIDNPSAC PDARETALGG KDELATATES TVEIEEPKKA KRSSKEEADL
Consensus  -SI-SYRTDI SM-DF-NSRD FG--DNMGA- PD-QET-L-G KDE--TTTE- T-E--E-KKA KRSSKEEADM

         *                    795
   Mouse  AYSAFLLQSS TIA.AQVHDG PQEA*
     Rat  AYSAFLFQSS TIA.AQVHDG PQEA*
  Bovine  AFTTFLLQAK NLASAATQNG PTEA*
   Human  AYKDFLLQSS TVA.AEAQDG PQEA*
  Rabbit  AYSAFLLQSN TIA.AEHQDG PKEA*
Consensus  AY--FLLQS- TIA-A---DG P-EA-
```

*FIGURE 3—Continued*

## C. Cleavage to Secretory Component

Between the fifth Ig domain and the transmembrane domain lies a short "stalk" region containing the proteolytic cleavage site used in separating SC from its transmembrane anchor (Fig. 2). Cleavage is thought to be catalyzed by a leupeptin-sensitive endoprotease residing in the apical plasma membrane (Musil and Baenziger, 1987; Breitfeld *et al.*, 1989; Solari *et al.*, 1989; Sztul *et al.*, 1993); however, the nature of this protease is currently unknown. Similarly, the precise site of cleavage within the stalk domain has remained elusive, due primarily to the "ragged" C-termini of SC purified from secretions (Eiffert *et al.,* 1984). Piskurich *et al.* (1995) have proposed a site N-terminal to a conserved glutamic acid residue in the consensus sequence, Phe–Ala–X–Glu (Fig. 3), where X is a polar or charged amino acid. Based on secondary structure predictions, this site is thought to lie within an $\alpha$ helix, preceded in every species except rabbit by a conserved proline-containing turn. Further work, perhaps involving site-specific mutagenesis, will be required to determine whether this is the true site of SC cleavage.

### D. Transmembrane Domain

The transmembrane domain of the pIgR is very highly conserved (79%), suggesting a possible role in the transmission of transmembrane signals in response to ligand binding. Although unoccupied receptors are transcytosed, recent evidence suggests that ligand binding enhances the rate of receptor transport (Song *et al.,* 1994). Mostov *et al.* (1984) have suggested that a conserved proline within the transmembrane domain, an uncommon feature in single-spanning membrane proteins (Brandl and Deber, 1986) may cause a kink in the predicted transmembrane $\alpha$ helix, and could amplify conformational changes induced by ligand binding. However, subsequent work has shown that mutagenesis of this proline has no observable effect on the behavior of either occupied or unoccupied receptors (J. E. Casanova and K. E. Mostov, unpublished observations). Regardless, recent evidence suggests that the binding of ligand, which is known to induce large conformational changes in SC (Bakos *et al.,* 1991b), can affect the behavior of the receptor (see below). It therefore remains possible that the conserved core transmembrane sequence functions in some signal-transducing capacity.

### III. Intracellular Transport

The cytoplasmic domains of many transmembrane proteins have been found to be required for their sorting and transport to appropriate cellular destinations. This process is particularly complex in epithelial cells, where the plasma membrane is subdivided into apical and basolateral domains with distinct and specialized functions. In most types of epithelia (hepatocytes are the exception) apical and basolateral membrane proteins are segregated from each other at the exit point from the Golgi apparatus, the trans-Golgi network (TGN) (Matlin and Simons, 1984; Rindler *et al.,* 1984) and transported to the appropriate surface in separate populations of carrier vesicles. Upon arrival at the cell surface, many types of receptor proteins are internalized by clathrin-mediated endocytosis. These internalized proteins enter an acidic, early endosomal compartment where further sorting takes place. Recycling receptors are returned to the cell surface from which they were internalized, other proteins are transported to lysosomes for degradation, and, in epithelia, still others, such as the pIgR, are packaged into transcytotic carrier vesicles for transport to the opposite cell surface. In hepatocytes, all plasma membrane proteins are transported together to the basolateral (sinusoidal) surface, and apical proteins reach the bile canaliculus via the transcytotic pathway (Bartles *et al.,* 1987).

How do proteins navigate their way through this complex labyrinth of subcellular compartments and membranes? Most proteins contain intrinsic structural features (often referred to as "sorting signals") that interact with the cellular sorting machinery. Such signals can consist of contiguous stretches of amino acids, noncontiguous residues that are brought together by protein folding, or post-translational modifications such as phosphorylation.

Most of what is known about the sorting and intracellular transport of the pIgR has been discovered using cell culture systems. Mostov and colleagues have developed a particularly useful system in which the pIgR is stably expressed in MDCK cells. When these cells are cultured on permeable filter supports, the pIgR functions as *in vivo,* transporting ligand from the basolateral to the apical cell surface (Mostov and Deitcher, 1986). The cells also contain an endogenous protease that catalyzes cleavage of the receptor to SC. This model system has allowed the identification and characterization of sorting signals by stable expression of mutant receptors and their subsequent analysis in polarized monolayer cultures.

Using this system, Mostov *et al.* (1986) demonstrated that the cytoplasmic domain of the pIgR was required for at least three stages of the transport pathway: (1) targeting of newly synthesized receptors to the basolateral cell surface; (2) clathrin-mediated endocytosis, and (3) subsequent sorting of internalized receptors into the transcytotic pathway. The cytoplasmic sequences required for each of these sorting steps have been identified and characterized and are described below.

## A. Basolateral Sorting

Initial mutagenesis experiments demonstrated that the basolateral sorting determinant resided within the first 17 amino acids of the cytoplasmic domain. A mutant receptor lacking 14 of these residues was transported directly to the apical cell surface, as was the mutant lacking the entire cytoplasmic domain. In contrast, a mutant containing only the first 17 amino acids and lacking the remainder of the cytoplasmic domain was transported basolaterally. To definitively demonstrate that this sequence contained a basolateral sorting signal, a chimeric protein was generated containing the extracellular domain of an apical membrane protein, placental alkaline phosphatase, and a cytoplasmic domain consisting of the 17-amino acid putative signal sequence. This chimeric protein was transported efficiently to the basolateral cell surface, demonstrating that the signal can function autonomously (Casanova *et al.,* 1991).

Further refinement of the signal sequence by alanine-scanning mutagenesis (Aroeti *et al.,* 1993) revealed an absolute requirement for three closely spaced amino acids, His[656], Arg[657], and Val[660] (Fig. 3). Replacement of any of these three residues with alanine resulted in the transport of newly synthesized receptors to both apical and basolateral surfaces in equivalent amounts, suggesting that they were no longer recognized by the cellular sorting machinery. Mutation of either Arg[655] or Tyr[668] to alanine also reduced the fidelity of basolateral sorting, but to a lesser extent. Mutagenesis of the remaining residues had no observable effect.

The secondary structure of a synthetic peptide corresponding to the signal sequence has been determined by two-dimensional NMR analysis (Aroeti *et al.*, 1993). An interesting result of these experiments was that the peptide was found to contain a $\beta$-turn spanning residues Arg[658], Asn[659], Val[660], and Asp[661], which was followed by a nascent helix. Similar $\beta$-turn structures have been found to be a feature of motifs required for clathrin-mediated endocytosis (Collawn *et al.*, 1990; Vaux, 1992). Endocytic signals of this type tend to have tyrosine or other aromatic residues at the 1 or 4 positions of the turn. Of the three residues identified by mutagenesis to be critical for sorting, His[656] and Arg[657] immediately precede the turn, and Val[660] occupies the 3 position. All of the residues in this region are completely conserved among species (except Arg[658], which is lysine in all species except rabbit).

Since the identification of the basolateral sorting signal in the pIgR, numerous other proteins have been identified that also contain basolateral sorting signals (Mostov *et al.*, 1992; Matter and Mellman, 1994). These signals appear to fall into two classes, those that overlap with endocytic signals, and those that do not. The pIgR clearly falls into the latter category, as the truncation mutant containing a functional basolateral sorting signal is not detectably endocytosed (Casanova *et al.*, 1991). Taken together, these findings suggest that $\beta$-turn structures may be a common feature of sorting signals, and that the nature of the amino acids composing or surrounding the turn may determine the specificity of interaction with the cellular sorting machinery.

## B. Endocytosis

Following its arrival at the basolateral cell surface, the pIgR is rapidly internalized via clathrin-mediated endocytosis. This process occurs constitutively and does not require ligand binding. As described above, association of proteins with clathrin-coated pits requires a functional endocytic signal. Two types of endocytic signals have been characterized to date, one which contains a characteristic $\beta$-turn including a tyrosine or other aromatic residue, and one containing two adjacent leucine residues which apparently does not involve a $\beta$ turn. The pIgR contains two tyrosine-based endocytic signals in its cytoplasmic domain, one centered on Tyr[668], the other on Tyr[734] (Phe in bovine pIgR). Each of these can mediate endocytosis independently of the other, although the distal signal is more efficient. Mutagenesis of both tyrosines simultaneously yields a receptor that is not detectably internalized (Okamoto *et al.*, 1992). As mentioned above, neither of these tyrosine-containing motifs is involved in basolateral sorting, as mutants in either residue (or both) are sorted to the basolateral surface as efficiently as the wild-type receptor.

## C. Postendocytic Sorting

Receptor molecules internalized from the cell surface enter early endosomes, which are a major crossroads of membrane traffic. All materials entering this compartment from the plasma membrane are sorted and transported to one of three destinations. Some proteins (e.g., LDL receptor) are recycled to the basolateral cell surface. Others (PDGF, EGF receptors) are transported to lysosomes for degradation. The pIgR (and other transcytosing molecules) are packaged into a separate class of carrier vesicles for transport to the apical cell surface. Ultrastructural studies using immunoelectron microscopy have shown that, in rat liver, the pIgR is concentrated in tubular extensions emerging from endosomes that presumably give rise to carrier vesicles (Geuze *et al.*, 1984).

One signal that has been identified that specifies sorting of the pIgR into the transcytotic pathway consists of a post-translational modification, phosphorylation of a single serine residue, $Ser^{664}$ (Fig. 3). In the MDCK system, mutation of this serine to alanine reduces incorporation of $^{32}P$ into the receptor by 80%, and dramatically reduces both the rate and the extent of receptor transcytosis (Casanova *et al.*, 1990). Conversion of the target serine to aspartic acid, which may mimic the negatively charged phosphoserine side chain, was found to enhance receptor transcytosis. This signal is at least partially autonomous, in that transplantation to a heterologous reporter protein enhances transcytosis of the chimera (placental alkaline phosphatase), although not to the same extent as native pIgR (Apodaca and Mostov, 1993). The location of $Ser^{664}$ immediately downstream of the $\beta$ turn in the basolateral sorting domain suggested that phosphorylation may function as a molecular switch, inactivating the basolateral signal upon arrival at the cell surface. This hypothesis is supported by the observation that, in pulse–chase experiments in rat liver, phosphorylated pIgR is not detectable in Golgi membranes, but is abundant in plasma membrane and endosomal fractions (Larkin *et al.*, 1986). Furthermore, it is the only form of the receptor in fractions enriched in transcytotic carrier vesicles (Sztul *et al.*, 1993).

A second, more distal phosphorylation site has been reported at $Ser^{726}$ (Hirt *et al.*, 1993). Mutation of this site to alanine was originally reported to result in a defect in basolateral sorting; however, subsequent work suggests that the major defect may be in endocytosis (Okamoto *et al.*, 1994). Internalization of receptors containing this mutation is reduced by 65% relative to wild-type controls, and all other aspects of receptor traffic appear to be normal (Okamoto *et al.*, 1994).

Recent evidence indicates that ligand-occupied receptors undergo more rapid transcytosis than do unoccupied receptors (Song *et al.*, 1994). Moreover, the presence of bound ligand is sufficient to overcome the inhibition of transcytosis imposed by the $Ala^{664}$ mutation. In other words, receptors to which IgA is bound are rapidly transcytosed whether $Ser^{664}$ is phosphorylated or not (Hirt *et al.*, 1993; Song *et al.*, 1994). One hypothesis that may account for this observation is that ligand binding induces a transmembrane conformational change that is mimicked by phosphorylation of the receptor at $Ser^{664}$.

## IV. ANOTHER STEP IN THE PATHWAY?

It has long been assumed that transcytotic vesicles, once formed, were transported directly to and fused directly with the apical plasma membrane. Some recent evidence, however, suggests that there may be yet another stop on the pathway. Using morphological methods, Barroso and Sztul (1994) and Apodaca et al. (1994) independently demonstrated that transcytosing material (anti-SC $Fab_2$ in the former case, dIgA in the latter) enters a compartment in the apical cytoplasm of MDCK cells en route to the cell surface. This compartment appears to be an apical endosome in that it is also accessible to apically internalized ligand (as well as nonspecific membrane markers). Based on these observations, both authors concluded that transcytosis is indirect, and occurs via an apical endosomal compartment. Delivery to the apical surface would then presumably be accomplished in vesicles recycling from this compartment to the apical cell surface.

In support of this model, Mazanec et al. (1992, 1995) have demonstrated that IgA internalized from the basolateral surface of MDCK monolayers can interact with intracellular viral proteins in infected cells. Monoclonal IgAs specific for either the hemagglutinin-neuraminidase (HN) of Sendai virus (Mazanec et al., 1992) or for the hemagglutinin of influenza virus (Mazanec et al., 1995) have been shown to colocalize with viral proteins in infected MDCK cells, and reduced the titer of intracellular virus 10- to 100-fold relative to nonspecific IgA or IgG. It is not yet clear whether intracellular IgA interacts with intact virions or prevents the assembly of viral coats, although the latter seems more likely. Similarly, the exact cellular location where transcytosing IgA comes into contact with viral proteins is not known. One possibility is that newly synthesized viral proteins pass through an endosomal compartment en route to the cell surface. Alternatively, viral infection may cause the diversion of transcytotic vesicles to virion-containing compartments. Clearly, further work will be necessary to clarify these issues.

## V. CONCLUSIONS

A great deal of progress has been made in the last 15 years in our understanding of the structure and function of the pIgR, yet many questions remain unresolved. How is the specificity for polymeric vs monomeric immunoglobulins achieved? What are the determinants in the $\alpha$ and $\mu$ chains that initiate noncovalent interaction with SC? At the cellular level, the machinery that recognizes and sorts the pIgR in the Golgi apparatus and in endosomes remains virtually unknown. Similarly, the kinase(s) that catalyze receptor phosphorylation and the protease responsible for SC formation are as yet uncharacterized. Given the rapid rate of progress in recent years, answers to these questions should soon be at hand.

# REFERENCES

Apodaca, G., and Mostov, K. E. (1993). Transcytosis of placental alkaline phosphatase-polymeric immunoglobulin receptor fusion proteins is regulated by mutations of ser664. *J. Biol. Chem.* **268,** 23712.

Apodaca, G., Katz, L. A., and Mostov, K. E. (1994). Receptor-mediated transcytosis of IgA in MDCK cells is via apical recycling endosomes. *J. Cell Biol.* **125,** 67–86.

Arnold, R. R., Cole, M. F., and Prince, S. J., and McGhee, J. R. (1977). Secretory IgM antibodies to *Streptococcus mutans* in subjects with selective IgA deficiency. *Clin. Immunol. Immunopathol.* **8,** 475–486.

Aroeti, B., Kosen, P. A., Kuntz, I. D., Cohen, F. E., and Mostov, K. E. (1993). Mutational and secondary structural analysis of the basolateral sorting signal of the polymeric immunoglobulin receptor. *J. Cell Biol.* **123,** 1149–1160.

Bakos, M. A., Kurosky, A., and Goldblum, R. M. (1991a). Characterization of a critical binding site for human polymeric Ig on secretory component. *J. Immunol.* **147,** 3419–3426.

Bakos, M. A., Kurosky, A., Woodard, C. S., Denney, R. M., and Goldblum, R. M. (1991b). Probing the topography of free and polymeric Ig-bound human secretory component with monoclonal antibodies. *J. Immunol.* **146,** 162–168.

Bakos, M. A., Kurosky, A., Czerwinski, E. W. and Goldblum, R. M. (1993). A conserved binding site on the receptor for polymeric Ig is homologous to CDR1 of Ig Vκ domains. *J. Immunol.* **151,** 1346–1352.

Bakos, M. A., Widen, S. G., and Goldblum, R. M. (1994). Expression and purification of biologically active domain I of the human polymeric immunoglobulin receptor. *Mol. Immunol.* **31,** 165–168.

Banting, G., Brake, B., Braghetta, P., Luzio, J. P., and Stanley, K. K. (1989). Intracellular targeting signals of polymeric immunoglobulin receptors are highly conserved between species. *FEBS Lett.* **254,** 177–183.

Barroso, M., and Sztul, E. S. (1994). Basolateral to apical transcytosis in polarized cells is indirect and involves BFA and trimeric G protein sensitive passage through the apical endosome. *J. Cell Biol.* **124,** 83–100.

Bartles, J. R., Ferraci, H. M., Stieger, B., and Hubbard, A. L. (1987). Biogenesis of the rat hepatocyte plasma membrane *in vivo:* Comparison of the pathways taken by apical and basolateral proteins using subcellular fractionation. *J. Cell Biol.* **105,** 1241–1251.

Beale, D., and Coadwell, J. (1987). Tertiary structures for the extracellular domains of the polyimmunoglobulin receptor (secretory component) derived by primary structure comparisons with immunoglobulins. *Comp. Biochem. Physiol.* **86B,** 365–372.

Brandl, C. R., and Deber, C. M. (1986). Hypothesis about the function of membrane-buried proline residues in transport proteins. *Proc. Natl. Acad. Sci. U.S.A.* **83,** 917–921.

Brandtzaeg, P. (1974). Mucosal and glandular distribution of immunoglobulin components: Differential localization of free and bound SC in secretory epithelial cells. *J. Immunol.* **112,** 1553–1559.

Brandtzaeg, P. (1975). Human secretory Immunoglobulin M: An immunochemical and immunhistochemical study. *Immunology* **29,** 559–570.

Brandtzaeg, P. (1985). Role of J chain and secretory component in receptor-mediated glandular and hepatic transport of immunoglobulins in man. *Scand. J. Immunol.* **22,** 111–146.

Brandtzaeg, P., and Prydz, H. (1984). Direct evidence for an integrated function of J chain and secretory component in epithelial transport of immunoglobulins. *Nature (London)* **311,** 71–73.

Breitfeld, P. P., Harris, J. M., and Mostov, K. M. (1989). Postendocytotic sorting of the ligand for the polymeric immunoglobulin receptor in Madin-Darby canine kidney cells. *J. Cell Biol.* **109,** 475–486.

Breitfeld, P. P., McKinnon, W. C., and Mostov, K. E. (1990). Effect of nocodazole on vesicular traffic to the apical and basolateral surfaces of polarized MDCK cells. *J. Cell Biol.* **111,** 2365–2373.

Casanova, J. E., Breitfeld, P. P., Ross, S. A., and Mostov, K. E. (1990). Phosphorylation of the polymeric immunoglobulin receptor required for its efficient transcytosis. *Science* **248,** 742–745.

Casanova, J. E., Apodaca, G., and Mostov, K. E. (1991). An autonomous signal for basolateral sorting in the cytoplasmic domain of the polymeric immunoglobulin receptor. *Cell (Cambridge, Mass.)* **66,** 65–75.

Chintalacharuvu, K. R., Tavill, A. S., Louis, L. N., Vaerman, J. P., Lamm, M. E., and Kaetzel, C. S. (1994). Disulfide bond formation between dimeric immunoglobulin A and the polymeric immunoglobulin receptor during hepatic transcytosis. *Hepatology (Baltimore)* **19,** 162–173.

Collawn, J. F., Stangel, M., Kuhn, L. A., Esekogwu, V., Jing, S., Trowbridge, I. S., and Tainer, J. A. (1990). Transferrin receptor internalization sequence YXRF implicates a tight turn as the structural recognition motif for endocytosis. *Cell (Cambridge, Mass.)* **63,** 1061–1072.

Coyne, R. S., Siebrecht, M., Peitsch, M. C., and Casanova, J. E. (1994). Mutational analysis of polymeric immunoglobulin receptor/ligand interactions: Evidence for the involvement of multiple CDR-like loops in receptor domain 1. *J. Biol. Chem.* **269,** 31620–31625.

Deitcher, D. L., and Mostov, K. E. (1986). Alternate splicing of rabbit polymeric immunoglobulin receptor. *Mol. Cell. Biol.* **6,** 2712–2715.

Eiffert, H., Quentin, E., Decker, J., Hillemeir, S., Hufschmidt, M., Klingmuller, D., Weber, M., and Hilschmann, N. (1984). Die primarstuktur der menschlichen freien sekretkomponente end die Anordnung der disulfide brucken. *Hoppe-Seyler's Z. Physiol. Chem.* **365,** 1489–1495.

Fallgreen-Gebauer, E., Gebauer, W., Bastian, A., Kratzin, H. D., Eiffert, H., Zimmermann, B., Karas, M., and Hischmann, N. (1993). The covalent linkage of secretory component to IgA. Structure of sIgA. *Biol. Chem. Hoppe-Seyler* **374,** 1023.

Fleury, S., Lamarre, D., Meloche, S., Ryu, S. E., Cantin, D., Hendrickson, W. A., and Sekaly, R.-P. (1991). Mutational analysis of the interaction between CD4 and class II MHC: Class II antigens contact CD4 on a surface opposite the gp120 binding site. *Cell* **66,** 1037–1049.

Frutiger, S., Hughes, G. J., Hanly, W. C., Kingzette, M., and Jaton, J.-C. (1986). The amino terminal domain of rabbit secretory component is responsible for noncovalent binding to immunoglobulin A dimers. *J. Biol. Chem.* **261,** 16673–16681.

Geuze, H. J., Slot, J. W., Strous, G. J. A. M., Peppard, J., von Figura, K., Hasilik, A., and Schwartz, A. L. (1984). Intracellular receptor sorting during endocytosis: Comparative immunoelectron microscopy of multiple receptors in rat liver. *Cell (Cambridge, Mass.)* **37,** 195–204.

Hanson, L. A. (1961). Comparative immunological studies of the immune globulins of human milk and of blood serum. *Int. Arch. Allergy Appl. Immunol.* **18,** 241–267.

Hendrickson, B. A., Conner, D. A., Ladd, D. J., Kendall, D., Casanova, J. E., Corthesy, B., Max, E., Neutra, M. R., Seidman, C. E., and Seidman, J. G. (1995). Altered hepatic transport of IgA in mice lacking J chain. *J. Exp. Med* in press.

Hirt, R. P., Hughes, G. J., Frutiger, S., Michetti, P., Perregaux, O., Poulin-Godefroy, O., Jeanguenat, N., Neutra, M. R., and Kraehenbuhl, J.-P. (1993). Transcytosis of the polymeric immunoglobulin receptor requires phosphorylation of serine 664 in the absence but not the presence of dimeric IgA. *Cell (Cambridge, Mass.)* **74,** 245.

Hunziker, W., Mâle, P., and Mellman, I. (1990). Differential microtubule requirements for transcytosis in MDCK cells. *EMBO J.* **9,** 3515–3525.

Krajci, P., Solberg, R., Sandberg, M., Oyen, O., Jahnsen, T., and Brandtzaeg, P. (1989). Molecular cloning of the human transmembrane secretory component (poly Ig receptor) and its mRNA expression in human tissues. *Biochem. Biophys. Res. Commun.* **158,** 783–789.

Krajci, P., Kvale, D., Tasken, K., and Brandtzaeg, P. (1992). Molecular cloning and exon–intron mapping of the gene encoding human transmembrane secretory component (the poly-Ig receptor). *Eur. J. Immunol.* **22,** 2309–2315.

Kuhn, L. C., and Kraehenbuhl, J.-P. (1982). The sacrificial receptor-translocation of polymeric IgA across epithelia. *Trends Biochem. Sci.* **7,** 299–302.

Kulseth, M. A., Krajci, P., Myklebost, O., and Rogne, S. (1995). Cloning and characterization of two forms of bovine polymeric immunoglobulin receptor. *DNA Cell Biol.* **14**, 251–256.

Larkin, J. M., Sztul, E. S., and Palade, G. E. (1986). Phosphorylation of the rat hepatic polymeric IgA receptor. *Proc. Natl. Acad. Sci. U.S.A.* **83**, 4759–4763.

Matlin, K. S., and Simons, K. (1984). Sorting of an apical membrane glycoprotein occurs before it reaches the cell surface in cultured epithelial cells. *J. Cell Biol.* **99**, 2131–2139.

Matter, K., and Mellman, I. (1994). Mechanisms of cell polarity: Sorting and transport in epithelial cells. *Curr. Opin. Cell Biol.* **6**, 545–554.

Mazanec, M. B., Kaetzel, C. S., Lamm, M. E., Fletcher, D., and Nedrud, J. G. (1992). Intracellular neutralization of virus by immunoglobulin A antibodies. *Proc. Natl. Acad. Sci. U.S.A.* **89**, 6901–6905.

Mazanec, M. B., Coudret, C. L., and Fletcher, D. R. (1995). Intracellular neutralization of influenza virus by immunoglobulin A anti-hemaglutinin monoclonal antibodies. *J. Virol.* **69**, 1339–1343.

Mostov, K. E., and Blobel, G. (1982). A transmembrane precursor of secretory component. *J. Biol. Chem.* **257**, 11816–11821.

Mostov, K. E., and Deitcher, D. L. (1986). Polymeric immunoglobulin receptor expressed in MDCK cells transcytoses IgA. *Cell (Cambridge, Mass.)* **46**, 613–621.

Mostov, K. E., Kraehenbuhl, J.-P., and Blobel, G. (1980). Receptor-mediated transcellular transport of immunoglobulin: Synthesis of secretory component as multiple and larger transmembrane forms. *Proc. Natl. Acad. Sci. U.S.A.* **77**, 7257–7261.

Mostov, K. E., Friedlander, M., and Blobel, G. (1984). The receptor for transepithelial transport of IgA and IgM contains multiple immunoglobulin-like domains. *Nature (London)* **308**, 37–43.

Mostov, K. E., de Bruyn Kops, A., and Deitcher, D. L. (1986). Deletion of the cytoplasmic domain of the polymeric immunoglobulin receptor prevents basolateral localization and endocytosis. *Cell (Cambridge, Mass.)* **47**, 359–364.

Mostov, K. E., Apodaca, G., Aroeti, B., and Okamoto, C. (1992). Plasma membrane protein sorting in polarized epithelial cells. *J. Cell Biol.* **116**, 577–583.

Musil, L., and Baenziger, J. (1987). Cleavage of membrane secretory component to soluble secretory component occurs on the cell surface of rat hepatocyte monolayers. *J. Cell Biol.* **104**, 1725–1733.

Okamoto, C. T., Shia, S. P., Bird, C., Mostov, K. E., and Roth, M. G. (1992). The cytoplasmic domain of the polymeric immunoglobulin receptor contains two internalization signals that are distinct from its basolateral sorting signal. *J. Biol. Chem.* **267**, 9925–9932.

Okamoto, C. T., Song, W., Bomsel, M., and Mostov, K. E. (1994). Rapid internalization of the polymeric immunoglobulin receptor requires phosphorylated serine 726. *J. Biol. Chem.* **269**, 15676.

Piskurich, J. F., Blanchard, M. H., Youngman, K. R., France, J. A., and Kaetzel, C. S. (1995). Molecular cloning of the mouse polymeric Ig receptor: Functional regions of the molecule are conserved among five mammalian species. *J. Immunol.* **154**, 1735–1747.

Rindler, M. J., Ivanov, I. E., Plesken, H., Rodriguez-Boulan, E., and Sabatini, D. D. (1984). Viral glycoproteins destined for apical or basolateral plasma membrane domains transverse the same Golgi apparatus during their intracellular transport in Madin-Darby canine kidney cells. *J. Cell Biol.* **98**, 1304–1319.

Salter, R. D., Benjamin, R. J., Wesley, P. K., Buxton, S. E., Garrett, T. P. J., Clayberger, C., Krensky, A. M., Norment, A. M., Littman, D. R., and Parham, P. (1990). A binding site for the T-cell coreceptor CD8 on the α3 domain of HLA A2. *Nature (London)* **345**, 41–46.

Sanders, S. K., Fox, R. O., and Kavathas, P. (1991). Mutations in CD8 that affect interactions with HLA Class I and monoclonal anti-CD8 antibodies. *J. Exp. Med.* **174**, 371–379.

Solari, R., Schaerer, E., Tallichet, C., Braiterman, L. T., Hubbard, A. L., and Kraehenbuhl, J.-P. (1989). Cellular location of the cleavage event of the polymeric immunoglobulin receptor and the fate of its anchoring domain in the rat hepatocyte. *Biochem. J.* **257**, 759.

Song, W., Bomsel, M., Casanova, J., Vaerman, J.-P., and Mostov, K. (1994). Stimulation of transcytosis of the polymeric immunoglobulin receptor by dimeric IgA. *Proc. Natl. Acad. Sci. U.S.A.* **91**, 163.

Sztul, E. S., Howell, K. E., and Palade, G. E. (1985). Biogenesis of the polymeric IgA receptor in rat hepatocytes. I. Kinetic studies of its intracellular forms. *J. Cell Biol.* **100,** 1248–1254.

Sztul, E., Colombo, M., Stahl, P., and Samanta, R. (1993). Control of protein traffic between distinct plasma membrane domains: Requirement for a novel 108,000 mw protein in the fusion of transcytotic vesicles with the apical plasma membrane. *J. Biol. Chem.* **268,** 1876–1885.

Thompson, R. A. (1970). Secretory piece linked to IgM in individuals deficient in IgA. *Nature (London)* **266,** 946–948.

Tomasi, T. B., Jr., Tan, E. M., Solomon, A., and Prendergast, R. A. (1965). Characteristics of an immune system common to certain external secretions. *J. Exp. Med.* **121,** 101–124.

Vaux, D. (1992). The structure of an endocytosis signal. *Trends Cell Biol.* **2,** 189–192.

Williams, A. F., and Barclay, A. N. (1988). The immunoglobulin superfamily: Domains for cell surface recognition. *Annu. Rev. Immunol.* **6,** 381–405.

*part*

# III

# MUCOSAL T LYMPHOCYTES AND LYMPHOCYTE MIGRATION

# Chapter 14

# Ligand Recognition by $\gamma\delta$ T Cells

Yueh-hsiu Chien

*Department of Microbiology and Immunology, Stanford University, Stanford, California 94305*

## I. Introduction

It has been just over a decade since the accidental discovery of the T-cell receptor (TCR) $\gamma$ chain gene during the search for TCR $\alpha$ chain (Saito *et al.*, 1984). Anti-peptide antisera eventually led to the identification of a novel subset of T cells bearing the $\gamma\delta$ TCR heterodimer (Brenner *et al.*, 1986; Bank *et al.*, 1986; Lanier *et al.*, 1987). Since this time, despite intense effort, the role(s) of $\gamma\delta$ T cell in the immune system is still not clear. Although $\gamma\delta$ T cells can be triggered to secrete lymphokines and mount cytolytic responses in many experimental systems, and they are found to predominate in some pathological situations where $\alpha\beta$ T cells are not very active, almost all of the well-defined cellular immune functions attributed to T cells are performed by $\alpha\beta$ T cells (reviewed in Haas *et al.*, 1993, Havran and Boismenu, 1994). Nevertheless, $\gamma\delta$ T cells are present in all vertebrate animals. Recent studies with mice that lack either $\alpha\beta$ or $\gamma\delta$ T cells show that infections can be cleared in both types of mice, but the mode of clearance is quite different (reviewed in Kaufman, 1994), suggesting that these two types of T cells are contributing to host immune competence differently. In addition, mice that have only $\alpha\beta$ T cells are immunocompromised when compared with mice that have both $\alpha\beta$ and $\gamma\delta$ T cells. This further indicates that $\gamma\delta$ T cells perform unique functions. In order to discern the function of $\gamma\delta$ T cells in the immune system it will be necessary to identify their recognition properties (likely targets and recognition requirements). Because $\alpha\beta$ T cells recognize peptides derived from degraded protein antigens in association with the MHC molecules, it has been commonly assumed that $\gamma\delta$ T cells follow the same pattern. However, even early on, it was clear that classical MHC molecules do not play major roles in $\gamma\delta$ T-cell recognition; it was proposed that nonclassical MHC, heat-shock proteins, or as-yet-unidentified surface molecules are playing the role(s). As self-presentation is difficult to assess, we decided to turn the question around and ask when $\gamma\delta$ T-cell recognition does involve MHC molecules, do MHC molecules play a similar role as in $\alpha\beta$ T-cell recognition; to what extent do the MHC bound peptides confer specificity, and what kind of antigen-processing pathway is required? The model systems we studied are the recognition of a mouse classical MHC class II molecule IE$^k$ by the $\gamma\delta$ T-cell clone LBK5 and the recognition of the nonclassical MHC molecule TL-T10 and T22 by G8 (Schild *et al.*, 1994).

## II. RECOGNITION OF IE$^k$ BY LBK5 DOES NOT REQUIRE A SPECIFIC PEPTIDE/MHC COMPLEX FORMED IN EITHER ENDOSOMAL OR LYSOSOMAL COMPARTMENTS

The majority of $\alpha\beta$ T cells that recognize protein antigens presented by class II molecules require endocytosis of exogenous proteins that are degraded in the endocytic compartments. Class II MHC molecules are assembled in the ER and travel through endosomes or endosome-like compartments to the cell surface, acquiring processed peptides along the way (Neefjes and Ploegh, 1992; Germain and Margulies, 1993). We tested if perturbations in this pathway would affect the ability of IE$^k$ to stimulate LBK5. IE$^k$ $\alpha$ and $\beta$ chains were expressed in mutant CHO cell lines with temperature-sensitive endosomal acidification defects of the End1, 2, and 3 complementation groups (Colbaugh and Draper, 1993). Upon shifting to the nonpermissive temperature, various lesions in the endocytic pathway are induced. The defects impair the ability of these cells to present protein antigens to $\alpha\beta$ T cells, but they do not affect the synthesis, the surface expression, or the ability of the IE$^k$ molecule to present exogenously acquired antigens. This is illustrated by the fact that all of the mutants show severely reduced presentation of cytochrome c protein to the $\alpha\beta$ T cells 2B4 and 5CC7. Stimulation of the $\alpha\beta$ alloreactive clone A1A10 is also impaired, but the level of surface IE$^k$ expression on these mutant cells is indistinguishable from that of wild-type IE$^k$-CHO cells at either the permissive (34°C) or nonpermissive (39°C) temperatures. At 39°C, all of the mutant CHO cells present exogenous peptide antigens and *Staphylococcus* enterotoxin A (SEA) as well as wild-type CHO cells (Table I and data not shown). Surprisingly, these mutations have no effect on LBK5 activation (Table I).

As some class II MHC-associated peptides may also be acquired in endocytic compartments other than endosomes, we tested whether a peptide/IE$^k$ complex formed in these other compartments might be required for LBK5 recognition by using CHO cells expressing glycanphophatidyl-inositol (GPI) linked IE$^k$ chimeras (Wettstein *et al.*, 1991) as stimulator cells. The rationale is that GPI-IE$^k$ molecules, similar to naturally occurring GPI linked proteins, are transported to the cell surface directly after exiting from the Golgi and do not recycle (Thomas *et al.*, 1990). Thus, they would not intersect with the acidic intracellular compartments such as lysosomes or endosomes. GPI-IE$^k$ expressing cells do not present exogenously added protein antigens to $\alpha\beta$ T cells nor do they stimulate alloreactive $\alpha\beta$ T cells (Fig. 1, data not shown, and Wettstein *et al.*, 1991). Nonetheless, LBK5 can respond to these cells almost as efficiently as to wild-type IE$^k$-CHO cells (Fig. 1).

*TABLE I*

T-CELL RESPONSES TO IE$^k$ EXPRESSED ON TEMPERATURE-SENSITIVE CHO CELL MUTANTS

|  | 2B4 peptide(αβ) | | 2B4 protein(αβ) | | A1A10(αβ) | | LBK5 (γδ) | |
| --- | --- | --- | --- | --- | --- | --- | --- | --- |
| Temp. (°C): | 34 | 39 | 34 | 39 | 34 | 39 | 34 | 39 |
| IE$^k$-CHO | + + + | + + + + | + + + | + + + + | + + | + + + | + + | + + + |
| IE$^k$-G8.1 (end1) | + + + | + + + + | + + | 0 | + | 0 | + + | + + + |
| IE$^k$-25.2.2 (end2) | + + + | + + + + | + + + | + | + | 0 | + + | + + + |
| IE$^k$-G7.1 (end3) | + + + | + + + + | + + | 0 | + | 0 | + + | + + + |

*Note.* The responses of each hybridoma to IE$^k$ expressed on CHO mutant cells are compared with responses elicited from IE$^k$ expressed on normal CHO cells. Each "+" indicates a fivefold difference in IL-2 or IL-3 production. 0 Indicates no detectable IL-2/IL-3 production. The IL-2 production for the 2B4 hybridoma in response to the MCC (moth cytochrom c) peptide 88–103 was 125 U/ml and to the PCC protein 90 U/ml, IL-3 production of A1A10 (an αβ allorective T-cell hybridoma) was 25 U/ml, and that of LBK5 45 U/ml.

These results indicate that peptide loading in endosomal and/or lysosomal compartments is not required for LBK5 stimulation.

During the biosynthesis of class II MHC molecules the invariant (Ii) chain transiently associates with the αβ heterodimer in the ER. It has been suggested that this interaction can influence the binding of peptides to MHC class II molecules (Germain and Margulies, 1993). It was shown that the introduction of the invariant chain in CHO-IE$^k$ cells enhances their ability to present protein antigens to αβ T cells, but the presence of the invariant chain has no effect on the ability of these stimulator cells to stimulate LBK5 (Fig. 1). Thus the presence of the invariant chain during the biosyntheses of IE$^k$ has no effect on LBK5 recognition. Together, these results indicate that the antigen-processing requirements for LBK5 activation are not sensitive to manipulations that would influence the repertoire of peptides loaded onto the IE$^k$ molecule.

### III. DEFECTS IN THE MHC CLASS I AND CLASS II PEPTIDE LOADING PATHWAY DO NOT AFFECT IE$^k$ RECOGNITION BY LBK5

To further test if peptide bound to IE$^k$ confers the specificity of LBK5, we tested if functional class I and class II antigen-processing pathways in the stimulator cells are necessary for the stimulation of LBK5. IE$^k$ was expressed in the mouse cell line RMA-S, which has a point mutation in the peptide transporter gene Ham-

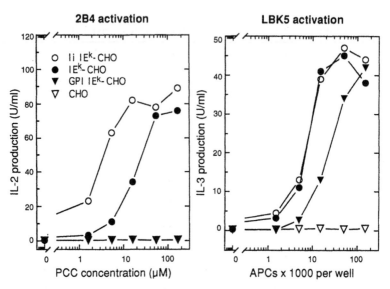

**FIGURE 1.** Stimulation of 2B4 and LBK5 with IE$^k$ expressing CHO cells. Stimulation of 2B4 and LBK5 with CHO cells expressing native IEk (IE$^k$-CHO), glycanphosphatidylinositol linked (GPI) IE$^k$ (GPI IE$^k$-CHO), native IEk together with invariant chain (Ii) p4I (Ii IE$^k$-CHO), and CHO cells. The response of 2B4 is measured by the production of IL2, that of LBK5 by the production of IL-3. 2B4 shows no response to CHO cells but the symbols are marked by the symbols from GPI IE$^k$-CHO cells.

2 (Attaya *et al.*, 1992) and is defective in class I-restricted pathway, the human cell line T2, which has a homozygous deletion in the H-2 region and is defective for both class I and II pathways (Cerundolo *et al.*, 1990), and their respective parental, nondefective lines, RMA and T1. Consistent with their antigen-processing defects, IE$^k$/RMA-S cells stimulated the $\alpha\beta$ alloreactive clone and presented cytochrome c peptide and the whole protein to 2B4, while IE$^k$/T2 cells could only present peptide (data not shown). In contrast, all transfectants were able to stimulate LBK5 comparably (Fig. 2A). These data show that the common class I and class II antigen-processing pathways are not necessary for LBK5's reactivity. This further illustrated that when LBK5 recognizes IE, the peptide bound to IE$^k$ does not confer specificity. Furthermore, addition of a specific peptide to the stimulator cells does not change their ability to stimulate LBK5.

## IV. LBK5 REACTIVITY CORRELATES DIRECTLY WITH THE AMOUNT OF SURFACE IE$^k$ EXPRESSION ON THE STIMULATOR CELLS

While these different IE$^k$-expressing cells can all stimulate LBK5, they appear to plateau at different levels. To determine if this reflects quantitative or qualitative differences between the IE$^k$ molecules, we compared the cell surface expression

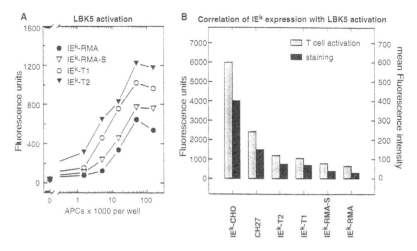

*FIGURE 2.* (A) Stimulation of LBK5 with native $IE^k$ expressed on RMA, RMA-S, T1, T2 cells. (B) Correlation of surface $IE^k$ expression with LBK5 responses. LBK5 cells expressing the NFAT-alkaline phosphatase gene were used. The fluorescence units represent measurements of NFAT-specific alkaline phosphates activity as described (Bram *et al.*, 1993). The mean fluorescence intensity represents the amount of surface $IE^k$ expression as measured by FACS staining. The same batch of cells was stained for surface $IE^k$ expression and tested for LBK5 activation at the same time.

of $IE^k$ on all stimulator cells by FACS and correlated this with their abilities to stimulate LBK5. As shown in Fig. 2B, LBK5 reactivity correlates directly with the amount of surface $IE^k$ expression on the stimulator cells.

## V. LBK5 RECOGNIZES IMMUNOPURIFIED $IE^k$ MOLECULES

It has been shown that presentation of bacterial superantigens by class II MHC molecules to $\alpha\beta$ T cells is independent of antigen processing (Yagi *et al.*, 1990). Since our experiments establish that neither class I nor class II antigen-processing pathways are required for the activation of LBK5, we sought to determine whether $IE^k$ is presenting a superantigen-like molecule to LBK5. Purified $IE^k$ molecules from the surface of the B-cell lymphoma CH27 were immobilized in microtiter wells (Kane *et al.*, 1989) and used to stimulate T cells. Immobilized $IE^k$ molecules and CH27 cells stimulate LBK5 to similar levels (Fig. 3). These results demonstrate that purified $IE^k$ alone is sufficient to activate LBK5.

## VI. $IE^k$ INTERACTS DIFFERENTLY WITH LBK5 THAN WITH $\alpha\beta$ T CELLS

Since our data indicate that LBK5 recognizes $IE^k$ with a variety of different peptides bound and most likely without a peptide as well, we next examined how this

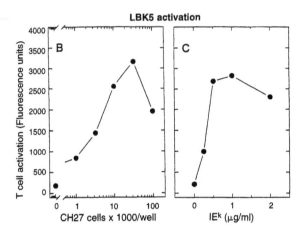

**FIGURE 3.** Stimulation of LBK5 with CH27 cells and platebound IE$^k$, LBK5 activation as measured by fluroescence units representing NFAT-specific alkaline phosphatase activity versus concentration of CH27 cells or purified IE$^k$ loaded into microtiter wells was plotted. Stimuatlion with plate bound IE$^k$ and CH27 cells were carried out in the same experiment.

recognition is achieved. To map the LBK5 epitope, we analyzed the response of LBK5 to a panel of 13 APC lines. Each line expresses a mutant IE$^k$ molecule with a single amino acid substitution at a residue predicted to be located on the MHC a helices and "pointing up" toward the $\alpha\beta$ TCR (Ehrich *et al.*, 1993). These assignments have been confirmed by the recently described X-ray crystal structure of the class II molecule, DR1 (Brown *et al.*, 1993). All of the APCs stain normally with more than six anti-IE monoclonal antibodies and bind peptides to the same extent as wild-type IE$^k$-CHO cells do. Stimulation of LBK5, two alloreactive $\alpha\beta$ T-cell hybridomas (A1A10, Ak44.1), and the presentation of peptides to more than 40 antigen-specific $\alpha\beta$ T cells by the mutant APCs were compared. The reactivity of all $\alpha\beta$ T cells surveyed is disrupted by mutations that are more centrally located around the peptide binding site (Fig. 4; Ehrich *et al.*, 1993; data not shown). However, none of the mutants which affect $\alpha\beta$ T-cell responses influence LBK5 reactivity. Only a glutamic acid to lysine change at position 79 near the extreme C-terminal end of the E$_\alpha$ $\alpha$ helix ablated LBK5 recognition. This mutant has no effect on any of more than 40 $\alpha\beta$ T cells tested (Ehrich *et al.* 1993; data not shown). Thus, the topology of $\alpha\beta$ vs $\gamma\delta$ T-cell recognition of the same IE molecule is likely to be quite different. Further analysis indicated that the specificity of LBK5 is influenced by the carbohydrate at $\alpha$82 as well as a polymorphic residue at $\beta$67, a residue that is solvent exposed (J. Hample and Y.-h. Chien, unpublished results). These results suggest that LBK5 recognizes IE$^k$ not from the "top" of the peptide–MHC complex, but from the "side," away from the peptide binding groove.

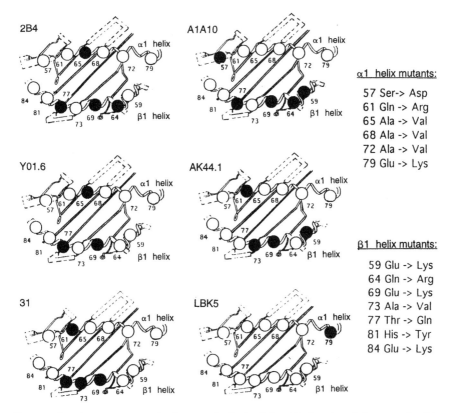

FIGURE 4. IE^k mutants and their effects on T-cell stimulation. The location of the mutated residues is depicted according to the model of Brown *et al.* (1993). The positions and amino acid substitutions of 13 IE^k mutants as well as the specificity of the hybridomas are as described (Ehrich *et al.*, 1993). Mutations at positions that showed more than a 1000-fold decrease in presentation efficiency to αβ T cells are shown in filled circles. For LBK5, the α79 mutation elicited no response from LBK5 at all APC concentrations tested. The dose-response curves of LBK5 to all the other mutants are indistinguishable from that of CHO cells expressing native IE^k molecules.

## VII. Antigen-Processing Requirements in Other Experimental Systems

Because γδ T cells that recognize classical MHC molecules are rare, we sought to test the generality of the LBK5 finding with another γδ T-cell clone, G8, whose reactivity was mapped to the MHC TL region. The ligands for G8 were identified by expression cloning and found to be the product of the nonclassical class I molecules T10 and the closely related T22 gene (94% identity) (Schild *et al.*, 1994; Weintraub *et al.*, 1994). As in the case of LBK5 described above, it was demonstrated that no conventional class I or class II antigen-processing pathways are required for TL recognition by the G8 clone. Again all variations in the ability of different stimulator cells to activate these $\gamma\delta$ T cells can be attributed solely to the level of their surface MHC expression (Fig. 5A). Also significant is the fact that G8 recognizes TL molecules expressed on Drosophila cells. *Drosophila melanogaster* does not have an immune system equivalent to that of mammals and appears to lack the factors necessary for any type of antigen processing and presentation (Fig. 5B).

The T10/T22 sequences have a 3-amino-acid deletion in the predicted $\alpha1$ $\alpha$ helix and a 13-amino-acid deletion in the $\alpha2$ helix when compared with MHC class I sequences. The amino acid residues following the 13-amino-acid deletion also do not have a helical propensity characteristic of classical MHC molecules. Therefore, even if the TL molecule folds similarly to classical MHC molecules, the $\alpha$ helix would be severely truncated on one side and the $\beta$ strand platform may be shortened (Ito *et al.*, 1990). In addition, T10 and T22 lack 4 of the 8 amino acids that are important for peptide binding by class I molecules (Teitell *et al.*, 1994). The addition of peptide libraries (7–9 amino acids long or shorter) does not augment the expression of TL on the surface of cells that are defective in the conventional antigen-processing pathway (H. Schild, M. Jackson, and Y.-h. Chien

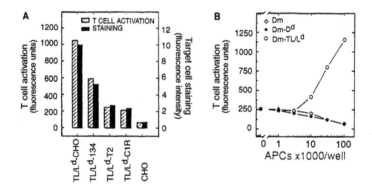

**FIGURE 5.** (A) Correlation of surface TL/L$^d$ expression on stimulator cells with G8 responses. (B) Stimulation of G8 with TL/L$^d$ expressed on Schneider's Drosophila cells. G8 cells expressing NFAT-alkaline phosphatase were used. 721.134 has a point mutation in one of the genes associated with class 1-restricted peptide transport (Spies and DeMars, 1991). C1R, derived from the human B-cell line Hmy2, is not defective in class I- or class II-restricted antigen processing (Zemmour *et al.*, 1992). The fluorescence unit represents measurement of NFAT-specific alkaline phosphatase activity as described in the legend to Fig. 1. The mean fluorescence intensity in (E) represents the amount of TL/L$^d$ expression as measured by FACS staining. The same batch of cells was stained for surface TL/L$^d$ expression and tested for G8 activation at the same time. Induction of expression of membrane-bound TL-L$^d$, staining of cells for flow cytometry, and the T-cell activation assay were carried out as described in Schild *et al.* (1994). As a control class I D$^b$ expressed on Drosophila cells and untransfected Drosophila cells were tested.

unpublished results). Further, peptide could not be eluted from T10 using standard methods (A. Kaliyaperumal, *et al.*, 1995). In addition, we have recently found that T10 and β2 microglobulin expressed in *Escherichia coli* are able to fold into stable complexes without exogenously added peptide. The folded material bound onto plastic plates can stimulate G8 to a similar extent as cells expressing TL10 (M. Crowley, N. Mavaddat, and Y.-h. Chien, manuscript in preparation). Thus, not only does G8 recognize T10 in the absence of peptide, but it also seems that TL10/22 does not bind peptide. At least one of the MHC-like molecules, the FcRn receptor, has a "closed" groove and thus is unable to bind peptides (Burmeister *et al.*, 1994).

The T22 molecule has also been identified as the ligand of another γδ T-cell clone, KN6 (Bonneville *et al.*, 1989). It is not clear if KN6 also recognizes T10, because the T10 gene assayed by Ito *et al.* (1990) is not functional. Similar to the results shown for G8, KN6 responded to T22-expressing cells from a variety of tissues as well as to T22-transfected cells deficient in the class I peptide transported (TAP1/TAP2). In an effort to evaluate the "peptide" requirements for KN6 recognition, the T22 gene was analyzed by mutagenesis (Moriwaki *et al.*, 1993). While some residues located on the "putative" peptide binding floor showed no effect, others reduced KN6 reactivity drastically, leading to the conclusion that a peptide is involved in the recognition. However, in these experiments the cell surface expression of the transfected gene was not monitored, and thus an alternative explanation is that these mutations prevented the proper expression of the protein. In fact, one of those mutations (residue 25 from Val to Phe) was generated independently and resulted in the loss of T22 surface expression (N. Mavaddat, M. Crowley, and Y.-h. Chien, unpublished results).

In addition to the LBK5 and G8, studies of another γδ T-cell clone, TgI4.4, specific for a herpes simplex virus type 1 transmembrane glycoprotein (gI), also indicates that the protein is recognized directly and required neither antigen processing nor presentation by other molecules (Sciammas *et al.*, 1994).

## VIII. Nonprotein Antigens Can Be Recognized by γδ T Cells

Recent studies of γδ T cells from healthy human peripheral blood and from patients with tuberculoid leprosy or rheumatoid arthritis that respond to heat-killed mycobacteria have identified the major stimulatory components to be phosphate-containing, nonpeptide molecules.

Schoel *et al.* (1994) identified the active component in mycobacterium as a nonprotein low-molecular-weight (1–3 kDa) compound that contains unusual carbohydrate and phosphate moieties. Constant *et al.* (1994) identified four distinct but related stimulating agents from *M. tuberculosis* (strain H37Rv), water-soluble extracts termed TUBag 1–4. TUBag 4 was identified as a 5'-triphosphorylated thymidine substituted at its γ-phosphate by an as yet to be characterized low-molecular-weight structure. TUBag 3 has a similar structure, but contains uridine instead of deoxythymidine. TUBag 1 and 2 are naturally occurring nonnucleotide minimal active fragments of TUBag 3 and 4. Tanaka *et al.* (1994, 1995) working with extracts from the same mycobacterial strain, identified isopentenyl pyrophosphate and related prenyl pyrophosphate derivatives as the major stimulatory component. They also found that synthetic alkenyl and prenyl derivatives of phosphate and pyrophosphate as well as $\gamma$-monoethyl derivatives of nucleoside and deoxynucleoside triphosphate stimulate particular $\gamma\delta$ T-cell clones, with the pyrophosphate and the TTP and UTP $\gamma$-derivatives being the most potent. Although the relative biological importance of these compounds remains to be determined, it is clear that a major class of stimulants are phosphate-containing nonpeptides. Another important finding is that all of these compounds can be found in both microbial and mammalian cells. It was suggested that these antigens can be produced by a number of pathogens as well as transformed, damaged, or stressed cells.

## IX. CDR3 Length Distributions of $\gamma\delta$ TCRs Are More Similar to That of Immunoglobulin Light and Heavy Chains Than to $\alpha\beta$ TCR

X-ray structural analysis of antibody–antigen complexes showed that one of the CDR3 loops (created by VDJ recombination) of Ig H and L chains is always involved in antigen contact. Similarly, the CDR3 of both $\alpha\beta$ TCR chains seem critical for peptide recognition. To search for a structural basis for the $\gamma\delta$ T-cell recognition, Rock *et al.* (1994) analyzed the CDR3 length distribution of all known antigen receptor polypeptides from mouse and humans. CDR3 lengths were tabulated using a computer program written in Pascal running on a VAX 6000-420 under VMS 5.4. After excluding sequence fragments without a complete CDR3 region, the program calculate CDR3 length as the distance from the J region-encoded GXG triplet (where G is glycine and X is any amino acid) to the nearest preceding V region-encoded cystein(C). Statistics were calculated on a Macintosh computer using StatView II (Abacus Concepts, Berkeley, CA). The variance formula used by StatView II is for an unbiased sample estimate, rather than for the population mean. The results are illustrated in Fig. 6.

For the $\alpha\beta$ TCR, the CDR3 length distributions are significantly constrained and are about equal in length. This probably reflects the requirements for $\alpha$ and $\beta$ chains of the TCR to contact the bound peptide. For Ig, CDR3 lengths for the light chains are short and constrained but those for the heavy chain are long and variable. This may reflect the fact that Ig recognize a variety of different antigenic surfaces, from small molecules to large pathogens. Surprisingly, for the $\gamma\delta$ TCR, the $\gamma$ chain is short and constrained and the $\delta$ chain is long and variable. Therefore, the $\gamma\delta$ TCR is more similar to that of Ig than that of $\alpha\beta$ TCR. This result further supports the finding that $\gamma\delta$ T cells recognize antigens very differently from $\alpha\beta$ T cells.

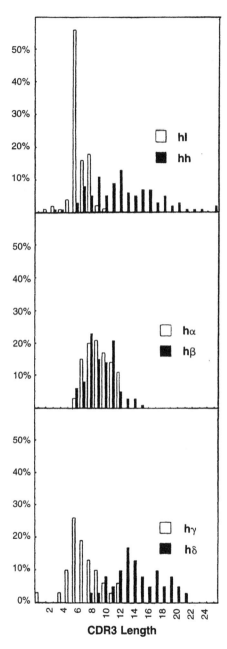

**FIGURE 6.** CDR3 lengths of antigen-specific immune receptor chains. Histograms showing percentages of CDR 3 sequences at given lengths in human chain families. hl, human Ig light chain; hh, human Ig heavy chain; h$\alpha$, human $\alpha$ TCR; h$\beta$, human $\beta$ TCR; h$\gamma$ TCR; h$\delta$, human $\delta$ TCR.

## X. $\gamma\delta$ T Cells—B-Cell-like Recognition Properties, T-Cell-like Signaling

Although $\gamma\delta$ TCR as a group may be more Ig-like in antigen recognition properties, the intracellular signaling mechanism of $\gamma\delta$ T cells may be closer to that of $\alpha\beta$ T cells. In particular, $\gamma\delta$ TCR, like $\alpha\beta$ TCR, need association with CD3 molecules for cell surface expression. Cross-linking of the engaged receptors is necessary for signaling. Cell surface antigens can be recognized as such, but recognition of soluble antigens such as the phosphate compounds requires an association with certain surface molecules to achieve multivalency under physiological conditions.

Another characteristic of antigen-specific $\alpha\beta$ T-cell stimulation is the requirement of a "second signal" through the "accessory" and/or "costimulatory" molecules. It appears that $\gamma\delta$ T cells may also depend on two or more signals for full activation (Haas *et al.*, 1993). However, $\gamma\delta$ T cells reside in a variety of different sites and express different types and quantities of surface molecules. It is conceivable that they may have different activation requirements.

## XI. Significance

The results discussed above suggest that $\gamma\delta$ T cells can respond to antigens that are not recognized by $\alpha\beta$ T cells, and that they are also able to respond to pathogens, damaged tissue, and cells directly and initiate immune response without the requirement for antigen processing or "professional" antigen-presenting cells. This would give $\gamma\delta$ T cells greater flexibility than the more classical type of $\alpha\beta$ T cell in mediating cellular immunity.

An understanding of the rules underlying antigen recognition and the characteristics of target antigens holds the key to understand $\gamma\delta$ T-cell function. The results discussed here are those of model systems but their extrapolations should provide an approach that may lead to a better appreciation of the roles of $\gamma\delta$ T cells in the immune system.

## References

Attaya, M., Jameson, S., Martinez, C. M., Hermel, E., Aldrich, C., Forman, J., Fischer Lindahl, K., Bevan, M. J., and Monaco, J. J. (1992). Ham-2 corrects the class I antigen-processing defect in RMA-S cells. *Nature (London)* 355, 647–649.

Bank, I., DePinho, R., Brenner, M., Cassimeris, J., Alt, F., and Chess, L. (1986). A functional T3 molecule associated with a novel heterodimer on the surface of immature human thymocytes. *Nature (London)* 322, 179–181.

Bonneville, M., Ito, K., Krecko, E., Itohara, S., Kappes, D., Ishida, I., Kanagawa, O., Janeway, C., Murphy, D., and Tonegawa, S. (1989). Recognition of a self major histocompatibility complex YTL region product by $\gamma\delta$ T-cell receptors. *Proc. Natl. Acad. Sci. U.S.A.* 86, 5928–5932.

Bram, R. J., Hung, D. T., Martin, P. K., Schreibert, S. L., and Crabtree, G. (1993). Identification of the immunophillins capable of mediating inhibition of signal transduction by cyclosporin A and FK506: Roles of calcineurin binding and cellular location. *Mol. Cell. Biol.* **13**, 4760–4769.

Brenner, M., McLean, J., Dialynas, D., Strominger, J., Smith, J., Owen, F., Seidman, J., Ip, S., Rosen, F., and Krangel, M. (1986). Identification of a putative second T-cell receptor. *Nature (London)* **322**, 145–149.

Brown, J. H., Jardetzky, T. S., Gorga, J. C., Stern, J. L., Urban, R. G., Strominger, J. L., and Wiley, D. C. (1993). Three-dimensional structure of the human Class II histocompatibility antigen HLA-DR1. *Nature (London)* **364**, 33–39.

Burmeister, W., Gastinel, L., Simister, N., Blum, M., and Bjorkman, P. (1994). Crystal structure at 2.2 A resolution of the MIIC-related neonatal Fc receptor. *Nature (London)* **372**, 336–343.

Cerundolo, V., Alexander, J., Anderson, K., Lamb, C., Cresswell, P., McMichael, A., Gotch, F., and Townsend, A. (1990). Presentation of viral antigen controlled by a gene in the major histocompatibility complex. *Nature (London)* **345**, 449–452.

Colbaugh, P. A., and Draper, R. K. (1993). Genetic analysis of membrane traffic in mamalian cells. "Endosomes and Lysosomes: A Dynamic Relationship." Jai Press, Greenwich, Connecticut.

Constant, P., Davodeau, F., Peyrat, M., Poquet, Y., Puzo, G., Bonneville, M., and Fournie, J. (1994). Stimulation of human gamma delta T cells by nonpeptidic mycobacterial ligands. *Science* **264**, 267–270.

Crowley, M., Mavaddat, N., and Chien, Y.-h. (1996). Manuscript in preparation.

Ehrich, E., Devaux, B., Rock, E. P., Jorgenson, J. L., Davis, M. M., and Chien, Y. (1993). T cell receptor interaction with peptide/Major Histocompatibility Complex (MHC) and superantigen/MHC ligands is dominated by antigen. *J. Exp. Med.* **178**, 713–722.

Germain, R. N., and Margulies, D. H. (1993). The biochemistry and cell biology of antigen processing and presentation. *Annu. Rev. Immunol.* **11**, 403–450.

Haas, W., Pereira, P., and Tonegawa, S. (1993). Gamma/delta cells. *Annu. Rev. Immunol.* **11**, 637–686.

Havran, W., and Boismenu, R. (1994). Activation and function of $\gamma\delta$ T cells. *Curr. Opin. Immunol.* **6**, 442–446.

Ito, K., Van Kear, L., Bonneville, M., Hsu, S., Murphy, D. B., and Tonegawa, S. (1990). Recognition of the product of a novel MHC TL region gene ($27^b$) by a mouse $\gamma\delta$ T cell receptor. *Cell (Cambridge, Mass.)* **62**, 549–561.

Kaliyaperumal, A., Falchetto, R., Cox, A., Dick, R., Chien, Y.-h., Matis, L., Hunt, D., and Bluestone, J. A. (1995). *J. Immunol.* **155**, 2379–2386.

Kane, K. P., Champoux, P., and Mescher, M. F. (1989). Solid-phase binding of class I and II MHC proteins: Immunoassay and T cell recognition. *Mol. Immunol.* **26**, 759–768.

Kaufmann S. (1994). Bacterial and protozoal infections in genetically disrupted mice. *Curr. Opin. Immunol.* **6**, 518.

Lanier, L., Federspiel, N., Ruitenberg, J., Phillips, J., Allison, J., Littman, D., and Weiss, A. (1987). The T cell antigen receptor complex expressed on normal peripheral blood CD4-CD8- T lymphocytes. *J. Exp. Med.* **165**, 1076–1094.

Moriwaki, S., Korn, B., Ichikawa, Y., van Kaer, L., and Tonegawa, S. (1993). Amino acid substitutions in the floor of the putative antigen-binding site of H-2T22 affect recognition by a gamma delta T-cell receptor. *Proc. Natl. Acad. Sci. U.S.A.* **90**, 11396–11400.

Neefjes, J. J., and Ploegh, H. L. (1992). Intracellular transport of MHC class II molecules. *Immunol. Today* **13**, 179–184.

Rock, E., Sibbald, P., Davis, M., and Chien, Y.-h. (1994). CDR3 length in antigen-specific immune receptors. *J. Exp. Med.* **179**, 323–328.

Saito, H., Kranz, D., Takagaki, Y., Hayday, A., Eisen, H., and Tonegawa, S. (1984). Complete primary structure of a heterodimeric T-cell receptor deduced from cDNA sequences. *Nature (London)* **309**, 757–762.

Schild, H., Mavaddat, N., Litzenberger, C., Ehrlich, E., Davis, M., Bluestone, J., Matis, L., Drapper,

R., and Chien, Y.-h. (1994). The nature of major histocompatibility complex recognition by $\gamma\delta$ T cells. *Cell (Cambridge, Mass.)* **76,** 29–37.

Schoel, B., Sprenger, S., and Kaufmann, S. (1994). Phosphate is essential for stimulation of V gamma 9V delta 2 T lymphocytes by mycobacterial low molecular weight ligand. *Eur. J. Immunol.* **24,** 1886–18892.

Sciammas, R., Johnson, R., Sperling, A., Brady, W., Linsley, P., Spear, P., Fitch, F., and Bluestone, J. (1994). Unique antigen recognition by a herpesvirus-specific TCR gamma delta cell. *J. Immunol.* **152,** 5392–5397.

Spies, T., and DeMars, R. (1991). Restored expression of major histocompatibility class I molecules by gene transfer of a putative peptide transporter. *Nature (London)* **351,** 323–324.

Tanaka, Y., Sano, S., Nieves, E., De Libero, G., Rosa, D., Modlin, R., Brenner, M., Bloom, B., and Morita, C. (1994). Nonpeptide ligands for human gamma delta T cells. *Proc. Natl. Acad. Sci. U.S.A.* **91,** 8175–8179.

Tanaka, Y., Morita, C., Tanaka, Y., Nieves, E., Brenner, M., and Bloom, B. (1995). Natural and synthetic non-peptide antigens recognized by human gamma delta T cells. *Nature (London)* **375,** 155–158.

Teitell, M., Cheroutre, H., Panwala, C., Holcombe, H., Eghtesady, P., and Kronenberg, M. (1994). Structure and function of H-2 T (Tla) region class I MHC molecules. *Crit. Rev. Immunol.* **14,** 1–27.

Thomas, J. R., Dwek, R. A., and Rademacher, T. W. (1990). Structure, biosynthesis, and function of glycosylphosphatidylinositols. *Biochemistry* **29,** 5413–5422.

Weintraub, B., Jackson, M., and Hedrick, S. (1994). Gamma delta T cells can recognize nonclassical MHC in the absence of conventional antigenic peptides. *J. Immunol.* **153,** 3051–3058.

Wettstein, D. A., Boniface, J. J., Reay, P. A., Schild, H., and Davis, M. M. (1991). Expression of a class II major histocompatability complex (MHC) heterodimer in a lipid-linked form with enhanced peptide/soluable MHC complex formation at low pH. *J. Exp. Med.* **174,** 219–228.

Yagi, J., Baron, J., Buxser, S., and Janeway, C. A. J. (1990). Bacterial proteins that mediate the association of a defined subset of T cell receptor:CD4 complexes with class II MHC. *J. Immunol.* **144,** 892–901.

Zemmour, J., Little, A.-M., Schendel, D. J., and Parham, P. (1992). The HLA-A,B "negative" mutant cell line C1R expresses a novel HLA-B35 allele, which also has a point mutation in the translation initiation codon. *J. Immunol.* **148,** 1941–1948.

# Chapter 15

# Development of Intestinal Intraepithelial Lymphocytes

Leo Lefrançois, Barbara Fuller, Sara Olson, and Lynn Puddington

*Department of Medicine, University of Connecticut Health Center, Farmington, Connecticut 06030*

## I. INTRODUCTION

Intraepithelial lymphocytes (IEL) of the small and large intestine comprise a specialized immune compartment presumably geared toward surveillance of the intestinal epithelial layer. One of the most intriguing aspects of IEL biology is the role of the thymus in their development (Lefrançois and Puddington, 1995). Whereas the vast majority of non-IEL T cells are derived from precursors that have matured and been selected in the thymus, small-intestinal IEL have unique requirements for the thymus in completing their developmental program (Lin *et al.*, 1993; Lefrançois and Olson, 1994; Wang and Klein, 1994). However, whether there is an absolute necessity for the thymus in IEL maturation has been questioned. Thus, thymectomized, irradiated bone marrow or fetal liver-reconstituted (ATXBM) mice contain IEL (Lefrançois *et al.*, 1990; Mosley *et al.*, 1990; Poussier *et al.*, 1992). In the mouse, $\alpha\beta$ T-cell receptor (TCR) and $\gamma\delta$ TCR cells each comprise roughly 50% of IEL (Lefrançois, 1991; Goodman and Lefrançois, 1989) and both of these subsets are present in ATXBM mice. Moreover, CD8$\alpha\alpha$ IEL, which contain $\gamma\delta$ TCR and $\alpha\beta$ TCR IEL and have been touted as the extrathymic IEL component (Rocha *et al.*, 1991), are produced in ATXBM mice but CD8$\alpha\beta$ $\alpha\beta$ TCR IEL are also generated (Poussier *et al.*, 1992). More recently, Rocha *et al.* (1994) showed that reconstitution of RAG2$^{-/-}$ mice with nude mouse bone marrow resulted in production of only CD8$\alpha\alpha$ IEL expressing either TCR type but in significantly lower numbers than found in euthymic mice. Furthermore, congenitally athymic nude mice contain ~5-fold fewer $\gamma\delta$ TCR IEL and few $\alpha\beta$ TCR IEL (Bandeira *et al.*, 1990; DeGeus *et al.*, 1990; Guy-Grand *et al.*, 1991). Taken together, these results suggest that the thymus is required for CD8$\alpha\beta$ IEL production and that it is involved in efficient production of all IEL. The reasons why ATXBM mice produce all IEL subsets is unclear but could be due to influence of the thymus on the intestine prior to thymectomy or due to effects of radiation on T-cell development.

*Essentials of Mucosal Immunology*

We have utilized neonatal thymectomy and thymus grafting as a means of studying the role of the thymus in IEL development (Lefrançois and Olson, 1994). In the case of thymus grafting, we tested whether the thymus is capable of producing IEL, rather than asking whether removal of the thymus affects IEL maturation. Overall, the results demonstrate that the thymus plays a dual role in IEL development: as a source of IEL precursors and as a source of as yet unidentified factors that aid IEL maturation.

## II. MATERIALS AND METHODS

### A. Mice

C57BL/6J, Balb/cJ, and CB6F$_1$ nude mice were obtained from Jackson Laboratories (Bar Harbor, ME). B6-Ly5.2 mice were obtained from Harlan. $\beta2^{-/-}$ mice were originally obtained from Dr. Rudolph Jaenisch (MIT) and are bred in our facility.

### B. mAbs

The following mAbs were used in this study: GL3, anti-$\gamma\delta$ TCR (Goodman and Lefrançois, 1989); H57.597, anti-$\alpha\beta$ TCR (Kubo et al., 1989); 3.168, anti-CD8 (Sarmiento et al., 1982); anti-CD4-PE (Becton–Dickinson, San Jose, CA); H35-17-2, anti-CD8$\beta$ (Goldstein et al., 1982), anti-Ly5.1 and anti-Ly5.2 (Shen, 1991).

### C. Neonatal Thymectomy

Within 24 hr of birth mice were thymectomized using suction according to the protocol of Sjokin et al. (1963).

### D. Grafting and Reconstitution Studies

Fetal and neonatal thymus lobes were grafted subcutaneously to adult nTx or SCID mice. B6-Ly5.2, C57BL/6J, or $\beta2^{-/-}$ (Ly5.1) mice were used as graft donor or recipient which allowed distinction between host- and graft-derived cells. IEL and LN cells were isolated 4–8 weeks after grafting and examined by fluorescence flow cytometry. Day 19 fetal intestine or fetal thymus (from B6-Ly5.1 mice) was grafted subcutaneously into thymectomized, irradiated (1100 rad) (Balb/c × B6-Ly5.2)F$_1$ mice that had been reconstituted with T-cell-depleted bone marrow from B6-Ly5.2 mice. Grafting was performed 3 weeks after reconstitution. For reconstitution of nude mice, (Balb/c × B6-Ly5.2)F$_1$ Day 13 fetal liver was injected intravenously into irradiated (1100 rad) (Balb/c × C57BL/6)F$_1$ nude mice.

## E. Isolation of IEL

IEL were isolated essentially as described previously (Goodman and Lefrançois, 1988). Briefly, the small intestines of individual mice were cut into 5-mm pieces and washed twice with medium. The washed intestinal pieces were then stirred at 37°C for 20 min in medium with the addition of 1 m$M$ dithioerythritol. This step was repeated, the resultant supernatants were filtered rapidly through nylon wool, and the filtrate was centrifuged through a 44%/67.5% Percoll gradient. The cells at the interface of the Percoll gradient were collected and prepared for flow cytometry.

## F. Isolation of LN Subsets

Inguinal, brachial, cervical, and mesenteric lymph nodes were removed and pooled and single-cell suspensions were prepared using a tissue homogenizer. The preparation was filtered through Nytex and the filtrate centrifuged to pellet the cells.

## G. Immunofluorescence Analysis

Lymphocytes were resuspended in PBS–0.2%BSA–0.1% NaN$_3$ (PBS/BSA/NaN$_3$) at a concentration of $1 \times 10^6$–$1 \times 10^7$ cells/ml followed by incubation at 4°C for 30 min with 100 $\mu$l of properly diluted mAb. The mAbs either were directly labeled with fluorescein isothiocyanate (FITC) and phycoerythrin (PE) or were biotinylated. For the latter, avidin–phycoerythrin (Av-PE) or avidin–Red 613 (Av-R613; BRL Life Technologies, Gaithersburg, MD) were used as secondary reagents for detection. After staining, the cells were washed twice with PBS/BSA/NaN$_3$ and relative fluorescence intensities were measured with a FACScan (Becton–Dickinson).

## III. Results and Discussion

In order to determine whether the thymus was necessary during early life for generation of IEL, mice were neonatally thymectomized (nTx). IEL and LN T cells were isolated 8 weeks later and analyzed for T cell receptor and coreceptor expression. Strikingly, $\gamma\delta$ TCR IEL were greatly reduced in nTx mice (Fig. 1). As expected, few mature T cells were present in lymph nodes of nTx mice. In addition to $\gamma\delta$ IEL depletion, a population of CD8$^+$TCR$^-$IEL was greatly increased in some nTx mice as compared to controls (Fig. 2). These results suggested that the thymus was providing signals to IEL or to the epithelium that were essential for normal $\gamma\delta$ and $\alpha\beta$ IEL maturation. The presence of putative immature IEL (TCR$^{low}$, CD8$^+$TCR$^-$), which are also present in nude mice, further implies that the later developmental stages of IEL were occurring in the intestine.

One interpretation of the result of nTx on the IEL compartment, particularly

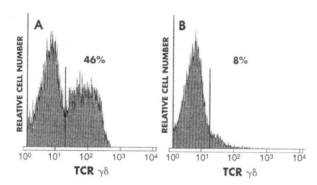

**FIGURE 1.** Neonatal thymectomy blocks γδTCR IEL production. C57BL/6J mice were sham-operated (A) or thymectomized (B) within 1 day after birth. IEL were isolated 20 weeks later and reacted with phycoerythrin-coupled GL3 (anti-TCRγδ). Relative intensities of individual cells were measured with a Becton–Dickinson FACScan. Gating using forward- and right-angle light scatter was used to include only the lymphocyte population based on staining with an anti-CD45 mAb (not shown). The bold vertical line in the histograms represents the demarcation between positive and negative staining as determined using an appropriately labeled irrelevant mAb.

with regard to γδ IEL, is simply that the thymus is the source of mature or immature IEL precursors (IELp). In order to test whether the thymus can produce IEL, we grafted fetal or neonatal thymus to immunodeficient hosts. B6-Ly5 congenic mice were utilized to allow tracking of graft- and host-derived cells. Grafting of B6-Ly5.1 neonatal thymus to B6-Ly5.2 mice resulted in production of a significant population of thymus-derived IEL (Fig. 3), as well as LN cells (data not shown). All $\alpha\beta$ TCR IEL subsets, including the so-called extrathymic subsets lacking Thy1 and CD8$\beta$, were generated from the thymus (Fig. 3; Lefrançois and Olson, 1994). In addition, γδ TCR IEL could be produced by the thymus. Although our original observations suggested that the early thymus could not produce γδ IEL (Lefrançois and Olson, 1994), the large number of grafted animals that we have now examined suggests that γδ IEL can be produced by the thymus from early fetal to neonatal periods. However, the production of $\alpha\beta$ TCR IEL by thymus grafts always outweighs γδ IEL production, sometimes exclusively.

The ability to generate CD4$^-$8$^+$ IEL from thymus grafts allowed us to determine whether intrathymic positive selection of IEL precursors (IELp) occurred (Fuller and Lefrançois, 1995). Thymus from B6-Ly5.2 MHC class I$^+$ mice was grafted to B6-Ly5.1 $\beta2^{-/-}$ mice, which lack MHC class I, and graft-derived cells were detected by expression of Ly5.2 (Fig. 4). Due to a lack of positive selection by MHC class I, $\beta2^{-/-}$ mice lack CD4$^-$8$^+$ $\alpha\beta$ TCR IEL and LN T cells (Fig. 4). Therefore, when grafted with MHC class I$^+$ thymus, if intrathymic selection of IELp occurs then we would expect to find CD4$^-$8$^+$ IEL and LN T cells in the grafted animals. $\alpha\beta$ TCR IEL from unmanipulated $\beta2^{-/-}$ mice contained 11% $\alpha\beta$ TCR cells and these were primarily CD4$^+$8$^+$ and CD4$^+$8$^-$ cells. Only 14%

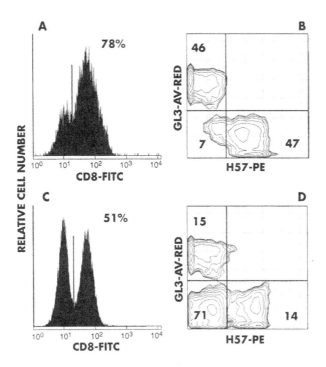

**FIGURE 2.** A population of CD8$^+$ TCR$^-$ IEL are present in nTx mice. IEL from sham-operated (A and B) or nTx (C and D) C57BL/6J mice were analyzed by three-color fluorescence flow cytometry for CD8, $\gamma\delta$ TCR, and $\alpha\beta$ TCR expression. Cells were reacted with 3.168-FITC (anti-CD8), H57-PE (anti-$\alpha\beta$ TCR), and GL3-biotin. The latter was detected with avidin-RED613 (BRL, Gaithersburg, MD). CD8$^+$ cells to the right of the bold vertical line in A and C were analyzed for $\gamma\delta$ TCR and $\alpha\beta$ TCR expression as shown in B and D.

of $\alpha\beta$ TCR IEL, which represented <2% of total IEL, were CD4$^-$8$^+$ and virtually all of these expressed the CD8$\alpha\alpha$ homodimer. CD4$^-$8$^+$ LN T cells were not detectable. These findings indicate that CD4$^-$8$^+$ $\alpha\beta$ TCR IEL required MHC class I for positive selection and conversely that CD4$^-$8$^+$ IEL did not. The latter result suggested that these cells either were derived from CD4$^+$8$^-$ IEL or perhaps were intermediates in IEL development. Thymus grafting resulted in an increase in $\alpha\beta$ TCR IEL to 60% of total IEL with the majority being graft-derived. However, graft-derived IEL, which were 90% $\alpha\beta$ TCR, contained only 5% CD4$^-$8$^+$ cells with the remainder largely CD4$^+$8$^+$ and CD4$^+$8$^-$ (Fig. 4). In contrast, the thymus grafts produced CD8$^+$ efficiently as well as CD4$^+$ LN T cells (Fig. 4). Similar results were obtained from analysis of many mice that have been grafted in this way. These results indicated that extrathymic MHC class I expression was necessary for positive selection of thymus-derived CD4$^-$8$^+$ IEL. Alternatively,

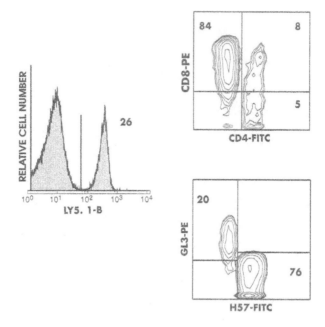

**FIGURE 3.** Neonatal thymus contains precursors for $\alpha\beta$ TCR and $\gamma\delta$TCR IEL. B6-Ly5.2 mice that had been neonatally thymectomized 6 weeks earlier were grafted subcutaneously with neonatal (<24 hr old) thymus lobes from C57BL/6 (Ly5.1) mice. Six weeks later IEL were isolated and reacted with mAbs specific for Ly5.1, CD8, and CD4 or $\gamma\delta$TCR (GL3) and $\alpha\beta$TCR (H57). The Ly5.1$^+$ cells were analyzed for either CD4 and CD8 (upper right panel) or $\gamma\delta$TCR and $\alpha\beta$TCR (lower right panel) by fluorescence flow cytometry.

extrathymic MHC class I is necessary for expansion of thymus-selected IEL upon arrival in the intestine. We are currently testing this hypothesis.

The controversy surrounding the involvement of the thymus in IEL development stems in part from apparently disparate results in ATXBM mice and nude mice. The former contain IEL, whereas nude mice have low numbers of $\gamma\delta$ IEL and few, if any, $\alpha\beta$ TCR IEL. The results from nude mice would suggest that all $\alpha\beta$ TCR IEL and a large portion of $\gamma\delta$ TCR IEL are thymus-dependent. However, there has been some discussion of whether the nude mouse is a good model of extrathymic development. This is due in part to the possibility that an early thymic rudiment may influence limited T-cell development. Additionally, with regard to IEL development, it is possible that the nude epithelial defect extends to the intestine. It is also possible that the absence of a thymus throughout life, as opposed to adult thymectomy, results in a long-term defect in nude mouse intestine that will not allow IEL development. In order to test this possibility we lethally irradiated and reconstituted nude mice with Day 13 fetal liver. Again, only donor fetal liver-derived cells were analyzed (Fig. 5). Small numbers of CD4$^+$8$^-$ and

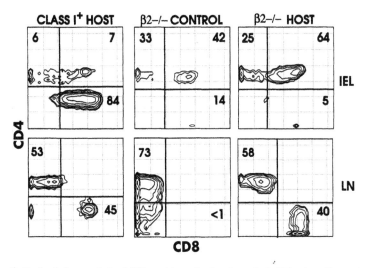

**FIGURE 4.** Lack of thymus-derived IEL positive selection in grafted $\beta2^{-/-}$ mice. Six-week-old nTx C57BL/6 or C57BL/6-$\beta2^{-/-}$ mice were grafted subcutaneously with B6-Ly5.2 neonatal thymus. LN T cells and IEL were isolated 8 weeks later and analyzed by three-color fluorescence flow cytometry with mAbs specific for Ly5.2 and CD4 and CD8. Populations were gated on the Ly5.2$^+$ subset and analyzed for CD4 and CD8 expression. In the grafted mice >90% of the donor IEL populations expressed $\alpha\beta$ TCR. For the $\beta2^{-/-}$ control the analysis was performed on $\alpha\beta$ TCR$^+$ cells.

CD4$^-$8$^+$ IEL were produced as well as a population of CD4$^-$8$^-$ non-T cells. Thus, TCR analysis showed that ~45% of IEL expressed either $\gamma\delta$ TCR or $\alpha\beta$ TCR. The TCR$^-$ population was not characterized further but contained ~15% sIg$^+$ cells. Therefore, a significant population of non-T, non-B cells was produced

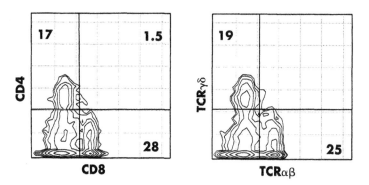

**FIGURE 5.** Reconstitution of IEL in nude mice. (Balb/c $\times$ C57BL/6)F$_1$ nude mice were irradiated (1100 rad) and reconstituted with $1 \times 10^7$ Day 13 (Balb/c $\times$ B6-Ly5.2)F$_1$ fetal liver cells. Twelve weeks later IEL were isolated and fetal liver-derived cells (Ly5.2$^+$) were examined for CD4, CD8, and TCR expression by fluorescence flow cytometry.

in these mice, which could represent IELp. These results indicate that the nude mouse intestine can support $\gamma\delta$ and $\alpha\beta$ IEL production, albeit limited. It should also be noted that in the absence of irradiation, no donor-derived IEL could be detected, despite the fact that few IEL are present in nude mice. This result indicated that IELp contained in fetal liver do not develop in the absence of irradiation in these experimental systems; this is also true for adult bone marrow IELp. This may be due to an inability to home to the gut in the absence of intestinal damage by irradiation, the production of radiation-induced factors that impinge on T-cell production, or a requirement for precursors to occupy the bone marrow for complete development. It should be noted that irradiation can induce immature thymocytes to differentiate to the $CD4^+8^+$ stage and can also induce $\beta$ TCR rearrangement in SCID mice (Danska *et al.*, 1994; Zuniga-Pflucker *et al.*, 1994). The potential untoward effects of radiation should be considered when discussing T-cell development in these model systems.

The ability of the intestine to act as a surrogate thymus has been suggested by experiments using ectopic intestinal grafts (Mosley and Klein, 1992). In that system, fetal intestine was grafted to irradiated, thymectomized, bone marrow-reconstituted mice. Curiously, 3 weeks after grafting with fetal intestine under the kidney capsule or subcutaneously, an apparently normal complement of CD4 and CD8 LN T cells appeared in these animals. T cells persisted in these mice for at least 11 weeks. Since the IEL compartment was not examined in that study, we sought to determine whether intestinal grafts could generate IEL. Our system was devised such that the source of all cells could be determined. Irradiated, thymectomized (Balb/c × B6-Ly5.2)F$_1$ mice were reconstituted with T-depleted bone marrow from B6-Ly5.2 mice. Three weeks later these mice received B6-Ly5.1 fetal intestine or fetal thymus grafts and 5 weeks after grafting IEL and LN cells were analyzed. Grafts were examined at the time of sacrifice and only mice in which the thymus or intestine grafts had obviously thrived were included in the analysis. Examination of lymphocytes for Ly5.1 and Ly5.2 expression simultaneously allows assignation of each cell to host, graft, or bone marrow derivation as shown in Fig. 6A. When ATXBM mice were grafted with fetal thymus, graft- and bone marrow-derived LN and IEL populations were detected. In LN, 15% of the cells were graft-derived and all expressed $\alpha\beta$ TCR (data not shown). Forty-five percent of IEL were graft-derived and the majority expressed $\alpha\beta$TCR, again demonstrating that the thymus can produce IEL. Neither LN or IEL from fetal intestine-grafted mice contained graft-derived cells, indicating that the fetal gut was not a source of T cell precursors. However, it is possible that gut-resident IELp were present in the graft but were unable to traffic out of the tissue following *in situ* development.

In order to determine whether the presence of thymus or intestine grafts directed T-cell development from bone marrow precursors, we examined TCR expression of the bone marrow-derived population (Fig. 6B). In fetal thymus-grafted mice, $\sim$11% of bone marrow-derived LN cells expressed $\alpha\beta$ TCR. This is a reasonable percentage given that complete reconstitution in a normal mouse generally requires at least 8 weeks. This analysis was performed 5 weeks after grafting, so

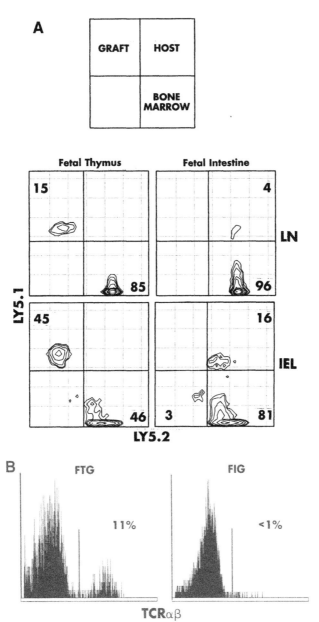

FIGURE 6. Fetal intestinal grafts do not support T cell production. (Balb/c × B6-Ly5.2)F$_1$ mice were irradiated and reconstituted with $2 \times 10^7$ T-cell-depleted B6-Ly5.2 bone marrow cells. Three weeks later, these mice received subcutaneous fetal thymus or fetal intestine grafts. Five weeks later IEL and LN cells were isolated and analyzed for Ly5.1, Ly5.2, and TCR expression by three-color fluorescence flow cytometry. (A) Expression of Ly5.1 and Ly5.2 on LN cells and IEL. (B) Expression of $\alpha\beta$ TCR on Ly5.1$^-$Ly5.2$^+$ LN cells from fetal thymus-grafted (FTG) or fetal intestine-grafted (FIG) mice.

the time until engraftment (i.e., vascularization) should also be taken into account. In contrast to the results obtained with thymus-grafted animals, no T cells were present in LN cells from fetal intestine-grafted mice (Fig. 6B). Thus, we find no evidence that ectopic intestinal grafts can direct T-cell development in the peripheral or intestinal lymphoid tissues.

The data now available indicate clearly that the thymus plays a pivotal role in IEL development. Removal of the thymus early in life disrupts severely the maturation and/or expansion of IEL subsets. This defect is long-term, indicating that although bone marrow contains IELp, such cells are unable to generate IEL in the absence of a thymus. However, thymus-derived IELp can repopulate the intestine in this system. Nevertheless, our results suggest that IELp may leave the thymus prior to TCR rearrangement and undergo positive selection in the intestine (Fig. 4 and Fuller and Lefrançois, 1995). Although arguments can be made against the use of the nude mouse as a model for athymic T cell development, in the case of IEL these mice may provide a valuable lesson. In the apparent complete absence of thymic influence due to a congenital defect, few $\alpha\beta$ IEL and low numbers of $\gamma\delta$ IEL develop *in vivo*. In models in which the thymus is removed during adulthood and the animals are irradiated and reconstituted, $\alpha\beta$ IEL and $\gamma\delta$ IEL develop. Thus, taken in the extreme, either the thymus provides factors that induce competence in the intestinal epithelium (or elsewhere) which subsequently allows IEL development, or the animal models employed are faulty. In any case, the main question that now confronts us is whether the unique developmental pathway of IEL provides the basis for specialized, organ-specific immunity.

ACKNOWLEDGMENTS

This work was supported by NIH Grants AI35917 and DK45260.

REFERENCES

Bandeira, A., Itohara, S., Bonneville, M., Burlen-Defranoux, O., Mota-Santos, T., Coutinho, A., and Tonegawa, S. (1990). Extrathymic origin of intestinal intraepithelial lymphocytes bearing T-cell antigen receptor $\gamma\delta$. *Proc. Natl. Acad. Sci. U.S.A.* **88**, 43–47.

Danska, J. S., Pflumio, F., Williams, C. J., Huner, O., Dick, J. E., and Guidos, C. J. (1994). Rescue of T cell-specific V(D)J recombination in SCID mice by DNA-damaging agents. *Science* **266**, 450–455.

DeGeus, B., Van den Enden, M., Coolen, C., Nagelkerken, L., Van der Heijden, P., and Rozing, J. (1990). Phenotype of intraepithelial lymphocytes in euthymic and athymic mice: Implications for differentiation of cells bearing a CD3-associated $\gamma\delta$ T cell receptor. *Eur. J. Immunol.* **20**, 291–298.

Fuller, B., and Lefrançois, L. (1995). Requirement for extrathymic class I histocompatibility antigens for positive selection of thymus-derived T lymphocytes. *J. Immunol.* in press.

Golstein, P., Goridis, C., Schmitt-Verhulst, A. M., Hayot, B., Pierres, A., Van Agthoven, A., Kaufmann, Y., Eshar, Z., and Pierres, M. (1982). Lymphoid cell surface interaction structures detected using cytolysis-inhibiting monoclonal antibodies. *Immunol. Rev.* **68**, 5.

Goodman, T., and Lefrançois, L. (1988). Expression of the $\gamma$-$\delta$ T-cell receptor on intestinal CD8 + intraepithelial lymphocytes. *Nature (London)* **333**, 855–858.

Goodman, T., and Lefrançois, L. (1989). Intraepithelial lymphocytes. Anatomical site, not T cell receptor form, dictates phenotype and function. *J. Exp. Med.* **170**, 1569–1581.

Guy-Grand, D., Cerf-Bensussan, N., Malissen, B., Malassis-Seris, M., Briottet, C., and Vassalli, P. (1991). Two gut intraepithelial CD8 + lymphocyte populations with different T cell receptors: A role for the gut epithelium in T cell differentiation. *J. Exp. Med.* **173**, 471–481.

Kubo, R., Born, W., Kappler, J. W., Marrack, P., and Pigeon, M. (1989). Characterization of a monoclonal antibody which detects all murine $\alpha\beta$ T cell receptors. *J. Immunol.* **142**, 2736.

Lefrançois, L. (1991). Phenotypic complexity of intraepithelial lymphocytes of the small intestine. *J. Immunol.* **147**, 1746–1751.

Lefrançois, L., and Olson, S. (1994). A novel pathway of thymus-directed T lymphocyte maturation. *J. Immunol.* **153**, 987–995.

Lefrançois, L., and Puddington, L. (1995). Extrathymic intestinal T cell development: Virtual reality? *Immunol. Today* **16**, 16–21.

Lefrançois, L., Mayo, J., and Goodman, T. (1990). Ontogeny of T cell receptor (TCR) $\alpha,\beta$+ and $\gamma,\delta$+ intraepithelial lymphocytes (IEL). *In* "Cellular Immunity and the Immunotherapy of Cancer" (M. T. Lotze and O. J. Finn, eds.), pp. 31–40. Wiley-Liss, New York.

Lin, T., Matsuzaki, G., Kenai, H., Nakamura, T., and Nomoto, K. (1993). Thymus influences the development of extrathymically derived intestinal intraepithelial lymphocytes. *Eur. J. Immunol.* **23**, 1968–1974.

Mosley, R. L., and Klein, J. R. (1992). Peripheral engraftment of fetal intestine into athymic mice sponsors T cell development: Direct evidence for thymopoietic function of murine small intestine. *J. Exp. Med.* **176**, 1365–1373.

Mosley, R. L., Styre, D., and Klein, J. R. (1990). Differentiation and functional maturation of bone marrow-derived intestinal epithelial T cells expressing membrane T cell receptor in athymic radiation chimeras. *J. Immunol.* **145**, 1369–1375.

Poussier, P., Edouard, P., Lee, C., Binnie, M., and Julius, M. (1992). Thymus-independent development and negative selection of T cells expressing T cell receptor $\alpha/\beta$ in the intestinal epithelium: Evidence for distinct circulation patterns of gut and thymus-derived T lymphocytes. *J. Exp. Med.* **176**, 187–199.

Rocha, B., Vassalli, P., and Guy-Grand, D. (1991). The V$\beta$ repertoire of mouse gut homodimeric $\alpha$ CD8 + intraepithelial lymphocytes reveals a major extrathymic pathway of T cell differentiation. *J. Exp. Med.* **173**, 483–486.

Rocha, B., Vassalli, P., and Guy-Grand, D. (1994). Thymic and extrathymic origins of gut intraepithelial lymphocyte populations in mice. *J. Exp. Med.* **180**, 681–686.

Sarmiento, M., Glasebrook, A. L., and Fitch, F. W. (1982). IgG or IgM monoclonal antibodies reactive with different determinants on the molecular complex bearing Lyt-2 antigen block T-cell mediated cytolysis in the absence of complement. *J. Immunol.* **125**, 2665.

Shen, F. W. (1991). Monoclonal antibodies to mouse lymphocyte differentiation alloantigens. *In* "Monoclonal Antibodies and T-Cell Hybridomas: Perspectives and Technical Advances" (U. Hammerling and J. F. Kearney, eds.), p. 25. Elsevier/North-Holland Publ., Amsterdam.

Sjokin, K., Dalmasso, A. P., Smith, J. M., and Martinez, C. (1963). Thymectomy in newborn and adult mice. *Transplantation* **1**, 521–525.

Wang, J., and Klein, J. R. (1994). Thymus–neuroendocrine interactions in extrathymic T cell development. *Science* **265**, 1860–1862.

Zuniga-Pflucker, J. C., Jiang, D., Schwartzberg, P. L., and Lenardo, M. J. (1994). Sublethal $\gamma$-radiation induces differentiation of CD4-/CD8- into CD4 + /CD8 + thymocytes without T cell receptor $\beta$ rearrangement in recombinase activation gene 2-/- mice. *J. Exp. Med.* **180**, 1517–1521.

# Chapter 16

# Intraepithelial γδ T Cell and Epithelial Cell Interactions in the Mucosal Immune System

Hiroshi Kiyono, Kohtaro Fujihashi, Masafumi Yamamoto, Takachika Hiroi, Michel Coste, Shigetada Kawabata, Prosper Boyaka, and Jerry R. McGhee

*Departments of Oral Biology and Microbiology, Immunobiology Vaccine Center, University of Alabama at Birmingham Medical Center, Birmingham, Alabama 35294; and Department of Mucosal Immunology, Research Institute for Microbial Diseases, Osaka University, Suita, Osaka 565, Japan*

## I. INTRODUCTION

The mucosa-associated tissues including the gastrointestinal (GI) tract are covered by epithelial cells which are situated along the intestinal crypt/villus axis and as such represent a dynamic continuum of enterocyte function. The intestinal epithelium represent a major surface of contact between ubiquitous environmental antigens of the GI tract lumen and the underlying mucosal immune system. Epithelial cells in the crypt of the villus are rapidly proliferating and are less differentiated (Cheng and Leblond, 1974; Quaroni and Isselbacher, 1985). In contrast, epithelial cells at the tip of villus are differentiated as matured cells possessing absorptive and digestive functions. It has been shown that intestinal epithelial cells express MHC class II molecules (Scott *et al.,* 1980; Bland, 1988) and can present soluble antigen to antigen-specific T cells (Bland and Warren, 1986; Mayer and Shlien, 1987; Kaiserlian *et al.,* 1989). These findings suggested that the epithelial cells could be an important antigen-presenting cell for controlling mucosal immune responses. Since a large number of CD3[+] T cells reside in the intestinal epithelium, it is logical to investigate molecular and cellular aspects of cell to cell interactions between intraepithelial T lymphocytes and epithelial cells for mucosal immune responses.

CD3[+] T cells situated in the mucosal epithelium are commonly termed intraepithelial lymphocytes (IELs). It has been estimated that one CD3[+] T cell can be found for every six epithelial cells (Ferguson and Parrot, 1972). Although IELs possess several unique characteristics when compared with CD3[+] T cells in other organized systemic lymphoid tissues, a most profound feature of IEL is the occurrence of high numbers of γδ T cells. Thus, it has been shown that 20–80%

*Essentials of Mucosal Immunology* Copyright © 1996 by Academic Press, Inc. All rights of reproduction in any form reserved.

of IELs expressed γδ heterodimer chains of T-cell receptor (TCR) dependent on the age, strain, and microenvironment (Bonneville *et al.*, 1988; Goodman and Lefrançois, 1988; Mosley *et al.*, 1991; Taguchi *et al.*, 1991; Fujihashi *et al.*, 1992). However, it is now generally agreed that approximately equal numbers of γδ and αβ T cells are seen in IELs isolated from young adult mice (Mosely *et al.*, 1991; Taguchi *et al.*, 1991; Fujihashi *et al.*, 1990). Despite the numerous attempts which have been made to understand thymic and extrathymic development of γδ T cells in murine IELs, very little information is currently available regarding the biological role of γδ T cells. However, it was recently shown that intraepithelial γδ T cells modulate growth and differentiation of epithelial cells (Boismenu and Havran, 1994; Komano *et al.*, 1995). Thus, these γδ T cells have been shown to produce keratinocyte growth factor which supports growth of cultured epithelial cells (Boismenu and Havran, 1994). Further, the disruption of TCRδ gene resulted in the reduction of epithelial cell turnover and the inhibition of MHC class II expression (Komano *et al.*, 1995). These findings clearly demonstrated the importance of cell to cell interactions between mucosal T lymphocytes and epithelial cells for the intestinal immune system. In this chapter, we summarize our recent observations which describe molecular aspects of mucosal γδ T cell and epithelial cell interactions via particular cytokines and their receptors. Further, we provide new evidence that mucosal γδ T cells can influence the CD4$^+$, αβ T-cell dependent IgA B-cell response.

## II. ROLE OF CYTOKINES FOR T-CELL GROWTH AND ACTIVATION

For the understanding of immunological function of intraepithelial γδ T cells, it is important to examine the interaction between cytokine and cytokine receptor(s) for γδ T cells. A large number of cytokines including IL-1, IL-2, IL-4, and IL-6 have been shown to influence growth, activation, and proliferation of T cells (Watson and Mochizuki, 1980; Mizel, 1982; Garman *et al.*, 1987; Grabstein *et al.*, 1987). Among these cytokines, IL-2 was originally described as a T-cell growth factor which can support T-cell development directly without a requirement for other interleukins (Watson and Mochizuki, 1980). Although IL-7 was originally named as a pre-B-cell growth factor (Namen *et al.*, 1988a,b) this 25-kDa interleukin has been shown to augment anti-CD3 and lectin-induced proliferative responses of mature T cells (Chazen *et al.*, 1989; Morrissey *et al.*, 1989; Armitage *et al.*, 1990). It was also shown that IL-7 play an important role in T-cell development since IL-7-specific mRNA was detected in murine thymus (Namen *et al.*, 1988a). In addition, IL-7 induced proliferation of fetal thymic T-cell precursors and thymocytes (Conlon *et al.*, 1989; Watson *et al.*, 1989; Fabbi *et al.*, 1992). Disruption of the IL-7 gene resulted in the 10- to 20-fold reductions of thymic and splenic T cells (von Freeden-Jeffry *et al.*, 1995). These findings demonstrate that IL-7 is an important growth factor for T lymphocytes. It has been proposed that IL-2 and IL-7 serve as complementary T cell activation factors for thymus-derived γδ T cells in addition to $\alpha\beta$ T cells (Okazaki *et al.*, 1989). Furthermore, a combination of IL-2 and IL-7 induced high proliferative responses in peritoneal γδ T cells isolated from *Listeria*-infected mice in the presence of peritoneal macrophages (Skeen and Ziegler, 1993). Taken together, it was of interest to explore cytokine communication pathways by IL-2 and IL-7 as an essential element for cell to cell interactions between intraepithelial T cells and epithelial cells.

## III. EXPRESSION OF IL-2R AND IL-7R BY MUCOSAL γδ T CELLS

It was originally reported that γδ T cells isolated from IEL are divided into two subsets based on the intensity of TCR expression (Tauchi *et al.*, 1992). When we isolated $CD3^+$ T cells from IEL of C3H/HeN mice for the analysis of γδ TCR expression, two distinct populations of γδ T cells were observed (Fig. 1). Forty to 50% of $CD3^+$ T cells were γδ T cells and contained approximately equal frequencies of $\gamma\delta^{Dim}$ (mean intensity of ~300) and $\gamma\delta^{Bright}$ (mean intensity of ~700) T cells (Table I). In order to characterize these two subsets of γδ T cells, $\gamma\delta^{Dim}$ and $\gamma\delta^{Bright}$ T cells were purified by flow cytometry. An aliquot of $\gamma\delta^{Dim}$ or $\gamma\delta^{Bright}$ T cells was then examined for the expression of IL-2 and IL-7 cytokine-specific receptors (R) since these two cytokines are thought to serve as complementary T-cell stimulation and growth factors (as discussed above). When the expression of these cytokine receptors was examined in $\gamma\delta^{Dim}$ and $\gamma\delta^{Bright}$ IELs, the former T cells expressed both IL-2R and IL-7R (Fujihashi *et al.*, 1996a). In contrast, $\gamma\delta^{Bright}$ T cells did not express receptors for IL-2 or IL-7 (Fig. 1). This finding was further supported by the analysis of mRNA expression for IL-2R and IL-7R using reverse-transcriptase PCR (RT-PCR). When RNA was isolated from intraepithelial $\gamma\delta^{Dim}$ or $\gamma\delta^{Bright}$ T cells, and examined for the respective cytokine receptor-specific PCR product, 700 and 302 bp of amplified messages which correspond to IL-2R and IL-7R, respectively, were found in the $\gamma\delta^{Dim}$ T cells but not the $\gamma\delta^{Bright}$ T cells (Fig. 2). These results provided new findings that $\gamma\delta^{Dim}$ IELs constitutively ex-

TABLE I

UNIQUE CHARACTERISTICS OF INTRAEPITHELIAL γδ T LYMPHOCYTES

| γδ T cells | Mean intensity of TCR expression | Cytokine receptor expression | | Cytokine-induced T-cell proliferation (cpm)[a] | | |
|---|---|---|---|---|---|---|
| | | IL-2R | IL-7R | IL-2 | IL-7 | IL-2 + IL-7 |
| γδ $TCR^{Dim}$ | 333 | + | + | 33,880 | 27,720 | 123,200 |
| γδ $TCR^{Bright}$ | 702 | − | − | 410 | 350 | 450 |

[a]The levels of [³H]thymidine incorporated in controls (cells only) were 308 ± 50 cpm.

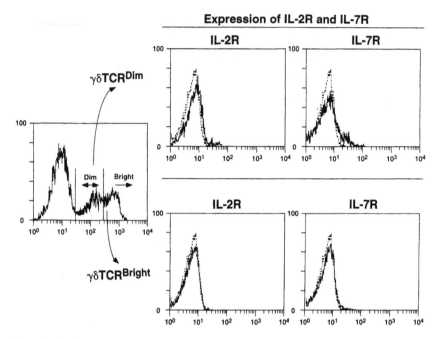

**FIGURE 1.** Expression of IL-2R and IL-7R on $\gamma\delta$ T-cell subsets isolated from IELs. $\gamma\delta$ T cells isolated from murine intestinal IELs were separated into two fractions based on the intensity of $\gamma\delta$TCR expression (e.g., $\gamma\delta^{Dim}$ and $\gamma\delta^{Bright}$ T cells). Flow cytometry analysis revealed that the $\gamma\delta^{Dim}$ T cells expressed both IL-2R and IL-7R while the $\gamma\delta^{Bright}$ T cells did not.

press both IL-2R and IL-7R, while $\gamma\delta^{Bright}$ T cells do not harbor either receptor (Fujihashi *et al.*, 1996a).

## IV. INDUCTION OF DNA REPLICATION IN INTRAEPITHELIAL $\gamma\delta$ T CELLS BY IL-2 AND IL-7

Since $\gamma\delta^{Dim}$ T cells express IL-2R and IL-7R (Figs. 1 and 2), it was important to test if this subset of IELs responds to exogenous IL-2 and/or IL-7. In the initial experiment, different concentrations of recombinant murine IL-2 (rmIL-2) (0.1–500 units/ml) and rmIL-7 (0.01–50 ng/ml) were added to the cultures containing CD3$^+$ IELs. Concentrations of 100 units and 5 ng per milliliter of recombinant IL-2 and IL-7 induced maximal proliferative responses. When splenic CD3$^+$ T cells and thymocytes from the same mice were tested under similar conditions, the former cells reacted to the high concentration of IL-2 (500 units/ml), while 50 ng/ml of IL-7 was also necessary to induce proliferative responses in cultures containing thymocytes. These results demonstrated that CD3$^+$ IELs were much more susceptible to stimulation signals provided by these cytokines than splenic

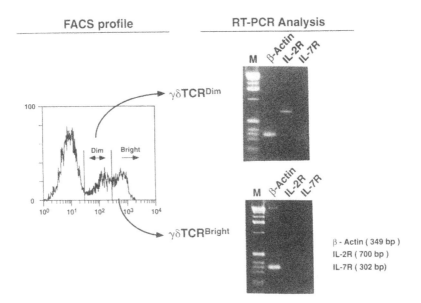

FIGURE 2. IL-2R- and IL-7R-specific mRNA expression by mucosal $\gamma\delta$ T cells. When RNA was isolated from FACS-purified $\gamma\delta^{Dim}$ and $\gamma\delta^{Bright}$ T cells and then examined by the respective cytokine-specific reverse transcriptase-PCR (RT-PCR), 700 and 302 bp of messages which correspond to IL-2R and IL-7R were only detected in the $\gamma\delta^{Dim}$ T cells.

CD3$^+$ T cells and thymocytes. When $\gamma\delta^{Dim}$ T cells were incubated with an optimal concentration of IL-2 (100 units/ml) or IL-7 (5 ng/ml), high levels of T-cell proliferative responses were noted (Table I). Further, cocultivation with IL-2 and IL-7 provided a synergistic effect for proliferation of $\gamma\delta^{Dim}$ T cells (Table I). On the other hand, $\gamma\delta^{Bright}$ T cells did not respond to either IL-2 or IL-7. These results indicated that intraepithelial $\gamma\delta^{Dim}$ T cells expressing IL-2R and IL-7R respond to exogenous IL-2 and IL-7 and lead to the high level of DNA replication and cell proliferation (Fujihashi *et al.*, 1996a).

## V. SOURCE OF IL-2 AND IL-7 FOR MUCOSAL $\gamma\delta$ T CELLS

Based on the results described above, IL-2 and IL-7 are essential cytokines for the activation and growth of intraepithelial $\gamma\delta^{Dim}$ T cells in mucosal epithelia. However, an important question regarding the source of these two cytokines in mucosa-associated tissues remains unanswered. One potential source of IL-7 for these mucosal $\gamma\delta^{Dim}$ T cells could be the epithelial cells. In this regard, it was suggested that the sources of the IL-7-specific mRNA could be thymic epithelial cells and/or thymic stromal cells, since the production of this cytokine by thymocytes was equivocal (Henney, 1989; Fabbi *et al.*, 1992). Our study further demonstrated that murine intestinal epithelial cells express IL-7-specific mRNA (Fujihashi *et al.,* 1996a). It was recently shown that human epithelial cells were also capable of producing IL-7 (Watanabe *et al.,* 1995). Taken together, cell to cell interactions between epithelial cells and $\gamma\delta^{Dim}$ IELs via IL-7 and IL-7R, respectively, could be an important cytokine communication for the activation of $\gamma\delta$ T cells in the intestinal epithelium. IL-2 produced by neighboring $\alpha\beta$ T cells in IELs would further augment IL-7-induced proliferation of $\gamma\delta^{Dim}$ T cells. Our recent results showed that IL-2 message was detected in intraepithelial $\alpha\beta$ T cells (Fujihashi *et al.,* 1996a). Further, our previous study indicated that CD4 bearing $\alpha\beta$ IELs are capable of producing IL-2 upon stimulation via the TCR–CD3 complex (Fujihashi *et al.,* 1993). Taken together, our findings suggested a triad of cell interactions among $\gamma\delta^{Dim}$ T cells, epithelial cells, and $\alpha\beta$ T cells through IL-2R and IL-7R expression, and IL-7 and IL-2 synthesis, respectively, for the stimulation and development of $\gamma\delta^{Dim}$ T cells in the intestinal epithelium (Fig. 3).

## VI. Regulatory Function of $\gamma\delta$ T Cells for IgA Responses

The mucosal immune system is a separate entity from the systemic immune system and is regulated by different subsets of lymphoid cells. As described above, the intestinal epithelium contains large numbers of $\gamma\delta$ T cells in addition to $\alpha\beta$ T cells. In addition, the lamina propria of small intestine also consists of higher numbers of $\gamma\delta$ T cells when compared with systemic lymphoid tissues (Aicher *et*

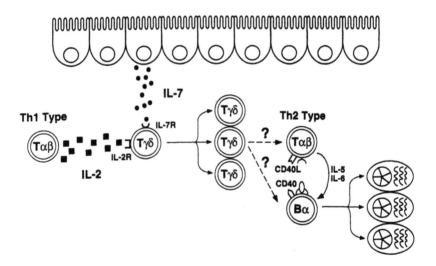

**FIGURE 3.** Two phases of triad cell interactions among $\gamma\delta$ T cells, $\alpha\beta$ T cells and epithelial cells for IgA B-cell responses.

*al.,* 1992). Despite the fact that mucosal $\gamma\delta$ T cells possess several unique features (Kiyono and McGhee, 1994), the immunobiological functions of this T-cell subset remain to be determined. Our previous studies have suggested that mucosal $\gamma\delta$ T cells are essential regulatory T cells for the induction and maintenance of IgA immune response under the influence of systemic unresponsiveness induced by prolonged oral administration of large doses of protein antigens (Fujihashi *et al.,* 1990, 1992). When $\gamma\delta$ T cells from mucosal effector sites (e.g., IEL) of orally tolerized mice were isolated and adoptively transfered to syngeneic mice with oral tolerance, the abrogation of systemic unresponsiveness was noted (Fujihashi *et al.,* 1992). This finding was the first indication that mucosal $\gamma\delta$ T cells possess an ability to regulate IgA responses. In addition, it was recently shown that $\gamma\delta$ T cells specifically downregulate antigen-specific IgE responses (McMenamin *et al.,* 1994, 1995). To this end, the $\gamma\delta$ T cells from mice or rats intranasally immunized with a 1% ovalbumin (OVA) aerosol selectively suppressed OVA-specific IgE responses. These findings suggested that $\gamma\delta$ T cells may play an important role for the downregulation of the IgE response in contrast to the upregulation of the IgA response.

Mutant mice lacking $\gamma\delta$ T cells have been produced by introducing germ-line mutations in the TCR$\delta$-chain gene (Itohara *et al.,* 1993). These TCR$\delta$-chain-deleted mice could provide a useful model to elucidate the exact role of $\gamma\delta$ T cells for the induction and regulation of mucosal IgA immune responses. Thus, we initially examined possible effects of TCR$\delta$ gene disruption by characterizing total numbers of IgM-, IgG-, and IgA-producing cells in mucosal associated and systemic tissues, and levels of IgM, IgG, and IgA titers in fecal extracts and serum obtained from TCR$\delta^{-/-}$ mice (Fujihashi *et al.,* 1996b). When the frequency of IgM-, IgG-, and IgA-producing cells were compared between spleen of TCR$\delta^{-/-}$ mice and their background strains [(129 $\times$ B6)F2], essentially identical numbers of IgM and IgG producing cells were seen. However, the numbers of IgA secreting cells in mucosa-associated tissues such as intestinal lamina propria of TCR$\delta^{-/-}$ mice were significantly lower than in control background mice (Fujihashi *et al.,* 1996b).

These observations were further confirmed by the assessment of fecal extracts and serum using isotype-specific ELISA. The level of IgA was reduced by approximately $\sim$80% in fecal extracts obtained from TCR$\delta$ gene disrupted mice when compared with normal background mice. In addition, serum IgA titers in TCR$\delta^{-/-}$ mice were also reduced. These results suggested that the depletion of $\gamma\delta$ T cells resulted in the reduction of IgA synthesis but did not affect IgM and IgG isotypes. It has been shown that $\alpha\beta$ T cells with CD4 phenotype producing Th2 cytokines (e.g., IL-5 and IL-6) are an essential T-cell subset for the induction and regulation of IgA responses. To this end, a significant reduction in IgA synthesis was noted in anti-CD4-treated and athymic mice (Guy-Grand *et al.,* 1975; Mega *et al.,* 1991). The CD4$^+$ T-cell-depleted mice harbored PP which were smaller with fewer germinal centers as well as low numbers of IgA-producing cells in the intestinal LP

(Mega *et al.,* 1991). Furthermore, our most recent and separate study showed that TCR$\beta^{-/-}$ mice contain almost no mucosal IgA-producing cells (Fujihashi *et al.,* manuscript in preparation). In order to maintain maximum IgA responses in mucosa-associated tissues, a triad cell communication among $\gamma\delta$ T cells, CD4$^+$ $\alpha\beta$ T cells, and IgA B cells may be a prerequisite (Fig. 3).

## VII. Summary

The results obtained by our study indicate that at least two phases of a triad of cell interactions are essential for the mucosal immune response. First, it was shown that epithelial cell-derived IL-7 and $\alpha\beta$ T-cell-secreted IL-2 are essential activation and growth signals for a subset of IL-7R- and IL-2R-positive $\gamma\delta$ T cells (Fig. 3). Thus, incubation of these intraepithelial $\gamma\delta$ T cells together with IL-2 and IL-7 resulted in high proliferative responses. For the second phase of cell interactions, $\gamma\delta$ T cells play an important immunoregulatory function for Th2-type CD4$^+$ $\alpha\beta$ T-cell-induced B-cell differentiation to IgA-producing cells. To this end, reduction of IgA-secreting cells was noted in TCR$\delta$ gene-disrupted mice. Thus, a triad cell interaction among $\gamma\delta$ T cells, $\alpha\beta$ Th2 cells, and IgA B cells is necessary for the maximum IgA responses (Fig. 3).

## Acknowledgments

This work was supported by NIH grants AI 35544, DE 09838, AI 18958, DK 44240, AI 35344, DE 08228, and DE 04217, by grants from the Ministry of Education, Science, Sports and Cultures and the Ministry of Health and Welfare, and by a grant from Asahi Chemical Co., Ltd. and Taisho Pharmaceutical Co. Ltd., in Japan. We thank Ms. Sheila Shaw for the preparation of the manuscript.

## References

Aicher, W. K., Fujihashi, K., Yamamoto, M., *et al.* (1992). Effects of the 1pr / 1pr mutation on T and B cell populations in the lamina propria of the small intestine, a mucosal effector site. *Int. Immunol.* **4,** 959–968.

Armitage, R. J., Namen, A. E., Sassenfeld, H. M., *et al.* (1990). Regulation of human T cell proliferation by IL-7. *J. Immunol.* **144,** 938–941.

Bland, P. (1988). MHC class II expression by the gut epithelium. *Immunol. Today* **9,** 174–178.

Bland, P. W., and Warren, L. G. (1986). Antigen presentation by epithelial cells of the rat small intestine. II. Selective induction of suppressor T cells. *Immunology* **58,** 9–14.

Boismenu, R., and Havran, W. L. (1994). Modulation of epithelial cell growth by intraepithelial $\gamma\delta$ T cells. *Science* **266,** 1253–1255.

Bonneville, M., Janeway, C. A., Jr., Ito, K., *et al.* (1988). Intestinal intraepithelial lymphocytes are a distinct set of $\gamma\delta$ T cells. *Nature (London)* **336,** 479–481.

Chazen, G. D., Pereira, G. M. B., LeGros, G., *et al.* (1989). Interleukin 7 is a T-cell growth factor. *Proc. Natl. Acad. Sci. U.S.A.* **86,** 5923–5927.

Cheng, H., and Leblond, C. (1974). Origin, differentiation and renewal of the four main epithelial cell types in the mouse small intestine. I. Columnar Cell. *Am. J. Anat.* **141,** 461–479.

Conlon, P. J., Morrissey, P. J., Nordan, R. P., *et al.* (1989). Murine thymocytes proliferate in direct response to interleukin-7. *Blood* **74**, 1368–1373.

Fabbi, M., Groh, V., and Strominger, J. L. (1992). IL-7 induces proliferation of CD3-/low CD4-, CD8- human thymocyte precursors by an IL-2 independent pathway. *Int. Immunol.* **4**, 1–5.

Ferguson, A., and Parrott, D. M. V. (1972). The effect of antigen deprivation on thymus-dependent and thymus-independent lymphocytes in the small intestine of mouse. *Clin. Exp. Immunol.* **12**, 477–488.

Fujihashi, K., Taguchi, T., McGhee, J. R., *et al.* (1990). Regulatory function for murine intraepithelial lymphocytes: Two subsets of CD3$^+$, T cell receptor-1$^+$ intraepithelial lymphocyte T cells abrogate oral tolerance. *J. Immunol.* **145**, 2010–2019.

Fujihashi, K., Taguchi, T., Aicher, W. K., *et al.* (1992). Immunoregulatory functions for murine intraepithelial lymphocytes: $\gamma/\delta$ T cell receptor-positive (TCR$^+$) T cells abrogate oral tolerance, while $\alpha/\beta$ TCR$^+$ T cells provide B cell help. *J. Exp. Med.* **175**, 695–707.

Fujihashi, K., Yamamoto, M., McGhee, J. R., *et al.* (1993). Function of $\alpha\beta$TCR$^+$ intestinal intraepithelial lymphocytes: Th1- and Th2—type cytokine production by CD4$^+$ CD8$^-$ and CD4$^+$ CD8$^-$ T cells for helper activity. *Int. Immunol.* **5**, 1473–1481.

Fujihashi, K., Kawabata, S., Hiroi, T., *et al.* (1995a). Interleukin 2 (IL-2) and Interleukin 7 (IL-7) reciprocally induce IL-7 and IL-2 receptors on $\gamma\delta$ T-cell receptor-positive intraepithelial lymphocytes. *Proc. Natl. Acad. Sci. USA* **93**, 3613–3618.

Fujihashi, K., McGhee, J. R., Kweon, M., *et al.* (1996b). $\gamma\delta$T cell-deficient mice have impaired mucosal immunoglobulin A responses. *J. Exp. Med.* **183**, 1929–1935.

Garman, R. D., Jacobs, K. A., Clark, S. C., *et al.* (1987). B-cell-stimulatory factor 2 (beta 2 interferon) functions as a second signal for interleukin 2 production by mature murine T cells. *Proc. Natl. Acad. Sci. U.S.A.* **84**, 7629–7633.

Goodman, T., and Lefrançois, L. (1988). Expression of the $\gamma\delta$ T-cell receptor on intestinal CD8$^+$ intraepithelial lymphocytes. *Nature (London)* **333**, 855–858.

Grabstein, K. H., Park, L. S., Morrissey, P. J., *et al.* (1987). Regulation of murine T cell proliferation by B cell stimulatory factor-1. *J. Immunol.* **139**, 1148–1153.

Guy-Grand, D., Griscelli, C., and Vassilli, P. (1975). Peyer's patches, gut IgA plasma cells and thymic function: Study in nude mice bearing thymic grafts. *J. Immunol.* **115**, 361–364.

Henney, C. S. (1989). Interleukin 7: Effects on early events in lymphopoiesis. *Immunol. Today* **10**, 170–173.

Itohara, S., Mombaerts, P., Lafaille, J., *et al.* (1993). T cell receptor $\gamma$ gene mutant mice: Independent generation of $\alpha\beta$ T cells and programmed rearrangements of $\gamma\delta$ TCR gene. *Cell (Cambridge, Mass.)* **72**, 337–348.

Kaiserlian, D., Vidal, K., and Revillard, J.-P. (1989). Murine enterocytes can present soluble antigens to specific class II-restricted CD4$^+$ T cells. *Eur. J. Immunol.* **19**, 1513–1516.

Kiyono, H. and McGhee, J. R. (1994) Mucosal immunology: Intraepithelial lymphocytes. *Adv. Host. Def. Mech.*, **9**, 1–204.

Komano, H., Fujiura, Y., Kawaguchi, M., *et al.* (1995). Homeostatic regulation of intestinal epithelia by intraepithelial $\gamma\delta$ T cells. *Proc. Natl. Acad. Sci. U.S.A.* **92**, 6147–6151.

McMenamin, C., Pimm, C., McKersey, M., *et al.* (1994). Regulation of IgE responses to inhaled antigen in mice by antigen-specific $\gamma\delta$ T cells. *Science* **265**, 1869–1871.

McMenamin, C., McKersey, M., Kuhnlein, P., *et al.* (1995). $\gamma\delta$ T cells down-regulate primary IgE responses in rats to inhaled soluble protein antigens. *J. Immunol.* **154**, 4390–4394.

Mayer, L., and Shlien, R. (1987). Evidence for function of Ia molecules on gut epithelial cells in man. *J. Exp. Med.* **166**, 1471–1483.

Mega, J., Bruce, M. G., Beagley, K. W., *et al.* (1991). Regulation of mucosal responses by CD4$^+$ T lymphocytes: Effects of anti-L3T4 treatment on the gastrointestinal immune system. *Int. Immunol.* **3**, 793–805.

Mizel, S. B. (1982). Interleukin 1 and T cell activation. *Immunol. Rev.* **63**, 51–72.

Morrissey, P. J., Goodwin, R. G., Nordan, R. P., *et al.* (1989). Recombinant interleukin 7, pre-B cell growth factor, has costimulatory activity on purified mature T cells. *J. Exp. Med.* **169**, 707–716.

Mosley, R. L., Whetsell, M., and Klein, J. R. (1991). Proliferative properties of murine intestinal intraepithelial lymphocytes (IEL): IEL expressing TCR $\alpha\beta$ or TCR $\gamma\delta$ are largely unresponsive to proliferative signals mediated via conventional stimulation of the CD3-TCR complex. *Int. Immunol.* **3**, 563–569.

Namen, A. E., Lupton, S., Hjerrild, K., *et al.* (1988a). Stimulation of B-cell progenitors by cloned murine interleukin-7. *Nature (London)* **333**, 571–573.

Namen, A. E., Schmierer, A. E., March, C. J., *et al.* (1988b). B cell precursor growth-promoting activity. Purification and characterization of a growth factor active on lymphocyte precursors. *J. Exp. Med.* **167**, 988–1002.

Okazaki, H., Ito, M., Sado, T., *et al.* (1989). IL-7 promotes thymocyte proliferation and maintains immunocompetent thymocytes bearing $\alpha\beta$ or $\gamma\delta$ T-cell receptors *in vitro*. *J. Immunol.* **143**, 2917–2922.

Quaroni, A., and Isselbacher, K. J. (1985). Study of intestinal cell differentiation with monoclonal antibodies to intestinal cell surface components. *J. Dev. Biol.* **111**, 267–279.

Scott, H., Solheim, B. G., Brandtzaeg, P., *et al.* (1980). HLA-DR-like antigens in the epithelium of the human small intestine. *Scand. J. Immunol.* **12**, 77–82.

Skeen, M. J., and Siegler, H. K. (1993). Intercellular interactions and cytokine responsiveness of peritoneal $\gamma\beta$ and $\gamma\delta$ T cells from *Listeria*-infected mice: synergistic effects of interleukin 1 and 7 on $\gamma\delta$ T cells. *J. Exp. Med.* **178**, 985–996.

Taguchi, T., Aicher, W. K., Fujihashi, K., *et al.* (1991). Novel function for intestinal intraepitheial lymphocytes. Murine CD3$^+$, $\gamma\delta$ TCR$^+$ T cells produce IFN-$\gamma$ and IL-5. *J. Immunol.* **147**, 3736–3744.

Tauchi, Y., Matsuzaki, G., Takimoto, H., *et al.* (1992). A new subpopulation of intestinal intraepithelial lymphocytes expressing high level of T cell receptor $\gamma\delta$. *Eur. J. Immunol.* **22**, 2465–2468.

von Freeden-Jeffry, U., Vieira, P., Lucian, L. A. *et al.* (1995) Lymphopenia in inerleukin (IL)-7 gene-deleted mice identifies IL-7 as a nonredundant cytokine. *J. Ex. Med.* **181**, 1519–1526.

Watanabe, M., Ueno, Y., Yajima, T., Iwao, Y., Tsuchiya, M., Ishikawa, H., Aiso, S., Hibi, T., and Ishii, H. (1995). Interleukin 7 is produced by human intestinal epithelial cells and regulates the proliferation of intestinal mucosal lymphocytes. *J. Clin. Invest.* **95**, 2945–2953.

Watson, J., and Mochizuki, D. (1980). Interleukin 2: A class of T cell growth factors. *Immunol. Rev.* **51**, 257–278.

Watson, J. D., Morrissey, P. J., Namen, A. E., *et al.* (1989). Effect of IL-7 on the growth of fetal thymocytes in culture. *J. Immunol.* **143**, 1215–1222.

# Chapter 17

# Lymphocyte–Epithelial Cross-Talk in the Intestine: Do Nonclassical Class I Molecules Have a Big Part in the Dialogue?

Beate C. Sydora,*·† Richard Aranda,†‡ Shabnam Tangri*·†‡ Hilda R. Holcombe,*·†
Victoria Camerini,†·§·1 A. Raul Castaño,¶ Jeffrey E. W. Miller,‖ Susanna Cardell,**
William D. Huse,‖ Per A. Peterson,¶ Hilde Cheroutre,*·† and Mitchell Kronenberg*·†

*Department of Microbiology and Immunology and †Molecular Biology Institute,
University of California, Los Angeles, Los Angeles, California 90095; ‡Department of Medicine,
Division of Digestive Diseases, UCLA School of Medicine, Los Angeles, California 90095;
§Department of Pediatrics, Division of Neonatology, UCLA School of Medicine, Los Angeles,
California 90095; ¶The R. W. Johnson Pharmaceutical Research Institute at Scripps Research
Institute, La Jolla, California 92037; ‖Ixsys Corporation, La Jolla, California 92037;
**Institut de Génétique et Biologie Moléculaire et Cellulaire, INSERM-CNRS,
Université Louis Pasteur, 67085 Strasbourg, France

This chapter focuses on the behavior and properties of nonclassical class I molecules expressed by mouse intestinal epithelial cells, and the possible role these molecules may have in the development and function of mouse intestinal intraepithelial lymphocytes (IEL).

## I. IEL DIFFER GREATLY FROM OTHER LYMPHOCYTE POPULATIONS

It has been known for many years that mucosal T cells, particularly those in the intestinal epithelium, have a phenotype distinct from that of other T-cell populations (Lefrancois, 1991; Camerini et al., 1993). A partial list of some of the markers and other functional properties that distinguish mouse small-intestinal IEL from T cells in spleen or lymph node is presented in Table I. IEL in the large intestine share some features in common with those in the small intestine, although there also are some significant differences between the two populations (Camerini et al., 1993; Ibraghimov and Lynch, 1994; Beagley et al., 1995; Boll et al., 1995). It is reasonable to suppose that intestinal epithelial cells are involved

---

[1] Current address: Division of Neonatology, Department of Pediatrics, University of Virginia, Charlottesville, VA 22908.

TABLE I

PHENOTYPIC AND FUNCTIONAL PROPERTIES OF MOUSE
SMALL-INTESTINAL IEL

| | Splenic T cells | Small IEL[a] |
|---|---|---|
| $\alpha\beta$ TCR | >95% | 50–60% |
| $\gamma\delta$ TCR | <5% | 40–50% |
| CD4/CD8 ratio | 2.5–3 | 0.1 |
| CD8 $\alpha\alpha$ homodimers | Not detectable | $\gamma\delta$ TCR: 90% $\alpha\beta$ TCR: 30–50% |
| CD4/CD8$\alpha\alpha$ double positives | Not detectable | Variable (4–30%) |
| CD28 | >95% | $\gamma\delta$ TCR: Not detectable $\alpha\beta$ TCR: 50–70% |
| CD2 | >95% | 10–20% |
| Thy1 | >95% | 40–50% |
| CD69 | <5% | 90% |
| CD62L (L selectin) | 90% | <5% |
| $\alpha_E\beta7$ | <5% | 80–90% |
| p150,95 | <5% | >90% |
| CD5 | 80% | $\gamma\delta$ TCR: Not detectable $\alpha\beta$ TCR: 50–70% |
| CD45RB[high] | | |
| CD4[+] | 40–80% | <5% |
| CD8[+] | 40–80% | 90% |
| Fresh cells are cytolytic | − | + |
| Activated MAP-K | − | + |
| TCR-induced proliferation | + (Vigorous) | ± (Limited) |

[a] Percentages for small intestinal IEL are only approximate, based upon the experience of the Kronenberg laboratory (Camerini et al., 1993, and unpublished data) and others in the field (Lefrancois, 1991; Rocha et al., 1995). The percentage CD2[+] IEL is for BALB/c mice; some other strains have a higher percentage of positive cells. The level of Thy1 expression is heterogenous, making the distinction of positive from negative cells difficult.

in part in the induction of the unique IEL phenotype. The recent demonstration that intestinal epithelial cells can produce several cytokines, either constitutively or following bacterial invasion (Eckmann et al., 1993), is consistent with the idea that epithelial cells are important for shaping the properties of IEL. Direct cell–cell contact, through expression of molecules like E-cadherin, which interacts with the $\alpha_E\beta_7$ integrin (Cepek et al., 1993), also is likely to be critical.

Intestinal epithelial cells may influence the phenotype and behavior of mature IEL residing in the intestine. In addition the results from some experiments suggest that IEL differentiate from immature precursors in the intestine itself (reviewed in Rocha *et al.*, 1995). There is also evidence to suggest that IEL recirculate little, if at all, once they are mature (Baca *et al.*, 1987; Poussier *et al.*, 1992). In summary, it is possible that the life history of many IEL, from the precursor stage to maturity, occurs entirely in the epithelial layer. If this were in fact true, then intestinal epithelial cells could influence the differentiation of IEL from immature TCR precursors, as well as having effects on more mature cells. IEL are complex, however, and they are likely to contain several distinct cell lineages. Evidence that some IEL can arise not from an extrathymic intestinal lineage, but from circulating, post-thymic T cells in the lymph node and spleen, comes from studies of the transfer of alloreactive thoracic duct lymphocytes into normal recipients (Sprent, 1976). Furthermore, when transferred to immunodeficient *scid/scid* (scid) mice, spleen and lymph node T cells can reconstitute the IEL population. We have employed this latter system extensively, in order to study the phenotypic changes that occur when lymph node or splenic T cells enter the intestinal compartment.

## II. LYMPH NODE AND SPLEEN CAN GIVE RISE TO IEL IN SCID MICE

### A. Expression of Homing Receptors and Activation Markers

The experimental system we have employed involves the intraperitoneal (ip) injection of $>10^5$ lymphocytes from spleen or lymph node into scid mice. The donor-derived lymphocytes are analyzed by flow cytometry and functional assays at least 6 weeks later. We employ a semisyngeneic transfer, in which lymphocytes from (C57BL/6 × BALB/c) F1 mice are transferred into C.B-17 scid mice. The F1 mice are H-$2^{b/d}$ heterozygotes at the MHC, while the C.B-17 mice are H-$2^d$, a congenic strain matched for BALB/c at most loci other than the Ig heavy chain locus.

   We have found that when transferred to scid recipients, unfractionated spleen and lymph node cells can extensively repopulate the host scid intestine, including IEL and lamina propria lymphocytes, with donor-derived T cells. In some but not all instances, the number of donor-derived T cells can be much greater than is found in normal, unmanipulated mice. It could be argued that this repopulation is largely artifactual, as a result of the "empty" lymphocyte compartment present in scid mice. Consistent with this hypothesis, the results from parabiotic mice suggest that T cells from lymph node and spleen enter the IEL compartment only in low numbers (Poussier *et al.*, 1992). A striking finding from these transfer experiments, however, is that the phenotype of the donor-derived lymphocytes is similar to that of some normal IEL subpopulations. In contrast to the original donor population, donor-derived cells that have colonized the intestinal epithelium have high levels of the activation marker CD69 and the integrin $\alpha_E\beta_7$ involved in epithelial cell adhesion. They also have low or undetectable levels of the lymph node homing receptor L selectin (CD62L), and they proliferate poorly in response to TCR-mediated signals (Sydora *et al.*, manuscript in preparation). These data suggest that normal, peripheral T cells did not simply fill the intestinal compartments in an aphysiologic manner.

There are small numbers of T cells in the starting population that express CD69 and $\alpha_E\beta_7$. It therefore is uncertain if the intestine is selectively inducing the expansion of lymphocytes from a preexisting subpopulation, or if it is inducing a phenotypic conversion in T cells that started out without expressing markers such as CD69 and $\alpha_E\beta_7$. The role of the epithelium in these processes of selective expansion or differentiation is likewise uncertain.

### B. CD4$^+$ T Cells Acquire CD8 under the Influence of the Intestinal Epithelium

It is noteworthy that scid recipients of lymph node or spleen cells have relatively large numbers of donor-derived, CD4/CD8 double-positive IEL. This is observed even when the starting population consists of sorted, CD4$^+$ single-positive cells (Fig. 1), similar results have been published by others (Morrissey *et al.*, 1995; Reimann and Rudolphi, 1995). The form of CD8 expressed by these double-positive IEL consists almost entirely of CD8 $\alpha\alpha$ homodimers (Morrissey *et al.*, 1995; Reimann and Rudolphi, 1995). These data argue for a true phenotypic conversion, at least with regard to this phenotype, rather than expansion of a preexisting cell population. The double-positive cells are detectable only in the epithelium of the small and large intestine; they cannot be detected either in the starting donor popu-

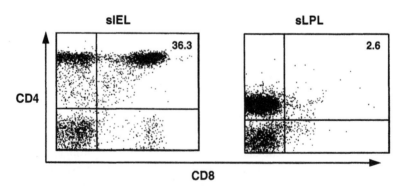

**FIGURE 1.** CD4/CD8 double-positive mucosal T cells originate from CD4 T cells. C.B-17 scid mice were injected ip with sorted CD4$^+$ spleen cells from (C57BL/6 × BALB/c)F1 mice, and the small-intestinal IEL (sIEL) and lamina propria lymphocytes (sLPL) of recipient mice were analyzed for K$^b$ (indicating donor origin), CD4, and CD8 by three-color flow cytometry. Following the dispase treatment needed to isolate LPL, CD4 and CD8 levels tend to be lower.

lation or in donor-derived cells that have homed to extraintestinal sites such as the spleen (R. Aranda, unpublished observations). In addition, there is a much higher percentage of these cells in the intestinal epithelium than in lamina propria (Fig. 1). Because this double-positive population is confined to the intestinal epithelium, these data strongly suggest that intestinal epithelial cells play an important role in the induction of CD8 expression by CD4 single-positive T cells, and/or in the selection of these double-positive cells. Because CD8 molecules are known to bind to the $\alpha 3$ domain of class I molecules (Salter *et al.*, 1990), these data further suggest that class I molecules could be an important element in the postulated cross talk between IEL and epithelial cells. The class I molecules responsible for any such effect may be either classical class I molecules or nonclassical class I molecules which also interact with CD8 (Teitell *et al.*, 1991; Sanders *et al.*, 1991).

## III. EXPRESSION OF NONCLASSICAL CLASS I MOLECULES IN THE INTESTINE

The hallmark of nonclassical class I molecules is their lack of polymorphism. Several nonclassical class I molecules are expressed in the intestine (Hershberg *et al.*, 1990; Bleicher *et al.*, 1990; Blumberg *et al.*, 1991; Wu *et al.*, 1991; Wang *et al.*, 1993). Some of these, such as the proteins encoded by the *T10/T22* gene pair, are expressed at the mRNA level in nearly all tissues (Ito *et al.*, 1990; Eghtesady *et al.*, 1992). For two nonclassical class I molecules, the thymus leukemia (TL) antigen and mouse CD1 (mCD1), the intestinal epithelium is a particularly prominent site of expression. For the TL antigen, the small intestinal epithelium is the sole sight where this class I molecule is expressed in all inbred mouse strains, although some inbred strains also express TL antigen on thymocytes and some other bone marrow-derived cells (reviewed in Teitell *et al.*, 1994). For mCD1, the results from immunohistochemical analysis indicate that intestinal epithelial cells are a major site of expression (Bleicher *et al.*, 1990). Although the results of Western blot analysis do not support this conclusion (Mosser *et al.*, 1991), Martin and colleagues were able to find mCD1 expression in Paneth cells (Lacasse and Martin, 1992). The remainder of this article therefore will focus on the properties of the TL antigen and mCD1, and our attempts to relate their unique properties and the expression of these molecules in the intestinal epithelium to the development of mouse IEL.

## IV. CD1 AND TL ANTIGEN STRUCTURE

Although the TL antigen and mCD1 are both nonpolymorphic molecules expressed by intestinal epithelial cells, from a structural point of view they are quite different from one another. The TL antigen is encoded in the *H-2T* region of the MHC, on chromosome 17, by the *T3^b* gene in *b* haplotype strains, and by the *T3^d* and the $T18^d$ genes in d haplotype strains (Chorney *et al.,* 1989; reviewed in Teitell *et al.,* 1994). The number and organization of *T*-region genes in the MHC of different mouse strains differ. Therefore, in mouse strains expressing haplotypes other than H-$2^b$ or H-$2^d$, the TL antigen is encoded by closely related (>95% sequence identity) alleles and pseudoalleles of *T3* and $T18^d$. It should be noted that the TL antigen, defined by a series of antisera and monoclonal antibodies, is quite divergent from several other *H-2T* encoded class I genes. Despite this, the products of some of these other genes, such as the *T10* and *T22* genes, unfortunately are sometimes also called TL antigens. mCD1 is encoded by a pair of closely related genes located on chromosome 3 (Bradbury *et al.,* 1991) (Fig. 1). The two genes, *CD1.1* and *CD1.2,* share approximately 90% sequence similarity for the $\alpha1$ and $\alpha2$ domains (Bradbury *et al.,* 1988; Balk *et al.,* 1991a). Both the TL antigen and the mCD1 protein molecules have the typical quarternary structure of an antigen-presenting class I molecule. They both form heterodimers at the cell surface in which a heavy chain of approximately 38–50 kDa interacts with the $\beta2$ microglobulin ($\beta2$m) light chain. The extracellular portion of the heavy chain consists of $\alpha1$, $\alpha2$, and $\alpha3$ domains, the $\alpha1$ and $\alpha2$ domains in the classical class I molecules form the groove in which the presented peptide resides (Bjorkman *et al.,* 1987a,b). The TL antigen has features which suggest that, like classical class I molecules, it could present nanomeric peptides. The conservation in the $\alpha1$ and $\alpha2$ domains is greater than 50% with classical class I molecules of the mouse, and those conserved class I amino acids that make hydrogen bond contacts with the peptide also are found in the TL antigen (Teitell *et al.,* 1994). TL antigen alloreactive T cells have been reported (Morita *et al.,* 1994). At this time, however, there is no evidence that definitively shows that the TL antigen can bind and present peptides. In contrast to the structure of the TL antigen, the mCD1 sequence does not show the presence of the conserved, class I peptide contact points, and mCD1 is rather distantly related to classical class I molecules in the $\alpha1$ and $\alpha2$ domains (Calabi and Milstein, 1986; Hughes, 1991).

## V. SURFACE EXPRESSION OF THE TL ANTIGEN AND mCD1 DOES NOT REQUIRE TAP

### A. A Peptide Transporter Is Required for Surface Expression of Classical Class I Molecules

In general, classical class I molecules can only be expressed in a native configuration at the surface of the cell if intracellular heavy chain has bound $\beta2$m and peptide has been loaded into the groove (Elliott *et al.,* 1991). The interactions of class I heavy chain with these two components occur in the endoplasmic reticulum (ER) of the cell before transport to the surface. Antigen processing occurs in the cytoplasm, and the cytosolic peptides generated by antigen processing are then transported into the ER for binding to class I molecules. This peptide transport is mediated by the transporter for antigen processing (TAP) (Monaco *et al.*, 1990; Spies and DeMars, 1991; Attaya *et al.*, 1992; Yang *et al.*, 1992). The TAP molecule is an ABC-type transporter, and it permits the ATP-dependent movement of peptides from the cytosol to the ER. The transporter is a heterodimer encoded by two genes, *TAP-1* and *TAP-2,* both located in the MHC (Monaco *et al.*, 1990; Spies and DeMars, 1991; Attaya *et al.*, 1992; Yang *et al.*, 1992). Cells which lack one or both of the TAP gene products are not able to express class I molecules at the cell surface at 37°C, although the peptide-free class I molecules in TAP-deficient cells are stable at lower temperatures (Ljunggren *et al.*, 1990).

## B. Analysis of TL Antigen and mCD1 Expression in TAP-Deficient Cells

We used TL antigen (*T18$^d$* gene) and mCD1 (*CD1.1* gene) expression constructs to transfect TAP-deficient cells, including TAP-2-deficient mouse RMA-S cells and TAP-1- and TAP-2-deficient *Drosophila melanogaster* tissue culture cells. Expression of the TL antigen and mCD1 was not reduced by culture at the nonpermissive (37°C) temperature when compared to the levels expressed following culture at room temperature (Holcombe *et al.*, 1995). Figure 2 shows results from RMA-S transfectants that express the TL antigen: surface expression of $K^b$ and $D^b$ molecules encoded by endogenous genes was significantly affected by culture at 37°C, while TL antigen expression levels were unchanged compared to the permissive, lower temperature. Similar results for the TL antigen have been obtained by others (Rodgers *et al.*, 1995). We also found mCD1 expression is TAP-independent in both RMA-S cells and insect cell transfectants (M. Teitell, H. Holcombe, A. Hagenbaugh, L. Brossay, M. J. Jackson, L. Pond, S. P. Balk, C. Terhorst, P. A. Peterson, and M. Kronenberg, manuscript submitted). The results of pulse-chase labeling studies support the flow cytometry data on TL antigen expression. The TAP mutation disrupted the normal trafficking of K and D molecules. In contrast, the TAP mutation in RMA-S cells did not alter the kinetics for the arrival of the TL antigen either at the Golgi apparatus or at the cell surface (Holcombe *et al.*, 1995).

The TAP-independence of TL antigen and mCD1 expression suggests that these class I proteins can be expressed as empty molecules on the cell surface, or alternatively, that they are loaded with peptide or some other ligand by a distinct pathway. It is logical to assume that invertebrate *D. melanogaster* cells lack any pathway specifically adapted for the loading of ligands into class I molecules, and therefore, that the mCD1 and TL molecules expressed on the surface or secreted by these cells are mostly empty. It remains formally possible, however, that some pathway, which is not specific for the loading of class I molecules, is used for loading mCD1 or TL antigen in these insect cells. An example of such a pathway is the TAP-independent generation of peptides in the ER by cleavage of the hydrophobic leader sequences from the N-termini of cell surface and secreted pro-

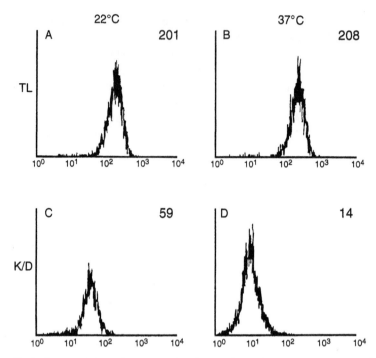

**FIGURE 2.** Surface expression of the TL antigen is not affected by the absence of TAP function. Staining of TL antigen ($TI8^d$) transfectants of TAP 2-deficient RMA-S cells for TL antigen and $K^b/D^b$ expression. Cells were cultured at the indicated temperatures, and the mean fluorescence units are indicated. Reproduced from the *Journal of Experimental Medicine*, 1995, 181, p. 1435, by copyright permission of the Rockefeller University Press.

teins (Henderson *et al.*, 1992; Wei and Cresswell, 1992), a process which takes place in all eukaryotic cells. We therefore carried out an extensive biochemical analysis of the soluble TL antigen/$\beta$2m complexes derived from insect cells. Bound peptides could not be detected by several methods including Edman degradation of acid-eluted purified TL antigen, which should have contained peptides, sequence of the entire TL heavy chain/$\beta$2m complex prior to acid elution, and mass spectrometry (Holcombe *et al.*, 1995). We conclude, therefore, that empty TL molecules, and perhaps mCD1 molecules as well, can reach the cell surface where they are stably expressed.

### C. What Might "Empty" TL Antigen and mCD1 Expression Mean for the Mucosal Immune System?

The TAP-independence of surface expression of the TL antigen and mCD1 distinguishes these nonclassical class I molecules from other class I molecules. This leads to the speculation that this TAP-independence, and the likelihood that these two nonclassical class I molecules can leave the ER and reach the cell surface without bound ligand, is somehow connected with the specialized function of these class I molecules in the mucosal immune system. There are several possible alternative speculations as to what such a specialized function in mucosal immunity might be. These are outlined in Figure 3. First, the TL antigen and mCD1 could be involved in sampling or uptake of luminal peptides for their ultimate presentation to cells of the systemic immune system by classical antigen-presenting molecules. For example, longer luminal peptides (symbolized by the adjacent black circles) could be taken up by mCD1, which binds long peptides (see below), and perhaps also by the TL antigen. These peptides could then be further processed in the epithelial cell to nonamers for presentation by classical class I (single black circle) or they could be represented by class II molecules. The peptides taken up by the epithelial cell in this way also could be transported across the epithelial cell into the lamina propria, and subsequently presented by either class I or class

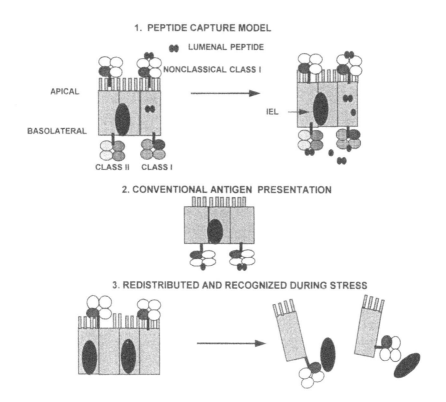

**FIGURE 3.** Models for the function of TAP-independent class I molecules in the mucosal immune system.

II molecules expressed there. This sampling or uptake mediated by either the TL antigen or mCD1 could play a role in the induction of immune responses, or in the induction of systemic oral tolerance to peptide antigens. If classical class I molecules are capable of presenting peptides originally brought into the intestinal epithelial cell by the TL antigen and mCD1, this would require the exit of the peptide from an endosomal compartment for entry of the peptide into a typical class I pathway for peptide presentation. Although this is not part of the standard model for class I presentation, macrophages have been shown to be capable of such a transfer, in that they can present endocytosed peptides in a TAP-dependent fashion (Kovacsovics-Bankowski and Rock, 1995). Peptide uptake for class II presentation also is possible, and it might make sense from a physiologic point of view, if the nonclassical class I molecules were expressed apically and class II molecules were not. In addition to expression on the apical surface, this model predicts a vesicular distribution of recycled TL antigen and mCD1 in the epithelial cells, following endocytosis of peptide–TL or peptide–mCD1 complexes. Second, the TL antigen and mCD1 might be more directly involved in antigen presentation to resident lymphocytes in the intestinal mucosa. More than 75% of the intestinal intraepithelial lymphocytes (IEL) are CD8 single-positive (Petit *et al.*, 1985; Lefrançois, 1991), and therefore most likely recognize peptide in the context of a class I molecule. It has been shown that the $\alpha 3$ domain of the TL antigen (Teitell *et al.*, 1991) and mCD1 (M. Teitell, H. Holcombe, A. Hagenbaugh, L. Brossay, M. J. Jackson, L. Pond, S. P. Balk, C. Terhorst, P. A. Peterson, and M. Kronenberg, manuscript submitted) can bind to CD8. In addition, the CD8$^+$ T-cell population in the intestine contains subpopulations that are specific to this site, such as the V$\gamma 5^+$ $\gamma\delta$ TCR$^+$ lymphocytes and the TCR $\alpha\beta$ T cells that express CD8 molecules composed of $\alpha\alpha$ homodimers instead of the more typical CD8 $\alpha\beta$ heterodimers (Jarry *et al.*, 1990; Lefrancois, 1991; Guy-Grand *et al.*, 1991). Together with the site-specific expression of the TL antigen and mCD1, this suggests that a subset of IEL might be TL antigen- or mCD1-specific. Evidence for recognition of human CD1d molecules by human CD8$^+$ IEL has been published (Balk *et al.*, 1991b), but a direct analysis of the specificity of mouse IEL is hampered by the extreme difficulty in growing IEL *in vitro* (Mosley *et al.*, 1991; Sydora *et al.*, 1993). This model does not have any particular requirements concerning the origin of the peptide or other ligand presented, or the intracellular distribution of the nonclassical class I molecule. It does require either a basolateral localization of the TL antigen or mCD1 on the cell surface, or a nonpreferential distribution in terms of basolateral and apical sides, as the IEL tend to be basolaterally located. Third, it is possible that the TL antigen and mCD1 function as markers of epithelial cell stress, and that the presence or absence of bound peptides or other ligands either is not required or is irrelevant to their function. According to this model, the TL antigen and mCD1 normally are located primarily apically, where they will be sequestered from basolateral IEL. Under conditions of stress or disruption of the epithelial cell tight junctions, apical TL antigen and mCD1 would be exposed to

IEL, which might have T-cell antigen receptors that are "hard wired" to recognize one of these class I molecules. Such a model is consistent with the view that $\gamma\delta$ T cells that recognize MHC are not dependent on bound peptides (Schild *et al.*, 1994). This model predicts an apical localization in normal epithelial cells and a relocalization under conditions of stress.

## VI. A STRUCTURAL MOTIF FOR PEPTIDE BINDING TO mCD1

### A. Bacteriophage Peptide Display Libraries Can Be Used To Determine Class I Binding Motifs

In an attempt to identify the structural requirements for peptide binding to mCD1, a bacteriophage peptide display library was screened with soluble mCD1 molecules. High levels of soluble mCD1–mouse $\beta2$ microglobulin complexes were produced in *D. melanogaster* cells (Castaño *et al.*, 1995). These mCD1 molecules were used to screen a codon-based, random peptide display library. Each M13 bacteriophage in the random peptide display library contains a different 22-amino-acid sequence at the mature N-terminus of the gene VIII coat protein. Forty-seven clones were selected from the library for their ability to bind mCD1. The alignment of the gene VIII N-terminal sequences of these selected clones shows a well-defined sequence motif consisting of an aromatic phenylalanine or tryptophan amino acid at anchor position 1 in 100% of the clones, an amino acid with a long aliphatic side chain (isoleucine, leucine, or methionine) at position 4 in 80% of the clones, and a tryptophan in position 7 in 75% of the clones (see Table II). Anchor position 1 could be found at a variety of positions in the 22-amino-acid sequence, most commonly at amino acid 5. These results suggest that mCD1 should have a peptide binding groove capable of binding the hydrophobic anchor

*TABLE II*

BINDING OF SYNTHETIC PEPTIDES TO mCD1 [a]

| Peptide | Sequence | $K_D$ | T-cell response |
|---------|----------|-------|-----------------|
|         | . . . .1 . . 4 . . 7 | | |
| p7 | ELWRNLRLWGYCMNLSNMPL | $9.3 \times 10^{-7}$ | Not done |
| p11 | LSFDWSELRRWGTWAAAEVFEL | $1.5 \times 10^{-7}$ | − |
| p18 | YEKPWQNLWDWGAEAFKDLID | $2.4 \times 10^{-7}$ | ± |
| p99 | YEHDFHHIREWGNHWKNFLAVM | $1.5 \times 10^{-7}$ | + |
| p99A1 | YEHDAHHIREWGNHWKNFLAVM | $2.0 \times 10^{-4}$ | − |
| p99A7 | YEHDFHHIREAGNHWKNFLAVM | $3.6 \times 10^{-5}$ | − |

[a] Anchor amino acids of the indicated synthetic peptides are in bold and the position numbers of the amino acids in the core binding motif are indicated on the top line. Cytotoxic T-cell responses of a line raised to a derivative of p99 are indicated. All data in the table are from Castaño *et al.* (1995).

amino acids of peptides. They further suggest that this groove, like that of class II molecules, might be open at the ends and therefore capable of accommodating longer peptides.

## B. Synthetic Peptides Bind to Soluble mCD1 Molecules

In order to confirm that binding of phage gene VIII fusion proteins in the display library corresponds to actual peptide binding, we carried out competition binding studies in which inhibition of binding of soluble mCD1 to $^{125}$I-labeled peptide p99 was measured. As can be seen from the data summarized in Table II, each of four synthetic peptides, which are derived from the sequences of different phage clones selected from the library, could compete for p99 binding. The calculated binding constants for mCD1 for these four peptides are approximately equivalent, in the range of $1.5-9.3 \times 10^{-7}$ $M$. Additional experiments using variants of the prototypical p99 peptide confirmed the requirement for the anchor amino acids, and for a peptide length much longer than the peptides that typically bind to classical class I molecules (Castaño *et al.*, 1995). For example, as shown in Table II, alanine substitution of anchor position 1 or 7 causes a drastic decrease in mCD1–peptide binding.

## C. Peptide or Nonpeptide Ligands for CD1

Recently it has been shown that human CD1b molecules can present nonpeptide ligands from bacteria, including lipids such as mycolic acids (Beckman *et al.*, 1994) and the lipoglycan lipoarabinomannan (LAM) (Sieling *et al.*, 1995). Direct binding of these compounds to CD1b molecules has not been demonstrated, although antigen presentation of nonpeptide ligands by CD1b is by far the most likely explanation for the T-cell functional studies that have been carried out. It is possible that the entire CD1 family of molecules is adapted and conserved primarily for the presentation of lipids. If this were true, peptide ligands capable of binding to mCD1 were identified only because the starting material used was a peptide display library. This hypothesis would require that the hydrophobic motif for mCD1 binding in some way mimics bacterial lipids, a hypothesis which lacks experimental validation at this time. Alternatively, it is possible that CD1 molecules bind a variety of hydrophobic molecules including peptides and nonpeptides. Finally, as suggested by others (Calabi *et al.*, 1989; Porcelli, 1995), there may be two categories of CD1 molecules. Type I molecules, including human CD1b, may bind primarily to lipids and glycolipids. Type two molecules, on the other hand, which include mCD1 and its homolog human CD1d, may bind primarily to peptides. In this regard, it should be noted that an evolutionary comparison of the $\alpha$1 and $\alpha$2 domain sequences of CD1 molecules justifies including the CD1d and mCD1-like molecules in one group and the CD1a, CD1b, and CD1c molecules in another (Hughes, 1991; Porcelli, 1995).

## VII. PEPTIDE-SPECIFIC AND mCD1-RESTRICTED T CELLS

### A. Peptide-Specific T Cells Are mCD1-Restricted

To assess the immunologic relevance of mCD1-peptide binding, we raised peptide-specific mCD1-restricted T-cell lines by immunizing C57BL/6 mice with mCD1 transfectants of the RMA-S cell line. The RMA-S transfectant cells were pre-loaded with a variant of the mCD1-binding p99 peptide (Castaño et al., 1995). Lymph node or spleen cells were removed from the immunized animals and re-stimulated in the presence of the peptide-loaded mCD1$^+$ RMA-S cells. In this way, several peptide-specific and mCD1-restricted T-cell lines were generated. The responding cells are $\alpha\beta$ TCR$^+$, CD8 $\alpha\beta^+$, and they require both surface mCD1 expression and antigenic peptide in order to respond to target cells. The response evoked includes cytotoxic T-cell activity (Castaño et al., 1995) and $\gamma$-interferon release (Table III). The results of three experimental approaches argue that the response is truly mCD1-restricted. First, partial blocking of cytolysis could be achieved with a rabbit anti-mCD1 antisera, but not with either control rabbit anti-sera or with mAbs specific for K and D molecules expressed by the target cells (Castaño et al., 1995). Second, recognition of mCD1 plus peptide is not MHC restricted: $b$ haplotype (RMA, RMA-S), $k$ haplotype (L cell), and $d$ haplotype (J774) targets that have been transfected with an mCD1 expression construct and pulsed with the appropriate peptide all can be recognized. Third, the reactive T lymphocytes can be stimulated to release $\gamma$-interferon by plate-bound mCD1 in the presence of the appropriate peptide, which plate-bound mCD1 alone did not stimulate (Table III).

### B. Peptide Bound to mCD1 Is Recognized by T Cells

We tested whether the mCD1-restricted T-cell lines were truly peptide-specific, or if they were just recognizing a conformational change in mCD1 that might be

*TABLE III*

PEPTIDE-SPECIFIC AND mCD1-RESTRICTED T-CELL RESPONSES

| Antigen presenting cell | Plate-bound CD1[a] | p99a peptide | $\gamma$-Interferon (units/ml) |
|---|---|---|---|
| RMA-S/CD1 | None | + | 63.8 |
| RMA-S/CD1 | None | None | 4.9 |
| J774/CD1 | None | + | 48.6 |
| None | + | None | 1.6 |
| None | + | + | 33.1 |

[a]Tissue culture wells were coated with the 7F11 mAb that recognizes the influenza virus hemagglutinin (HA), and then with soluble mCD1 molecules from insect cells that have a carboxyl terminal HA epitope tag.

caused by the binding of any peptide with adequate affinity for mCD1. We assayed a T-cell line raised against a p99-related peptide for its ability to react with mCD1⁺RMA-S targets that were loaded with either p11 or p18. The sequences of these peptides and the results are summarized in Table II. All three peptides, p11, p18, and p99, have a good anchor motif, although they have little other sequence in common, and the affinity of all three peptides for mCD1 is similar (Table II). Despite this, the p11 synthetic peptide did not stimulate the lytic activity of mCD1-reactive T-cells, while p18 had a low degree of cross-reactivity (Castaño *et al.*, 1995). In addition, when mCD1⁺RMA-S cells were first prepulsed with p11 and then given a p99-related peptide, the recognition of p99 presented by mCD1 was greatly reduced. The results provide support for the idea that all of the peptides bind to the same site on mCD1. In addition, they suggest that peptide–mCD1 recognition is similar to peptide–class I or –class II recognition, and that in addition to anchor amino acids that contact the mCD1 molecule, other amino acid side chains of the peptide may make important contacts with the mCD1-restricted TCRs.

### C. CD1 Autoreactive T Cells

An additional group of T cells in the mouse, those that express the NK1.1 surface marker, appears to be autoreactive for mCD1 (Bendelac *et al.*, 1995). Unlike the peptide-specific cells described above, NK 1.1⁺ T cells are either CD4⁺ or CD4/ CD8 double negative. This distinct population of T cells requires β2m but probably not TAP for its development (Adachi *et al.*, 1995). The NK 1.1⁺ T cells are selected by thymocytes or some other hematopoietic cells rather than thymic epithelium (Bendelac *et al.*, 1994; Ohteki and MacDonald, 1994; Adachi *et al.*, 1995), they express relatively invariant TCRs composed of a Vβ2, Vβ7, or Vβ8.2 β chain and a Vα14-Jα281 α chain (Adachi *et al.*, 1995), and they stimulate prodigious quantities of IL-4 following stimulation (Yoshimoto and Paul, 1994). It has been shown that several hybridomas from this population respond to CD1.1 transfectants, and that a bulk population of NK1.1⁺ thymocytes had a similar reactivity (Bendelac *et al.*, 1995). These data, combined with the relatively limited TCR repertoire of these cells, lead to the suggestion that most NK1.1⁺ T cells are CD1 autoreactive. It is not known if a particular ligand, peptide or nonpeptide, must be bound by CD1 for this reactivity to occur.

Cardell and co-workers have identified another group of seven mCD1-specific T cells by analyzing T-cell hybridomas made from the relatively small number of CD4⁺ T cells remaining in the periphery of class II-deficient mice (Cardell *et al.*, 1995). Some (>15%) of the residual CD4⁺ T cells in class II-deficient mice express NK1.1 (Cardell *et al.*, 1995), and like the NK1.1⁺ T cells described by Bendelac and co-workers (1995), seven of the large group of T-cell hybridomas derived from this population are apparently mCD1 autoreactive. The TCR V regions expressed by the CD1-autoreactive T cells are diverse, and they do not include the ones typical of the NK 1.1 population in normal mice. These data suggest that the population of $CD4^+$ and double-negative mCD1-reactive T cells normally is a complex one, containing cells that express a predominant TCR and cells that express diverse TCRs. Alternatively, the population analyzed by Cardell *et al.,* (1995) may for some reason only be found in class II-deficient mice.

## VIII. MUCOSAL LYMPHOCYTES SHOW UNIQUE REQUIREMENTS FOR THEIR SELECTION

### A. Expression of the TL Antigen and mCD1 Does Not Require TAP but Does Require β2m

The experiments described in the preceding sections show that the TL antigen and mCD1 do not require functional TAP molecules for surface expression. In addition they show that mCD1 molecules are antigen-presenting molecules that can present a class of peptides that are distinct from those presented by classical class I molecules, on account of both their length and their highly hydrophobic anchor motifs. Conspicuously absent, however, are any data showing that either of these molecules is important for the development of IEL. The difficulty in stimulating IEL to proliferate *in vitro* (Mosley *et al.,* 1991; Sydora *et al.,* 1993) has resulted in an inability to raise mouse IEL-derived cell lines of defined specificities. We therefore took a genetics-based approach to determine if nonclassical class I molecules are necessary for IEL development. Thymocytes from class I-deficient mice, including $β2m^{-/-}$ and Tap $1^{-/-}$ mice (Koller *et al.,* 1990; Van Kaer *et al.,* 1992), were analyzed for surface expression of nonclassical class I molecules by flow cytometry. By this assay, we found that expression of both the TL antigen and mCD1 is highly dependent on the presence of β2m (B. C. Sydora, L. Brossay, A. Hagenbaugh, M. Kronenberg, and H. Cheroutre, in press). Similar results were obtained when R1.E, a β2m variant of the $TL^+R1.1$ cell line, was analyzed for TL-antigen expression (Hyman and Stallings, 1976), or when these β2m-deficient R1.E cells were transfected with an mCD1 expression construct and analyzed for surface CD1 expression (M. Teitell, H. Holcombe, A. Hagenbaugh, L. Brossay, M. J. Jackson, L. Pond, S. P. Balk, C. Terhorst, P. A. Peterson, and M. Kronenberg, submitted for publication). In contrast, previously published data on human CD1d and mCD1 suggested that these molecules were at least partly β2m-independent (Balk *et al.,* 1994). This discrepancy may depend on the cell type analyzed, as the cells that did not require β2m for detectable CD1 expression include intestinal epithelial cells and melanoma cells (Balk *et al.,* 1994), while thymocytes clearly do require β2m for surface CD1 expression. In $TAP^{-/-}$ mice, the levels of TL antigen and mCD1 expression on thymocytes were not reduced compared to wild-type mice. This result also agrees with the results from the analysis of transfectants of TAP-deficient cells as outlined in Section V. In summary, unlike classical class I molecules, *in vitro* and *in vivo* expression of the TL antigen and mCD1 does not require TAP, although it either absolutely requires $\beta$2m (TL antigen), or requires it to a significant extent (mCD1).

## B. Some $\alpha\beta$ TCR$^+$, CD8$^+$ IEL Do Not Require TAP for Their Development

Given that the surface expression of the TL antigen and mCD1 does not require a functional TAP molecule, while surface expression of classical class I molecules does, we tested if the development of IEL is likewise TAP-independent. A previous analysis of IEL in $\beta$2m$^{-/-}$ mice showed that $\alpha\beta$ TCR$^+$, CD8 single-positive IEL were virtually absent in these mice, including those IEL that express CD8 $\alpha\alpha$ homodimers and those IEL that express CD8 $\alpha\beta$ heterodimers (Correa *et al.,* 1992). The numbers of $\gamma\delta$ TCR$^+$, CD8$^+$ IEL were not affected in $\beta$2m$^{-/-}$ mice (Correa *et al.,* 1992). If some $\alpha\beta$ TCR$^+$ CD8 single-positive IEL depend on either the TL antigen or mCD1 for their development, then they should be present in TAP-deficient mice. This is exactly what was found (B. C. Sydora, L. Brossay, A. Hagenbaugh, M. Kronenberg, and H. Cheroute, in press). As shown in Table IV, in the lymph node of either $\beta$2m$^{-/-}$ or TAP$^{-/-}$ mice, appreciable numbers of CD8-positive T cells cannot be found. In contrast, there is a significant population of $\alpha\beta$ TCR$^+$, CD8 single-positive IEL only in the TAP-deficient mice, but not in $\beta$2m-deficient mice. Compared to control mice, TAP$^{-/-}$ mice have 16% the normal number of $\alpha\beta$ TCR$^+$, CD8 single-positive IEL, while $\beta$2m$^{-/-}$ mice have 1% the normal number (B. C. Sydora, L. Brossay, A. Hagenbaugh, M. Kronenberg, and H. Cheroute, in press). These TAP-independent IEL are predominantly but not exclusively CD8 $\alpha\alpha^+$, and they express a diverse repertoire of TCRs not enriched for those V$\beta$ genes characteristic of the mCD1-autoreactive NK1.1$^+$ T-cell population.

These data implicate a requirement for either TL antigen or mCD1 expression for the development of IEL. There are, however, alternative interpretations for the presence of $\alpha\beta$ TCR$^+$, CD8 single-positive IEL in TAP-deficient mice. For exam-

*TABLE IV*

T-CELL POPULATIONS IN CLASS I-DEFICIENT MICE

| Mouse Strain | $\alpha\beta$ TCR$^+$, CD8$^+$ | | $\gamma\delta$TCR+ IEL |
|---|---|---|---|
| | Lymph node | IEL | |
| Control ($n=5$) | $20 \pm 3$ | $31 \pm 2$ | $35 \pm 9$ |
| $\beta$2m$^{-/-}$ ($n=5$) | $0.3 \pm 0.2$ | $1 \pm 1$ | $54 \pm 6$ |
| TAP$^{-/-}$ ($n=7$) | $0.8 \pm 0.2$ | $7 \pm 2$ | $45 \pm 9$ |

*Note.* The percentage positive cells for the indicated populations, $\pm$ standard deviation, is indicated.

ple, the positive selection of IEL might require only very low levels of classical class I molecule expression. Using flow cytometry, we could not detect surface expression of $K^b$ on cells from either mutant mouse strain, but there are some data suggesting that the level of expression is slightly higher in TAP$^{-/-}$ mice than in $\beta2m^{-/-}$ mice. It also could be hypothesized that the level of class I expression is less critical for IEL development than the type of peptides or other ligands bound. For example, the selection of IEL could be dependent on peptides loaded into classical class I molecules by a TAP-independent pathway, such as the cleavage of hydrophobic leader peptides in the ER (Henderson *et al.*, 1992; Wei and Cresswell, 1992).

### C. Do Double-Positive IEL Require Class I Molecules?

A second, striking result from comparison of the IEL in $\beta2m^{-/-}$ and TAP$^{-/-}$ mice came from analysis of the $\alpha\beta$ TCR$^+$ CD4/CD8 double-positive population. This population was unaffected by the TAP mutation, but surprisingly, the numbers of CD4/CD8 double-positive cells were reduced 10-fold in $\beta2m^{-/-}$ mice. The double positives may be precursors of mature single-positive IEL which are developing in the gut. In this case, by analogy with the double-positive thymocytes, one would not predict that the either $\beta2m$ or TAP deficiency would have an effect on double-positive IEL number. However, if precursors are being selected in the intestine, different rules may apply than for the thymus. A second view holds that the double-positive IEL arise from conventional, thymus-derived, CD4$^+$ single-positive T cells that have homed to the gut and acquired CD8 under the influence of the intestinal milieu. Consistent with this, as noted above, some CD4 single-positive T cells acquire CD8 $\alpha\alpha$ homodimers in the intestinal epithelium following transfer to scid recipients (Morrissey *et al.*, 1995; Reimann and Rudolphi, 1995). It is not known why the absence of $\beta2m$ but not the absence of TAP would have an effect on the number of these cells, although it is possible that interaction of CD8 $\alpha\alpha$ with TAP-independent class I molecules in the gut gives the double-positive IEL a signal that increases their survival time or time of residence in the intestine.

### IX. CONCLUSIONS

In summary, IEL have a phenotype that is distinct from other T-cell populations, and these lymphocytes may be the product of a separate, thymus-independent lineage. If such a lineage exists, it would be likely that the intestinal epithelium plays a major role in its development. It is also possible, however, that some IEL are derived from thymus-derived T cells. This is evidenced by the ability of conventional CD4$^+$ cells to home to the gut epithelium in scid mice, and to acquire characteristics of the T cells that normally reside in the intestine. The acquisition of some markers by these cells, such as the expression of CD8 $\alpha\alpha$ homodimers, is highly specific to IEL, implicating a role for the epithelial cells in inducing this phenotypic change in T cells. It is reasonable to speculate that class I molecules in the gut may play a role in the induction or the selection of gut cells expressing CD8.

We have shown that nonpolymorphic class I molecules expressed in the intestine have unique properties, most notably, their lack of a requirement for TAP in order to be expressed on the cell surface. This lack of a TAP requirement may provide some insight into the specialized function of the TL antigen and mCD1 in the mucosal immune system. We also have demonstrated that mCD1 can function as an antigen-presenting molecule, and that it presents peptide antigens distinct from those presented by classical class I molecules.

Evidence that the TL antigen and/or mCD1 are important restriction elements for IEL is only indirect, and as discussed in Section V, these class I molecules could have other functions, such as transport of luminal peptides into epithelial cells, or they could be recognized directly in a peptide-independent fashion by $\gamma\delta$ IEL or some other population. It is notable that a population of $\alpha\beta$ TCR$^+$ CD8 single-positive IEL requires $\beta$2m but not TAP, similar to the requirements for surface expression of the TL antigen and mCD1. These data definitively establish that the requirements for the selection and/or accumulation of these $\alpha\beta$ TCR$^+$ CD8 IEL in the intestine are distinct from those for other $\alpha\beta$ TCR$^+$, CD8 populations in spleen and lymph node. In addition, although only correlative, the data strongly implicate a role for nonclassical class I molecules in the development of these IEL.

## ACKNOWLEDGMENTS

We thank Mr. David Ng for help with the preparation of the manuscript. Supported by National Institutes of Health Grants RO1 CA52511 (M.K. and H.C.), PO1 DK46763 (M.K. and R.A.), K11 AI 01213 (H.R.H.), a grant from the Crohn's and Colitis Foundation of America (B.C.S.), grants from the Jonsson Cancer Center Foundation and the Jaye Haddad Foundation (S.T.), a grant from the Ministerio de Educación y Ciencia of Spain (A.R.C.), and the Swedish Natural Science Research Council (S.C.).

## REFERENCES

Adachi, Y., Koseki, H., Zijlstra, M., and Taniguchi, M. (1995). Positive selection of invariant V$\alpha$ 14$^+$ T cells by non-major histocompatibility complex-encoded class I-like molecules expressed on bone marrow-derived cells. *Proc. Natl. Acad. Sci. U.S.A.* **92,** 1200–1204.

Attaya, M., Jameson, S., Martinez, C. K., Hermel, E., Aldrich, C., Forman, J., Lindahl, K. F., Bevan, M. J., and Monaco, J. J. (1992). Ham-2 corrects the class I antigen-processing defect in RMA-S cells. *Nature (London)* **355,** 647–649.

Baca, M. E., Mowat, A. M., MacKenzie, S., and Parrott, D. M. (1987). Functional characteristics of intraepithelial lymphocytes from mouse small intestine. III. Inability of intraepithelial lymphocytes to induce a systemic graft-versus-host reaction is because of failure to migrate. *Gut* **28,** 1267–1274.

Balk, S. P., Bleicher, P. A., and Terhorst, C. (1991a). Isolation and expression of cDNA encoding the murine homologues of CD1. *J. Immunol.* **146,** 768–774.

Balk, S. P., Ebert, E. C., Blumenthal, R. L., McDermott, F. V., Wucherpfennig, K. W., Landau, S. B., and Blumberg, R. S. (1991b). Oligoclonal expansion and CD1 recognition by human intestinal intraepithelial lymphocytes. *Science* **253**, 1411–1415.

Balk, S. P., Burke, S., Polischuk, J. E., Frantz, M. E., Yang, L., Porcelli, S., Colgan, S. P., and Blumberg, R. S. (1994). Beta 2-microglobulin-independent MHC class Ib molecule expressed by human intestinal epithelium. *Science* **265**, 259–262.

Beagley, K. W., Fujihashi, K., Lagoo, A. S., Lagoo-Deenadaylan, S., Black, C. A., Murray, A. M., Sharmanov, A. T., Yamamoto, M., McGhee, J. R., and Elson, C. O. (1995). Differences in intraepithelial lymphocyte T cell subsets isolated from murine small versus large intestine. *J. Immunol.* **154**, 5611–5619.

Beckman, E., Porcelli, S. A., Morita, C. T., Behar, S. M., Furlong, S. T., and Brenner, M. B. (1994). Recognition of a lipid antigen by CD1-restricted $\alpha\beta^+$ T cells. *Nature (London)* **372**, 691–694.

Bendelac, A., Killeen, N., Littman, D. R., and Schwartz, R. H. (1994). A subset of CD4$^+$ thymocytes selected by MHC class I molecules. *Science* **263**, 1774–1778.

Bendelac, A., Lantz, O., Quimby, M. E., Yewdell, J. W., Bennink, J. R., and Brutkiewicz, R. R. (1995). CD1 recognition by mouse NK1$^+$ T lymphocytes. *Science* **268**, 863–865.

Bjorkman, P. J., Saper, M. A., Samraoui, B., Bennett, W. S., Strominger, J. L., and Wiley, D. C. (1987a). Structure of the human class I histocompatibility antigen, HLA-A2. *Nature (London)* **329**, 506–512.

Bjorkman, P. J., Saper, M. A., Samraoui, B., Bennett, W. S., Strominger, J. L., and Wiley, D. C. (1987b). The foreign antigen binding site and T cell recognition regions of class I histocompatibility antigens. *Nature (London)* **329**, 512–518.

Bleicher, P. A., Balk, S. P., Hagen, S. J., Blumberg, R. S., Flotte, T. J., and Terhorst, C. (1990). Expression of murine CD1 on gastrointestinal epithelium. *Science* **250**, 679–682.

Blumberg, R. S., Terhorst, C., Bleicher, P., McDermott, F. V., Allan, C. H., Landau, S. B., Trier, J. S., and Balk, S. P. (1991). Expression of a nonpolymorphic MHC class I-like molecule, CD1D, by human intestinal epithelial cells. *J. Immunol.* **147**, 2518–2524.

Boll, G., Rudolphi, A., Spiess, S., and Reimann, J. (1995). Regional specialization of intraepithelial T cells in the murine small and large intestine. *Scand. J. Immunol.* **41**, 103–113.

Bradbury, A., Belt, K. T., Neri, T. M., Milstein, C., and Calabi, F. (1988). Mouse CD1 is distinct from and co-exists with TL in the same thymus. *EMBO J.* **7**, 3081–3086.

Bradbury, A., Milstein, C., and Kozak, C. A. (1991). Chromosomal localization of Cd1d genes in the mouse. *Somatic Cell Mol. Genet.* **17**, 93–96.

Calabi, F., and Milstein, C. (1986). A novel family of human major histocompatibility complex-related genes not mapping to chromosome 6. *Nature (London)* **323**, 540–543.

Calabi, F., Jarvis, J. M., Martin, L., and Milstein, C. (1989). Two classes of CD1 genes. *Eur. J. Immunol.* **19**, 285–292.

Camerini, V., Panwala, C., and Kronenberg, M. (1993). Regional specialization of the mucosal immune system. Intraepithelial lymphocytes of the large intestine have a different phenotype and function than those of the small intestine. *J. Immunol.* **151**, 1765–1776.

Cardell, S., Tangri, S., Chan, S., Kronenberg, M., Benoist, C., and Mathis, D. (1995). CD1-restricted CD4$^+$ T cells in Major Histocompatibility Complex Class II-deficient mice. *J. Exp. Med.* **182**, 993–1004.

Castaño, A. R., Tangri, S., Miller, J. E., Holcombe, H. R., Jackson, M. R., Huse, W. D., Kronenberg, M., and Peterson, P. A. (1995). Peptide binding and presentation by mouse CD1. *Science* **269**, 223–226.

Cepek, K. L., Parker, C. M., Madara, J. L., and Brenner, M. B. (1993). Integrin alpha E beta 7 mediates adhesion of T lymphocytes to epithelial cells. *J. Immunol.* **150**, 3459–3470.

Chorney, M. J., Mashimo, H., Bushkin, Y., and Nathenson, S. G. (1989). Characterization of the thymus leukemia (TL) product encoded by the BALB/c T3c gene by DNA-mediated gene transfer. Comparison to the T13c product and BALB/c leukemia TL. *J. Immunol.* **143**, 3762–3768.

Correa, I., Bix, M., Liao, N. S., Zijlstra, M., Jaenisch, R., and Raulet, D. (1992). Most gamma delta T cells develop normally in beta 2-microglobulin-deficient mice. *Proc. Natl. Acad. Sci. U.S.A.* **89,** 653–657.

Eckmann, L., Kagnoff, M. F., and Fierer, J. (1993). Epithelial cells secrete the chemokine interleukin-8 in response to bacterial entry. *Infect. Immun.* **61,** 4569–4574.

Eghtesady, P., Brorson, K. A., Cheroutre, H., Tigelaar, R. E., Hood, L., and Kronenberg, M. (1992). Expression of mouse T1a region class I genes in tissues enriched for gamma delta cells. *Immunogenetics* **36,** 377–388.

Elliott, T., Cerundolo, V., Elvin, J., and Townsend, A. (1991). Peptide-induced conformational change of the class I heavy chain. *Nature (London)* **351,** 402–406.

Guy-Grand, D., Cerf-Bensussan, N., Malissen, B., Malassis-Seris, M., Briottet, C., and Vassalli, P. (1991). Two gut intraepithelial CD8⁺ lymphocyte populations with different T cell receptors: a role for the gut epithelium in T cell differentiation. *J. Exp. Med.* **173,** 471–481.

Henderson, R. A., Michel, H., Sakaguchi, K., Shabanowitz, J., Appella, E., Hunt, D. F., and Engelhard, V. H. (1992). HLA-A2.1-associated peptides from a mutant cell line: a second pathway of antigen presentation. *Science* **255,** 1264–1266.

Hershberg, R., Eghtesady, P., Sydora, B., Brorson, K., Cheroutre, H., Modlin, R., and Kronenberg, M. (1990). Expression of the thymus leukemia antigen in mouse intestinal epithelium. *Proc. Natl. Acad. Sci. U.S.A.* **87,** 9727–9731.

Holcombe, H. R., Castano, A. R., Cheroutre, H., Teitell, M., Maher, J. K., Peterson, P. A., and Kronenberg, M. (1995). Nonclassical behavior of the thymus leukemia antigen: Peptide transporter-independent expression of a nonclassical class I molecule. *J. Exp. Med.* **181,** 1433–1443.

Hughes, A. L. (1991). Evolutionary origin and diversification of the mammalian CD1 antigen genes. *Mol. Biol. Evol.* **8,** 185–201.

Hyman, R., and Stallings, V. (1976). Characterization of a TL⁻ variant of a homozygous TL⁺ mouse lymphoma. *Immunogenetics* **3,** 75–84.

Ibraghimov, A. R., and Lynch, R. G. (1994). Heterogeneity and biased T cell receptor alpha/beta repertoire of mucosal CD8⁺ cells from murine large intestine: Implications for functional state. *J. Exp. Med.* **180,** 433–444.

Ito, K., Van Kaer, L., Bonneville, M., Hsu, S., Murphy, D. B., and Tonegawa, S. (1990). Recognition of the product of a novel MHC TL region gene (27b) by a mouse gamma delta T cell receptor. *Cell (Cambridge, Mass.)* **62,** 549–561.

Jarry, A., Cerf-Bensussan, N., Brousse, N., Selz, F., and Guy-Grand, D. (1990). Subsets of CD3⁺ (T cell receptor alpha/beta or gamma/delta) and CD3- lymphocytes isolated from normal human gut epithelium display phenotypical features different from their counterparts in peripheral blood. *Eur. J. Immunol.* **20,** 1097–1103.

Koller, B. H., Marrack, P., Kappler, J. W., and Smithies, O. (1990). Normal development of mice deficient in beta 2M, MHC class I proteins, and CD8⁺ T cells. *Science* **248,** 1227–1230.

Kovacsovics-Bankowski, M., and Rock, K. L. (1995). A phagosome-to-cytosol pathway for exogenous antigens presented on MHC class I molecules. *Science* **267,** 243–246.

Lacasse, J., and Martin, L. H. (1992). Detection of CD1 mRNA in Paneth cells of the mouse intestine by *in situ* hybridization. *J. Histochem. Cytochem.* **40,** 1527–1534.

Lefrançois, L. (1991). Phenotypic complexity of intraepithelial lymphocytes of the small intestine. *J. Immunol.* **147,** 1746–1751.

Ljunggren, H. G., Stam, N. J., Ohlen, C., Neefjes, J. J., Hoglund, P., Heemels, M. T., Bastin, J., Schumacher, T. N., Townsend, A., and Karre, K. (1990). Empty MHC class I molecules come out in the cold. *Nature (London)* **346,** 476–480.

Monaco, J. J., Cho, S., and Attaya, M. (1990). Transport protein genes in the murine MHC: Possible implications for antigen processing. *Science* **250,** 1723–1726.

Morita, A., Takahashi, T., Stockert, E., Nakayama, E., Tsuji, T., Matsudaira, Y., Old, L. J., and Obata,

Y. (1994). TL antigen as a transplantation antigen recognized by TL-restricted cytotoxic T cells. *J. Exp. Med.* **179**, 777–784.

Morrissey, P. J., Charrier, K., Horovitz, D. A., Fletcher, F. A., and Watson, J. D. (1995). Analysis of the intra-epithelial lymphocyte compartment in SCID mice that received co-isogenic CD4$^+$ T cells. Evidence that mature post-thymic CD4$^+$ T cells can be induced to express CD8 alpha *in vivo*. *J. Immunol.* **154**, 2678–2686.

Mosley, R. L., Whetsell, M., and Klein, J. R. (1991). Proliferative properties of murine intestinal intraepithelial lymphocytes (IEL): IEL expressing TCR $\alpha\beta$ or TCR $\gamma\delta$ are largely unresponsive to proliferative signals mediated via conventional stimulation of the CD3-TCR complex. *Int. Immunol.* **3**, 563–569.

Mosser, D. D., Duchaine, J., and Martin, L. H. (1991). Biochemical and developmental characterization of the murine cluster of differentiation 1 antigen. *Immunology* **73**, 298–303.

Ohteki, T., and MacDonald, H. R. (1994). Major histocompatibility complex I related molecules control the development of CD4$^+$ 8$^-$ and CD4$^-$ 8$^-$ subsets of natural killer 1.1$^+$ T cell receptor-$\alpha/\beta^+$ cells in the liver of mice. *J. Exp. Med.* **180**, 699–704.

Petit, A., Ernst, P. B., Befus, A. D., Clark, D. A., Rosenthal, K. L., Ishizaka, T., and Bienenstock, J. (1985). Murine intestinal intraepithelial lymphocytes I. Relationship of a novel Thy-1-,Lyt-1-,Lyt-2$^+$, granulated subpopulation to natural killer cells and mast cells. *Eur. J. Immunol.* **15**, 211–215.

Porcelli, S. A. (1995). The CD1 family: A third lineage of antigen presenting molecules. *Adv. Immunol.* **59**, 1–98.

Poussier, P., Edouard, P., Lee, C., Binnie, M., and Julius, M. (1992). Thymus-independent development and negative selection of T cells. *J. Exp. Med.* **176**, 187–199.

Reimann, J., and Rudolphi, A. (1995). Co-expression of CD8 alpha in CD4$^+$ T cell receptor alpha beta$^+$ T cells migrating into the murine small intestine epithelial layer. *Eur. J. Immunol.* **25**, 1580–1588.

Rocha, B., Guy-Grand, D., and Vassalli, P. (1995). Extrathymic T cell differentiation. *Curr. Opin. Immunol.* **7**, 235–242.

Rodgers, J. R., Mehta, V., and Cook, R. G. (1995). Surface expression of beta 2-microglobulin-associated thymus-leukemia antigen is independent of TAP2. *Eur. J. Immunol.* **25**, 1001–1007.

Salter, R. D., Benjamin, R. J., Wesley, P. K., Buxton, S. E., Garrett, T. P., Clayberger, C., Krensky, A. M., Norment, A. M., Littman, D. R., and Parham, P. (1990). A binding site for the T-cell co-receptor CD8 on the alpha 3 domain of HLA-A2. *Nature (London)* **345**, 41–46.

Sanders, S. K., Giblin, P. A., and Kavathas, P. (1991). Cell–cell adhesion mediated by CD8 and human histocompatibility leukocyte antigen G, a nonclassical major histocompatibility complex class 1 molecule on cytotrophoblasts. *J. Exp. Med.* **174**, 737–740.

Schild, H., Mavaddat, N., Litzenberger, C., Ehrich, E. W., Davis, M. M., Bluestone, J. A., Matis, L., Draper, R. K., and Chien, Y. H. (1994). The nature of major histocompatibility complex recognition by gamma delta T cells. *Cell (Cambridge, Mass.)* **76**, 29–37.

Sieling, P. A., Chatterjee, D., Porcelli, S. A., Prigozy, T. I., Mazzaccaro, R. J., Soriano, T., Bloom, B. R., Brenner, M. B., Kronenberg, M., Brennan, P. J., and Modlin, R. L. (1995). CD1-restricted T cell recognition of microbial lipoglycan antigens. *Science* **269**, 227–230.

Spies, T., and DeMars, R. (1991). Restored expression of major histocompatibility complex class I molecules by gene transfer of a putative peptide transporter. *Nature (London)* **351**, 323–324.

Sprent, J. (1976). Fate of H2-activated T lymphocytes in syngeneic hosts. I. Fate in lymphoid tissues and intestines traced with $^3$H-thymidine, $^{125}$I-deoxyuridine and $^{51}$chromium. *Cell. Immunol.* **21**, 278–302.

Sydora, B. C., Mixter, P. F., Holcombe, H. R., Eghtesady, P., Williams, K., Amaral, M. C., Nel, A., and Kronenberg, M. (1993). Intestinal intraepithelial lymphocytes are activated and cytolytic but do not proliferate as well as other T cells in response to mitogenic signals. *J. Immunol.* **150**, 2179–2191.

Teitell, M., Mescher, M. F., Olson, C. A., Littman, D. R., and Kronenberg, M. (1991). The thymus leukemia antigen binds human and mouse CD8. *J. Exp. Med.* **174,** 1131–1138.

Teitell, M., Cheroutre, H., Panwala, C., Holcombe, H., Eghtesady, P., and Kronenberg, M. (1994). Structure and function of *H-2T(Tla)* Region Class I MHC Molecules. *Crit. Rev. Immunol.* **14,** 1–27.

Van Kaer, L., Ashton-Rickardt, P. G., Ploegh, H. L., and Tonegawa, S. (1992). TAP1 mutant mice are deficient in antigen presentation, surface class I molecules, and CD4–8$^+$ T cells. *Cell (Cambridge, Mass.)* **71,** 1205–1214.

Wang, Q., Geliebter, J., Tonkonogy, S., and Flaherty, L. (1993). Expression of the *Q2* gene of the MHC in thymus and intestinal epithelial cells. *Immunogenetics* **38,** 370–372.

Wei, M. L., and Cresswell, P. (1992). HLA-A2 molecules in an antigen-processing mutant cell contain signal sequence-derived peptides. *Nature (London)* **356,** 443–446.

Wu, M., Van Kaer, L., Itohara, S., and Tonegawa, S. (1991). Highly restricted expression of the thymus leukemia antigens on intestinal epithelial cells. *J. Exp. Med.* **174,** 213–218.

Yang, Y., Fruh, K., Chambers, J., Waters, J. B., Wu, L., Spies, T., and Peterson, P. A. (1992). Major histocompatibility complex (MHC)-encoded HAM2 is necessary for antigenic peptide loading onto class I MHC molecules. *J. Biol. Chem.* **267,** 11669–11672.

Yoshimoto, T., and Paul, W. E. (1994). CD4positive NK1.1positive T cells promptly produce interleukin 4 in response to *in vivo* challenge with anti-CD3. *J. Exp. Med.* **179,** 1285–1295.

# Chapter 18

# Lamina Propria Lymphocytes: A Unique Population of Mucosal Lymphocytes

Maria T. Abreu-Martin and Stephan R. Targan

*Inflammatory Bowel Disease Center, Cedars-Sinai Medical Center,
Los Angeles, California 90048*

## I. INTRODUCTION

The gastrointestinal immune system is organized to permit efficient and effective transfer of lumenal information resulting in an appropriate immune response. An "appropriate" intestinal immune response can be defined loosely as one that protects against pathogens while allowing the absorption of complex nutrients without injury to the epithelium. The complex regulation of intestinal mucosal lymphocytes which maintains this precarious balance is still being elucidated. This chapter highlights unique aspects of T-cell regulation within the lamina propria lymphocyte (LPL) compartments as compared with lymphocytes in the periphery and intraepithelial lymphocytes (IEL). In general, LPL are thymically derived, highly activated lymphocytes with predominantly T-helper 2 (Th2) cell phenotype. LPL activation is distinct from that of classical memory T cells in their CD2/CD28 predominance which likely contributes to limiting T-cell receptor (TCR)/CD3-mediated signals in the mucosa. Antigen (Ag) presentation in the gut may involve nonclassical, nonpolymorphic class I-like molecules expressed by epithelial cells which may positively select extrathymically derived lymphocyte populations as well as tolerize self-reactive lymphocytes. These special features of the mucosal immune system are integrated to downregulate immune responses to ubiquitous lumenal Ags.

## II. ORGANIZATION OF GALT

As is true of the bowel wall, the mucosal immune system, also known as gut-associated lymphoreticular tissue (GALT), can be divided into layers. The first layer consists of IEL which reside within the epithelium itself, above the basement membrane. Beneath this layer, in the lamina propria located between the epithelium and submucosa, reside the LPL. Finally, the afferent limb of the gastrointestinal immune system consists of organized lymphoid tissue in the form of Peyer's patches (PP) found predominantly in the small bowel and appendix, solitary lymphoid nodules present in the colon and ileum, and mesenteric lymph nodes (MLN) (James, 1991). The phenotype and function of the LPL compartment is addressed first in this chapter, followed by a discussion of unique features of the intestinal immune system involving several components of GALT.

## III. PHENOTYPE OF LAMINA PROPRIA T CELLS

The study of both human and murine LPL has been facilitated by methods of enzymatic digestion of freshly isolated intestinal mucosa (Comer *et al.*, 1986; Van der Heijden and Stok, 1987). LPL are approximately 40 to 90% T cells and of those approximately 65 to 80% of CD3$^+$ cells are also CD4$^+$ (Beagley and Elson, 1992) (see Table I). The ratio of CD4$^+$ to CD8$^+$ cells in the lamina propria is similar to that found in peripheral blood (65 to 35%) (James *et al.*, 1986; James, 1991; Senju *et al.*, 1991). In contrast to the extrathymic derivation of IEL, lamina propria T-cell ontogeny involves the thymus followed by induction in the PP and the lymphoid follicles within the mucosa. Naive T cells enter mucosal lymphoid follicles, encounter Ag, enter the peripheral circulation, and home back to the lamina propria (Jalkanen *et al.*, 1989; Jalkanen, 1991; Zeitz *et al.*, 1991).

As in peripheral blood (PB), approximately 95% of the T cells bear an $\alpha\beta$ TCR complex (Ullrich *et al.*, 1990; Fujihashi *et al.*, 1994). Compared to the 40% of IEL that express the $\gamma\delta$ TCR, only 3% of CD3$^+$ LPL express this form of TCR (Ullrich *et al.*, 1990). Although peripheral blood lymphocytes (PBL) and LPL share several common phenotypic features, LPL differ in their apparent maturational state compared with PBL. Cell surface markers and functional assays dem-

*TABLE I*

PHENOTYPIC MARKERS OF INTRAEPITHELIAL LYMPHOCYTES
AND LAMINA PROPRIA LYMPHOCYTES COMPARED WITH PERIPHERAL
BLOOD LYMPHOCYTES

| Cell surface markers | IEL (%) | LPL (%) | PBL (%) |
|---|---|---|---|
| CD4$^+$ | 20 | 65 | 65 |
| CD8$^+$ | 80 | 35 | 35 |
| $\alpha\beta$ TCR | 50 | 95 | 95 |
| $\gamma\delta$ TCR | 50 | 3 | 3 |
| HML-1 ($\alpha^E\beta^7+$) | 90 | 30–40 | 0 |
| CD25 ($\alpha$-chain IL-2R) | 15–30 | 15–30 | <5 |
| CD45R0$^+$ | 85 | 65–95 | 30–50 |
| CD45RA$^+$ | 15–20 | 10–22 | 60–90 |

*Note.* References: (James *et al.*, 1986; Cerf-Bensussan *et al.*, 1987; James, 1991; Senju *et al.*, 1991; Schieferdecker *et al.*, 1992; Targan *et al.*, 1995).

onstrate that $CD4^+$ lamina propria T cells are predominantly of memory phenotype. Approximately 66–96% of LPL express the CD45RO form of the CD45 molecule with the minority (10–22%) expressing the CD45RA form. This pattern is consistent with these T cells being of "memory" phenotype (Schieferdecker *et al.*, 1990; Senju *et al.*, 1991; Targan *et al.*, 1995). By contrast, CD45RO is expressed on 30–50% of PB T cells and CD45RA on 30–50%, suggesting an even distribution of memory and naive phenotypes. Both $CD45RO^+$ lamina propria and PB T cells express CD2 and its ligand CD58 (Schieferdecker *et al.*, 1992). Targan *et al.*, (1995) have found a slight increase in CD2 receptor number on LPL compared with PBL.

Approximately half of the $CD8^+$ lamina propria subset express the CD28 molecule associated with cytolytic function (James *et al.*, 1986). This is similar to the percentage found in PB $CD8^+$ cells. The percentage of $CD8^+$ LPL expressing the CD11 phenotype associated with suppressor–effector function is the same or lower than PBL (James *et al.*, 1986; 1987). Thus, lamina propria T cells differ from PB T cells in having predominantly the phenotypes of memory and cytolytic T cells. These characterizations of T cells should be readdressed more precisely in the context of T-lymphocyte cytokine production, i.e., Th1-, Th2-, and Th0-like subsets.

### A. Lamina Propria Lymphocytes Express a Higher Percentage of Activation Markers

Compared with PB lymphocytes, lamina propria T cells more frequently express cell surface markers associated with activated cells. This finding is probably the result of the continuous antigenic and mitogenic challenge of the intestinal environment. Studies of lamina propria T cells from monkeys compared with PB lymphocytes, splenic lymphocytes, and mesenteric lymphocytes reveal that LPL express a significantly higher percentage of interleukin-2 receptor-positive ($IL-2R^+$) cells as well as messenger RNA for IL-2R (Zeitz *et al.*, 1988; Schieferdecker *et al.*, 1990, 1992). Both $CD4^+$ and $CD8^+$ lamina propria T cells demonstrate this increased IL-2R expression. Exogenous IL-2 causes increased proliferation of lamina propria T cells compared with other lymphocytes and increased helper function by $CD4^+$ cells but does not enhance $CD8^+$ suppressor function. This finding suggests that suppressor function may be regulated differently than helper function (James and Graeff, 1987). Again, these studies do not address differences in cytokine secretory patterns such as an upregulation of Th2 compared with Th1 responses.

Other activation markers found on lamina propria T cells include MHC class II, transferrin receptors, and the 4F2 lymphocyte activation antigens (Zeitz *et al.*, 1988; Peters *et al.*, 1989; Schreiber *et al.*, 1991; Senju *et al.*, 1991). Approximately 40% of LPL express the $\alpha^E\beta^7$ integrin recognized by the HML-1 mAb (described below). Although not normally expressed on PBL, $\alpha^E\beta^7$ can be induced on PB T cells by mitogens, phorbolester, Ag, and rIL-2, again suggesting that T-cell activation leads to expression of this Ag (Schieferdecker *et al.*, 1990). More recently, TGF$\beta$ has been shown to increase expression of $\alpha^E\beta^7$ (Kilshaw and Murant, 1991; Parker *et al.*, 1992). Thus, $\alpha^E\beta^7$ seems to be an additional activation marker found on a subset of previously activated T cells in the lamina propria which can be induced *in vitro* by different activation signals on PBL.

## B. Homing of Lymphocytes to the Lamina Propria

Unlike PBL and IEL, the nature of the ligand–receptor interactions directing LPL to home back to the mucosa is unclear. Flow cytometric analysis of human lamina propria T cells reveals that the majority of CD4$^+$ cells are negative for expression of the primate homolog of MEL-14, the Leu-8 antigen (James *et al.*, 1986; James *et al.*, 1987; Kanof *et al.*, 1988). MEL-14 serves as a murine homing receptor for peripheral lymph nodes and is expressed on a majority of PBL; thus, Leu-8-expressing lymphocytes are diverted to peripheral nodes rather than the mucosa (Berg *et al.*, 1991). The CD45RO$^+$ LPL subset has diminished expression of CD29, the $\beta$ chain of VLA antigens, and CD11a/CD18, $\alpha$ and $\beta$ chain of LFA-1, compared with PB T cells (Schieferdecker *et al.*, 1990, 1992). Thus, the phenotypic features commonly attributed to classical memory cells in the periphery are modified for the specialized function of lamina propria T cells.

A recognized marker found on more than 90% of human IEL is the Ag recognized by the human mucosal lymphocyte 1 (HML-1) mAb. This marker is also expressed on 40% of LPL, predominantly within the CD8$^+$ population but on less than 2% of PBL (Cerf-Bensussan *et al.*, 1987) (Schieferdecker *et al.*, 1990). Immunoprecipitation of the membrane protein yields a noncovalent heterodimer composed of an $\alpha$ and $\beta$ chain characteristic of the integrin superfamily of adhesion molecules and is referred to as the $\alpha^E\beta^7$ integrin (Yuan *et al.*, 1991; Parker *et al.*, 1992). The $\beta7$ chain is also found in association with the $\alpha4$ chain, $\alpha4\beta7$, in mouse. TGF$\beta$ dramatically increases the expression of the HML-1 Ag on IEL but not LFA-1 expression (Parker *et al.*, 1992). Other cytokines including IFN$\gamma$, IL-1, and IL-4 do not have this effect. Therefore, TGF$\beta$, a cytokine produced by epithelial cells and PP lymphocytes, can alter the expression of lymphocyte adhesion molecules to facilitate mucosal homing.

The endothelial receptor for the $\alpha^4\beta^7$ molecule is thought to be the mucosal vascular addressin MadCAM-1 expressed on high endothelial venules of PP, mesenteric lymph nodes, and endothelium of gut mucosa (Berlin *et al.*, 1993; Briskin *et al.*, 1993). IEL are further diverted to the epithelium by virtue of the adhesion molecule E-cadherin expressed by epithelial cells, which interacts specifically with $\alpha^E\beta^7$ (Cepek *et al.*, 1994). Finally, the *in vivo* relevance of $\alpha^4\beta^7$ expression has been shown in a primate model of colitis (Podolsky *et al.*, 1993). Cotton-top tamarins develop a spontaneous chronic colitis with periodic acute inflammation. Administration of Ab against the $\alpha^4$ integrin chain significantly reduces the histologic inflammation. These findings suggest that the $\alpha^4$ integrin chain may also be important for homing of lymphocytes to the lamina propria. Finally, LPL may express unique adhesion molecules that facilitate their homing to the mucosa or lymphocytes, once in the mucosa, lose expression of the above described adhesion molecules.

## IV. FUNCTION OF LAMINA PROPRIA T CELLS

### A. Cytokine Production by Lamina Propria T Cells: Providing B-Cell Help (Table II)

As with other mucous membranes, the predominant type of immunoglobulin (Ig) secreted by the B lymphocytes of the gut is IgA, accounting for 70–90% of all Ig present in normal intestinal mucosa (Brandtzaeg et al., 1985, 1989; Strober and Harriman, 1991; Beagley and Elson, 1992). Preservation of an IgA-predominant humoral response is important because IgA traps potential antigens in the lumen before they elicit an immune response and IgA does not bind complement. Indeed, IgA deficiency is associated with an increase in autoimmune diseases, suggesting that lumenal IgA is an important barrier to unwanted Ag exposure (Liblau and

TABLE II

FUNCTIONAL FEATURES

| Function | IEL | LPL | PP |
|---|---|---|---|
| Cytokine production | Cd4$^+$: IL-4, IL-5, IL-6>> IFN$\gamma$ CD8$^+$: IFN$\gamma$>>IL-5, IL-6 $\gamma\delta^+$: IFN$\gamma$, TGF$_\beta$, TNF$\alpha$, IL-5 | IL-4, IL-5>>IFN$\gamma$ | TGF$_\beta$, little IFN$\gamma$, IL-5 |
| B-cell help | Yes: CD4$^+$ subset (not CD8$^+$) | Yes: terminal differentiation of sIgA$^+$B cells | Yes: induction of IgA isotype switch |
| Cytotoxic T-cell activity | + + + + | + + | + + |
| Preferential activation pathway(s) | ↓ Proliferation to TCR stimuli; ↑ IL-2 secretion with CD2 stimulation | ↓ Proliferation and cytokine secretion to TCR stimuli; ↑ proliferation and cytokine secretion with CD2 (± CD28) stimulation (IFN$\gamma$, TNF$\alpha$, IL-2, IL-4) | |

Note. References: (Ebert, 1989; James et al., 1990; Pirzer et al., 1990; Taguchi et al., 1990; Mosley et al., 1991; Qiao et al., 1991; Ohteki and MacDonald, 1993; Targan et al., 1995).

Bach, 1992). In functional assays of lamina propria helper function, investigators have demonstrated that lamina propria T cells have marked helper effect in Ig production by T-depleted LPL. This is especially true if one measures IgA production (Smart *et al.*, 1988). Indeed, lamina propria T cells can provide help for IgA and IgM synthesis by T-depleted PB mononuclear cells but do not provide significant help in IgG production. These data suggest that lamina propria T cells are skewed toward providing help for IgA synthesis and do not require mitogenic activation for this function. This latter finding may be because of a heightened state of activation of LPL as well as a higher proportion of CD4$^+$/Leu-8$^-$ cells in LPL compared with PBL (Kanof *et al.*, 1987; Kanof *et al.*, 1988). As one might expect, CD8$^+$ LPL suppress Ig synthesis by B cells, but do so to a similar extent as CD8$^+$ PBL (James *et al.*, 1985; Lee *et al.*, 1988).

Much of the observed effect of T cells is mediated through the regulated secretion of cytokines by T helper cells. These cytokines can be divided into Th1 cytokines (IFN$\gamma$, IL-2, TNF$\alpha$) and Th2 cytokines (IL-4, IL-5, IL-10) which are associated with cell-mediated immunity and humoral immunity, respectively. The generation of secretory IgA in the gut is the combined result of T helper cytokines responsible for the isotype switch from IgM to IgA in the PP and the cytokines leading to IgA secretion by surface IgA$^+$ (sIgA$^+$) cells in the LPL (Cebra *et al.*, 1991). Whereas Th1 cytokines support IgG2a synthesis in B-cell cultures, Th2 cytokines support IgA, IgG1, and IgE responses (Coffman *et al.*, 1988; Xu-Amano *et al.*, 1992a). Transforming growth factor-$\beta$ (TGF$_\beta$) (Spalding and Griffin, 1986; Coffman *et al.*, 1989; Sonoda *et al.*, 1989; Lebman *et al.*, 1990a,b; Sonoda *et al.*, 1992), derived from both T cells and nonlymphoid cells, and IL-5 (Bond *et al.*, 1987; Coffman *et al.*, 1987; Murray *et al.*, 1987; Beagley *et al.*, 1988), derived from Th2 cells, are involved in enhancing the heavy-chain isotype switch from IgM to IgA in mucosal B lymphocytes. Terminal differentiation of sIgA$^+$-positive B cells to IgA-secreting plasma cells is predominantly regulated by IL-5 and IL-6 with synergistic contribution by IL-2 and IL-4 (Harriman *et al.*, 1988; Beagley *et al.*, 1989, 1991; Kunimoto *et al.*, 1989; Fujihashi *et al.*, 1991).

Based on the above observations, one would expect that lamina propria T cells are Th2-like cells. James *et al.* (1990) has demonstrated that inactivated lymphocytes do not have detectable levels of cytokine messenger RNA. After activation with phorbol myristate acetate (PMA) and ionomycin, high levels of IL-4 and IL-5 mRNA were detected in LPL and mesenteric lymph node but not in PBL, spleen, or peripheral nodes (James *et al.*, 1990). LPL also demonstrated high expression of IL-2 and IFN$\gamma$. Using ELISPOT assays, Taguchi *et al.* (1990) have demonstrated that CD4$^+$ cells freshly isolated from PP have relatively few IFN$\gamma$ and IL-5-secreting cells compared with LPL and IEL. Of these subsets, LPL had the highest number of cells spontaneously secreting IL-5. While in IEL equal numbers of IFN$\gamma$ and IL-5 secreting cells were seen, the ratio of IL-5- to IFN$\gamma$-secreting cells in LPLs was 3:1.

The same studies performed in mice which had been orally immunized with

SRBC results in a high frequency of IL-5-secreting CD4$^+$ cells in PP whereas intraperitoneal immunization results in a high frequency of IFN$\gamma$-secreting CD4$^+$ cells in the spleen (Xu-Amano et al., 1992b). Functionally, it would seem that although both Th1- and Th2-type cytokines are produced by LPL the overall effect is Th2-predominant and achieves IgA rearrangement and secretion.

### B. Altered LPL Cytokine Production under Inflammatory Conditions of the Bowel

In health, Th2 cytokine secretion predominates in lamina propria T cells and facilitates IgA synthesis by lamina propria B cells as well as serving other immunoregulatory functions. Several groups have analyzed LPL cytokine production in Crohn's disease and ulcerative colitis in an effort to understand etiologic factors in human intestinal inflammation. IL-2, IFN$\gamma$, and TNF$\alpha$ production by lamina propria mononuclear cells has been found to be increased in patients with Crohn's disease, but not in patients with ulcerative colitis (Mullin et al., 1992; Breese et al., 1993, 1994; Sartor, 1994). These findings suggest that T helper cells in the lamina propria of Crohn's disease have a Th1 predominance compared with ulcerative colitis and control lamina propria which have a Th2 predominance.

Using genetic manipulation or severe combined immunodeficient (scid) mice reconstitution studies, much information about intestinal inflammation and lamina propria lymphocyte function has been gained. Investigators reconstituted scid mice with purified CD4$^+$ lymph node T cells which were sorted on the basis of their expression of the CD45RB Ag into a CD45RB$^{hi}$ and CD45RB$^{lo}$ cells (Morrissey et al., 1993); scid mice received CD4$^+$/CD45RB$^{hi}$, CD4$^+$/CD45RB$^{lo}$, or whole lymph node cells. Interestingly, the scid mice that received CD45RB$^{hi}$/CD4$^+$ T cells developed a wasting disease that was not seen in scid mice that received the CD4$^+$/CD45RB$^{lo}$ cells or whole lymph node cells. This wasting disease was associated with hyperplasia of the intestinal mucosa and lymphoid cell accumulation in the lamina propria consistent with intestinal inflammation. Further studies using this model have found that transfer of CD4$^+$/CD45RB$^{hi}$ cells results in transfer of Th1-predominant cells based on their pattern of cytokine secretion (Powrie et al., 1994). An increase in IFN$\gamma$ and TNF$\alpha$ production was found. Indeed, the wasting disease could be abrogated or attenuated by neutralizing Abs to IFN$\gamma$ and TNF$\alpha$, respectively.

Three types of mice have been genetically engineered to develop intestinal inflammation as a result of disrupting cytokine genes or T-cell receptor genes. Knockout mice with a disruption in the IL-2 gene develop a disease very similar to ulcerative colitis with colonic bleeding and ulceration (Sadlack et al., 1993). These mice have increased numbers of IgA- and IgG1-secreting cells and increased numbers of activated B cells, both in peripheral blood and in the intestinal mucosa. This may occur as a result of unregulated Th2-type cells but all the immunologic derangements have not been fully characterized. In addition to histologic colitis, these animals produce anti-colon antibodies. It is unclear if these antibodies develop in the late stages of colitis or occur prior to overt disease as a result of failed tolerance to self-Ags. Genetically engineered mice that are deficient in IL-10 develop chronic enterocolitis involving the gut from duodenum to colon (Kuhn et al., 1993). Although IL-10-deficient mice have a normal Ab response to systemic immunization, they are unable to generate a Th2 immune response to nematode infection. IL-10 is a cytokine produced by Th2 cells and macrophages which inhibits Th1 cell development and downregulates Th1 cytokine responses (Fiorentino et al., 1991a,b; Powrie et al., 1993). Therefore, the most notable immunologic derangement is their inability to suppress Th1 immune responses, and their enterocolitis is thought to be from overproduction of Th1 cytokines by antigenically stimulated T cells and macrophages. Of interest is the observation that animals kept in a pathogen-free environment have much attenuated disease. These data taken together point to the precarious balance that exists within the mucosal environment to continuously downregulate excessive or "unbalanced" Th1 and Th2 cytokine production. Antigenic stimulation, specifically with bacterial Ags, serves as the trigger, however, to incite deregulated inflammation in what is likely a genetically predetermined environment.

## V. REGULATION OF LAMINA PROPRIA T CELLS

The normal histology of the lamina propria contains lymphocytes, plasma cells, and macrophages with a paucity of polymorphonuclear cells. It is not until the normal architecture of the intestinal tract is distorted by immune cells and damage occurs to the epithelium that the intestine is said to be inflamed (Lewin et al., 1989). As described above, these resident lymphocytes are in a heightened state of activation without causing mucosal damage. Why, then, do these LPL not cause perpetual pathologic inflammation? This delicate balance is achieved because LPL activation is tempered by development of tolerance to food-born antigens and bacterial species. In the next section, we will examine unique features of LPL activation compared with PBL.

### A. Activation Pathways in Lamina Propria T Cells

Several surprises exist in measures of LPL responses based on its predominant memory phenotype compared with classical CD45RO$^+$ memory T cells. Peripheral memory T cells proliferate and secrete cytokines in response to recall Ag or stimulation through the TCR. Lamina propria T cells, however, show diminished proliferative responses to recall Ag in vitro, stimulation via the TCR/CD3 complex, and protein kinase C activators (Pirzer et al., 1990; Qiao et al., 1991). In Cynomolgus monkeys immunized rectally with Chlamydia trachomatis (Zeitz et al., 1988), lymphocytes isolated from PB, spleen, and mesenteric nodes proliferate in response to *C. trachomatis* Ags but not lamina propria T cells. Neither removal of CD8$^+$ suppressor T cells nor Ag presentation by peripheral monocytes restored a proliferative response in lamina propria T cells. Lamina propria T cells from infected animals were, however, able to provide antigen-specific help for polyclonal immunoglobulin synthesis by immune B lymphocytes after stimulation with *C. trachomatis* Ags. Thus, humoral immunity is preserved but cell-mediated immunity is restricted.

The proposed effect of downregulated, antigen-specific responses by lamina propria T cells is to prevent clonal expansion of T cells directed against harmless dietary antigens. In this way, pathologic mucosal inflammation is prevented. If this hypothesis is correct, chronic idiopathic inflammation of the bowel such as that seen in Crohn's disease or ulcerative colitis may be secondary to an impaired downregulatory mechanism. Qiao *et al.* (1994) measured the proliferative responses of lamina propria T cells to Ag receptor stimulation in patients with Crohn's disease and ulcerative colitis compared with normal controls. Lamina propria T cells from patients with Crohn's disease and ulcerative colitis had increased proliferation to anti-CD3 stimulation compared with controls. Thus, lamina propria T cells from patients with chronic intestinal inflammation lose their physiologic unresponsiveness to lumenal antigens and can be stimulated to proliferate *in vitro* with microbial Ags.

By contrast, lamina propria T cells have enhanced proliferation and cytokine production in response to CD2 and CD28 stimulation (Pirzer *et al.*, 1990; Qiao *et al.*, 1991, 1993; Targan *et al.*, 1995). This CD2-predominant activation of lamina propria T cells cannot be explained solely on the basis of differences in CD2 expression between lamina propria T cells and PB T cells, although there is a slight increase in LPL CD2 expression (Schieferdecker *et al.*, 1992; Targan *et al.*, 1995). The CD2 receptor which interacts with LFA-3 (CD58) acts as an accessory activation pathway to the TCR complex and activates many of the same second signal pathways including inositol 1,4,5-triphosphate generation, DAG generation, tyrosine protein kinase activity, and phosphorylation of the TCR ζ-chains (Pantaleo *et al.*, 1987; Monostori *et al.*, 1990; Samelson *et al.*, 1990). Unlike CD2, CD28 (Tp44) stimulation alone has very little signal transduction effect but can synergize with TCR/CD3 stimulation to augment lymphocyte proliferation and cytokine secretion (Weiss *et al.*, 1986; Lindstein *et al.*, 1989; Thompson *et al.*, 1989). This latter effect is due to stabilization of cytokine mRNA transcripts (Lindstein *et al.*, 1989).

Although lamina propria T cells require alternative receptor-mediated stimuli to proliferate and secrete cytokines. These findings suggest differences in postreceptor signaling in lamina propria T cells. In support of this signal transduction hypothesis, lamina propria T-cell activation with immobilized anti-CD3 results in low amounts of intracellular inositol 1,4,5-triphosphate generation and no free calcium increase when compared with PB T lymphocytes (Qiao *et al.*, 1991). In a comparison with PB T cells, Targan *et al.*, have shown that stimulation of lamina propria T cells with ligation of CD2 results in significantly greater production of IFN$\gamma$, IL-2, IL-4, and TNF$\alpha$ (Fig. 3 in Targan *et al.,* 1995). Coligation of lamina propria T cells with anti-CD28 exaggerates CD2 over CD3 predominance in LPL cytokine production. Targan *et al.* (1995) are the first to find a consistent and unique phosphorylation pattern following CD2 stimulation compared with CD3. This study found that LPL activation with CD2 ligation correlated with tyrosine phosphorylation of a 72-kDa protein which was not seen following CD3 ligation of LPL or with CD2 ligation of PBL. At present, the 72-kDa protein has not been identified. These provocative data support that lamina propria T cells represent a distinct subset of previously activated T cells whose cell surface receptors and postreceptor signaling apparatus are altered to accommodate different activation signals.

It is unclear where and what type of inductive process lamina propria T cells undergo that changes their activation pathway, because lamina propria T cells originate from the same pool of thymically conditioned lymphocytes as PB lymphocytes. Qiao *et al.* (1991) have demonstrated that exposure of PB T lymphocytes to supernatant from intestinal mucosa for 60 hr can change their activation pattern to a pattern similar to freshly isolated lamina propria T cells, i.e., CD2/CD28-predominant activation and diminished CD3 activation. Studies of the mucosal supernatant suggest that the substance(s) responsible for this lamina propria-specific effect are small, nonprotein molecules with oxidative properties (Qiao *et al.,* 1993). Targan *et al.* (1995) have reproduced the phenotype of lamina propria T cells using a model of PBL cocultured with an irradiated B-cell line, Daudi, in the presence of IL-2. These cells develop functional characteristics similar to LPL with CD2 predominance. Moreover, these lamina propria-like T cells stimulated via CD2 develop a tyrosine phosphorylation pattern similar to freshly isolated LPL with 72-kDa phosphorylation. Addition of TGF$\beta$ to both LPL and lamina propria-like cells in culture maintained or enhanced CD2 predominance and decreased CD3 responses (Deem and Targan, 1995). Unlike the studies by Qiao, supernatants from Daudi cells plus IL-2 could not reproduce the LPL phenotype, implying that cell contact is required for the shift in phenotype. Thus in both models described above, PBL have the potential to differentiate into cells with LPL features which suggests that LPL may be a more differentiated form of PBL.

An interesting hypothesis has emerged from the study of LPL with regard to T cell–B cell interactions. The studies performed in our laboratories suggest that lamina propria B cells play a significant role in regulating lamina propria T cells. The ligands for CD2, CD28,LFA-3, and B7-1/B7-2 are found on B cells. These ligands can act synergistically to activate lamina propria T cells in a noncognate fashion (Linsley *et al.,* 1991; Sen *et al.,* 1992). Lamina propria T cells that are anergic to stimulation delivered through the TCR (as in the *C. trachomatis proctitis* model) may be reactivated to proliferate and secrete cytokines to provide B-cell help or secrete cytotoxic cytokines to selectively kill infected epithelial cells in the presence of B cells (Deem *et al.,* 1991; Abreu-Martin *et al.,* 1995). Further support for this hypothesis is the critical role of B-cell contact in transforming PB T cells to lamina propria-like T cells with a CD2-predominant phenotype.

## B. The Unique Relationship of Lamina Propria Lymphocytes and Intestinal Epithelial Cells

LPL responses are regulated not only by ligand–receptor interactions with other lymphocytes but also by intestinal epithelial cells (IEC). In addition to the participation of IEC in Ag presentation (described below), cytokines secreted by IEC have direct effects on lymphocytes. IL-8 secreted by IEC augments the inflammatory response through the recruitment of polymorphonuclear cells and lymphocytes to a site of bacterial invasion (Mukaida and Matsushima, 1992; Eckmann *et al.*, 1993; Mitsuyama *et al.*, 1994; Abreu-Martin *et al.*, 1995). Watanabe *et al.* (1995) have described another cytokine secreted by IEC which may have an important regulatory effect on mucosal lymphocytes. IL-7 is a cytokine produced by stromal cells in bone marrow, thymus, spleen, liver, and kidney which supports the growth of lymphoid precursors of both B-cell and T-cell lineages (Namen *et al.*, 1988; Chazen *et al.*, 1989; Goodwin *et al.*, 1989; Morrissey *et al.*, 1989). Studies of the expression of IL-7 in the intestinal mucosa have revealed that IL-7 mRNA and protein are expressed in colonic epithelial cells and epithelial goblet cells and that IL-7 receptors are expressed by both LPL and IEL (Watanabe *et al.*, 1995). Recombinant IL-7 stimulated a significant increase in LPL proliferation but inhibited anti-CD3 stimulated LPL proliferation, whereas these two stimuli were synergistic in PBL proliferation. While IL-7 alone caused an increase in PBL cell numbers, it did not stimulate DNA synthesis, suggesting that the effect of IL-7 is different on PBL than on LPL. Thus, IL-7 may be a trophic factor for lamina propria T cells which simultaneously limits the ability of LPL to respond to antigenic stimulation via the TCR.

Antigen-presenting cells (APCs) in the intestinal mucosa include classical APCs such as macrophages, B cells, and dendritic cells (Liu and MacPherson, 1994) and nonclassical APCs such as IEC (Mayer *et al.*, 1992). There is a growing body of research demonstrating that mucosal T cells recognize and respond to Ag in the context of classical and nonclassical restriction elements expressed by the intestinal epithelium. Several groups have demonstrated that murine, rat, and human IEC express class II MHC molecules and can present protein Ags and elicit Ag-specific T-cell responses *in vitro* (Bland and Warren, 1986a,b; Mayer and Shlien, 1987; Kaiserlian *et al.*, 1989). The inflammatory cytokines IFNγ and TNFα increase class I and class II MHC expression on epithelial cells (Guy-Grand and Vassalli, 1986). Mayer and Shlien (1987) have demonstrated that IEC are capable of taking up soluble antigen, processing it, and presenting it to Ag-primed T cells. Antibodies against Ia molecules inhibit the MLR elicited by IEC, suggesting that an MHC-restricted response occurs between lymphocytes and IEC (Bland and Warren, 1986a,b; Mayer and Shlien, 1987).

Ag presentation by IEC to LPL also serves an immunoregulatory function. IEC preferentially activate the suppressor subset of PB T cells characterized by $CD8^+$/ $CD28^-$/cells (Bland and Warren, 1986a,b; Mayer and Shlien, 1987). This induction of Ag nonspecific suppressor function may serve to tonically downregulate mucosal immune responses and facilitate the development of tolerance to ubiquitous intestinal Ags. This suppressor–inducer function of IEC is defective in chronic intestinal inflammation. Freshly isolated enterocytes from patients with Crohn's disease or ulcerative colitis failed to induce $CD8^+$ suppressor activity and preferentially stimulated $CD4^+$ helper T cells (Mayer and Eisenhardt, 1990). Thus, in these human diseases characterized by a failure to downregulate the intestinal immune response, there is evidence for pathologic Ag presentation by IEC and consequently pathologic immunoregulation.

Studies of the specific interaction of IEC with LPL have demonstrated that CD8 is necessary for LPL response in allogeneic MLR using IEC as APC (Panja et al., 1993). Surprisingly, however, Ab's against class I MHC molecules do not inhibit the ability of IEC to stimulate allogeneic MLR. Bleicher et al., (1990) have described the expression of a family of MHC class I-like molecules on gastrointestinal tract epithelium in the mouse referred to as CD1 molecules. Studies in human tissues corroborated that a specific member of the CD1 family, CD1d, is expressed on the majority of IEC (Blumberg et al., 1991). CD1d coprecipitates with $\beta2$-microglobulin in IEC. Sieling et al. (1995) have described the intracellular processing and presentation of bacterial wall lipoglycans in the context of CD1b to $\alpha\beta$ TCR T cell. Castano et al. (1995) have also demonstrated the ability of the CD1 molecule to bind appropriate peptides and generate an Ag-specific T-cell response. The functional relevance of CD1d in epithelial–T-cell interactions has been demonstrated (Panja et al., 1993). Antibodies against CD1d or CD8 inhibited PB T-cell proliferation in allogeneic mixed cell cultures using IEC. These Ab's did not, however, inhibit proliferation when the responding cell was LPL, suggesting that additional ligands are important.

Panja et al. (1994) have found that LPLs preferentially proliferate in response to IEC in comparison to other allogeneic, class II-expressing, professional APCs. This is in contrast to PB T cells which preferentially proliferate in response to professional APCs in an allogeneic MLR. Moreover, Abs against several class II MHC molecules fail to inhibit proliferation of LPL in response to IEC but inhibit proliferation of PB T cells in response to IEC and professional APCs. Proliferation of LPL only occurred in allogeneic IEC mixed-cell cultures and not in autologous IEC mixed-cell cultures. This finding suggests that LPL proliferation is not due to memory T-cell activation in response to ubiquitous lumenal Ags on IEC or to nonpolymorphic adhesion molecules such as LFA-3. These data taken together support the conclusion that LPLs recognize a polymorphic restriction element on IEC that is not class II MHC, class I MHC, or CD1. This IEC determinant is currently under investigation but will be an important clue to the unique interaction between the gastrointestinal immune system and the epithelium it defends.

Another nonclassical, nonpolymorphic class I molecule that may be involved in Ag presentation in the gut is the thymus leukemia (TL) antigen, which is encoded in the T region of the mouse MHC by the T3 and T18 genes (Teitell *et al.*, 1994). The TL Ag is expressed primarily by IEC and thymocytes. Analysis of the α1 and α2 domains of the TL Ag show homology with the peptide binding site of classical class I molecules. Although Ag presentation by IEC in the context of the TL Ag has not been demonstrated, this nonpolymorphic determinant may act as an additional selection factor for CD8[+] IEL and LPL.

## VI. SUMMARY

The dual evolutionary pressures on the gastrointestinal tract, absorption of nutrients and exclusion of microbiologic pathogens, has resulted in a complex and precise gastrointestinal immune system to accomplish these goals. Lamina propria lymphocytes are characterized by their reduced ability to respond to TCR stimulation with recall Ags but preferential activation via CD2/CD28 stimulation. Diminished CD3 activation may be due to IL-7 production by intestinal epithelial cells, whereas enhanced CD2 activation may be due to lamina propria B cell contact factors. Although both Th1 and Th2 cytokines are necessary to maintain mucosal homeostasis, spontaneous and induced Th2 cytokine production predominates in health and provides B-cell help for plasma cell differentiation.

## REFERENCES

Abreu-Martin, M. T., Vidrich, A., Lynch, D. H., and Targan, S. R. (1995). Divergent induction of apoptosis and IL-8 secretion in HT-29 cells in response to TNF-α and ligation of Fas antigen. *J. Immunol.* **155,** 4147–4154.

Beagley, K. W., and Elson, C. O. (1992). Cells and cytokines in mucosal immunity and inflammation. *Gastroenterol. Clin. North Am.* **21,** 347–366.

Beagley, K. W., Eldridge, J. H., Kiyono, H., Everson, M. P., Koopman, W. J., Honjo, T., and McGhee, J. R. (1988). Recombinant murine IL-5 induces high rate IgA synthesis in cycling IgA-positive Peyer's patch B cells. *J. Immunol.* **141,** 2035–2042.

Beagley, K. W., Eldridge, J. H., Lee, F., Kiyono, H., Everson, M. P., Koopman, W. J., Hirano, T., *et al.* (1989). Interleukins and IgA synthesis. Human and murine interleukin 6 induce high rate IgA secretion in IgA-committed B cells. *J. Exp. Med.* **169,** 2133–2148.

Beagley, K. W., Eldridge, J. H., Aicher, W. K., Mestecky, J., Di Fabio, S., Kiyono, H., and McGhee, J. R. (1991). Peyer's patch B cells with memory cell characteristics undergo terminal differentiation within 24 hours in response to interleukin-6. *Cytokine* **3,** 107–16.

Berg, M., Murakawa, Y., Camerini, D., and James, S. P. (1991). Lamina propria lymphocytes are derived from circulating cells that lack the Leu-8 lymph node homing receptor. *Gastroenterology* **101,** 90–99.

Berlin, C., Berg, E. L., Briskin, M. J., Andrew, D. P., Kilshaw, P. J., Holzmann, B., Weissman, I. L., *et al.* (1993). Alpha 4 beta 7 integrin mediates lymphocyte binding to the mucosal vascular addressin MAdCAM-1. *Cell (Cambridge, Mass.)* **74,** 185–195.

Bland, P. W., and Warren, L. G. (1986a). Antigen presentation by epithelial cells of the rat small intestine. I. Kinetics, antigen specificity and blocking by anti-Ia antisera. *Immunology* **58,** 1–7.

Bland, P. W., and Warren, L. G. (1986b). Antigen presentation by epithelial cells of the rat small intestine. II. Selective induction of suppressor T cells. *Immunology* **58,** 9–14.

Bleicher, P. A., Balk, S. P., Hagen, S. J., Blumberg, R. S., Flotte, T. J., and Terhorst, C. (1990). Expression of murine CD1 on gastrointestinal epithelium. *Science* **250,** 679–682.

Blumberg, R. S., Terhorst, C., Bleicher, P., McDermott, F. V., Allan, C. H., Landau, S. B., Trier, J. S., and Balk, S. P. (1991). Expression of a nonpolymorphic MHC class I-like molecule, CD1D, by human intestinal epithelial cells. *J. Immunol.* **147,** 2518–2524.

Bond, M. W., Shrader, B., Mosmann, T. R., and Coffman, R. L. (1987). A mouse T cell product that preferentially enhances IgA production. II. Physicochemical characterization. *J. Immunol.* **139,** 3691–3696.

Brandtzaeg, P., Valnes, K., Scott, H., Rognum, T. O., Bjerke, K., and Baklien, K. (1985). The human gastrointestinal secretory immune system in health and disease. *Scand. J. Gastroenterol. Suppl.* **114,** 17–38.

Brandtzaeg, P., Halstensen, T. S., Kett, K., Krajci, P., Kvale, D., Rognum, T. O., Scott, H., and Sollid, L. M. (1989). Immunobiology and immunopathology of human gut mucosa: Humoral immunity and intraepithelial lymphocytes. *Gastroenterology* **97,** 1562–1584.

Breese, E., Braegger, C. P., Corrigan, C. J., Walker-Smith, J. A., and MacDonald, T. T. (1993). Interleu-kin-2- and interferon-gamma-secreting T cells in normal and diseased human intestinal mucosa. *Immunology* **78,** 127–131.

Breese, E. J., Michie, C. A., Nicholls, S. W., Murch, S. H., Williams, C. B., Domizio, P., Walker-Smith, J. A., and MacDonald, T. T. (1994). Tumor necrosis factor alpha-producing cells in the intestinal mucosa of children with inflammatory bowel disease. *Gastroenterology* **106,** 1455–1466.

Briskin, M. J., McEvoy, L. M., and Butcher, E. C. (1993). MAdCAM-1 has homology to immunoglob-ulin and mucin-like adhesion receptors and to IgA1. *Nature (London)* **363,** 461–464.

Castano, A. R., Tangri, S., Miller, J. E., Holcombe, H. R., Jackson, M. R., Huse, W. D., Kronenberg, M., and Peterson, P. A. (1995). Peptide binding and presentation by mouse CD1 [see comments]. *Science* **269,** 223–226.

Cebra, J. J., George, A., and Schrader, C. E. (1991). A microculture containing TH2 and dendritic cells supports the production of IgA by clones from both primary and IgA memory B cells and by single germinal center B cells from Peyer's patches. *Immunol. Res.* **10,** 389–392.

Cepek, K. L., Shaw, S. K., Parker, C. M., Russell, G. J., Morrow, J. S., Rimm, D. L., and Brenner, M. B. (1994). Adhesion between epithelial cells and T lymphocytes mediated by E-cadherin and the alpha E beta 7 integrin. *Nature (London)* **372,** 190–193.

Cerf-Bensussan, N., Jarry, A., Brousse, N., Lisowska-Grospierre, B., Guy-Grand, D., and Griscelli, C. (1987). A monoclonal antibody (HML-1) defining a novel membrane molecule present on human intestinal lymphocytes. *Eur. J. Immunol.* **17,** 1279–1285.

Chazen, G. D., Pereira, G. M. B., LeGros, G., Gillis, S., and Shevach, E. M. (1989). Interleukin 7 is a T-cell growth factor. *Proc. Natl. Acad. Sci. U.S.A.* **86,** 5923–5927.

Coffman, R. L., Shrader, B., Carty, J., Mosmann, T. R., and Bond, M. W. (1987). A mouse T cell product that preferentially enhances IgA production. I. Biologic characterization. *J. Immunol.* **139,** 3685–3690.

Coffman, R. L., Seymour, B. W., Lebman, D. A., Hiraki, D. D., Christiansen, J. A., Shrader, B., Cherwinski, H. M., *et al.* (1988). The role of helper T cell products in mouse B cell differentiation and isotype regulation. *Immunol. Rev.* **102,** 5.

Coffman, R. L., Lebman, D. A., and Shrader, B. (1989). Transforming growth factor beta specifically enhances IgA production by lipopolysaccharide-stimulated murine B lymphocytes. *J. Exp. Med.* **170,** 1039–1044.

Comer, G. M., Ramey, W. G., Kotler, D. P., and Holt, P. R. (1986). Isolation of intestinal mononuclear cells from colonoscopic biopsies for immunofluorescence analysis by flow cytometry. *Dig. Dis. Sci.* **31,** 151–156.

Deem, R. L., and Targan, S. R. (1995). The role of transforming growth factor beta (TGF-beta) in molding the activation state of lamina propria (LP) T cells. *Gastroenterology* **108,** A.

Deem, R. L., Shanahan, F., and Targan, S. R. (1991). Triggered human mucosal T cells release tumour necrosis factor-alpha and interferon-gamma which kill human colonic epithelial cells. *Clin. Exp. Immunol.* **83,** 79–84.

Ebert, E. C. (1989). Proliferative responses of human intraepithelial lymphocytes to various T-cell stimuli. *Gastroenterology* **97,** 1372–1381.

Eckmann, L., Jung, H. C., Schurer-Maly, C., Panja, A., Morzycka-Wroblewska, E., and Kagnoff, M. F. (1993). Differential cytokine expression by human intestinal epithelial cell lines: Regulated expression of interleukin 8. *Gastroenterology* **105,** 1689–1697.

Fiorentino, D. F., Zlotnick, A., Mosmann, T. R., Howard, M., and O'Garra, A. (1991a). IL-10 inhibits cytokine production by activated macrophages. *J. Immunol.* **147,** 3815–3822.

Fiorentino, D. F., Zlotnick, A., Vieira, P., Mosmann, T. R., Howard, M., Moore, K. W., and O'Garra, A. (1991b). IL-10 acts on the antigen presenting cell to inhibit cytokine production by Th1 cells. *J. Immunol.* **146,** 3444–3451.

Fujihashi, K., McGhee, J. R., Lue, C., Beagley, K. W., Taga, T., Hirano, T., Kishimoto, T., *et al.* (1991). Human appendix B cells naturally express receptors for and respond to interleukin 6 with selective IgA1 and IgA2 synthesis. *J. Clin. Invest.* **88,** 248–252.

Fujihashi, K., Yamamoto, M., McGhee, J. R., and Kiyono, H. (1994). Function of alpha beta TCR+ and gamma delta TCR+ IELs for the gastrointestinal immune response. *Int. Rev. Immunol.* **11,** 1–14.

Goodwin, R. G., Lupton, S., Schmierer, A., Hjerrild, K. J., Jerzy, R., Clevenger, W., Gillis, S., *et al.* (1989). Human interleukin-7: Molecular cloning and growth factor activity on human and murine B-lineage cells. *Proc. Natl. Acad. Sci. U.S.A.* **86,** 302–306.

Guy-Grand, D., and Vassalli, P. (1986). Gut injury in mouse graft-versus-host reaction. Study of its occurrence and mechanisms. *J. Clin. Invest.* **77,** 1584–1595.

Harriman, G. R., Kunimoto, D. Y., Elliott, J. F., Paetkau, V., and Strober, W. (1988). The role of IL-5 in IgA B cell differentiation. *J. Immunol.* **140,** 3033–3039.

Jalkanen, S. (1991). Lymphocyte traffic to mucosa-associated lymphatic tissues. *Immunol. Res.* **10,** 268–270.

Jalkanen, S., Nash, G. S., De los Toyos, J., MacDermott, R. P., and Butcher, E. C. (1989). Human lamina propria lymphocytes bear homing receptors and bind selectively to mucosal lymphoid high endothelium. *Eur. J. Immunol.* **19,** 63–68.

James, S. P. (1991). Mucosal T-cell function. *Gastroenterol. Clin. North Am.* **20,** 597–612.

James, S. P., and Graeff, A. S. (1987). Effect of IL-2 on immunoregulatory function of intestinal lamina propria T cells in normal non-human primates. *Clin. Exp. Immunol.* **70,** 394–402.

James, S. P., Fiocchi, C., Graeff, A. S., and Strober, W. (1985). Immunoregulatory function of lamina propria T cells in Crohn's disease. *Gastroenterology* **88,** 1143–1150.

James, S. P., Fiocchi, C., Graeff, A. S., and Strober, W. (1986). Phenotypic analysis of lamina propria lymphocytes. Predominance of helper-inducer and cytolytic T-cell phenotypes and deficiency of suppressor-inducer phenotypes in Crohn's disease and control patients. *Gastroenterology* **91,** 1483–1489.

James, S. P., Graeff, A. S., and Zeitz, M. (1987). Predominance of helper-inducer T cells in mesenteric lymph nodes and intestinal lamina propria of normal nonhuman primates. *Cell. Immunol.* **107,** 372–383.

James, S. P., Kwan, W. C., and Sneller, M. C. (1990). T cells in inductive and effector compartments of the intestinal mucosal immune system of nonhuman primates differ in lymphokine mRNA expression, lymphokine utilization, and regulatory function. *J. Immunol.* **144,** 1251–1256.

Kaiserlian, D., Vidal, K., and Revillard, J. P. (1989). Murine enterocytes can present soluble antigen to specific class II-restricted CD4+ T cells. *Eur. J. Immunol.* **19,** 1513–1516.

Kanof, M. E., Strober, W., and James, S. P. (1987). Induction of CD4 suppressor T cells with anti-Leu-8 antibody. *J. Immunol.* **139,** 49.

Kanof, M. E., Strober, W., Fiocchi, C., Zeitz, M., and James, S. P. (1988). CD4 positive Leu-8 negative helper-inducer T cells predominate in the human intestinal lamina propria. *J. Immunol.* **141,** 3029–3036.

Kilshaw, P. J., and Murant, S. J. (1991). Expression and regulation of beta 7(beta p) integrins on mouse lymphocytes: Relevance to the mucosal immune system. *Eur. J. Immunol.* **21,** 2591–2597.

Kuhn, R., Lohler, J., Rennick, D., Rajewsky, K., and W. Muller (1993). Interleukin-10-deficient mice develop chronic enterocolitis [see comments]. *Cell (Cambridge, Mass.)* **75,** 263–274.

Kunimoto, D. Y., Nordan, R. P., and Strober, W. (1989). IL-6 is a potent cofactor of IL-1 in IgM synthesis and of IL-5 in IgA synthesis. *J. Immunol.* **143,** 2230–2235.

Lebman, D. A., Lee, F. D., and Coffman, R. L. (1990a). Mechanism for transforming growth factor beta and IL-2 enhancement of IgA expression in lipopolysaccharide-stimulated B cell cultures. *J. Immunol.* **144,** 952–959.

Lebman, D. A., Nomura, D. Y., Coffman, R. L., and Lee, F. D. (1990b). Molecular characterization of germ-line immunoglobulin A transcripts produced during transforming growth factor type beta-induced isotype switching. *Proc. Natl. Acad. Sci. U.S.A.* **87,** 3962–3969.

Lee, A., Sugerman, H., and Elson, C. O. (1988). Regulatory activity of the human CD8⁺ cell subset: A comparison of CD8⁺ cells from the intestinal lamina propria and blood. *Eur. J. Immunol.* **18,** 21–27.

Lewin, K. J., Riddell, R. H., and Weinstein, W. M. (eds.) (1989). "Gastrointestinal Pathology and Its Clinical Implications," Inflammatory Bowel Diseases. Igaku-Shoin, New York.

Liblau, R. S., and Bach, J. F. (1992). Selective IgA deficiency and autoimmunity. *Int. Arch. Allergy Immunol.* **99,** 16–27.

Lindstein, T., June, C. H., Ledbetter, J. A., Stella, G., and Thompson, C. B. (1989). Regulation of lymphokine messenger RNA stability by a surface-mediated T cell activation pathway. *Science* **244,** 339–343.

Linsley, P. S., Brady, W., Grosmaire, L., Aruffo, A., Damle, N. K., and Ledbetter, J. A. (1991). Binding of the B cell activation antigen B7 to CD28 costimulates T cell proliferation and interleukin 2 mRNA accumulation. *J. Exp. Med.* **173,** 721–730.

Liu, L. M., and MacPherson, G. G. (1994). The role of dendritic cells in the uptake and presentation of oral antigens. *Adv. Exp. Med. Biol.* **355,** 81–86.

Mayer, L., and Eisenhardt, D. (1990). Lack of induction of suppressor T cells by intestinal epithelial cells from patients with inflammatory bowel disease. *J. Clin. Invest.* **86,** 1255–1260.

Mayer, L., and Shlien, R. (1987). Evidence for function of Ia molecules on gut epithelial cells in man. *J. Exp. Med.* **166,** 1471–1483.

Mayer, L., Panja, A., Li, Y., Siden, E., Pizzimenti, A., Gerardi, F., and Chandswang, N. (1992). Unique features of antigen presentation in the intestine." *Ann. N.Y. Acad. Sci.* **664,** 39–46.

Mitsuyama, K., Toyonaga, A., Sasaki, E., Watanabe, K., Tateishi, H., Nishiyama, T., Saiki, T., *et al.* (1994). IL-8 as an important chemoattractant for neutrophils in ulcerative colitis and Crohn's disease. *Clin. Exp. Immunol.* **96,** 432–436.

Monostori, E., Desai, D., Brown, M. H., Cantrell, D. A., and Crumpton, M. J. (1990). Activation of human T lymphocytes via the CD2 antigen results in tyrosine phosphorylation of T cell antigen receptor zeta-chains. *J. Immunol.* **144,** 1010–1014.

Morrissey, P. J., Goodwin, R. G., Nordan, R. P., Anderson, D., Grabstein, K. H., Cosman, D., Sims, J., *et al.* (1989). Recombinant interleukin 7, pre-B cell growth factor, has costimulatory activity on purified mature T cells. *J. Exp. Med.* **169,** 706–716.

Morrissey, P. J., Charrier, K., Braddy, S., Liggitt, D., and Watson, J. D. (1993). CD4⁺ T cells that express high levels of CD45RB induce wasting disease when transferred into congenic severe combined immunodeficient mice. Disease development is prevented by cotransfer of purified CD4⁺ T cells. *J. Exp. Med.* **178,** 237–244.

Mosley, R. L., Whetsell, M., and Klein, J. R. (1991). Proliferative properties of murine intestinal intraepithelial lymphocytes (IEL): IEL expressing TCR alpha beta or TCR tau delta are largely unresponsive to proliferative signals mediated via conventional stimulation of the CD3-TCR complex. *Int. Immunol.* **3,** 563–569.

Mukaida, N., and Matsushima, K. (1992). Regulation of IL-8 production and the characteristics of the receptors for IL-8. *Cytokines* **4**, 41–53.

Mullin, G. E., Lazenby, A. J., Harris, M. L., Bayless, T. M., and James, S. P. (1992). Increased interleukin-2 messenger RNA in the intestinal mucosal lesions of Crohn's disease but not ulcerative colitis. *Gastroenterology* **102**, 1620–1627.

Murray, P. D., McKenzie, D. T., Swain, S. L., and Kagnoff, M. F. (1987). Interleukin 5 and interleukin 4 produced by Peyer's patch T cells selectively enhance immunoglobulin A expression. *J. Immunol.* **139**, 2669–2674.

Namen, A. E., Lupton, S., Hjerrild, K., Wignall, J., Mochizuki, D. Y., Schmierer, A. E., Mosley, B., *et al.* (1988). Stimulation of B-cell progenitors by cloned murine interleukin-7. *Nature (London)* **333**, 571–575.

Ohteki, T., and MacDonald, H. R. (1993). Expression of the CD28 costimulatory molecule on subsets of murine intestinal intraepithelial lymphocytes correlates with lineage and responsiveness. *Eur. J. Immunol.* **23**, 1251–1255.

Panja, A., Blumberg, R. S., Balk, S. P., and Mayer, L. (1993). CD1d is involved in T cell–intestinal epithelial cell interactions. *J. Exp. Med.* **178**, 1115–1119.

Panja, A., Barone, A., and Mayer, L. (1994). Stimulation of lamina propria lymphocytes by intestinal epithelial cells: Evidence for recognition of nonclassical restriction elements. *J. Exp. Med.* **179**, 943–950.

Pantaleo, G., Olive, D., Poggi, A., Pozzan, T., Moretta, L., and Moretta, A. (1987). Antibody-induced modulation of the CD3/T cell receptor complex causes T cell refractoriness by inhibiting the early metabolic steps involved in T cell activation. *J. Exp. Med.* **166**, 619–624.

Parker, C. M., Cepek, K. L., Russell, G. J., Shaw, S. K., Posnett, D. N., Schwarting, R., and Brenner, M. B. (1992). A family of beta 7 integrins on human mucosal lymphocytes. *Proc. Natl. Acad. Sci. U.S.A.* **89**, 1924–1928.

Peters, M. G., Secrist, H., Anders, K. R., Nash, G. S., Rich, S. R., and MacDermott, R. P. (1989). Normal human intestinal B lymphocytes. Increased activation compared with peripheral blood. *J. Clin. Invest.* **83**, 1827–1833.

Pirzer, U. C., Schurmann, G., Post, S., Betzler, M., and Meuer, S. C. (1990). Differential responsiveness to CD3-Ti vs. CD2-dependent activation of human intestinal T lymphocytes. *Eur. J. Immunol.* **20**, 2339–2342.

Podolsky, D. K., Lobb, R., King, N., Benjamin, C. D., Pepinsky, B., Sehgal, P., and deBeaumont, M. (1993). Attenuation of colitis in the Cotton-top tamarin by anti-$\alpha$4 integrin monoclonal antibody. *J. Clin. Invest.* **92**, 372–380.

Powrie, F., Leach, M. W., Mauze, S., Menon, S., Caddle, L. B., and Coffman, R. L. (1994). Inhibition of Th1 responses prevents inflammatory bowel disease in *scid* mice reconstituted with CD45RBhi CD4[+] T cells. *Immunity* **1**, 553–562.

Powrie, F., Menon, S., and Coffman, R. L. (1993). Interleukin-4 and interleukin-10 synergize to inhibit cell-mediated immunity *in vivo*. *Eur. J. Immunol.* **23**, 2223–2229.

Qiao, L., Schurmann, G., Betzler, M., and Meuer, S. C. (1991). Activation and signaling status of human lamina propria T lymphocytes. *Gastroenterology* **101**, 1529–1536.

Qiao, L., Schurmann, G., Autschbach, F., Wallich, R., and Meuer, S. C. (1993). Human intestinal mucosa alters T-cell reactivities. *Gastroenterology* **105**, 814–819.

Qiao, L., Golling, M., Autschbach, F., Schurmann, G., and Meuer, S. C. (1994). T cell receptor repertoire and mitotic responses of lamina propria T lymphocytes in inflammatory bowel disease. *Clin. Exp. Immunol.* **97**, 303–308.

Sadlack, B., Merz, H., Schorle, H., Schimpl, A., Feller, A. C., and Horak, I. (1993). Ulcerative colitis-like disease in mice with a disrupted interleukin-2 gene [see comments]. *Cell (Cambridge, Mass.)* **75**, 253–261.

Samelson, L. E., Fletcher, M. C., Ledbetter, J. A., and June, C. H. (1990). Activation of tyrosine phosphorylation in human T cells via the CD2 pathway. Regulation by the CD45 tyrosine phosphatase. *J. Immunol.* **145**, 2448–2454.

Sartor, R. B. (1994). Cytokines in intestinal inflammation: Pathophysiological and clinical considerations. *Gastroenterology* **106**, 533–539.

Schieferdecker, H. L., Ullrich, R., Weiss-Breckwoldt, A. N., Schwarting, R., Stein, H., Riecken, E. O., and Zeitz, M. (1990). The HML-1 antigen of intestinal lymphocytes is an activation antigen. *J. Immunol.* **144**, 2541–2549.

Schieferdecker, H. L., Ullrich, R., Hirseland, H., and Zeitz, M. (1992). T cell differentiation antigens on lymphocytes in the human intestinal lamina propria. *J. Immunol.* **149**, 2816–2822.

Schreiber, S., MacDermott, R. P., Raedler, A., Pinnau, R., Bertovich, M. J., and Nash, G. S. (1991). Increased activation of isolated intestinal lamina propria mononuclear cells in inflammatory bowel disease [see comments]. *Gastroenterology* **101**, 1020–1030.

Sen, J., Bossu, P., Burakoff, S. J., and Abbas, A. K. (1992). T cell surface molecules regulating noncognate B lymphocyte activation. Role of CD2 and LFA-1. *J. Immunol.* **148**, 1037–1042.

Senju, M., Wu, K. C., Mahida, Y. R., and Jewell, D. P. (1991). Two-color immunofluorescence and flow cytometric analysis of lamina propria lymphocyte subsets in ulcerative colitis and Crohn's disease. *Dig. Dis. Sci.* **36**, 1453–1458.

Sieling, P. A., Chatterjee, D., Porcelli, S. A., Prigozy, T. I., Mazzaccaro, R. J., Soriano, T., Bloom, B. R., *et al.* (1995). CD1-restricted T cell recognition of microbial lipoglycan antigens [see comments]. *Science* **269**, 227–230.

Smart, C. J., Trejdosiewicz, L. K., Badr-el-Din, S., and Heatley, R. V. (1988). T lymphocytes of the human colonic mucosa: functional and phenotypic analysis. *Clin. Exp. Immunol.* **73**, 63–69.

Sonoda, E., Matsumoto, R., Hitoshi, Y., Ishii, T., Sugimoto, M., Araki, S., Tominaga, A., *et al.* (1989). Transforming growth factor beta induces IgA production and acts additively with interleukin 5 for IgA production. *J. Exp. Med.* **170**, 1415–1420.

Sonoda, E., Hitoshi, Y., Yamaguchi, N., Ishii, T., Tominaga, A., Araki, S., and Takatsu, K. (1992). Differential regulation of IgA production by TGF-beta and IL-5: TGF-beta induces surface IgA-positive cells bearing IL-5 receptor, whereas IL-5 promotes their survival and maturation into IgA-secreting cells. *Cell Imunol.* **140**, 158–172.

Spalding, D. M., and Griffin, J. A. (1986). Different pathways of differentiation of pre-B cell lines are induced by dendritic cells and T cells from different lymphoid tissues. *Cell (Cambridge, Mass.)* **44**, 507–515.

Strober, W., and Harriman, G. R. (1991). The regulation of IgA B-cell differentiation. *Gastroenterol. Clin. North Am.* **20**, 473–494.

Taguchi, T., McGhee, J. R., Coffman, R. L., Beagley, K. W., Eldridge, J. H., Takatsu, K., and Kiyono, H. (1990). Analysis of Th1 and Th2 cells in murine gut-associated tissues. Frequencies of CD4+ and CD8+ T cells that secrete IFN-gamma and IL-5. *J. Immunol.* **145**, 68–77.

Targan, S. R., Deem, R. L., Liu, M., Wang, S., and Nel, A. (1995). Definition of a lamina propria T cell responsive state. Enhanced cytokine responsiveness of T cells stimulated through the CD2 pathway. *J. Immunol.* **154**, 664–675.

Teitell, M., Cheroutre, H., Panwala, C., Holcombe, H., Eghtesady, P., and Kronenberg, M. (1994). Structure and function of H-2 T (Tla) region class I MHC molecules. *Crit. Rev. Immunol.* **14**, 1–27.

Thompson, C. B., Lindsten, T., Ledbetter, J. A., Kunkel, S. L., Young, H. A., Emerson, S. G., Leiden, J. M., and June, C. H. (1989). CD28 activation pathway regulates the production of multiple T-cell-derived lymphokines/cytokines. *Proc. Natl. Acad. Sci. U.S.A.* **86**, 1333–1337.

Ullrich, R., Schieferdecker, H. L., Ziegler, K., Riecken, E. O., and Zeitz, M. (1990). Gamma delta T cells in the human intestine express surface markers of activation and are preferentially located in the epithelium. *Cell. Immunol.* **128**, 619–627.

Van der Heijden, P. J., and Stok, W. (1987). Improved procedure for the isolation of functionally active lymphoid cells from the murine intestine. *J. Immunol. Methods* **103**, 161–167.

Watanabe, M., Ueno, Y., Yajima, T., Iwao, Y., Tsuchiya, M., Ishikawa, H., Aiso, S., *et al.* (1995).

Interleukin 7 is produced by human intestinal epithelial cells and regulates the proliferation of intestinal mucosal lymphocytes. *J. Clin. Invest.* **95,** 2945–2953.

Weiss, A., Manger, B., and Imboden, J. (1986). Synergy between the T3/antigen receptor complex and Tp44 in the activation of human T cells. *J. Immunol.* **137,** 819–825.

Xu-Amano, J., Beagley, K. W., Mega, J., Fujihashi, K., Kiyono, H., and McGhee, J. R. (1992a). Induction of T helper cells and cytokines for mucosal IgA responses. *Adv. Exp. Med. Biol.* **327,** 107–117.

Xu-Amano, J., Aicher, W. K., Taguchi, T., Kiyono, H., and McGhee, J. R. (1992b). Selective induction of Th2 cells in murine Peyer's patches by oral immunization. *Int. Immunol.* **4,** 433–445.

Yuan, Q., Jiang, W. M., Hollander, D., Leung, E., Watson, J. D., and Krissansen, G. W. (1991). Identity between the novel integrin beta 7 subunit and an antigen found highly expressed on intraepithelial lymphocytes in the small intestine. *Biochem. Biophys. Res. Commun.* **176,** 1443–1449.

Zeitz, M., Greene, W. C., Peffer, N. J., and James, S. P. (1988). Lymphocytes isolated from the intestinal lamina propria of normal nonhuman primates have increased expression of genes associated with T-cell activation. *Gastroenterology* **94,** 647–655.

Zeitz, M., Schieferdecker, H. L., Ullrich, R., Jahn, H. U., James, S. P., and Riecken, E. O. (1991). Phenotype and function of lamina propria T lymphocytes. *Immunol. Res.* **10,** 199–206.

# Chapter 19

# Cytokine Gene Knockout Mice—Lessons for Mucosal B-Cell Development

Alistair J. Ramsay,* Shisan Bao,† Kenneth W. Beagley,‡ Sarah J. Dunstan,§
Alan J. Husband,† Manfred Kopf,¶ Klaus I. Matthaei,* Ian A. Ramshaw,*
Richard A. Strugnell,§ Ian G. Young,* and Xiaoyun Tan*

*The John Curtin School of Medical Research, The Australian National University, Canberra,
Australia 0200; †Department of Veterinary Pathology, University of Sydney, Sydney, Australia 2006;
‡Discipline of Pathology, University of Newcastle, Newcastle, Australia 2300;
§Department of Microbiology, University of Melbourne, Melbourne, Australia 3052;
and ¶Basel Institute for Immunology, CH-4005 Basel, Switzerland

## I. INTRODUCTION

Immune responses at mucosal surfaces are characterized by the production and secretion of antibodies of the IgA isotype which represent a "first line of defense" against colonization by many pathogens (Mestecky and McGhee, 1987). Most of the IgA-producing cells originate in mucosa-associated lymphoid tissues (MALT), such as Peyer's patches in the intestine, where they encounter antigen. Subsequently, they disseminate via draining lymph and blood circulation to mucosal effector sites where IgA production occurs (Craig and Cebra, 1971). While the induction of mucosal IgA responses is known to be dependent on cognate help provided by CD4$^+$ T cells in MALT (Kawanishi et al., 1983), factors important in the subsequent development of these responses have not been well-defined. It is clear, however, that cytokines, soluble factors secreted by T cells and other immunocytes, play major roles at different stages of the mucosal immune response.

Cytokines are involved in communication between cells of the immune system and are critical in determining both the type and the magnitude of immune responses. The observation that different subsets of CD4$^+$ T helper cells produce different spectra of cytokines has provided a likely explanation for the key role played by these cells in immunoregulation (Mossman and Coffman, 1989). Thus, whether the immune response is driven toward humoral or cell-mediated immunity is determined, in part, by the profile of cytokines produced by CD4$^+$ T helper cell subpopulations. One subset (Th1) secretes interleukin-2 (IL-2), interferon-$\gamma$ (IFN-$\gamma$), and tumor necrosis factor-$\alpha$ (TNF$\alpha$) and promotes cell-mediated immunity

247

(CMI), which is considered to be important in immune defense against intracellular parasites such as viruses. Another population (Th2) secretes IL-4, IL-5, IL-6, and IL-10, factors which, *in vitro,* preferentially induce antibody responses, with selective stimulation of IgG1, IgE, and IgA isotypes. Cytokines also influence the development of these different T cell subpopulations. For example, the Th2-derived factors IL-4 and IL-10 inhibit the development of Th1 cells *in vitro,* while IFNγ produced by Th1 cells suppresses the Th2 response. The range of potential immune responses to an infectious agent may therefore be tightly regulated by cytokines produced by T cells.

Cytokine production at mucosae is apparently biased toward Th2 responses (Taguchi *et al.,* 1990), which may be an important factor in the predominance of IgA antibodies in these tissues. In this chapter, we will review evidence in support of this concept from *in vitro* and *in vivo* studies and describe how our recent work with mice rendered deficient for Th2-type cytokines sheds further light on the role of these factors in mucosal immunoregulation. Some implications of this work for improved mucosal vaccination strategies will also be discussed.

## II. Cytokines in Mucosal B-Cell Development— *In Vitro* and *In Vivo* Studies

A large number of *in vitro* and *in vivo* studies have supported a major role for the Th2-type cytokines, particularly IL-4, IL-5, and IL-6, in the development of mucosal IgA reactivity. Certainly, Th2 cells have been isolated at high frequency from mucosal tissues (Taguchi *et al.,* 1990; Xu-Amano *et al.,* 1992). There is also a clear predominance of cells expressing mRNA for Th2 cytokines in the murine small bowel, with IL-4 and IL-5 predominating in Peyer's patches and these factors, along with IL-6, also abundantly expressed in the lamina propria at sites of IgA production (Bao *et al.,* 1993). In contrast, mRNA for the Th1 factor IFNγ, thought to downregulate IgA secretion, was detected only near the muscularis.

*In vitro,* IL-4 promotes switching to IgA in murine B-cell lines (Lin *et al.,* 1991; Wakatsuki and Strober, 1993) and has been widely regarded as an essential factor for the development of surface (S)IgA$^+$ cells from S-IgA$^-$ cells, perhaps in conjunction with transforming growth factor beta (TGFβ) (Ehrhardt *et al.,* 1992). This factor is also thought to be an IgA switch factor in humans (Islam *et al.,* 1991). In contrast, murine IL-5 has no activity on S-IgA$^-$ B cells, but has been shown to increase IgA reactivity of activated mucosal S-IgA$^+$ B cells, either alone (Beagley *et al.,* 1988) or in synergy with IL-4 (Murray *et al.,* 1987), IL-6 (Kunimoto *et al.,* 1989), or TGF$_β$ (Coffman *et al.,* 1989). Thus, IL-5, while not apparently promoting a switch to IgA, acts as a S-IgA$^+$ B cell terminal differentiation factor. There is, however, no direct evidence that IL-5 normally plays such a role during IgA production *in vivo,* although, as outlined above, it has recently been shown that T cells which secrete IL-5, thereby corresponding to the Th2 type, are present at high frequency in IgA effector sites of murine mucosal tissues.

In addition, vector-expressed IL-5 selectively enhances antigen-specific IgA reactivity in murine lungs following local immunization (Ramsay and Kohonen-Corish, 1993).

It is now accepted that IL-6, a multifunctional cytokine originally identified for its ability to induce B-cell terminal differentiation (Okada *et al.,* 1983), also markedly and selectively enhances IgA production *in vitro* by isotype-committed B cells but not S-IgA⁻ B cells (Beagley *et al.,* 1989). In this respect, IL-6 appears to be a significantly more potent factor than IL-5. The *in vivo* relevance of these findings has not been determined, but the presence in mucosal tissues of T cells, macrophages, and other cells capable of IL-6 production *in vitro* (Fujihashi *et al.,* 1991; Mega *et al.,* 1992), and the broad distribution of cells containing IL-6 mRNA in intestinal mucosa (Bao *et al.,* 1993), are consistent with the idea that this factor is important in regulating the effector stage of IgA responses. The proposed influence of IL-4, IL-5, and IL-6 on mucosal IgA immunoregulation, based on these data, is summarized in Fig. 1.

The recent development of technologies whereby specific mutations may be introduced into the germline has allowed the generation of strains of mice in which particular genes have been inactivated (Capecchi, 1989). The availability of strains rendered deficient for IL-4, IL-5, or IL-6 production has allowed us to examine the induction and development of mucosal immune responses in the absence of each of these factors. This work will be described below following an · outline of the generation and initial phenotypic studies of these animals.

## III. Generation and Phenotypic Analysis of Cytokine Gene-Targeted Mice

Mice deficient for IL-4, IL-5, or IL-6 were generated using homologous recombination in embryonic stem cells with conventional gene targeting techniques. Each

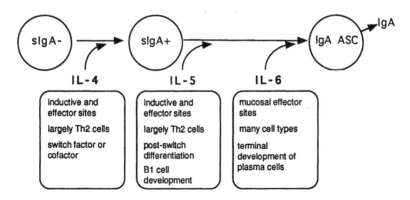

FIGURE 1. The proposed activities of IL-4, IL-5, and IL-6 in mucosal B-cell development.

of these strains developed normally; however, specific phenotypic changes were observed in each case when comparisons were made with wild-type control mice.

The IL-4-deficient mice had normal numbers of peritoneal B1 cells and B2 cells in the bone marrow, spleen, and lymph nodes (Kopf et al., 1993). Numbers of T cells and their distribution of typical surface markers were also unaltered. However, the development of Th2 cells in these animals and their ability to secrete IL-5 and IL-10 in response to helminth infestation were markedly impaired. Serum levels of IgG1 and IgE antibodies were, respectively, diminished and absent in IL-4-deficient mice.

IL-5-deficient mice showed normal lymphoid development and their production of cytokines other than IL-5 was not affected by the mutation (Kopf et al., 1996). The major phenotypic change in these mice was an inability to mount eosinophilia in response to parasite infestation or in a model of allergic lung disease, preventing the development of disease in the latter case (Foster et al., 1996)

Mice lacking IL-6 (IL-6$^{-/-}$) had normal levels of B cells but a reduction in total T-cell numbers and failed to mount optimal responses to injury or infection (Kopf et al., 1994). In particular, although total serum immunoglobulin levels were similar in IL-6$^{-/-}$ mutants and their wild-type littermates, the mutants had impaired serum IgG antibody responses following virus infection and succumbed to intracellular parasites such as *Listeria monocytogenes* and vaccinia virus. Their secretion of cytokines other than IL-6 appeared not to be affected.

These mice provided an ideal opportunity to assess the *in vivo* relevance of IL-4, IL-5, and IL-6 for mucosal IgA responses.

## IV. Mucosal Immune Responses in IL-4-Deficient Mice

*In vitro* evidence suggested that IL-4 may be an important switch factor for the production of S-IgA$^+$ B cells from S-IgM$^+$/S-IgA$^-$ B cells (Lin et al., 1991: Wakatsuki and Strober, 1993). The absence of IL-4, therefore, and the resultant downregulation of the Th2 phenotype in IL-4-deficient mice might suggest that they would be impaired in their ability to produce mucosal IgA antibodies. However, neither IgA antibody levels in lung lavage nor numbers of IgA-secreting cells in the lungs or small-intestinal lamina propria differed in IL-4$^{-/-}$ mice or wild-type mice that had not been deliberately immunized (Table 1). These results clearly showed that the ability of mucosal B cells to undergo switching to IgA production was not dependent on the presence of IL-4. Nevertheless, IL-4$^{-/-}$ mice had significantly smaller and fewer small intestinal Peyer's patches than wild-type mice with very poor germinal center development (not shown), a finding also reported by Vajdy et al. (1994). These workers found that IL-4 deficiency resulted in a marked inability to mount intestinal IgA responses following oral immunization with soluble proteins in the face of a strong response to cholera toxin given as a component of the inoculum. This deficiency appeared to be due to a failure of IL-4$^{-/-}$ mice to

### TABLE I
NORMAL IgA LEVELS IN IL-4$^{-/-}$ MICE

| Mice | Lung lavage IgA (mg/ml, ELISA) | Lung IgA ASC (ELISPOT) | Gut IgA ACC (IF cells/cm) |
|---|---|---|---|
| IL-4$^{+/+}$ | 106 ± 28 | 1406 ± 112 | 1605 ± 41 |
| IL-4$^{-/-}$ | 97 + 21 | 1367 ± 210 | 1580 ± 62 |

*Note.* Standard ELISA was performed on lung lavage fluid, ELISPOT on lung cell digests (Ramsay and Kohonen-Corish, 1993), and immmunofluorescent staining on sections of small-intestinal tissue (Ramsay *et al.,* 1994) using unimmunized mice. Figures represent mean ± SEM for groups of four mice.

mount antigen-specific Th2 cells and B cells required to induce germinal center activity in the gut.

Thus, the importance of IL-4 for the development of the Th2 subset and the immune responses driven by these cells is further illustrated in the context of the mucosal IgA response, at least to soluble antigen, and for the normal development of MALT. An important caveat, however, is that the genetic background of the animals under study may have a major influence on the results obtained in this system. For example, while the above-mentioned work was performed using IL-4$^{-/-}$ mice bred on a C57B1/6 × 129/Sv background, those on a C57B1/6 background appear to have relatively normal Peyer's patch development and responsiveness. Clarification of the importance of genetic factors in establishing the phenotype of gene-targeted mice awaits further investigation. It is clear, nevertheless, that isotype switching and mucosal IgA production can occur in the absence of IL-4.

## V. MUCOSAL IMMUNE RESPONSES IN IL-5-DEFICIENT MICE

It was apparent that IL-5-deficient mice displayed little defect in their ability to mount mucosal IgA responses (Fig. 2), despite *in vitro* evidence that IL-5 promotes the development of sIgA$^+$ mucosal B cells and the predominance of cells secreting this factor at mucosae. Numbers of IgA$^+$-staining cells in the small intestinal lamina propria were similar in IL-5$^{-/-}$ and wild-type mice that had not been deliberately immunized. We then treated these mice with a range of immunogens to further explore the effects of IL-5-deficiency on mucosal IgA reactivity. No significant differences were found in small intestinal IgA responses in IL-5$^{-/-}$ and wild-type mice following local immunization with ovalbumin (Fig. 2). In order to examine antiviral mucosal responses, we used recombinant vaccinia virus (rVV) constructs encoding the gene for the hemagglutinin (HA) glycoprotein of

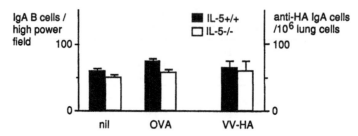

**FIGURE 2.** The mucosal IgA response in IL-5$^{-/-}$ mice. Small-intestinal tissues from unimmunized mice or from those given local inocula of ovalbumin (OVA) were stained by immunofluorescence for IgA$^+$ cells. Lung tissues from mice given intranasal inocula of VV encoding influenza HA (VV-HA) were assayed for HA-specific IgA cells by ELISPOT. All procedures were performed as described elsewhere (Ramsay et al., 1994). Values shown are for groups of four mice ± SEM.

influenza virus (VV-HA-TK). Lung IgA responses against the HA antigen were similar in IL-5-deficient and wild-type mice given intranasal inocula of the virus (Fig. 2). Finally, specific lung antibody responses were also measured following sublethal intranasal infection with influenza virus and were found not to be affected by IL-5-deficiency (not shown).

There is evidence that IL-5 influences the development of the B1 cell subset which is characterized largely by expression of the CD5 marker (Vaux et al., 1990). We therefore analyzed this population in both the peritoneal cavity and the small-intestinal lamina propria of IL-5$^{-/-}$ mice by fluorescence activated cell sorter. Cells from the former site are thought to supply a significant proportion of intestinal IgA$^+$ cells. While there was a small but significant decrease in IgA$^+$/CD5$^+$ peritoneal B cells in IL-5-deficient mice, such cells were present in equal numbers in the small intestine (not shown).

Overall, while IL-5 is apparently produced in abundance in mucosal tissues and may be used to stimulate mucosal IgA responses, its absence *in vivo* has no obvious deleterious effects on IgA production.

## VI. MUCOSAL IMMUNE RESPONSES IN IL-6-DEFICIENT MICE

We have reported that IL-6 deficiency results in a marked reduction in numbers of IgA-producing cells at mucosae and grossly deficient responses to conventional B-cell antigens such as soluble proteins and viruses (Ramsay et al., 1994). We have further suggested that IL-6 may be less important for the development of IgA-producing B1 cells, which apparently respond to a different set of antigens than conventional B2 cells, and which are present in greater numbers in IL-6$^{-/-}$ mice than in wild-type mice (Beagley et al., 1995). Here, we will summarize these data and describe new work supporting the concept that IL-6 may be an important factor for the development of conventional mucosal B-cell responses.

In the absence of deliberate immunization, IL-6$^{-/-}$ mice had substantially fewer IgA plasma cells in their small intestines and lungs (Fig. 3) and mesenteric lymph nodes (MLN, not shown) compared to wild-type mice. Qualitative differences were also apparent, in that IgA-positive cells stained much less intensely in the mutants. The paucity of IgA plasma cells in IL-6$^{-/-}$ mice was consistent with the distribution of IL-6 mRNA in intestines as determined by *in situ* hybridization, in that while IL-6 mRNA was broadly distributed throughout the lamina propria of wild-type mice, no signal was detected in IL-6$^{-/-}$ mice (Ramsay *et al.*, 1994).

Overall, the small intestines of IL-6-deficient mice had 50–60% fewer IgA-staining cells than wild-type mice and the majority of these cells stained diffusely compared to those in the latter. An explanation for this difference may lie in the observation that over 40% of murine intestinal IgA cells (50% in humans) are thought to be B1 cells, many of which are CD5$^{+}$, deriving from the peritoneal cavity rather than MALT (Pecquet *et al.*, 1992). We have shown that there is a population of IgA precursors originating from the peritoneal cavity in wild-type mice which do not respond to IL-6 by secreting IgA (Beagley *et al.*, 1995). These cells may be distinguished from conventional Peyer's patch-derived B cells by their expression of the CD5 marker. We have also found that small-intestinal IgA cells in IL-6$^{-/-}$ mice display a higher level of CD5 expression than in wild-type mice. Together, these data suggest that there is an IL-6-independent subset of in-testinal IgA plasma cells in normal mice derived from peritoneal cavity precursors and that this subset may account for the residual numbers of S-IgA$^{+}$ cells in IL-6$^{-/-}$ mice.

Support for this proposition comes from our experiments using a recombinant *Salmonella typhimurium* construct encoding the C-fragment of tetanus toxin, a strong conventional B-cell antigen. Specific IgA levels against tetanus toxoid in IL-6$^{-/-}$ mice orally immunized with this construct were 10-fold lower than in wild-type mice (S. J. Dunstan, A. J. Ramsay, and R. A. Strugnell, unpublished data). In

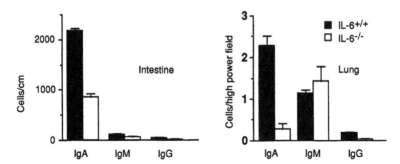

**FIGURE 3.** Numbers of IgA plasma cells in small intestines and lungs of IL-6$^{-/-}$ mice. Tissues were stained by immunofluorescence as described elsewhere (Ramsay *et al.*, 1994). Values shown are for groups of four mice ± SEM.

contrast, strain differences in IgA responses mounted against the bacterial lipopolysaccharide (a B1 antigen) were far less marked.

We next determined the consequences of IL-6 deficiency on the development of mucosal antibody responses to other conventional B-cell antigens. When immunized locally with ovalbumin, IL-6$^{-/-}$ mice mounted deficient intestinal IgA-specific responses (not shown). We then studied responses to virus infection in IL-6$^{-/-}$ and wild-type mice. For this, we employed recombinant vaccinia virus (rVV) constructs encoding the gene for the hemagglutinin (HA) glycoprotein of influenza virus (VV-HA-TK) and monitored the production of anti-HA antibody and numbers of HA-specific antibody secreting cells (ASC) in lungs following intranasal immunization. Whereas wild-type mice given VV-HA-TK mounted strong, specific IgA and IgG responses by Day 8 or 15, IL-6$^{-/-}$ mice did not develop significant numbers of ASC following virus infection (Fig. 4). This suggests that IL-6 plays an important role in the development of mucosal antibody responses to virus infection.

In an attempt to restore responsiveness, we next used rVV encoding HA together with the gene for murine IL-6 (VV-HA-IL-6) to reconstitute the expression of IL-6 in the lung (Fig. 5). Recombinant VV constructs encoding genes for foreign proteins produce these factors in a highly localized manner at sites and levels determined by the extent of virus replication (Ramshaw *et al.*, 1992; Ramsay *et*

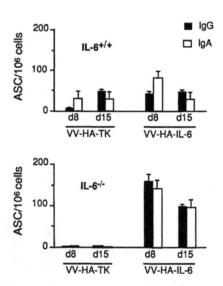

FIGURE 4. The antiviral IgA and IgG responses in lungs of IL-6$^{-/-}$ mice. Mice were given intranasal inocula of control virus (VV-HA-TK) or virus expressing IL-6 (VV-HA-IL-6) and numbers of HA-specific plasma cells were monitored 8 and 15 days later by ELISPOT (Ramsay *et al.*, 1994). Values shown are for groups of five mice ± SEM.

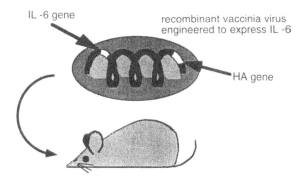

**FIGURE 5.** Intranasal immunization of mice with rVV encoding HA and IL-6.

*al.,* 1993). The ability of IL-6$^{-/-}$ mice to mount sustained mucosal antibody responses was fully restored following local administration of rVV expressing IL-6 (Fig. 4). This was not the case when the mutants were given rVV encoding IL-4 or IL-5, despite the *in vitro* evidence that these factors also promote mucosal antibody responses. While vector-encoded IL-6 promoted the development of lung IgA precursor cells, which are of mucosal origin, it clearly also provided proliferative signals for plasma cell precursors entering the lung from systemic immune sites, as shown by the restoration of IgG responses in IL-6$^{-/-}$ mice (Fig. 4). In addition, while ELISA titers of HA-specific IgA and IgG antibodies were negligible in bronchial lavage fluids from IL-6$^{-/-}$ mice given VV-HA-TK, strong responses, similar to those found in wild-type mice, were detected in IL-6$^{-/-}$ mice given VV-HA-IL-6 (not shown). These findings provide strong evidence that IL-6 plays a major role in the development of mucosal antibody responses to virus infection.

## VII. MUCOSAL IgA IMMUNITY IN Th2 CYTOKINE-DEFICIENT MICE—A SUMMARY

A wealth of data from *in vitro* and *in vivo* studies has suggested that Th2 cytokines are important mediators in mucosal B-cell development and IgA production. IL-4 was thought to be an important factor or cofactor for the switch of sIgM$^+$ B cells to S-IgA$^+$ cells, probably in the MALT, but apparently this factor also is expressed strongly in mucosal effector tissues such as the intestinal lamina propria. IL-5 producing T cells are found in MALT and effector tissues, while IL-6, produced by a multiplicity of cell types, is expressed strongly outside MALT in effector sites. These factors are not thought to be involved in isotype switching but are potent *in vitro* stimulators of the development and terminal differentiation of S-IgA$^+$ B cells, particularly IL-6. In addition, IL-5 has been thought to play an important role in B1 cell development.

Our studies in cytokine-deficient mice have confirmed some of these findings but have suggested that Th2 factors may not be crucial for some of the other functions attributed to them. It should be noted, however, that the immune systems of these mutant mice have developed in the absence of the deleted factor. Where no observable effect of the deficiency under examination is seen, it is possible that compensatory mechanisms, which may not normally be called upon to perform a particular function, may have come into play. It was clear from the work of our group and others that significant levels of IgA production occurred in the absence of IL-4, demonstrating that this factor is not crucial for IgA isotype switching. However, IL-4 was clearly important for the normal development of the intestinal IgA response to soluble protein antigen and, apparently, the optimal development of functional MALT. In contrast, IL-5 deficiency appeared to have little effect on the development of mucosal B1 or B2 cells or their IgA responsiveness. While this factor may indeed promote IgA B-cell development, it is clearly not a critical mediator. IL-6 appears to play a more important role, probably in the terminal differentiation of antibody-secreting plasma cells. Conventional mucosal IgA B cell responses were markedly impaired in IL-6$^{-/-}$ mice, which also mounted deficient IgG responses to protein and viral antigens at both mucosal and systemic sites. B1 development appeared normal, however, and it is possible that these cells may account for the majority of mucosal IgA-producing immunocytes in the absence of IL-6.

## VIII. Implications for Mucosal Vaccination

Our findings in cytokine-deficient mice suggest that IL-6 functions *in vivo* in the development of mucosal IgA responses. It is likely that IL-6 promotes the development of IgA$^+$ B cells arriving in the submucosa following their exposure to antigen in the organized mucosal lymphoid tissues. In addition to its ability to reconstitute responses in IL-6-deficient mice, vector-expressed IL-6 was seen to enhance specific IgA and IgG ASC numbers three- to fourfold in normal mice by Day 8 after infection (Fig. 4). This factor may, therefore, be a useful vaccine adjuvant for mucosal immune responses which are characteristically short-lived and often difficult to induce.

This, in fact, represents an example of an approach to vaccination taken by our group at The John Curtin School of Medical Research (A.J.R. and I.A.R.), i.e., to encode the genes for vaccine antigens along with those for cytokines such as IL-6 in infectious recombinant virus vectors (Ramshaw *et al.*, 1992; Ramsay *et al.*, 1993; Leong *et al.*, 1994). Various attempts previously have been made to modify the immune response by the administration of recombinant cytokines. This work has been hampered, however, by the short half-life of these factors *in vivo* and by difficulties in targeting recombinant material to sites of immune reactivity, with very high, and consequently nonphysiological concentrations required for observable effects. In contrast, during replication *in vivo*, our virus constructs produce the encoded factor which is secreted from infected cells, i.e., the extent and sites of virus replication determine the level and sites of production of the cytokine, which appears to act in a highly localized manner. Using this system, we have studied the immunoregulatory and antiviral properties of a number of factors. Our findings suggest that expression of selected cytokines may allow manipulation of the microenvironment to favor development of appropriate protective immune responses and, where required, suitable attenuation of the vector.

A major factor in the efficacy of infectious virus vaccines is their ability to replicate and persist in the host for several days, allowing prolonged and enhanced production of desired antigens in host cells. Vaccinia and other poxvirus vectors now being developed have the capacity to carry enough heterologous DNA to encode single or multiple genes for immunogenic proteins and allow faithful transcription and translation from inserted genes and appropriate post-translational processing and transport (Moss and Flexner, 1987). Vaccinia also stimulates good cell-mediated and humoral immunity, is highly stable, and has been successful as a vaccine in the eradication of smallpox.

To study the influence of both IL-5 and IL-6 on the development of antiviral mucosal antibody responses *in vivo,* we immunized mice intranasally with rVV encoding these factors. When lung sections were examined by immunofluorescent staining, far larger numbers of IgA ASC, clustered at foci of rVV infection, were seen in normal mice given VV-HA-IL-5 or VV-HA-IL-6 than in those given control virus (not shown). When we monitored the development of lung immunocytes secreting antibodies specific for the coexpressed HA glycoprotein by ELISPOT assay, we saw significantly greater numbers of anti-HA IgA ASC in the lungs of mice given VV-HA-IL-5 than in those given the control virus (Ramsay and Kohonen-Corish, 1993). The elevated response was first detected on Day 10 after infection and peaked on Day 14, at fourfold greater than control levels. This had declined by Day 21, although anti-HA IgA ASC were found at significantly higher levels at this stage than in mice given control virus, and was still present on Day 28, by which time responses in the control group had fallen below detectable levels. In contrast, essentially similar patterns of specific IgG reactivity were found and there was no evidence of enhanced systemic reactivity. The ability of monoclonal antibodies specific for mIL-5 to abolish the elevated response confirms that this factor was responsible for upregulating anti-HA IgA levels. We also used an ELISA to measure anti-HA IgA antibody levels in lung lavage fluids and found fourfold increases in IgA titers in mice given rVV expressing IL-5 by 28 days postinfection, and IL-6 at both 21 and 28 days. The titers presumably reflected the greater numbers of HA-specific IgA ASC found in lungs between Days 10 and 21 and were of similar magnitude to the ASC responses. Thus, both IL-5 (notwithstanding our findings in IL-5-deficient mice) and IL-6, when expressed *in vivo* as components of replicating rVV, are effective stimulators of antigen-specific mucosal IgA responses.

A major concern about the use of VV as a vaccine vector for humans is that of safety. Another poxvirus with a restricted host range, fowlpoxvirus (FPV), is currently being tested as a vaccine vector and appears to be safe, as determined in laboratory animals and humans (Cox *et al.*, 1993). The advantage of FPV over VV as a delivery vector is that FPV replication is blocked in mammalian cells; however, foreign genes under the control of early promoters are still expressed, resulting in presentation of heterologous protein to the immune system (Somogyi *et al.*, 1993). This makes the virus potentially extremely safe but, nonetheless, highly immunogenic. We therefore studied the capacity of rFPV to deliver IL-6 for the purposes of enhancing IgA responses (Leong *et al.*, 1994). As seen with rVV, marked differences in mucosal antibody responses were found in mice given intranasal inocula of rFPV constructs. Strong IgA responses were found in the lungs of mice given FPV-HA-IL-6 by 1 week after immunization whereas no responses were detected in mice given control virus (Table II). Peak IgA responses (Week 4) were three- to fourfold higher in mice given FPV-HA-IL-6 than in controls. Reactivity was greatly elevated when mice were boosted with FPV-HA-IL-6 or challenged with a sublethal dose of wild-type influenza virus (Table II).

*TABLE II*

PRIMARY AND RECALL MUCOSAL ANTI-HA ANTIBODY RESPONSES IN MICE
GIVEN rFPV

| Time | Immunization with | Number of anti-HA ASC/$10^6$ lung cells | |
| --- | --- | --- | --- |
| | | IgG | IgA |
| Primary responses | | | |
| Week 1 | FPV-HA | 22.6 | 0.0 |
| | FPV-HA-IL6 | 114.0 | 60.7 |
| Week 3 | FPV-HA | 14.0 | 28.0 |
| | FPV-HA-IL6 | 41.4 | 98.6 |
| Week 4 | FPV-HA | 13.5 | 20.0 |
| | FPV-HA-IL6 | 45.3 | 81.2 |
| Boosting at 3 weeks after immunization | | | |
| Week 1 | FPV-HA | 34.3 | 33.3 |
| | FPV-HA-IL6 | 262.2 | 469.7 |
| Challenge at 3 weeks after immunization | | | |
| Week 1 | FPV-HA | 34.3 | 33.3 |
| | FPV-HA-IL6 | 312.2 | 569.7 |

*Note.* Groups of four mice were given $10^7$ PFU virus intranasally and anti-HA ASC were determined at time intervals as indicated. At Week 3 postimmunization, some mice were given a booster, similar to the priming dose, or were challenged with a sublethal dose ($10^{-3}$ HAU) of wild-type influenza virus intranasally. Recall antibody responses were determined 1 week later.

FPV-HA-IL-6 also induced significantly greater numbers of antigen-specific lung IgG ASC than control virus, which were also greatly augmented upon boosting or challenge (Table II). These are findings of potential importance for the development of strategies to enhance recall antibody responses to vaccine antigens.

Our approach may also be useful for stimulating mucosal immunity to a wide range of vector-encoded antigens, including HIV glycoprotein. In this respect, further experiments are underway using a range of other established vectors engineered to encode cytokine genes, including adenovirus and *Salmonella,* which may be more suitable for immunization by the oral route. We are also investigating the systemic and mucosal delivery of nucleic acid vaccines encoding cytokines for enhanced mucosal priming. The expression of cytokine genes may prevent complications associated with the inadvertent vaccination of immunodeficient individuals by attenuating the vaccine vector. Of particular importance, it should also be possible, with the appropriate choice of cytokines, to design a vaccine that selectively enhances desirable primary immune responses and primes for appropriate responses upon exposure to infectious antigen.

## REFERENCES

Bao, S., Goldstone, S., and Husband, A. J. (1993). Localisation of IFN-$\gamma$ and IL-6 in murine intestine by *in situ* hybridisation. *Immunology* **80,** 666–670.

Beagley, K. W., Eldridge, J. H., Kiyono, H., Everson, M. P., Koopman, W. J., Honjo, T., and McGhee, J. R. (1988). Recombinant murine IL-5 induces high rate IgA synthesis in cycling IgA-positive Peyer's patch B cells. *J. Immunol.* **141,** 2035–2042.

Beagley, K. W., Eldridge, J. H., Lee, F., Kiyono, H., Everson, M. P., Koopman, W. J., Hirano, T., Kishimoto, T., and McGhee, J. R. (1989). Interleukins and IgA synthesis: Human and murine IL-6 induce high rate IgA secretion in IgA-committed B cells. *J. Exp. Med.* **169,** 2133–2148.

Beagley, K. W., Bao, S., Ramsay, A. J., Eldridge, J. H., and Husband, A. J. (1995). IgA production by peritoneal cavity B cells is IL-6-independent: Implications for intestinal IgA responses. *Eur. J. Immunol.* **25,** 2123–2126.

Capecchi, M. R. (1989). Altering the genome by homologous recombination. *Science* **244,** 1288–1292.

Coffman, R. L., Lebman, D. A., and Shrader, B. (1989). Transforming growth factor $\beta$ specifically enhances IgA production by lipopolysaccharide-stimulated murine B lymphocytes. *J. Exp. Med.* **170,** 1039–1044.

Cox, W. I., Tartaglia, J., and Paoletti, E. (1993). Induction of cytotoxic T lymphocytes by recombinant canarypox (ALVAC) and attenuated vaccinia (NYVAC) viruses expressing the HIV-1 envelope glycoprotein. *Virology* **195,** 845–850.

Craig, S. W., and Cebra, J. J. (1971). Peyer's patches: An enriched source of precursors for IgA-producing immunocytes in the rabbit. *J. Exp. Med.* **134,** 188–200.

Ehrhardt, R. O., Strober, W., and Harriman, G. R. (1992). Effects of transforming growth factor (TGF)-$\beta 1$ on IgA isotype expression. TGF-$\beta 1$ induces a small increase in sIgA$^+$ cells regardless of the method of B cell activation. *J. Immunol.* **148,** 3830–3836.

Foster, P. S., Hogan, S. P., Ramsay, A. J., Matthaei, K. I., and Young, I. G. (1996). IL-5 deficiency abolishes eosinophilia, hyperreactivity and lung damage in a mouse asthma model. *J. Exp. Med.* **183,** 195–201.

Fujihashi, K., McGhee, J. R., Lue, C., Beagley, K. W., Taga, T., Hirano, T., Kishimoto, T., Mestecky,

J., and Kiyono, H. (1991). Human appendix B cells naturally express receptors for and respond to interleukin 6 with selective IgA1 and IgA2 synthesis. *J. Clin. Invest.* **88,** 248–252.

Islam, K. B., Nilsson, L., Sideras, P., Hammarstrom, L., and Smith, C. I. (1991). TGF-beta-1 induces germline transcripts of both IgA subclasses in human B lymphocytes. *Int. Immunol.* **3,** 1099–1106.

Kawanishi, H., Saltzman, L., and Strober, W. (1983). Mechanisms regulating IgA class-specific immunoglobulin production in murine gut-associated lymphoid tissues. I. T cells derived from Peyer's patches that switch sIgM cells to sIgA cells *in vitro. J. Exp. Med.* **157,** 433–450.

Kopf, M., Le Gros, G., Bachmann, M., Lamers, M., Bluethmann, H., and G. Kohler. (1993). Disruption of the murine IL-4 gene blocks Th2 cytokine responses. *Nature (London)* **362,** 245–248.

Kopf, M., Baumann, H., Freer, G., Freudenberg, M., Lamers, M., Kishimoto, T., Zinkernagel, R., Bluethmann, H., and Kohler, G. (1994). Impaired immune and acute phase responses in interleukin-6-deficient mice. *Nature (London)* **368,** 339–342.

Kopf, M., Brombacher, F., Hodgkin, P. D., Ramsay, A. J., Millbourne, E. A., Dai, W. J., Ovington, K. S., Behm, C. A., Kohler, G., Young, I. G., and Matthaei, K. I. (1996). IL-5-deficient mice have a developmental defect in CD5$^+$ B cells and lack eosinphilia but have normal antibody and cytotoxic T cell responses. *Immunity* **4,** 15–24.

Kunimoto, D. Y., Nordan, R. P., and Strober, W. (1989). IL-6 is a potent cofactor of IL-1 in IgM synthesis and of IL-5 in IgA synthesis. *J. Immunol.* **143,** 2230–2235.

Leong, K. H., Ramsay, A. J., Boyle, D. B., and Ranshaw, I. A. (1994). Selective induction of immune responses by cytokines expressed in recombinant fowlpox virus. *J. Virol.* **68,** 8125–8130.

Lin, Y., Shockett, P., and Stavnezer, J. (1991). Regulation of the antibody class switch to IgA. *Immunol. Res.* **10,** 376–380.

Mega, J., McGhee, J. R., and Kiyono, H. (1992). Cytokine- and Ig-producing T cells in mucosal effector tissues: Analysis of IL-5- and IFN-gamma-producing T cells, T cell receptor expression, and IgA plasma cells from mouse salivary gland-associated tissues. *J. Immunol.* **148,** 2030–2039.

Mestecky, J., and McGhee, J. R. (1987). Immunoglobulin A (IgA): Molecular and cellular interactions involved in IgA biosynthesis and immune response. *Adv. Immunol.* **40,** 153–245.

Moss, B., and Flexner, C. (1987). Vaccinia virus expression vectors. *Annu. Rev. Immunol.* **5,** 305.

Mossman, T. R., and Coffman, R. L. (1989). TH1 and TH2 cells: Different patterns of lymphokine secretion lead to different functional properties. *Annu. Rev. Immunol.* **7,** 145–173.

Murray, P. D., McKenzie, D. T., Swain, S. L., and Kagnoff, M. F. (1987). Interleukin 5 and interleukin 4 produced by Peyer's patch T cells selectively enhance immunoglobulin A expression. *J. Immunol.* **139,** 2669–2674.

Okada, M., Sakaguchi, N., Yoshimura, N., Hara, H., Shimizu, K., Yoshida, N., Yoshizaki, K., Kishimoto, S., Yamamura, Y., and Kishimoto, T. (1983). B cell growth factors and B cell differentiation factor from human T hybridomas. Two distinct kinds of B cell growth factor and their synergism in B cell proliferation. *J. Exp. Med.* **157,** 583–590.

Pecquet, S. S., Ehrat, C., and Ernst, P. B. (1992). Enhancement of mucosal antibody responses to Salmonella typhimurium and the microbial hapten phosphorylcholine in mice with X-linked immunodeficiency by B-cell precursors from the peritoneal cavity. *Infect. Immun.* **60,** 503–509.

Ramsay A. J., and Kohonen-Corish, M. (1993). Interleukin-5 expressed by a recombinant virus vector enhances specific mucosal IgA responses *in vivo. Eur. J. Immunol.* **23,** 3141–3145.

Ramsay A. J., Ruby, J., and Ramshaw, I. A. (1993). A case for cytokines as antiviral effector molecules. *Immunol. Today* **14,** 155–157.

Ramsay, A. J., Husband, A. J., Ramshaw, I. A., Bao, S., Matthaei, K., Kohler, G., and Kopf, M. (1994). The role of interleukin-6 in mucosal IgA responses *in vivo. Science* **264,** 561–563.

Ramshaw, I. A., Ruby, J., Ramsay, A. J., Ada, G. L., and Karupiah, G. (1992). Expression of cytokines by recombinant vaccinia viruses: A model for studying cytokines in virus infections *in vivo. Immunol. Rev.* **127,** 157–182.

Somogyi, P., Frazier, J., and Skinner, M. A. (1993). Fowlpox virus host range restriction: Gene expression, DNA replication and morphogenesis in nonpermissive mammalian cells. *Virology* **197,** 439–444.

Taguchi, T., McGhee, J. R., Coffman, R. L., Beagley, K. W., Eldridge, J. H., Takatsu, K., and Kiyono, H. (1990). Analysis of Th1 and Th2 cells in murine gut-associated tissues. Frequencies of CD4[+] and CD8[+] T cells that secrete IFN-g and IL-5. *J. Immunol.* **145,** 68–77.

Vajdy, M., Kosco-Vilbois, M. H., Kopf, M., Kohler, G., and Lycke, N. (1994). Impaired mucosal immune responses in interleukin 4-targeted mice. *J. Exp. Med.* **181,** 41–53.

Vaux, D. L., Lalor, P. A., Cory, S., and Johnson, G. R. (1990). *In vivo* expression of interleukin 5 induces an eosinophilia and expanded Ly-1B lineage populations. *Int. Immunol.* **2,** 965–971.

Wakatsuki, Y., and Strober, W. (1993). Effect of downregulation of germline transcripts on immuno-globulin A isotype differentiation. *J. Exp. Med.* **178,** 129–138.

Xu-Amano, J., Kiyono, H., Jackson, R. J., Staats, H. F., Fujihashi, K., Burrows, P. D., Elson, C. O., Pillai, S., and McGhee, J. R. (1992). Helper T cell subsets for immunoglobulin A responses: oral immunization with tetanus toxoid and cholera toxin as adjuvant selectively induces Th2 cells in mucosa associated tissues. *J. Exp. Med.* **172,** 921–929.

# Chapter 20

# Adhesion Molecules on Mucosal T Lymphocytes

Alexandre Benmerah,* Natacha Patey,† and Nadine Cerf-Bensussan*

*Développement Normal et Pathologique du Système Immunitaire, INSERM U429, and †Department of Pathology, Hôpital Necker-Enfants Malades, 75743 Paris, France

## I. INTRODUCTION

The intestinal mucosa contains numerous T cells distributed in the lamina propria and in the epithelium (intraepithelial lymphocytes: IEL) which, together with IgA plasma cells, form the effector limb of the gut lymphoid-associated system. Studies in rodents suggest that mucosal T cells can be divided into two subsets. One subset of thymodependent CD3$^+$ $\alpha\beta$ TCR$^+$ lymphocytes derives, as IgA plasma cells, from blastic precursors sensitized to intraluminal antigens in Peyer's patches, circulates within a hemolymphatic cycle, and homes back into the intestinal mucosa (Guy-Grand and Vassalli, 1986; Guy-Grand et al., 1991). The majority of CD4$^+$ T cells remains in lamina propria whereas the majority of CD8$^+$ and a small number of CD4$^+$ T cells cross the basement membrane and distribute in between epithelial cells. In the intestinal mucosa, Peyer's patch-derived T cells can be activated by a new contact with the relevant antigen presented by lamina propria dendritic cells and probably in the epithelium by enterocytes. CD4$^+$ lamina propria T cells may favor the final differentiation of IgA plasma cells and control the local inflammatory response. Intraepithelial T cells secrete lymphokines and are strongly cytotoxic (reviewed in Cerf-Bensussan et al., 1993). A second subset of mucosal T lymphocytes derives from bone marrow precursors and migrates into the intestinal mucosa where they acquire, independently of the thymus, an $\alpha\beta$ or a $\gamma\delta$ T-cell receptor, an unusual CD3 complex containing the Fc$\epsilon$RI$\gamma$ chain, the CD8$\alpha$, chain and perhaps the CD8$\beta$ chain. These thymoindependent lymphocytes localize in the gut epithelium, have a repertoire distinct from that of thymodependent T cells, and exhibit cytotoxic properties. However, the mechanisms involved in their differentiation, local expansion, and activation as well as their function(s) in mucosal defenses are not known (reviewed in Rocha et al., 1995).

Intestinal T cells, as other lymphocytes, express a vast array of adhesion molecules. Recent studies have allowed definition of the nature of the adhesion molecules expressed by intestinal T lymphocytes, to demonstrate their role in mucosal homing and to delineate some of their functions in the interactions of intestinal T lymphocytes with the local partners of the immune response.

## II. NATURE OF ADHESION MOLECULES EXPRESSED BY MUCOSAL T LYMPHOCYTES

Adhesion molecules on lymphocytes belong to several structural families.

### A. Selectins

Selectins are 80- to 140-kDa single-chain integral membrane glycoproteins. Their main structural feature is an external N-terminal lectin-like domain responsible for their binding to complex sugars identical or related to sLe$^x$. They play a major role in homing by favoring the initial step of loose and reversible interactions between circulating cells and endothelial cells. Three selectins have been individualized, L-, E-, and P-selectins (reviewed in McEver *et al.*, 1995). L-selectin is expressed by small mature lymphocytes, monocytes, and polymorphonuclear cells (PMNs) whereas E- and P-selectins are expressed by inflammatory endotheliums. L-selectin allows the binding of lymphocytes to sugars identical or related to sLe$^x$ decorating mucin-like proteins expressed by endothelial cells: Glycam-1 on high endothelial venules (HEV) in peripheral lymph nodes, CD34 on all blood vessels, and MadCAM-1 on HEV in Peyer's patches and mesenteric lymph nodes (Berg *et al.*, 1993; Hemmerich *et al.*, 1994). Thereby, L-selectin is important for lymphocyte migration in peripheral and mesenteric lymph nodes as well as in Peyer's patches. However, L-selectin is shed from the lymphocyte cell surface during cell activation (Kahn *et al.*, 1994; McEver *et al.*, 1995) and is absent from most mucosal T cells (Salmi *et al.*, 1995; Schmitz *et al.*, 1988). In addition, lamina propria flat endothelium is thought to express a form of MadCAM-1 devoided of L-selectin-binding carbohydrates (Berlin *et al.*, 1995). Thus, L-selectin should not play an important role in intestinal homing to normal mucosa. Accordingly, anti-L-selectin antibodies do not block adhesion of lamina propria blasts on intestinal endothelium (Salmi *et al.*, 1995).

### B. Immunoglobulin Superfamily

The immunoglobulin superfamily is a large family of molecules made of variable numbers of paired or unpaired Ig domains, each Ig domain being composed of 90–100 amino acids arranged in a sandwich of two sheets of anti-parallel β strands and usually stabilized by a disulfide bond at its center. Several membrane receptors expressed by T cells belong to this family. They recognize complementary receptors on the surface of endothelial cells or of antigen presenting cells (APC) which may belong to the same family of proteins or to another family, the integrins (reviewed in Springer, 1990). Some proteins, such as CD3, CD28, CD4, and CD8, have a role in antigen recognition and signal transduction but do not efficiently participate in lymphocyte adhesion since their affinity for their ligand is too low. Others, such as CD2 and the intercellular adhesion molecules (ICAMs), have a role in lymphocyte adhesion (Fig. 1).

## 1. CD2

CD2 is a 50-kDa glycoprotein made of two immunoglobulin-like domains followed by a transmembrane sequence and a COOH-terminal cytoplasmic region of 116 or 117 residues. CD2 is expressed on all T cells and NK cells and binds CD58 (LFA-3), a 40- to 70-kDa, broadly distributed glycoprotein made of two immunoglobulin domains (reviewed in Bierer and Burakoff, 1989), and CD59, another broadly distributed glycoprotein of 18–20 kDa (Hahn *et al.,* 1992). The role of CD2 in lymphocyte adhesion is demonstrated by the inhibitory effect of anti-CD2 antibodies on the formation of conjugates between T cells and APC or between cytotoxic T lymphocytes and their targets (Bierer and Burakoff, 1989). The affinity of the CD2/CD58 interactions has been estimated to be in the range of $10^6 \, M^{-1}$. Electron microscopic measurements of intermembrane distance predict that interactions between CD2 and LFA-3 take place within a short intermembrane distance of 13 nm or less (Springer, 1990). In addition to its role in cell adhesion, CD2 transduces intracytoplasmic signals which synergize with signals

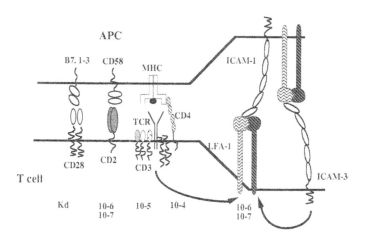

**FIGURE 1.** Schematical representation of the interactions between antigen-presenting cells (APC) and T cells. The arrows indicate that a signal given to T cells via the CD3–TCR complex or via ICAM-3 increases the avidity of LFA-1 for its ICAM-1 ligand and thus strengthens adhesion and interactions between APC and T cells.

given via CD3-TCR. Crosslinking of CD2 induces rise in cytoplasmic-free calcium, inositol phosphate, and diacylglycerol mobilization, tyrosine phosphorylation of the $\zeta$ chain of CD3 (Spruyt et al., 1991).

In the human intestinal mucosa, most if not all intestinal T cells express CD2 (Jarry et al., 1990; unpublished observations). The CD2 ligand, CD58/LFA3, is expressed by many lamina propria cells, including cells of the histiomonocytic lineage and is also strongly expressed by enterocytes (unpublished observations). The interaction of CD2 with CD58 may thus play a role not only in the interactions of lymphocytes with APC in lamina propria but also in the interactions of intraepithelial lymphocytes with enterocytes.

### 2. ICAM-1 and ICAM-3

Two intercellular adhesion molecules, ICAM-1 (CD54) and ICAM-3 (CD50), are expressed by lymphocytes. They are ligands for the $\beta2$ integrins, LFA-1, expressed by all leukocytes and MAC, expressed by polymorphonuclears cells and histiomonocytic cells (see below). Expression of ICAM-1 (CD54) is induced by inflammatory cytokines (IL1, TNF$\alpha$, $\gamma$-interferon) on numerous cell types, including macrophages, endothelial cells, and activated lymphocytes. ICAM-3 is constitutively expressed on lymphocytes and monocytes. Via their interactions with their lymphocyte ligand LFA-1, these two molecules play a major role in lymphocyte adhesion (reviewed in Springer, 1990; Campanero et al., 1993).

In tissue sections of normal intestine, ICAM-1 is expressed on endothelial cells and large cells resembling macrophages. In inflamed intestinal mucosa, such as in graft rejection, there is a diffuse and intense staining of most lamina propria cells. In contrast, even in inflamed mucosa, its expression is detected neither on IEL nor on epithelial cells (Fromont et al., 1995). These in situ studies contrast with in vitro studies of intestinal epithelial cell lines which suggest that ICAM-1 can be expressed by epithelial cells particularly after exposure to $\gamma$-interferon (Kvale et al., 1992). ICAM-3 is strongly expressed by lamina propria and intraepithelial lymphocytes (unpublished observations).

### C. Integrins

Integrins are integral membrane glycoproteins made of two different noncovalently bound $\alpha$ and $\beta$ subunits of approximately 120–180 and 90–120 kDa, respectively. Eight $\beta$ chains (with 37–75% homology) and 14 $\alpha$ chains (with 25–65% homology) have been identified. One $\beta$ chain can associate with different $\alpha$ chains, allowing definition of several subfamilies depending on the utilized $\beta$ chain. Some $\alpha$ chains (particularly $\alpha4$) can also associate with several $\beta$ chains. Integrins mediate adhesion of cells to extracellular matrix proteins (in which several binding sites have been precisely identified) and/or cell–cell adhesion via counterreceptors which generally belong to the immunoglobulin superfamily. The external N-terminal domains of the $\alpha$ and $\beta$ chains interact to form the ligand binding site. The intracytoplasmic domains of the $\beta$ chain are connected with cytoskeleton proteins such as $\alpha$-actinin, vinculin, and talin and with signaling molecules. Through these connections, integrins participate in a bidirectional dialog across the cell membrane which modulates their binding avidity and/or results in signal transduction (reviewed in Hynes, 1992; Clark and Brugge, 1995).

Avidity of integrins for their ligand is modulated by both extracellular and intracellular signals. At the basal state, integrins bind to their ligands with a relatively low affinity. Following binding to their ligands or cell activation, their avidity for their ligands can be multiplied more than 100 times (Hynes, 1992). These changes result from a redistribution of the integrin in the areas of cell contact regulated by the interactions of the intracytoplasmic domain of the $\beta$ chain with cytoskeleton proteins, as well as from conformational changes of the integrins which may be regulated via the intracytoplasmic domain of the $\alpha$ chain (Clark and Brugge, 1995). Besides their function in adhesion, integrins participate in signal transduction. Thus, activation of integrins can stimulate several tyrosine kinases, particularly the pp125$^{FAK}$, some tyrosine phosphatases, the phosphoinositide, and the RAS-MAP kinases pathways. The nature of the signaling pathways seem to vary for the different integrins and in the different cell types (reviewed in Clark and Brugge, 1995).

The $\beta$1, $\beta$2, and $\beta$7 integrins are expressed by lymphocytes and play a role in their migration and activation.

## 1. LFA-1

LFA-1 ($\alpha L \beta 2$ or CD11a/CD18) is expressed on all leukocytes. By interacting with its ICAM-1 and ICAM-3 ligands, LFA-1 contributes to lymphocyte activation by APC, to T and B cell interactions and to interactions of killer lymphocytes with their target cells (Springer, 1990). By interacting with its ICAM-1 and ICAM-2 ligands (the latter constitutively expressed by all endothelial cells), LFA-1 mediates adhesion strengthening to endothelium and diapedesis of lymphocytes, monocytes, and PMNs in many sites (Springer, 1994). LFA-1 has a higher binding avidity for ICAM-1 than for its other ligands. Moreover, its binding avidity for ICAM-1 can be modulated by many stimuli, some of which may be important *in vivo*. Thus, in T cells, activation of the CD3–TCR pathway induces a transient increase in the avidity of LFA-1 which favors specific contacts between T cells and APC or target cells (Dustin and Springer, 1989). Binding of ICAM-3 on T cells by LFA-1 on APC activates T cell p56$^{lck}$ and p59 $^{fyn}$ tyrosine kinases (Juan *et al.*, 1994). This signal increases the avidity of the LFA-1 molecule expressed by lymphocytes for its other ligand ICAM-1 present on APC (Campanero *et al.*, 1993), thereby promoting the interactions of T cells with APC and the exchange of specific signals (Fig. 1).

In the intestinal mucosa, LFA-1 is strongly expressed by all lamina propria T cells and macrophages (unpublished observations). It is also expressed by IELs, albeit at a lower level (Jarry *et al.*, 1990). As indicated above, ICAM-1 and -3 are expressed by most if not all lamina propria mononuclear cells, ICAM-1 and -2 by intestinal endothelial cells. In contrast, ICAM-1, -2, and -3 are not expressed by epithelial cells. The distribution of LFA-1 and of its ligands suggests that LFA-1 plays an important role in the interactions of lamina propria but not of intraepithelial lymphocytes with their local microenvironment.

### 2. VLA-4

VLA-4($\alpha4\beta1$ or CD49d/CD29) is expressed on most circulating lymphocytes and monocytes. It is a matrix receptor for an alternatively spliced fragment of fibronectin, a cellular ligand for VCAM-1, a molecule of the Ig superfamily expressed by activated endothelial cells and APC as well as a receptor for invasin, an outer membrane protein of *Yersinia pseudotuberculosis* (Masumoto and Hemler, 1993). Experimental studies indicate that VLA-4 plays a role in T-cell activation, in T-cell-mediated killing, and in lymphocyte homing to sites of chronic inflammation (Van Seventer *et al.*, 1991; Lobb and Hemler, 1994). In the intestine, lamina propria lymphocytes express $\alpha4$ and $\beta1$ (Salmi *et al.*, 1995). Expression of $\beta1$ is variable on IEL but is generally low or absent (Jarry *et al.*, 1988). VCAM-1 is expressed on large lamina propria cells (Fromont *et al.*, 1995), suggesting that VLA-4/VCAM-1 may play a role in the interactions of lamina propria lymphocytes with mucosal APC. In contrast, VCAM-1 expression by endothelial cells is weak and inconstant in normal individuals and is not detected in inflamed mucosa (Fromont *et al.*, 1995; Koizumi *et al.*, 1992), suggesting that VCAM-1 does not have an important role in the migration into the intestinal mucosa. Accordingly, anti-$\beta1$ antibodies have no effect on the binding of lamina propria lymphoblasts to mucosal endothelial cells (Salmi *et al.*, 1995).

### 3. $\alpha4\beta7$

The $\alpha4\beta7$ integrin is expressed by lymphocytes and monocytes. Its expression, as that of $\alpha4\beta1$, increases following lymphocyte activation. In human peripheral blood, it is expressed by most newborn T lymphocytes and by approximately 50% of T cells (Erle *et al.*, 1994). Its expression is very high in the human intestinal lamina propria lymphocytes but is approximately 10 times less on IEL, (Salmi *et al.*, 1995; personal observations). Similar to $\alpha4\beta1$, $\alpha4\beta7$ can bind fibronectin and VCAM-1 (Postigo *et al.*, 1993). However, its main ligand is MadCAM-1, a protein containing three immunoglobulin domains and one mucin-like domain, which is expressed by HEV in Peyer's patches and mesenteric lymph nodes and by the flat endothelium in lamina propria. Recent studies indicate that the interactions of $\alpha4\beta7$ and MadCAM-1 play a major role in lymphocyte homing to Peyer's patches and lamina propria (Berlin *et al.*, 1993; Erle *et al.*, 1994). In mice and in humans, TGF$_\beta$ downregulates $\alpha4$ expression and induces expression of another integrin $\alpha$ chain, $\alpha$E, which associates with $\beta7$ to form a distinct integrin, $\alpha$E$\beta7$ (Kilshaw and Murant, 1991; Parker *et al.*, 1992).

## 4. αEβ7 (CD103)

The $\alpha_E\beta7$ (CD103) integrin was initially defined by the HML-1 monoclonal antibody in humans (Cerf-Bensussan *et al.*, 1987) and by the M290 monoclonal antibody in mice (Kilshaw *et al.*, 1990). It is strongly expressed by IEL in the gut epithelium as well in other epitheliums (Cerf-Bensussan *et al.*, 1987, 1988) and appears on human peripheral T cells, particularly CD8$^+$, after several days of activation (Schiefferdecker *et al.*, 1990). It is also expressed by tumoral IEL in enteropathy-associated T-cell lymphomas (Spencer *et al.*, 1988) and in Mycosis fungoides (Simonitsch *et al.*, 1994). Finally, studies in rats (Cerf-Bensussan *et al.*, 1986) and in chicken (Haury *et al.*, 1993) suggest that the $\alpha_E\beta7$ integrin is also present on IELs in these species. The restricted distribution of $\alpha_E\beta7$/CD103 is likely related to the large production of TGF$\beta$ by epithelial cells (Barnard *et al.*, 1993) and by some activated T cells (Lucas *et al.*, 1990).

Recent work has demonstrated that CD103 mediates the binding of IEL to epithelial cells (Cepek *et al.*, 1993; Benmerah *et al.*, 1994; Roberts and Kilshaw, 1994). Furthermore, its epithelial ligand has been identified as the E-cadherin (Cepek *et al.*, 1994), an epithelial membrane protein previously known for its role in homophilic interactions between epithelial cells, in epithelial morphogenesis and formation of adherent junctions (Takeichi, 1991). It is interesting to observe that IELs may bind to a form of E-cadherin distinct from that involved in the formation of the adherent junctions. Indeed, to ensure adhesion between epithelial cells, E-cadherin must associate with several intracytoplasmic proteins, the $\alpha$- and $\beta$-catenins which connect the intracytoplasmic domain of E-cadherin with actin-based cytoskeleton (Kemler, 1993). In contrast, the association of E-cadherin with $\alpha$-catenin and cytoskeleton does not seem to be required for lymphoepithelial interactions since adhesion of lymphocytes via CD103 was normal on an $\alpha$-catenin-deficient epithelial cell line (Benmerah and Cerf-Bensussan, unpublished observations).

Experiments in animals suggest that the interactions of $\alpha_E\beta7$/CD103 on IELs and E-cadherin on epithelial cells do not play a role in lymphocyte homing into the epithelial layer (Cerf-Bensussan *et al.*, 1988, Haury *et al.*, 1993). However, these interactions may perhaps promote exchange of signals between the two cell types. On the one hand, E-cadherin is involved in the control of several epithelial functions including epithelial cell growth (Peifer, 1993). IEL may perhaps transduce, via CD103, signals modulating epithelial functions. On the other hand, E-cadherin may provide signals regulating IEL's activation. The observation that several anti-CD103 antibodies strongly enhance activation of human gut IELs via the CD3-TcR pathway sustains this hypothesis (Sarnacki *et al.*, 1992).

Besides its function in lymphoepithelial interactions, the CD103 integrin may have a role in lymphocyte interactions. Thus, one anti-CD103 antibody, HML-4 induces a strong homotypic aggregation of CD103$^+$ lymphocytes which is mediated via CD103 and may involved homophilic CD103–CD103 interactions (Benmerah *et al.*, 1994). The physiological role of CD103-mediated adhesion between lymphocytes remains to be investigated. *In vitro* studies suggest that homotypic aggregation is associated with the transduction of an activating signal into lymphocytes (Sarnacki *et al.,* 1992; unpublished observations). Such interactions may become important in inflamed epitheliums, as in celiac disease when the epithelium is overcrowed by IEL.

## D. Proteoglycan/Cartilage-Link Protein CD44

CD44 (H-CAM, Pgp-1) is a single-chain molecule of the proteoglycan family expressed on a wide range of cells in multiple variant isoforms generated by alternative splicing, by multiple N- and O-glycosylations and covalent linkage to chondroitin-sulfate. On hematopietic cells, including lymphocytes, the predominant form has an extracellular domain encoded by seven exons. The 37-kDa protein core is heavily N- and O-glycosylated to yield a 85- to 100-kDa mature protein. Variant forms with an extracellular domain encoded by additional exons can be observed, particularly after lymphocyte activation which also enhances the level of CD44 expression (reviewed in Stauder and Günthert, 1995).

The major ligand for CD44 is hyaluronic acid, but other components of the extracellular matrix, like fibronectin, collagen, and a sulfated proteoglycan, have been described as ligands for CD44. The avidity of the various isoforms of CD44 for hyaluronic acid is variable and increases in lymphocytes following activation of protein kinase C which interacts with the cytoplasmic tail of CD44 (Lesley *et al.,* 1992).

A growing number of functions have been assigned to CD44. In lymphocytes, CD44 may serve an accessory role in T-cell activation (reviewed in Stauder and Günthert, 1995). In addition, CD44 is involved in lymphocyte homing. Thus, CD44 expression by lymphocytes was correlated with their ability to bind HEV and an anti-CD44 polyclonal antibody blocked lymphocyte binding to peripheral, synovial, and mucosal HEV (reviewed in Salmi and Jalkanen, 1991). The effect of CD44 may be to enhance lymphocyte contact with HEV, which synthethize hyaluronic acid, and to favor retention in tissues. CD44 may also favor diapedesis since studies of CD44-transfected melanomatous cells have shown induction of cell mobility by the hematopietic form of CD44 (Thomas *et al.,* 1992). Endothelial CD44 may also contribute to lymphocyte homing since, *in vitro,* CD44 can present chemokines such as MIP1$\beta$ to lymphocytes. This chemokine activates the high-avidity conformation of integrins, probably via a G-protein-linked receptor, and thus stimulates lymphocyte adhesion (Tanaka *et al.,* 1993). Finally, besides a general function in lymphocyte migration, CD44 may more specifically enhance mucosal homing. Thus, one anti-CD44 monoclonal antibody, Hermes-3, specifically blocked binding to mucosal HEV. Furthermore, CD44 purified from lymphocytes but not from epithelial cells bound to the MadCAM-1 mucosal addressin, an interaction which was blocked by Hermes 3 via a domain distinct from the hyaluronate-binding site (reviewed in Salmi and Jalkanen, 1991).

## III. FUNCTIONS OF ADHESION MOLECULES EXPRESSED BY MUCOSAL T LYMPHOCYTES

### A. Functions of Adhesion Molecules in Homing of PP-Derived Blasts into the Intestinal Mucosa

Homing of lymphocytes into the intestinal mucosa is reviewed in another chapter and will be only considered briefly. *In vitro* studies showed that antibodies against CD44, LFA-1, and $\alpha 4\beta 7$ could partially block the adhesion of human intestinal lymphoblasts on intestinal endothelium (Salmi *et al.,* 1995). *In vivo* studies in rodents have confirmed the partial inhibitory effect of anti-LFA-1 and anti$\alpha 4\beta 7$ antibodies on lymphocyte homing into the intestine (Hamann *et al.,* 1994). Recent work indicates that $\alpha 4\beta 7$ can replace L-selectin (absent of most intestinal lymphocytes; see above) and support the initial step of loose and reversible attachment of lymphocytes on MadCAM-1$^+$ lamina propria venules (Berlin *et al.,* 1995). $\alpha 4\beta 7$, and probably LFA-1, then contribute to the second step of firm adhesion which precedes diapedesis and extravasation. The role of CD44 remains less well understood (see above).

### B. Functions of Adhesion Molecules in the Migration of T Lymphocytes in the Gut Epithelium

The mechanisms involved in the preferential localization of CD8$^+$ T cells and in the migration of some lymphoid precursors into the epithelium remain unknown. As indicated above, there is no evidence for a role for the CD103 integrin. Lamina propria lymphocytes and, at a lesser level, IEL express $\alpha 4\beta 1$ and $\alpha 4\beta 7$, two receptors for fibronectin. They express CD44, a receptor for hyaluronic acid, fibronectin, and collagen. Some IEL also express $\alpha 1\beta 1$, another integrin which is a receptor for collagen (Hynes, 1992; unpublished observations). These receptors may favor interactions of intestinal lymphocytes with the epithelial basement membrane rich in fibronectin, collagen, and hyaluronic acid and thus promote lymphocyte entrance into the epithelium. In addition, the gut epithelium, as other epitheliums, may secrete chemotactic factors able to activate the integrins and to promote the lymphocyte movement across the basement membrane. The production by intestinal epithelial cell lines of many chemokines including IL-8 (Eckmann *et al.,* 1993) and, moreover, MIP1$\alpha$ and -$\beta$, known for their chemoattractant activity toward T cells (Tanaka *et al.,* 1993, Yang *et al.,* 1995), supports this hypothesis (Fig. 2).

### C. Role of Adhesion Molecules in Activation and Functions of Lamina Propria Lymphocytes

After migration in the intestinal mucosa, the effector functions of Peyer's patch-derived lamina propria T cells are triggered by a new contact with the sensitizing

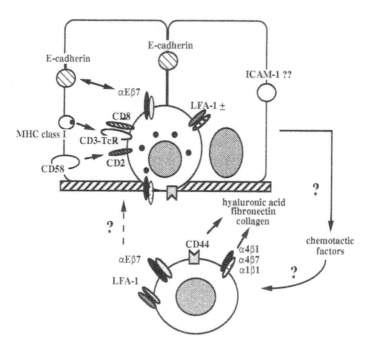

**FIGURE 2.** Hypothetical model of lymphoepithelial interactions.

antigen. The mechanisms which control the activation of intestinal T lymphocytes are not known. In the intestinal lamina propria, a large number of cells with the phenotypic and functional characteristics of macrophages and dendritic cells have been demonstrated (Bland and Kambarage, 1991; Pavli *et al.,* 1993). The role of adhesion molecules in the activation of lamina propria T cells by lamina propria APC has not been investigated specifically but is probably comparable to their role in other lymphoid organs. As indicated above, lamina propria T cells express CD2, CD50/ICAM-3, and LFA-1 and thus can interact with CD58/LFA-3, CD54/ICAM-1, and CD50/ICAM-3 expressed on lamina propria APC to favor specific contacts between the CD3/TcR complex of T cells and the antigenic peptides presented by MHC molecules on APC (Fig. 1). As previously discussed, these interactions not only promote cell contacts but also allow the transduction of accessory signals which synergize with specific signals transduced via the CD3–TCR complex. Activation of lamina propria T cells, mainly CD4[+], triggers the release of lymphokines able to enhance the local production of immuglobulins or to stimulate the inflammatory response of lamina propria macrophages, polymorphonuclears, mast cells, and endothelial cells necessary to prevent dissemination of infectious agents. In addition, lamina propria contains some cytotoxic CD8[+] T cells which may contribute to the elimination of macrophages infected by viruses or intracellular bacteriae. Adhesion of T cells on their infected targets can be mediated via the interactions of CD2 with CD58/LFA-3 and of LFA-1 with ICAM-1/CD54 (Shaw *et al.*, 1986).

## D. Role of Adhesion Molecules in Activation and Functions of Intraepithelial Lymphocytes

The normal gut epithelium contains no or very few conventional APC susceptible to present antigen to IEL. This function may be at least partially fulfilled by enterocytes. Indeed, a number of specific signals could be delivered in the epithelial layer to the CD3–TCR complex of IELs. Enterocytes express class I MHC antigens and thus could present peptides derived from viruses or intracellular bacteriae to CD8$^+$ thymodependent $\alpha\beta$ IEL (Shawar *et al.*, 1994) (Fig. 2). Villi enterocytes (and in certain circumstances crypt enterocytes) express class II MHC molecules, which may allow presentation of enterotoxins (unpublished observations) and perhaps of other soluble antigens to IEL (reviewed in Bland and Kambarage, 1991). Finally, recent work suggests that specific signals may be delivered to IEL by class I-like molecules, some of which are specifically expressed by the gut epithelium (Panja *et al.*, 1993; Shawar *et al.*, 1994) or even by small components independently of any MHC presentation in the case of $\gamma\delta$ IEL (Constant *et al.*, 1994). Conversely, epithelial cells infected by virus or damaged by enterotoxins can likely become targets for cytotoxic IEL (reviewed in Cerf-Bensussan *et al.*, 1993). Several adhesion molecules may favor these lymphoepithelial interactions (Fig. 2). The CD2 molecule on IELs could interact with LFA-3/CD58 on epithelial cells. In contrast, interactions between LFA-1 and CD54/ICAM-1, which play a major role in the periphery, may not take place or have only a minor role in the intestinal epithelium. As discussed above, LFA-1 is expressed by IEL, albeit often at a low level. Furthermore, it is difficult to detect *in situ* expression of ICAM-1 on epithelial cells. We suggest that the interactions of CD103 on IEL and E-cadherin on epithelial cells substitute in the intestinal epithelium for the LFA-1/ICAM-1 interactions. Anti-CD103 antibodies, which block adhesion of IEL on epithelial cells, also blocks the cytotoxicity of IEL against epithelial cells (Roberts *et al.*, 1993, Roberts and Kilshaw, 1994), indicating that CD103 is important to allow the contact of IEL with their epithelial targets. Furthermore, an accessory signal may be transduced via CD103 into lymphocytes, a signal which synergized with the specific signal given via CD3–TCR. Thus, one anti-CD103 antibody obtained against mouse IELs triggered the cytotoxicity of IEL (Lefrançois *et al.*, 1994). Furthermore, anti-CD103 antibodies used to mimic the effect of E-cadherin strongly potentialized the activation of IEL through the CD3–TcR pathway (Sarnacki *et al.*, 1992).

## IV. CONCLUSION

Experimental studies have allowed delineation of some of the unusual homing and functional properties of gut-associated lymphocytes. A large number of adhesion molecules likely to participate in the interactions of gut lymphocytes with their microenvironment have been identified. However, it must be emphasized that the precise role of each of these molecules at the various steps of the intestinal immune response remains largely hypothetical. The large number of antibodies now available against these molecules represents useful tools to identify molecules crucial for recruitment and/or activation of gut lymphocytes and thus to identify possible targets for immunointervention in intestinal diseases related to immune disorders.

## REFERENCES

Barnard, J. A., Warwick, G. J., and Gold, L. I. (1993). Localization of transforming growth factor $\beta$ isoforms in the normal murine small intestine and colon. *Gastroenterology* **105**, 67–73.

Benmerah, A., Badrichani, A., Ngohou, K., Mégarbané, B., Bègue, B., Cerf-Bensussan, N. (1994). Homotypic aggregation of CD103 ($\alpha E\beta 7$)$^+$ lymphocytes by an anti-CD103 antibody, HML-4. *Eur. J. Immunol.* **24**, 2243–2249.

Berg, E. L., McEvoy, L. M., Berlin, C., Bargatze, R. F., and Butcher, E. C. (1993). L-selectin-mediated lymphocyte rolling on MadCAM-1. *Nature (London)* **366**, 695–698.

Berlin, C., Berg, E., Briskin, M. J., Andrew, D. P., Kilshaw, P. J., Holzmann, B. Weissman, I. L., Hamann, A., and Butcher, E. C. (1993). $\alpha 4\beta 7$ integrin mediates lymphocyte-binding to the mucosal vascular addressin MadCAM-1. *Cell (Cambridge, Mass.)* **74**, 185–195.

Berlin, C., Bargatze, R. F., Campbell, J. J., von Andrian, U. H., Szabo, M. C., Hasslen, S. R., Nelson, R. D., Berg, E. L., Erlandsen, S. L., and Butcher, E. C. (1995). $\alpha 4$ integrins mediate lymphocyte attachment and rolling under physiologic flow. *Cell (Cambridge, Mass.)* **80**, 413–422.

Bierer, B. E., and Burakoff, S. J. (1989). T-lymphocyte-activation: The biology and function of CD2 and CD4. *Immunol. Rev.* **111**, 267–294.

Bland, P. W., and Kambarage, D. M. (1991). Antigen handling by the epithelium and lamina propria macrophages. *Gastroenterol. Clin. North Am.* **20**, 577–596.

Campanero, M. R., del Pozo, M. A., Sanchez-Mateos, P., Hernandez-Caselles, T., Craig, A., Pulido, R., and Sanchez-Madrid, F. (1993). ICAM-3 interacts with LFA-1 and regulates the LFA-1/ICAM-1 cell adhesion pathway. *J. Cell Biol.* **123**, 1007–1016.

Cepek, K. L., Parker, C. M., Madara, J. L., and Brenner, M. B. (1993). Integrin $\alpha E\beta 7$ mediates adhesion of T lymphocytes to epithelial cells. *J. Immunol.* **150**, 3459–3470.

Cepek, K. L., Shaw, S. K., Parker, C. M., Russell, G. J., Morrow, J. S., Rimm, D. R., and Brenner, M. B. (1994). Adhesion between epithelial cells and T lymphocytes mediated by E-cadherin and an integrin, $\alpha E\beta 7$. *Nature (London)* **372**, 190–193.

Cerf-Bensussan, N., Guy-Grand, D., Lisowska-Grospierre, B., Griscelli, C., and Bhan, A. K. (1986). A monoclonal antibody specific for rat intestinal lymphocytes. *J. Immunol.* **136**, 76–82.

Cerf-Bensussan, N., Jarry, A., Brousse, N., Lisowska-Grospierre, B., Guy-Grand, D., and Griscelli, C. (1987). A monoclonal antibody (HML-1) defining a novel membrane molecule present on human intestinal lymphocytes. *Eur. J. Immunol.* **17**, 1279–1285.

Cerf-Bensussan, N., Jarry, A., Gnéragbé, T., Brousse, N., Lisowska-Grospierre, B., Griscelli, C., and Guy-Grand, D. (1988). Monoclonal antibodies specific for intestinal lymphocytes. *Monogr. Allergy* **24**, 167–172.

Cerf-Bensussan, N., Cerf, M., and Guy-Grand, D. (1993). Gut intraepithelial lymphocytes and gastrointestinal diseases. *Curr. Opin. Gastroenterol.* **9**, 953–962.

Clark, E. A., and Brugge, J. S. (1995). Integrins and signal transduction pathways: The road taken. *Science* **268**, 233–238.

Constant, P., Davodeau, F., Peyrat, M.-A., Poquet, Y., Puzo, G., Bonneville, M., and Fournié, J-J. (1994). Stimulation of human γδ T cells by nonpeptidic mycobacterial ligands. *Science* **264**, 267–270.

Dustin, L. M., and Springer, T. A. (1989). T-cell receptor cross-linking transiently stimulates adhesiveness through LFA-1. *Nature (London)* **341**, 619–623.

Eckmann, L., Jung, H. C., Schürer-Maly, C., Panja, A., Morzycka-Wroblewska, E., and Kagnoff, M. (1993). Differential cytokine expression by human intestinal epithelial cell lines: Regulated expression of interleukin 8. *Gastroenterology* **105**, 1689–1697.

Erle, D. J., Briskin, M. J., Butcher, E. C., Garcia-Pardo, A. I., and Tidswell, M. (1994). Expression and function of the MadCAM-1 receptor integrin α4β7, on human leukocytes. *J. Immunol.* **153**, 517–528.

Fromont, G., Cerf-Bensussan, N., Patey, N., Canioni, D., Rambaud, C., Goulet, O., Révillon, Y., Ricour, C., and Brousse, N. (1995). Small bowell transplantation in children: An immunohistochemical study. *Gut* in press.

Guy-Grand, D., and Vassalli, P. (1986). Gut injury in graft-versus-host disease. Study of its occurence and mechanisms. *J. Clin. Invest.* **77**, 1584–95.

Guy-Grand, D., and Vassalli, P. (1986). Gut injury in graft-versus-host disease. Study of its occurence and mechanisms. *J. Clin. Invest.* **77**, 1584–95.

Guy-Grand, D., Cerf-Bensussan, N., Malissen, B., Malassis-Seris, M., Briottet, C., and Vassalli, P. (1991). Two gut intraepithelial CD8+ lymphocyte populations with different T cell receptors: A role for the gut epithelium in T cell differentiation. *J. Exp. Med.* **173**, 471–481.

Hahn, W. C., Menu, E., Bothwell, A. L. M., Sims, P. J., and Bierer, B. E. (1992). Overlapping but nonidentical binding sites on CD2 for CD58 and a second ligand CD59. *Science* **256**, 1805–1807.

Hamann, A., Andrew, D. P., Jablonski-Westrich, D., Holzmann, B., and Butcher, E. C. (1994). Role of α4-integrins in lymphocyte homing to mucosal tissues *in vivo*. *J. Immunol.* **152**, 3282–3293.

Haury, M., Kasahara, Y., Schall, S., Bucy, R. P., and Cooper, M. D. (1993). Intestinal lymphocytes in the chicken express an integrin-like antigen. *Eur. J. Immunol.* **23**, 313–319.

Hemmerich, S., Butcher, E. C., and Rosen, S. D. (1994). Sulfatation-dependent recognition of high endothelial venules (HEV)-ligands by L-selectin and MECA 79, an adhesion-blocking monoclonal antibody. *J. Exp. Med.* **180**, 2219–2226.

Hynes, R. O. (1992). Integrins: versatility, modulation, and signaling in cell adhesion. *Cell (Cambridge, Mass.)* **69**, 11–25.

Jarry, A., Cerf-Bensussan, N., Brousse N., Guy-Grand D., Muzeau F., and Potet, F. (1988). Same peculiar subset of HML-1+ lymphocytes present within normal intestinal epithelium is associated with tumoral epithelium of gastrointestinal carcinomas. *Gut* **29**, 1632–1638.

Jarry, A., Cerf-Bensussan, N., Brousse, N., Selz, F., and Guy-Grand, D. (1990). Subsets of CD3+(TCRαβ or TCRγδ) and CD3- lymphocytes isolated from normal human gut epithelium differ from their PBL counterparts. *Eur. J. Immunol.* **20**, 1097–1103.

Juan, M., Vinals, O., Pino-Otin, M. R., Places, L., Martinez-Caceres, E., Barcelo, J. J., Miralles, A., Vilella, R., de la Fuente, M. A., Vives, J., Yagüe, J., and Gaya, A. (1994). CD50 (intercellular adhesion adhesion molecule 3) stimulation induces calcium mobilization and tyrosine phosphorylation through p59fyn and p56lck in Jurkat T cell line. *J. Exp. Med.* **179**, 1747–1756.

Kahn, J., Ingraham, R. H., Shirley, F., Migaki, G. I., and Kishimoto, T. K. (1994). Membrane proximal cleavage of L-selectin: Identification of the cleavage site and a 6 kD transmembrane peptide fragment of L-selectin. *J. Cell Biol.* **125**, 461–470.

Kemler, R. (1993). From cadherins to catenins: Cytoplasmic protein interactions and regulation of cell adhesion. *Trends Genet.* **9**, 317–321.

Kilshaw, P. J., and Murant, S. J. (1990). A new surface antigen on intraepithelial lymphocytes in the intestine. *Eur. J. Immunol.* **20,** 2201–2207.

Kilshaw, P. J., and Murant, S. (1991). Expression and regulation of β7(βp) integrins on mouse lymphocytes: relevance to the mucosal immune system. *Eur. J. Immunol.* **21,** 2591–2596.

Koizumi, M., King, N., Lobb, R., Benjamin, C., and Podolsky, D. K. (1992). Expression of vascular adhesion molecules in inflammatory bowel disease. *Gastroenterology* **103,** 840–847.

Kvale, D., Krajci, P., and Brantzaeg, P. (1992). Expression and regulation of adhesion molecules ICAM-1 (CD54) and LFA-3 (CD58) in human intestinal epithelial cell lines. *Scand. J. Immunol.* **35,** 666–676.

Lefrançois, L., Barrett, T. A., Havran, W. L., and Puddington, L. (1994). Developmental expression of the αIELβ7 integrin on T cell receptor γδ and T cell receptor αβ T cells. *Eur. J. Immunol.* **24,** 635–640.

Lesley, J., He, Q., Miyake, K., Hamann, A., and Kincade, P. W. (1992). Requirements for hyaluronic acid binding by CD44: A role for the cytoplasmic domain and activation by antibody. *J. Exp. Med.* **175,** 257–266.

Lobb, R. R., and Hemler, M. E. (1994). The pathophysiologic role of α4 *in vivo*. *J. Clin. Invest.* **94,** 1722–1728.

Lucas, C., Bald, L. N., Fendly, B. M., Mora-Worms, M., Figari, I. S., Patzer, E. J., and Palladino, M. A. (1990). The autocrine production of transforming growth factor-β1 during lymphocyte activation. *J. Immunol.* **145,** 1415–1422.

Masumoto, A., and Hemler, M. E. (1993). Mutation of putative divalent cation sites in the α4 subunit of the integrin VLA-4: Distinct effects on adhesion to CS1/fibronectin, VCAM-1, and invasin. *J. Cell Biol.* **123,** 245–253.

McEver, R. P., Moore, K. L., and Cummings, R. D. (1995). Leukocyte trafficking mediated by selectin–carbohydrate interactions. *J. Biol. Chem.* **270,** 11025–11028.

Panja, A., Blumberg, R. S., Balk, S. P., and Mayer, L. (1993). CD1d is involved in T cell–intestinal epithelial cell interactions. *J. Exp. Med.* **178,** 1115–1119.

Parker, C. M., Cepek, K. L., Russell, G. J., Shaw, S. K., Posnett, D. N., Schwarting, R., and Brenner, M. B. (1992). A family of β7 integrins on human mucosal lymphocytes. *Proc. Natl. Acad. Sci. U.S.A.* **89,** 1924–1928.

Pavli, P., Hume, A., van der Pole, E., and Doe, W. F. (1993). Dendritic cells, the major antigen-presenting cells of the human colonic lamina propria. *Immunology* **78,** 132–141.

Peifer, M. (1993). Cancer, catenins, and cuticle pattern: A complex connection. *Science* **262,** 1667–1668.

Postigo, A. A., Sanchez, M. P., Lazarovits, A. I., Sanchez-Madrid, F., and De Landazuri, M. O. (1993). Alpha 4 beta 7 integrin mediates B cell binding to fibronectin and vascular cell adhesion molecule-1. Expression and function of alpha 4 integrins on human B lymphocytes. *J. Immunol.* **151,** 2471–83.

Roberts, A. I., O'Connell, S. M., and Ebert, E. C. (1993). Intestinal intraepithelial lymphocytes bind to colon cancer cells by HML-1 and CD11a. *Cancer Res.* **53,** 1608–1611.

Roberts, K., and Kilshaw, S. J. (1994). The mucosal T cell integrin αM290β7 recognizes a ligand on mucosal epithelial cell lines. *Eur. J. Immunol.* **23,** 1630–1635.

Rocha, B., Guy-Grand, D., and Vassalli, P. (1995). Extrathymic T cell differentiation. *Curr. Opin. Immunol.* **7,** 235–242.

Salmi, M., and Jalkanen, S. (1991). Regulation of lymphocyte traffic to mucosa-associated lymphatic tissues. *Gastroenterol. Clin. North Am.* **20,** 495–510.

Salmi, M., Andrew, D. P., Butcher, E. C., and Jalkanen, S. (1995). Dual binding capacity of mucosal immunoblasts to mucosal and synovial endothelium in humans: Dissection of the molecular mechanisms. *J. Exp. Med.* **181,** 137–149.

Sarnacki, S., Bègue, B., Buc, H., Le Deist, F., and Cerf-Bensussan, N. (1992). Enhancement of CD3-induced activation of human intestinal intraepithelial lymphocytes by stimulation of the β7-containing integrin defined by HML-1 antibody. *Eur. J. Immunol.* **22,** 2887–2892.

Schiefferdecker, H. L., Ullrich, R., Weiss-Breckwoldt, A. N., Schwarting, R., Stein, H., Riecken, E.-O., and Zeitz, M. (1990). The HML-1 antigen of intestinal lymphocytes is an activation antigen. *J. Immunol.* **144,** 2541–2549.

Schmitz, M., Nunez, D., and Butcher, E. C. (1988). Selective recognition of mucosal lymphoid high endothelium by gut intraepithelial lymphocytes. *Gastroenterology* **94,** 576–581.

Shaw, S., Luce, G. E. C., Quinones, R., Gress, R. E., and Springer, T. A. (1986). Two antigen-dependent adhesion pathways used by human cytotoxic T cell clones. *Nature (London)* **323,** 262–265.

Shawar, S. M., Vyas, J. M., Rodgers, J. R., and Rich, R. R. (1994). Antigen presentation by major histocompatibility complex class I-b molecules. *Annu. Rev. Immunol.* **12,** 839–880.

Simonitsch, I., Volc-Platzer, B., Mosberger, I., and Radaszkiewciz, T. (1994). Expression of monoclonal antibody HML-1 defined αEβ7 integrin in cutaneous T cell lymphoma. *Am. J. Pathol.* **145,** 1148–1158.

Spencer, J., Cerf-Bensussan, N., Jarry, A., Brousse N., Guy-Grand, D., Krajewski, A., and Isaacson, P. (1988). Enteropathy-associated T cell lymphoma (malignant histiocytosis of the intestine) is recognized by a monoclonal antibody (HML-1) that defines a membrane molecule on human mucosal lymphocytes. *Am. J. Pathol.* **132,** 1–5.

Springer, T. A. (1990). Adhesion receptors of the immune system. *Nature (London)* **346,** 425–434.

Springer, T. (1994). Traffic signals for lymphocyte recirculation and leukocyte emigration: The multistep paradigm. *Cell (Cambridge, Mass.)* **76,** 301–314.

Spruyt, L. L., Glennie, M. J., Beyers, A. D., and Williams, A. F. (1991). Signal transduction by the CD2 antigen on T cells and natural killer cells: Requirement for expression of a functional T cell receptor or binding of antibody Fc to the Fc receptor. *J. Exp. Med.* **174,** 1407–1415.

Stauder, R., and Günthert, U. (1995). CD44 isoforms. Impacts on lymphocyte activation and differentiation. *Immunologist* **3,** 78–83.

Takeichi, M. (1991). Cadherin cell adhesion receptors as a morphogenetic regulator. *Science.* **251,** 1451–1455.

Tanaka, Y., Adams, and D. H., Shaw, S. (1993). Proteoglycans on endothelial cells present adhesion-inducing cytokines to leukocytes. *Immunol. Today* **14,** 111–115.

Thomas, L., Byers, H. R., Vink, J., and Stamenkovic, I. (1992). CD44H regulates tumor cell migration on hyaluronate-coated substrate. *J. Cell Biol.* **118,** 971–977.

Van Seventer, G. A., Newman, W., Shimizu, Y., Nutman, T. B., Tanaka, Y., Horgan, K. J., Gopal, T. V., Ennis, E., O'Sullivan, D., Grey, H., and Shaw, S. (1991). Analysis of T cell stimulation by superantigen plus major histocompatibility complex class II molecules or by CD3 monoclonal antibody: Costimulation by purified adhesion ligands VCAM-1, ICAM-1, but not ELAM-1. *J. Exp. Med.* **174,** 901–913.

Yang, S. K., Eckmann, L., and Kagnoff, M. (1995). Colon epithelial cells express a broad array of chemokines. *Clin. Immunol. Immunopathol.* **76,** S20 (Abstract).

*Chapter 21*

---

# Intestinal Epithelial Cell-Derived Interleukin-7 as a Regulatory Factor for Intestinal Mucosal Lymphocytes

Mamoru Watanabe,* Yoshitaka Ueno,* and Toshifumi Hibi[*,†]

*Department of Internal Medicine, School of Medicine, Keio University, Tokyo 160, Japan; and †Keio Cancer Center, Tokyo 160, Japan*

## I. INTRODUCTION

The intestinal mucosa is continuously exposed to a variety of foreign antigens. Intestinal mucosal lymphocytes, the intraepithelial lymphocytes (IELs), and lamina propria lymphocytes (LPLs), located adjacent to the intestinal lumen and mucosal barrier, may initiate local immune responses to those exogenous antigens (Taguchi *et al.*, 1991; Barrett *et al.*, 1992; Kerckhove *et al.*, 1992), monitor intestinal enterocytes, and respond to nonpolymorphic molecules expressed on the surface of epithelial cells (Balk *et al.*, 1991; Panja *et al.*, 1993). Recent studies have demonstrated that interactions between mucosal lymphocytes and intestinal epithelial cells are crucial for maintaining mucosal immunity. In fact, Blumberg *et al.* have reported that CD1d expressed on intestinal epithelial cells was shown to be an important ligand for CD8[+] mucosal T-cell–epithelial cell interactions (Balk *et al.*, 1991). The mucosal lymphocytes may serve a critical role in the mucosal immune system by providing immune surveillance of epithelial cells (Janeway *et al.*, 1988). However, little is known about the precise mechanism by which functional differentiation and proliferation of these cells occurs in the intestinal mucosa. Although recent studies have shown that cytokines released from mucosal mononuclear cells may affect intestinal epithelial cell differentiation (Sadlack *et al.*, 1993; Kuhn *et al.*, 1993), the signals originating from epithelial cells that may regulate mucosal lymphocytes are yet to be defined. It has been reported that mucosal lymphocytes proliferate minimally to mitogens or stimulation through the CD3 pathway. This *in vitro* hyporesponsiveness of mucosal lymphocytes is supposed to be due to the absence of essential growth factor.

Interleukin-7 (IL-7) is a stromal cell-derived pleiotropic cytokine with lymphoid precursor cell growth-promoting activity (Namen *et al.*, 1988; Goodwin *et al.*, 1989; Morrissey *et al.*, 1989; Chazen *et al.*, 1989; Welch *et al.*, 1989; Armitage *et al.*, 1990). Our recent studies have demonstrated IL-7 mRNA expression and IL-7 protein production in the intestinal epithelial cells (Watanabe *et al.*, 1993, 1995). These results, in concert with the findings that IL-7 receptors are expressed by mucosal lymphocytes (Watanabe *et al.*, 1993, 1995; Marasco *et al.*, 1995; Fujihashi *et al.*, 1995, 1996), suggest that IL-7 regulates the proliferation of the intestinal mucosal lymphocytes. This review focuses on intestinal epithelial cell-derived IL-7 as a regulatory factor for the intestinal mucosal lymphocytes.

## II. INTERLEUKIN-7 AS A REGULATORY FACTOR FOR PERIPHERAL T CELLS

IL-7 was originally described as a growth factor for precursor B cells (Namen *et al.*, 1988; Goodwin *et al.*, 1989; Morrissey *et al.*, 1989). Subsequent *in vitro* studies have demonstrated that IL-7 is also a potent costimulus for both murine and human, immature and mature cells of the T-cell lineage in the thymus (Chazen *et al.*, 1989; Welch *et al.*, 1989; Armitage *et al.*, 1990; Goodwin and Namen, 1991; Appasamy, 1993). In mouse, abundant IL-7 mRNA expression has been demonstrated in bone marrow stromal cells, thymus, spleen, liver, kidney, and keratinocytes (Namen *et al.*, 1988; Heufler *et al.*, 1993; Wiles *et al.*, 1992). However, in the human tissues, the localization of IL-7 expression is not yet clearly defined. Recent studies have shown that IL-7 is expressed in human thymus, spleen, and keratinocytes (Goodwin and Namen, 1991; Appasamy *et al.*, 1993; Heufler *et al.*, 1993), though a potential role of IL-7 in peripheral lymphoid tissues remains unclear.

Morrissey *et al.* (1989) have found that IL-7 could stimulate proliferation, IL-2 receptor expression, and IL-2 production by mature lymph node T cells. Human peripheral blood T cells proliferate in response to IL-7 after being stimulated with anti-CD3 antibody or mitogens in short-duration cultures. IL-7 was sufficient to promote growth without costimulation of other cytokines in long-term cultures. Many other investigators have also confirmed the costimulatory effects of IL-7 on peripheral mature T-cell proliferation (Armitage *et al.*, 1990; Londei *et al.*, 1990). Moreover, IL-7 enhances the generation of peripheral cytotoxic T cell (Alderson *et al.*, 1990) and lymphokine-activated killer cells (Alderson *et al.*, 1990; Stotter *et al.*, 1991), and induces proinflammatory cytokine secretion and tumoricidal activity of peripheral blood monocytes (Alderson *et al.*, 1991).

It has been shown that IL-7 induces an increase in $\alpha\beta$ TCR$^+$CD4$^-$CD8$^-$ T cells in the lymph node and spleen of athymic nude mice (Kenai *et al.*, 1993). IL-7 has also been shown to be an essential cofactor for V(D)J rearrangement of the T-cell receptor $\beta$ gene in precursor T cells (Muegge *et al.*, 1993). Moreover, recent evidence of an extrathymic pool of $\alpha\beta$ TCR$^+$ mucosal lymphocytes in the gut suggests that intestinal epithelial cells may share some differentiation-inducing capacities with thymic epithelial cells, leading to *in situ* T-cell receptor rearrangement of extrathymically derived T cells (Rocha *et al.*, 1991). These results suggested a potential role of IL-7 in peripheral lymphoid tissues.

### III. NORMAL HUMAN INTESTINAL EPITHELIAL CELLS EXPRESS IL-7 mRNA AND PRODUCE IL-7 PROTEIN

We have shown that normal human and murine intestinal epithelial cells express IL-7 mRNA and produce IL 7 protein (Watanabe *et al.*, 1995). Reverse-transcription PCR analysis using human IL-7-specific primers demonstrated IL-7 mRNA expression in normal human colonic tissues. Southern blot hybridization using IL-7-specific probe confirmed the expression of IL-7 mRNA in the human colonic mucosa (Fig. 1). IL-7 mRNA expression was detected in the colon, and a detectable expression of IL-7 was found at other sites in the gastrointestinal tract. In our PCR and Southern blot analysis, IL-7 mRNA was not readily detectable in the normal human thymus tissues as previously reported (Goodwin and Namen, 1991).

To assess the localization of IL-7 mRNA in the intestinal mucosa, we used *in situ* hybridization, which clearly yielded IL-7 mRNA expression in the intestinal epithelial cells (Fig. 2) (Watanabe *et al.*, 1995). All intestinal epithelial cells stained positively, but the strongly positive-staining cells are intestinal goblet cells in the mucosa. Immunohistochemical analysis using an anti-human IL-7 mAb confirmed IL-7 protein expression in the human intestinal epithelial cells and intestinal goblet cells in normal intestinal mucosal tissues (Fig. 3). We then assessed the IL-7 mRNA expression in human colonic epithelial cell lines that can be induced to assume distinctive phenotype. Southern blotting analysis demonstrated that IL-7 mRNA was expressed in the 18-N2 subclone of HT29 in parallel with goblet

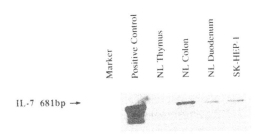

**FIGURE 1.** Southern blot hybridization demonstrated the expression of IL-7 mRNA in the normal human intestinal mucosa. IL-7 mRNA expression was detected in the colon, but was only barely detectable at other sites in the gastrointestinal tract. Note that IL-7 mRNA was not readily detectable in the normal human thymus tissues as reported, in contrast to the constitutive G3PDH mRNA. PCR products were blotted onto nylon membrane and hybridized with IL-7 gene-specific cDNA oligonucleotide probe labeled with digoxigenin. The specificity of the amplified bands for IL-7 was validated by their predicted size (681 bp). Markers represent 100-bp DNA ladder. SK-HEP-1, the cell line that was used to clone the cDNA for the human IL-7, served as a positive control.

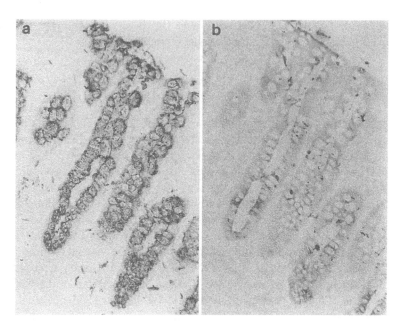

*FIGURE 2.*  *In situ* hybridization demonstrated the expression and localization of IL-7 mRNA in the human intestinal epithelial cells. Phase contrast micrograph of a human colonic mucosa following colorimetric detection of hybridized digoxigenin-labeled human IL-7 oligonucleotide antisense (a) and sense (as a negative control) (b) probes. IL-7 mRNA was expressed in the colonic epithelial cells and epithelial goblet cells in the intestinal mucosa.

cell phenotypic features such as the expression of mucin glycoprotein and typical morphological features (Podolsky *et al.*, 1993). IL-7 mRNA expression could be detected in relatively small amounts in the HT29-18-N2 line before phenotypic differentiation, but the expression level was significantly increased after emergence of the colonic goblet cell phenotype. IL-7 mRNA expression in the HT29-18-N2 line was significantly increased after interferon-$\gamma$ stimulation. In contrast, the Caco-2 cell line did not express IL-7 mRNA after induction of the enterocytic phenotype or interferon-$\gamma$ stimulation. These results indicated that IL-7 mRNA expression is selectively associated with the goblet cell differentiation among various cell lines. All these results suggested that IL-7 protein is produced by intestinal epithelial cells, and the epithelial goblet cells are the likely major source of IL-7 in their tissues.

Coste *et al.* (1995) showed the differential expression of IL-7 by intestinal epithelial cells isolated from tip and crypt portions of villi. Increased IL-7 expression was noted in the crypt epithelial cells compared with the tip epithelium. This finding is consisted with our finding as the epithelial goblet cells are enriched in the crypt portion of intestinal villi.

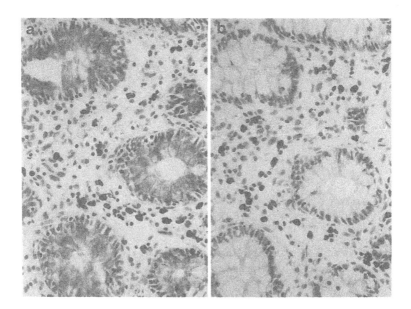

FIGURE 3. Immunohistochemical analysis using rabbit anti-human IL-7 Ab confirmed IL-7 protein expression in the human intestinal epithelial cells and epithelial goblet cells. The reactivity of anti-human IL-7 IgG Ab (10 μg/ml)(a), but not control rabbit IgG (10 μg/ml) (b) is confined to the colonic epithelial cells in the normal human intestinal mucosal tissues. Note that biotin-conjugated goat anti-rabbit Ab alone did not show the reactivity.

## IV. NORMAL HUMAN INTESTINAL MUCOSAL LYMPHOCYTES EXPRESS IL-7 RECEPTOR ON THE CELL SURFACE

How does locally produced IL-7 regulate mucosal lymphocytes? Localization of the IL-7 receptor, like that of IL-7 itself, is not well defined in the human tissues (Park *et al.*, 1990; Goodwin *et al.*, 1990; Benjamin *et al.*, 1994). IL-7 functional high-affinity receptor is a heterodimeric complex of two chains, the IL-7 receptor/p90 and the common gamma chain (γc, p64) (Appasamy, 1993). We have shown that IL-7 receptor was expressed in the human intestinal epithelial cell lines and intestinal epithelial cells in the human tissues by Southern blot (Fig. 4) and *in situ* hybridization (Watanabe *et al.*, 1995). Interestingly, human colonic epithelial cell lines Caco-2, COLO205, and HT29-N2 expressed IL-7 receptor mRNA. However, HT29-18-N2 expressed no detectable expression of IL-7 receptor when it produced IL-7 protein. Reinecker and Podolsky (1995) have demonstrated that human colonic epithelial cells express functional IL-7 receptor sharing a common γc chain of the IL-2 receptor. The other group also found the expression of p90 and p64 chains of the IL-7 receptor in the human colonic epithelial cell line (Marasco *et al.*, 1995).

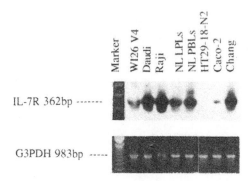

**FIGURE 4.** Southern blot hybridization demonstrated the IL-7 receptor mRNA expression in freshly isolated LPLs from human intestinal mucosa. The specificity of the amplified bands for IL-7 receptor mRNA was validated by their predicted size (362 bp). Markers represent 100-bp DNA ladder. WI-26 VA4, the cell line that was used to clone the cDNA for the human IL-7 receptor, served as a positive control. Human B-cell lymphoma cell lines Daudi and Raji and human hepatocyte cell line Chang expressed IL-7 receptor mRNA. Interestingly, human colonic epithelial cell line Caco-2 also expressed IL-7 receptor mRNA. However, human colonic epithelial cell line HT29-18-N2 showed no detectable expression of IL-7 receptor. For internal standard, amplified bands for G3PDH were used.

Since IL-7 has been shown previously to stimulate the growth of T-cell progenitors in mouse thymus and fetal liver (Namen *et al.,* 1988), we sought to determine whether locally produced IL-7 in the intestinal mucosa affects mucosal lymphocytes. We studied IL-7 receptor expression in the mucosal lymphocytes (Watanabe *et al.,* 1995). Immunohistochemical analysis demonstrated that both LPLs and IELs in the normal human colonic mucosa express the receptor for IL-7. We also used *in situ* hybridization, which yielded IL-7 receptor mRNA expression in the intestinal mucosal lymphocytes and intestinal epithelial cells in normal colonic mucosa. We then isolated mucosal lymphocytes from human colonic tissue, and studied the expression of IL-7 receptor mRNA and cell surface expression of IL-7 receptor. PCR and Southern blot analysis demonstrated IL-7 receptor mRNA in the LPLs of normal intestinal mucosa. The cell surface expression of IL-7 receptor by mucosal lymphocytes was confirmed using flow cytometric analysis of freshly isolated LPLs. On the contrary, IL-7 receptor was not found in freshly isolated PBLs, though those PBLs were shown to express IL-7 mRNA by Southern blot hybridization. Previous studies have shown that IL-7 stimulates the proliferation of human mature T cells only after exogenous stimulation in short-term culture (Welch *et al.,* 1989; Armitage *et al.,* 1990). Our result, in concert with these findings, suggests that IL-7 receptor protein on the cell surface is not expressed by resting PBLs, but rather is expressed by those PBLs after activation. Therefore, our results indicate that mucosal lymphocytes may be activated with continuous stimulation by a number of microbial or self antigens, and express IL-7 receptor.

Marasco *et al.* (1995) showed that mRNA transcripts for IL-7 receptor/p90 and $\gamma\delta$/p64 were expressed in human intestinal lamina propria mononuclear cells from biopsy samples of normal controls and patients with ulcerative colitis. Fujihashi *et al.* (1996) have demonstrated that a subset of murine intestinal $\gamma\delta$IELs, especially cells with dim expression of $\gamma\delta$ TCR$^+$ ($\gamma\delta^{Dim}$ T cells), constitutively expressed IL-7 receptor. IL-7 receptor expression on these $\gamma\delta$ T cells in the intestinal epithelium was induced by stem cell factor, a ligand for c-kit.

## V. IL-7 REGULATES THE PROLIFERATION OF INTESTINAL MUCOSAL LYMPHOCYTES

Subsequently, functional activity of IL-7 receptor was assessed by the utility of exogenous recombinant IL-7 to stimulate the growth of freshly isolated intestinal mucosal lymphocytes. We have demonstrated that rIL-7 alone stimulates a significant increase in DNA synthesis, and causes an eventual increase in cell recovery of isolated mucosal lymphocytes (Watanabe *et al.,* 1995). Unexpectedly, rIL-7 inhibited anti-CD3 mAb-induced DNA synthesis and proliferative responses of LPLs in a dose-dependent fashion. The numbers of cells in LPL cultures after stimulation with rIL-7 and anti-CD3 mAb were significantly decreased, compared with those in the culture with rIL-2 alone, rIL-7 alone, or rIL-7 and mitogens. These results differed significantly from those seen in proliferative responses of PBLs. IL-7 acted synergistically with anti-CD3 stimulation for the induction of the proliferation of human mature T cells and tumor-infiltrating lymphocytes from renal cell carcinoma (Sica *et al.,* 1993). Since previous studies have also shown that IL-7 is not directly mitogenic on peripheral blood T cells in short-term culture (Armitage *et al.,* 1990), our results suggest that IL-7 acts quite differently on mucosal and peripheral lymphocytes. It is possible that IL-7 may inhibit the proliferation of mucosal cells following certain stimulation.

The surface expression of lymphocyte-associated molecules was assessed on rIL-7-stimulated LPLs in the normal human intestinal mucosa by flow cytometry. These cells were 95% $\alpha\beta$ TCR$^+$, 5% $\gamma\delta$ TCR$^+$, 60%CD8a$^+$, and 40% CD4, no different from the phenotype of freshly isolated normal LPLs as reported. Interestingly, cell surface expression of CD3 in LPLs stimulated with anti-CD3 mAB + rIL-7 was significantly decreased compared with that in LPLs stimulated with anti-CD3 mAb alone. Relative mean fluorescence of CD3 expression in anti-CD3 mAb + IL-7-stimulated LPLs was decreased, though that of $\alpha\beta$ TCR$^+$ expression was unchanged. This result also contrasted with the case of freshly isolated PBLs where mean fluorescence of CD3 expression was increased in anti-CD3 mAb + IL-7-stimulated PBLs compared with that in anti-CD3 mAb-stimulated LPLs. This result is comparable to the findings that rIL-7 inhibited anti-CD3 mAb-induced DNA synthesis and proliferative responses of freshly isolated LPLs but not PBLs.

Bilenker *et al.* (1995) have demonstrated that IL-7 stimulates both IELs and

LPLs directly through an IL-2 pathway, suggesting that these cells are activated memory cells. IL-7 is shown to support all phenotypes of intestinal mucosal lymphocytes, whether these cells express the $\alpha\beta$ or $\gamma\delta$ TCR, CD4, or CD8 on the cell surface. This contrasts with T cells in the thymus and skin, where $\gamma\delta$ TCR$^+$ cells are preferentially stimulated (Fabbi et al., 1992; Uehira et al., 1993).

## VI. IL-7 and Human Inflammatory Bowel Disease

The importance of IL-7 as a mediator of local inflammatory responses remains unclear. Recent evidence suggests that IL-7 upregulates the expression of macrophage-derived cytokines such as IL-8, TNF, IL-1, and IL-6 and may function as an important proinflammatory cytokine (Standiford et al., 1992).

We have demonstrated the presence of the factor in the serum from patients with ulcerative colitis (UC) that exerted effects on mouse thymus (Watanabe et al., 1987). This factor was prepared from the serum of UC patients by a combination of gel filtration and anion exchange chromatography. This serum factor, when injected into experimental mouse in vivo, remarkably enhanced the cell growth and phenotypic changes of T cells in the thymus. This was unique to the UC serum since the administration of the serum fractions from normal controls or from patients with other colonic diseases including Crohn's disease did not effect the cell number and phenotypes of T cell in the mouse thymus.

To ascertain that serum factor from UC patients alters cell growth and phenotypes of intrathymic T cell in the microenvironment of thymus, we used in vitro mouse thymus organ culture system. The serum factor from UC exerted effects on organ-cultured embryo mouse thymus. A marked increase in cell growth was observed in thymus lobe cultures with medium containing the serum factor from UC. This result represents a direct demonstration that serum factor from UC enhances intrathymic T-cell proliferation without an influx of lymphoid precursor cells. Two-color FACS analysis revealed the increase in the proportion of CD4$^+$CD8$^-$ cells and CD4$^-$CD8$^-$ with the decrease in the proportion of CD4$^+$CD8$^+$ by addition of UC serum factor to the fetal thymus organ culture. Interestingly, majority of T cells in the organ culture with the serum factor of UC were brightly stained Thy-1$^+$ cells. In this culture, the number of Thy-1$^+$CD25$^+$ cells was increased. The addition of IL-2 to organ-culture of fetal thymus inhibited the development of Thy-1$^+$CD4$^+$CD8$^-$ cells. It is suggested that the alteration of the microenvironment by including growth factors in fetal organ cultures reveals a series of alternative differentiation pathways that are normally masked by more dominant pathway. Although the precise mechanisms of the effects by the serum factor have not been clarified yet, it was confirmed that the serum factor of UC patients alters the intrathymic differentiation process of T cells in mouse thymus. We purified the serum factor of UC and sequenced amino acid of the purified protein (Watanabe et al., 1996a). The serum factor from UC that alters intrathymic T-cell proliferation and differentiation in organ-cultured mouse thymus is, unexpectedly, human IL-7 itself. In mouse, abundant IL-7 mRNA expression has been demonstrated in thymus stromal cells, bone marrow stromal cells, spleen, liver, kidney, and keratinocytes. However, in the human tissues, the localization of IL-7 expression is not yet clearly defined. Human thymus tissues express only a detectable amount of IL-7 mRNA as others have previously reported, in sharp contrast to the case for the mouse thymus, where the highest IL-7 mRNA expression occurs in the thymus (Goodwin and Namen, 1991). Our demonstration that Southern blot hybridization demonstrated increased IL-7 mRNA expression in the intestinal epithelial cells is, therefore, quite interesting.

A possible role for IL-7 in mucosal inflammation has been suggested recently by our finding of altered IL-7 mRNA expression in the colonic epithelium in inflamed mucosa of patients with ulcerative colitis (Watanabe *et al.,* 1996b). Interestingly, IL-7 receptor expression was quite marked in the mucosal lymphocytes in severely inflamed colonic mucosa from patients with ulcerative colitis. These results favor the idea that IL-7 produced by intestinal epithelial cells may be involved in mucosal inflammation.

## VII. CONCLUSIONS

A major limitation in understanding the pathogenesis responsible for the mucosal injury observed in human inflammatory bowel disease has been the lack of animal models that possess the pathohistologic features of human disease. However, a series of valuable new models that spontaneously arise in gene knockout mice add significantly to our understanding of the mechanisms that lead to chronic intestinal inflammation and injury (Sadlack *et al.,* 1993; Kuhn *et al.,* 1993; Strober and Ehrhardt, 1993). Although none of the gene-disrupted mice are identical to the patients, they clearly show that T-cell abnormalities can preferentially manifest as chronic, noninfectious intestinal inflammation.

We have demonstrated the immune regulation through the IL-7 system in the intestinal mucosa of the mouse as well as that of the human. Murine intestinal epithelial cells in the small intestine and colonic mucosa express and produce IL-7. Murine IELs and LPLs express IL-7 receptor, and locally produced IL-7 is shown to be a growth and inhibitory factor for mucosal lymphocytes. We are studying the alteration of mucosal IL-7-mediated immune regulation in gene-disrupted and transgenic mice (Uehira *et al.,* 1993; Strober and Ehrhardt, 1993; Perchon *et al.,* 1994; Freeden-Jeffry *et al.,* 1995). These studies may lead to an understanding of the pathogenesis of human inflammatory intestinal disease.

### ACKNOWLEDGMENTS

The authors express special thanks to Professors Masaharu Tsuchiya, Sadakazu Aiso, Hiromichi Ishikawa, Sumiaki Tsuru, Sonoko Habu, and Hiromasa Ishii for critical comments, and to Drs. Noriaki

Watanabe, Yasushi Iwao, Haruhiko Ogata, Tatsuhiko Hayashi, Makoto Ohara, Yasuo Hosoda, Atsushi Hayashi, Nagamu Inoue, and Tomoharu Yajima for technical assistance. This study was supported in part by Grants-in-Aid from the Japanese Ministry of Education, Culture and Science, the Japanese Ministry of Health and Welfare, and Keio University.

## REFERENCES

Alderson, M. R., Sassenfeld, H. M., and Widmer, M. B. (1990). Interleukin-7 enhances cytolytic T lymphocyte generation and induces lymphokine-activated killer cells from human peripheral blood. *J. Exp. Med.* **172,** 577–587.

Alderson, M. R., Tough, T. W., Ziegler, S. F., and Grabstein, K. H. (1991). Interleukin-7 induces cytokine secretion and tumoricidal activity by human peripheral blood monocytes. *J. Exp. Med.* **173,** 923–930.

Armitage, R. J., Namen, A. E., Sassenfeld, H. M., and Grabstein, K. H. (1990). Regulation of human T cell proliferation by IL-7. *J. Immunol.* **144,** 938–941.

Appasamy, P. M. (1993). Interleikin-7: Biology and potential clinical applications. *Cancer Invest.* **11,** 487–499.

Balk, S. P., Ebert, E. C., Blumenthal, R. L., McDermott, F. V., Wucherpfenning, K. W., Landau, S. B., and Blumberg, R. S. (1991). Oligoclonal expansion and CD1 recognition by human intestinal intraepithelial lymphocytes. *Science* **253,** 1411–1415.

Barrett, T. A., Gajewski, T. F., Danielpour, D., Chang, E. B., Beagley, K. W., and Bluestone, J. A. (1992). Differential function of intestinal intraepithelial lymphocyte subsets. *J. Immunol.* **149,** 1124–1130.

Benjamin, D., Sharma, V., Knoblock, T. J., Armitage, R. J., Dayton, M. A., and Goodwin, R. G. (1994). B cell IL-7. Human B cell lines constitutively secrete IL-7 and express IL-7 receptors. *J. Immunol.* **152,** 4749–4757.

Bilenker, M., Roberts, A. T., Brolin, R. E., and Ebert, E. V. (1995). Interleukin-7 activates intestinal lymphocytes. *Dig. Dis. Sci.* **40,** 1744–1749.

Chazen, G. D., Pereira, G. M. B., LeGros, G., Gillis, S., and Shevach, E. M. (1989). Interleukin 7 is a T-cell growth factor. *Proc. Natl. Acad. Sci. U.S.A.* **86,** 5923–5927.

Coste, M., Boyaka, P. N., Kawabata S., Fujihashi K., Yamamoto M., Mcghee, J. R., and Kiyono, H. (1995). Differential expresseion of IL-7 by epithelial cells isolated from and crypt portions of intestinal villi. *Clin. Immunol. Immunopathol.* **76,** 27.

Fabbi, M., Groh, V., and and Strominger, J. L. (1992). IL-7 induces proliferation of CD3-/low CD4-CD8-human thymocyte precursors by an IL-2 independent pathway. *Int. Immunol.* **4,** 1–5.

Freeden-Jeffry, V. U., Viera, P., Lucian, L. A., McNeil, T., Burdach, S. E. G., and Murray, R. (1995). Lymphopenia in interleukin (IL)-7 gene-deleted mice identifies IL-7 as a nonredundant cytokine. *J. Exp. Med.* **181,** 1519–1526.

Fujihashi, K., Yamamoto, M., Kusumi, A., McGhee, J. R., and Kiyono, H. (1995). Stem cell factor upregulates IL-7 receptor expression on $\gamma\delta$ T cells in intestinal epithelium. *Clin. Immunol. Immunopathol.* **76:** 39.

Fujihashi, K., Kawabata, S., Hiroi, T., Yamamoto, M., McGhee, J. R., Nishikawa, S., and Kiyono, H. (1996). IL-2 and IL-7 reciprocally induce IL-7 and IL-2 receptors on $\gamma\delta$ TCR$^+$ intraepithelial lymphocytes. *Proc. Natl. Acad. Sci. U.S.A.* **93,** 3613–3618.

Goodwin, R. G., Lupton, S., Schmierer, A., Hjerrild, K. J., Jerzy, R., Clevenger, W., Gillis, S., Cosman, D., and Namen, A. E. (1989). Human interleukin 7: Molecular cloning and growth factor activity on human and murine B-lineage cells. *Proc. Natl. Acad. Sci. U.S.A.* **86,** 302–306.

Goodwin, R. G., Friend, D., Ziegler, S. F., Jerzy, R., Falk, B. A., Gimpel, S., Cosman, D., Dower, S. K., March, C. J., Namen, A. E., and Park, L. S. (1990). Cloning of the human and murine interleukin-7 receptors; demonstration of a soluble form and homology to a new receptor superfamily. *Cell (Cambridge, Mass.)* **60,** 941–951.

Goodwin, R. G., and Namen, A. E. (1991). Interleukin-7. "The Cytokine Handbook" pp. 191–200. Academic Press, San Diego.

Heufler, C., Topar, G., Grasseger, A., Stanzl, U., Koch, F., Romani, N., Namen, A. E., and Schuler, G. (1993). Interleukin 7 is produced by murine and human keratinocytes. *J. Exp. Med.* **178,** 1109–1114.

Janeway, C. A., Jr., Jones, B., and Hayday, A. (1988). Specificity and function of T cells bearing γ receptors. *Immunol. Today* **9,** 73–76.

Kenai, H., Matsuzaki, G., Nakamura, T., Yoshikai, Y., and Nomoto, K. (1993). Thymus-derived cytokine(s) including interleukin-7 induce increase of T cell receptor $\alpha/\beta$ + CD4-CD8- T cells which are extrathymically differentiated in athymic nude mice. *Eur. J. Immunol.* **23,** 1818–1825.

Kerckhove, C. V., Russell, G. J., Deusch, K., Reich, K., Bhan, A. K., DerSimonian, H., and Brenner, M. B. (1992). Oligoclonality of human intestinal intraepithelial T cells. *J. Exp. Med.* **175,** 57–63.

Kuhn, R., Loher, J., Rennick, D., Rajewsky, K., and Muller, W. (1993). Interleukin-10-deficient mice develop chronic enterocolitis. *Cell(Cambridge, Mass.)* **75,** 263–274.

Londei, M., Verhoef, A., Hawrylowicz, C., Groves, J., Berardinis, P. D., and Feldmann, M. (1990). Interleukin 7 is a growth factor for mature human T cells. *Eur. J. Immunol.* **20,** 425–428.

Marasco, R., Marasco, O., Morrone, G., Monteleone, G., Luzza, F., Venuta, S., and Pallone, F. (1995). m-RNA for interleukin 7 receptor (IL-7) chains in human intestinal lamina propria mononuclear cells (LPMC) and in the Caco-2 human colon carcinoma cell line. *Clin. Immunol. Immunopathol.* **76,** 69.

Morrissey, P. J., Goodwin, R. G., Nordan, R. P., Anderson, D., Grabstein, K. H., Cosman, D., Sims, J., Lupton, S., Acres, B., and Reed, S. G. (1989). Recombinant interleukin 7, pre-B cell growth factor, has costimulatory activity on purified mature T cells. *J. Exp. Med.* **169,** 707–716.

Muegge, K., Vila, M. P., and Durum, S. K. (1993). Interleukin-7: A cofactor for V(D)J rearrangement of the T cell receptor $\beta$ gene. *Science* **261,** 93–95.

Namen, A. E., Lupton, S., Hjerrild, K., Wignall, J., Mochizuki, D. Y., Schmierer, A. E., Mosley, B., March, C. J., and Urdal, D. L. (1988). Stimulation of B-cell progenitors by cloned murine interleukin-7. *Nature (London)* **333,** 571–573.

Panja, A., Blumberg, R. S., Balk, S. P., and Mayer, L. (1993). CD1d is involved in T cell-intestinal epithelial cell interactions. *J. Exp. Med.* **178,** 1115–1119.

Park, L. S., Friend, D. J., Schmierer, A. E., Dower, S. K., and Namen, A. E. (1990). Murine interleukin (IL-7) receptor. Characterization on an IL-7-dependent cell line. *J. Exp. Med.* **171,** 1073–1089.

Perchon, J. J., Morrissey, K. H., Grabsteim, K. H., Ramsdell, F. J., Eugene, M., Glinika, B. C., Park, L. S., Ziegler, S. F., and Williams, D. E. (1994). Early lymphocyte expansion is severely impaired in interleukin 7 receptor-deficient mice. *J. Exp. Med.* **180,** 1955–1960.

Podolsky, D. K., Lynch-Devaney, K., Stow, J. L., Oates, P., Murgue, B., DeBeaumont, M., Sands, B. E., and Mahida, Y. R. (1993). Identification of human intestinal trefoil factor. Goblet cell-specific expression of a peptide targeted for apical secretion. *J. Biol. Chem.* **268,** 6694–6702.

Reinecker, H. K., and Podolsky, D. K. (1995). Human intestinal epithelial cells express functional cytokine receptors sharing the common γc chain of the interleukin 2 receptor. *Proc. Natl. Acad. Sci. U.S.A.* **92,** 8353–8357.

Rocha, B., Vassali, P., and Guy-Grand, D. (1991). The V$\beta$ repertoire of mouse gut homodimeric a CD8+ intraepithelial T cell receptor $\alpha/\beta$ + lymphocytes reveals a major extrathymic pathway of T cell differentiation. *J. Exp. Med.* **173,** 483–486.

Sadlack, B., Merz, H., Schorle, H., Schimpl, A., Feller, A. C., and Horak, I. (1993). Ulcerative colitis-like disease in mice with a disrupted interleukin-2 gene. *Cell (Cambridge, Mass.)* **75,** 253–261.

Sica, D., Rayman, P., Stanley, J., Edinger, M., Tubbs, R. R., Klein, E., Bukowski, R., and Finke, J. H. (1993). Interleukin 7 enhances the proliferation and effector function of tumor-infiltrating lymphocytes from renal-cell carcinoma. *Int. J. Cancer* **53,** 941–947.

Standiford, T. J., Strieter, R. M., Allen, R. M., Burdick, M. D., and Kunkel, S. T. (1992). IL-7 up-regulates the expression of IL-8 from resting and stimulated human blood monocytes. *J. Immunol.* **149,** 2035–2039.

Stotter, H., Custer, M. C., Bolton, E. S., Guedez, L., and Lotze, M. T. (1991). IL-7 induces human lymphokine-activated killer cell activity and is regulated by IL-4. *J. Immunol.* **146,** 150–155.

Strober, W., and Ehrhardt, R. O. (1993). Chronic intestinal inflammation: An unexpected outcome in cytokine or T cell receptor mutant mice. *Cell (Cambridge, Mass.)* **75,** 203–205.

Taguchi, T., Aicher, W. K., Fujuhashi, K., Yamamoto, M., McGhee, J. R., Bluestone, J. A., and Kiyono, H. (1991). Novel function for intraepithelial lymphocytes: Murine CD3+, γ TCR T cells produce IFN-and IL-5. *J. Immunol.* **147,** 3736–3744.

Uehira, M., Matsuda, H., Hikita, I., Sakata, T., Fujiwara, H., and Nishimoto, H. (1993). The development of dermatitis infiltrated by γδ T cells in IL-7 transgenic mice. *Int. Immunol.* **5,** 1619–1627.

Watanabe, M., Aiso, S., Hibi, T., Watanabe, N., Iwao, Y., Yoshida, T., Asakura, H., Tsuru, S., and Tsuchiya, M. (1987). Alteration of T cell maturation and proliferation in the mouse thymus induced by serum factors from patients with ulcerative colitis. *Clin. Exp. Immunol.* **68,** 596–604.

Watanabe, M., Ono, A., Hibi, T., Aiso, S., and Tsuchiya, M. (1993). Immune reguratory defects in ulcerative colitis. "Current Topics in Mucosal Immunology," pp. 3–10. Excerpta Medica, Amsterdam.

Watanabe, M., Ueno, Y., Yajima, T., Iwao, Y., Tsuchiya, M., Ishikawa, H., Aiso, S., Hibi, T., and Ishii, H. (1995). Interleukin-7 is produced by human intestinal epithelial cells and regulates the proliferation of intestinal mucosal lymphocytes. *J. Clin. Invest.* **95,** 2945–2953.

Watanabe, M., Watanabe, N., Iwao, Y., Ogata, H., Tsuchiya, M., Ishii, H., Aiso, S., Oomori, T., Habu, S., and Hibi, T. (1996a). Interleukin 7 that induces T cell proliferation in organ-cultured mouse thymus is increased in the serum from patients with ulcerative colitis. Submitted for publication.

Watanabe, M., Ueno, Y., Hayashi, T., Ishii, H., and Hibi, T. (1996b). The expression of interleukin-7 mRNA and protein is decreased in the inflamed colonic mucosa from patients with ulcerative colitis. Submitted for publication.

Welch, P. A., Namen, A. E., Goodwin, R. G., Armitage, R., and Cooper, M. D. (1989). Human IL-7: A novel T cell growth factor. *J. Immunol.* **143,** 3562–3567.

Wiles, M. V., Ruiz, P., and Imhof, B. A. (1992). Interleukin-7 expression during mouse thymus development. *Eur. J. Immunol.* **22,** 1037–1042.

# Chapter 22

# Defects in T-Cell Regulation: Lessons for Inflammatory Bowel Disease

Stephen J. Simpson,* Georg A. Holländer,† Emiko Mizoguchi,‡ Atul K. Bhan,‡
Baoping Wang,* and Cox Terhorst*

*Division of Immunology, Beth Israel Hospital, †Division of Pediatric Oncology,
Dana Farber Cancer Institute, and ‡Department of Pathology, Massachusetts General Hospital,
Harvard Medical School, Boston, Massachusetts 02115

## I. THE GROWING LIST OF NEW MODELS FOR INFLAMMATORY BOWEL DISEASE

The intestinal mucosa is a rich source of components ready to generate very effective immune responses to the large number of pathogenic organisms that find their way into the intestine. This powerful arsenal of effector cytokines and cells can pose a considerable risk if not kept under very tight control, as is clearly illustrated by the severe intestinal pathology that often accompanies human inflammatory bowel disease (IBD). IBD encompasses two related conditions, ulcerative colitis (UC) and Crohn's disease (CD), that are thought to arise as immunopathological manifestations of a variety of initiating and predisposing factors (Podolsky 1991a,b). The usefulness of experimental animal models for IBD has long been appreciated. However, the recent emergence of a new generation of rodent IBD models born from refined and novel approaches to the manipulation of the immune system has generated new excitement in the field IBD research.

Models for IBD have, until recently, relied on the spontaneous development of disease within certain animal strains or species. One of the best characterized of these is the C3H/HeJ mouse. Although colitis in the C3H/Hej mouse was originally noted to develop with only sporadic occurance, the reproducibility of disease in these animals is now high, with the establishment of a colitis-susceptible pedigree (C3H/HeJ[Bir]) at the Jackson Laboratories (Sundberg et al., 1994). Other studies of IBD in animals have examined forms of inducible colitis by administration of agents such as acetic acid or dextran sodium sulfate to rodents, providing a cheap and reproducible means of studying intestinal inflammation (Sartor, 1995). One of the limitations of this approach, however, is that it does not allow for the potential study of spontaneous immunopathological initiating factors in IBD.

*Essentials of Mucosal Immunology*

Some of the first of the new spontaneous IBD models appeared as the unexpected consequence of targeted mutations of regulatory T-cell cytokine genes, including IL-2 (Sadlack *et al.*, 1993), IL-10 (Kühn *et al.*, 1993), and TGF$\beta$ (Shull *et al.*, 1992; Kulkarni *et al.*, 1993). The development of colitis in these animals was significant since it underscored the importance of cytokine-mediated regulation of pathogenic T cells. The studies of cytokine-deficient mice were complemented by others that demonstrated the importance of specific T-cell subsets in maintaining homeostasis within the mucosal lymphoid compartment. Thus, it was found that the genetic disruption of the $\alpha$ and $\beta$ TCR genes or class II MHC genes, which lead to the blockade of $\alpha\beta$ T-cell and CD4$^+$ T-cell development, respectively, also resulted in colitis in these animals (Mombaerts *et al.*, 1993). Other investigations, utilizing cellular manipulation of the immune system, enabled the further definition of specific subpopulations of normal CD4$^+$ T cells, defined by the cell surface expression of CD45RB, that possessed the capacity to prevent or to induce colitis on transfer into SCID mice (Powrie *et al.*, 1993, 1994a; Morrissey *et al.*, 1993).

Experiments from our laboratory on tg$\epsilon$26 mice (discussed in detail in Section II) directly demonstrated the importance of correct thymic T-cell selection for the development of regulatory CD4$^+$ T-cell subsets able to prevent induction of colitis (Holländer *et al.*, 1995a,b). The role of MHC molecules in selecting T cells with the capacity to cause a variety of immunopathological phenomena, including colitis, was elegantly demonstrated by studies of rats carrying a transgenic human class I molecule (HLA-B27) (Hammer *et al.*, 1990; see chapter by Taurog in this volume). The most recent additions to the list of rodent IBD models were mice with disruption to the G-protein signaling subunit, G$\alpha$i-2 (Rudolph *et al.*, 1995). The development of IBD in G$\alpha$i-2$^{null}$ mice may offer some new perspectives on the intracellular signaling mechanisms critical for correct T-cell immunoregulation.

## II. Colitis in Bone Marrow-Reconstituted tg$\epsilon$26 Mice

Mice transgenic for the human CD3-$\epsilon$ gene, designated tg$\epsilon$26 mice, display very early arrest in T-cell development that results in a complete T-cell and NK-cell deficiency (Wang *et al.*, 1994, 1995). Importantly, the absence of early T-cell precursors in these animals prevents the induction of a normal thymic microenvironment. Although normal *wt* bone marrow, competent to generate T-cell precursors, could restore the thymic structure of fetal or newborn thymi, transplantation of adult tg$\epsilon$26 mice with normal T-cell-depleted bone marrow cells resulted neither in the reconstitution of the architecture of the thymic stroma nor in normal T-cell ontogeny (Holländer *et al.*, 1995a).

Five to eight weeks after transplantation, 100% of bone marrow-transplanted tg$\epsilon$26 mice developed a lethal wasting syndrome accompanied by severe colitis.

Histological analysis of colons of bone marrow-reconstituted, but not untransplanted tgε26 mice, revealed an inflammatory bowel disease that involved the mucosa and submucosa. Typical features of this disease included hyperplasia, elongation, distortion and branching of crypts, and a loss of the normal mucin-producing goblet cells. Crypt abscesses could also be found frequently, especially in animals with severe inflammation. The disease in transplanted tgε26 mice was also characterized consistently by a substantial mononuclear infiltrate, comprising mostly neutrophils and lymphocytes.

Most striking in the tgε26 colitis model was a massive predominance of CD4$^+$ T cells (up to 95% of CD3$^+$ T cells), in both the intraepithelial compartment and the lamina propria of the colon. By definition of high expression of the activation markers CD69 and CD44, and low CD45RB and L-selectin expression (Bottomly et al., 1989; Lee et al., 1990; Bradley et al., 1992), both peripheral and intestinal CD4$^+$ T cells from bone marrow-transplanted tgε26 mice appeared to be of an activated or memory phenotype. Furthermore, fluorocytometric analysis after intracytoplasmic cytokine staining revealed that a large number of CD4$^+$ T cells from diseased bone marrow-transplanted tgε26 mice produced IFNγ (Simpson et al., 1995b). Interestingly, this was much more striking in colonic CD4$^+$ T cells than in those from the lymph node or spleen, suggesting local activation of CD4$^+$ T cells within the colon. Transplanted, but not unmanipulated, tgε26 mice also had very high levels of TNFα in their sera. Intracytoplasmic staining studies have revealed a small though significant number of colonic CD4$^+$ T cells positive for TNFα in colitic transplanted tgε26 mice. However, the relative paucity of these cells suggested that macrophages were in fact the most likely predominant source of this cytokine (Simpson et al., 1995b).

Using adoptive transfer of purified T-cell subpopulations from bone marrow-transplanted tgε26 mice, into immunodeficient RAG$^{null}$ mice, we confirmed that CD4$^+$ T cells alone were sufficient to cause colitis (Holländer et al., 1995b). However, the findings from previous studies of TCR$^{null}$ mice also suggested that γδ T cells may contribute to colitis (Mombaerts et al., 1993). To elucidate whether γδ TCR$^+$ T cells could in fact cause IBD, we engrafted tgε26 mice with bone marrow from different T-cell-deficient mice. Tgε26 mice transplanted with bone marrow from TCRβ$^{null}$ or TCRα$^{null}$ and TCRδ$^{null}$ donors developed colitis with a high incidence (Simpson et al., 1995b). Fluorocytometric and immunohistological examination of peripheral lymph nodes and spleen and colon tissue sections revealed the presence of large numbers of γδT cells in these animals. In contrast, none of the mice transplanted with bone marrow from TCRβ$^{null}$ × TCRδ$^{null}$ or RAG$^{null}$ (Mombaerts et al., 1992) bone marrow developed colitis.

Although the characteristics of disease observed in histological sections from each of the TCR$^{null}$ transplanted tgε26 mice were very similar to those observed in the original bone marrow-reconstituted tgε26 mice, we observed a clear gradation in severity of inflammation, ranging from very mild to severe. Furthermore, overt clinical signs of disease in TCRβ$^{null}$- and TCRα$^{null}$-transplanted tgε26 mice generally appeared later than in mice transplanted with *wt* bone marrow. Nevertheless, these data demonstrate that $\gamma\delta$ T cells were able to cause colitis in transplanted tg$\epsilon$26 mice.

The pathogenic potential of T cells generated within the tg$\epsilon$26 thymus strongly suggested that either a failure of negative selection of autoagressive T cells or a failure of positive selection of a regulatory T-cell subsets might have been responsible. To test this, we transplanted fetal thymuses under the kidney capsules of adult tg$\epsilon$26 mice prior to bone marrow grafting. Although thymocytes were observed in both the transplanted thymus and the orthotopic thymus, the orthotopic thymus remained structurally abnormal and supported the ontogeny of small numbers of cells. In contrast, the fetal thymus acquired a normal stromal architecture and sustained normal T-cell development (Holländer *et al.*, 1995a). Furthermore, no signs of colitis were evident in any of the mice that received successful thymus grafts (Holländer *et al.*, 1995b). These experiments provided a clear illustration of the importance of a normal thymic microenvironment for the development of regulatory $\alpha\beta$ T cells sufficient to prevent colitis in transplanted tg$\epsilon$26 mice.

## III. COMPARISON OF DISEASE IN DIFFERENT IBD MODELS

The IBD observed in each of the rodent models so far studied share a number of common features that relate closely to human IBD, including alterations of crypt architecture, formation of crypt abcesses, goblet cell depletion, and extensive mononuclear cell infiltrate. Moreover, frequent differences in the extent of infiltration, the nature of some of the inflammatory lesions, (e.g., the formation of ulceratons), and the regions of the intestine that were affected also constituted characteristics often observed in human IBD (Podolsky, 1991a,b). For example, mucosal inflammation in the IL-2$^{null}$ mice, transplanted tg$\epsilon$26 mice, $\alpha\beta$ TCR$^{null}$ mice, HLA-B27 transgenic rat, and TGF$\beta^{null}$ mice was superficial and resembled human UC. In contrast, regions of inflammation in CD45RB transferred SCID mice and IL-10$^{null}$ mice were more transmural and sometimes affected the distall small bowel, features that more closely resembled Crohn's disease (Sartor, 1995; Podolsky, 1991a,b). As suggested by Sartor (1995) it is likely that although the initiating and predisposing factors in each animal model and in human IBD may be quite disparate, the resulting pathology observed in each case is probably mediated by a limited array of effector cytokines and cells (Sartor, 1994, 1995; MacDermott and Stenson, 1988).

## IV. IMMUNOPATHOLOGY OF IBD

### A. Th1 vs Th2 T-Cell Responses

A feature common to all the murine models of IBD studied to date, with the exception of TCR$\beta \times \delta^{null}$ mice, is that T cells were required for development as well as for regulation of disease. The finding that mice completely deficient in T cells (i.e., TCR$\beta \times \delta^{null}$ mice) developed IBD appears at odds with two other examples of T-cell (but not B-cell)-deficient animals; neither *nude* mice nor unmanipulated tg$\epsilon$26 mice develop spontaneous signs of IBD. Furthermore, tg$\epsilon$26 mice transplanted with TCR $\beta^{null} \times \delta^{null}$ bone marrow showed no signs of disease (Simpson *et al.*, 1995b), and even those in the original report developed, at worst, only mild disease with less than 50% penetrance within the colony (Mombaerts *et al.*, 1993). Although this issue has yet to be resolved, the prevailing picture places T cells at the center of pathogenesis in most forms of rodent IBD, raising the question of which type of T-cell responses account for pathology in each model.

The initial response to the reports of IBD in the IL-2$^{null}$, TCR$^{null}$, and IL-10$^{null}$ mice was that a dichotomy must exist in the mechanism of disease in these animals (Strober and Ehrhardt, 1993). The reasoning for this was that since IL-2 production is a hallmark in differentiated Th1 cells and that IL-10 is a signature cytokine for Th2 cells, the absence of either of these would shunt the general T-cell phenotype toward the opposite T helper subset. Consequently, a predominance of Th2 like cells in IL-2$^{null}$ colitis and a predominance of Th1-like cells in IL-10$^{null}$ mice would be apparent. Thus, it was envisaged that different diseases with a similar histopathology would be caused principally by either of two mechanisms. In IL-2$^{null}$ mice disease would result from a humoral, antibody-mediated mechanism driven by IL-4-secreting cells. Similarly, the prediction in mice with a severe T-cell deficiency (i.e., $\alpha\beta$ TCR$^{null}$ mice) has been that colitis developed primarily via unrestrained B-cell reactivity resulting from an absence of T-cell help (Mombaerts *et al.*, 1993). Conversely, colitis in IL-10$^{null}$ mice would be driven by a cell-mediated response, in which IFN$\gamma$ and TNF would play principal roles.

It appears from more recent data that the mechanisms operational in the pathogenesis of IBD in these rodent models may be more complex than originally hypothesized. Thus, IL-10$^{null}$ mice do indeed possess a strongly biased Th1-like response made evident by high IFN$\gamma$ production (Kühn *et al.*, 1993). However, there was also evidence for some hyperresponsive B-cell activity in IL-10$^{null}$ mice as measured by elevated serum levels of IgG subclasses and IgA. Antibodies reactive with colonic tissue or luminal bacterial antigens were detected in IL-2$^{null}$ and TCR$^{null}$ mice, respectively, suggesting B-cell involvement in these forms of IBD. However, direct evidence suggests that the role of B cells is, at most, secondary in IL-2$^{null}$ colitis, since IL-2$^{null}$ $\times$ Jh$^{null}$ mice which lack mature B cells nevertheless develop colitis (Ma *et al.*, 1995). In view of these findings and the lack of data on adoptive transfer of disease with B cells or serum from colitic mice, the role of B cells in rodent IBD needs further clarification.

The involvement of Th1 responses in initiating IBD was illustrated by experiments in which normal peripheral CD4$^+$, CD45RB$^{lo}$ (memory) T cells were shown to regulate the activity of pathogenic CD4$^+$, CD45RB$^{hi}$ (naive) T cells after transfer into SCID mice (Powrie *et al.*, 1993, 1994a). In the absence of CD45RB$^{lo}$ cells, CD45RB$^{hi}$ cells became inappropriately activated and homed to the intestinal mucosa, where they initiated a strong inflammatory response, characterized by high IFN$\gamma$ and TNF$\alpha$ production and the aquisition of a CD4RB$^{lo}$ phenotype (Powrie *et al.*, 1994b). In a similar study, Rudolphi and colleagues demonstrated that unseparated intestinal CD4$^+$ T cells from normal mice (which, unlike peripheral CD4$^+$ T cells, comprise high numbers of both CD45RB$^{lo}$ and CD45RB$^{hi}$ cells), preferentially homed to the intestinal mucosa and induced IBD on transfer into SCID mice (Rudolphi *et al.*, 1994). These latter experiments are of significance since they demonstrate that CD45RB$^{lo}$ CD4$^+$ T cells of the normal intestinal mucosa are distinct from nonpathogenic CD45RB$^{lo}$ CD4$^+$ regulatory T cells found in the peripheral lymphoid organs (Morrissey *et al.*, 1993; Powrie *et al.*, 1993, 1994a). These findings also illuminate potentially important differences in the mechanisms of peripheral and intestinal T-cell regulation.

In IL-2$^{null}$ mice, large numbers of CD4$^+$ T cells were found with a CD45RB$^{lo}$ and L-selectin$^{lo}$ phenotype, resembling those observed in colitic SCID mice after transfer of CD45RB$^{hi}$ cells (Simpson *et al.*, 1995a; Morrissey *et al.*, 1993; Powrie *et al.*, 1993, 1994a,b). Preliminary data from our laboratory using intracytoplasmic staining also revealed that a significant number of colonic CD4$^+$ T cells in IL-2$^{null}$ mice produced IFN$\gamma$. By similar criteria, Th1-dominated responses were also apparent in several other rodent IBD models, including transplanted tg$\epsilon$26 mice, TGF$\beta^{null}$ mice, and the transgenic HLA$\beta$27 rat.

## B.  $\gamma\delta$ T Cells in IBD

Evidence from our studies of tg$\epsilon$26 mice transplanted with TCR$\alpha^{null}$ and TCR$\beta^{null}$ bone marrow, and the original report of the $\alpha\beta$ TCR$^{null}$ colitis, suggest that $\gamma\delta$ T cells in sufficient numbers can mediate colitis (Simpson *et al.*, 1995b; Mombaerts *et al.*, 1993). In both cases, colitis in the absence of $\alpha\beta$ T cells correlated with a large expansion in the number of $\gamma\delta$ T cells, which may have simply resulted from "space-filling" of the lymphoid compartment, or because of a lack of specific $\alpha\beta$T-cell regulation. $\gamma\delta$ T cells are known to be significant producers of IFN$\gamma$, and we have preliminary data, using intracytoplasmic staining, that suggests this may be case in bone marrow-transplanted tg$\epsilon$26 mice.

In light of the above findings it is curious that athymic *nude* mice, which possess (thymus independent) $\gamma\delta$ T cells and lack $\alpha\beta$ T cells, do not develop IBD. The answer to this may be that *nude* mice cannot, by definition, develop thymus-dependent $\gamma\delta$ T cells. In contrast, in both forms the $\alpha\beta$ TCR$^{null}$ mice and $\alpha\beta$ TCR$^{null}$ transplanted tg$\epsilon$26 mice, large numbers of presumably thymus-derived $\gamma\delta$ T cells were observed in both the periphery and the intestine (Simpson *et al.*, 1995b). It is therefore apparent that in the presence of a thymus, but in the absence of $\alpha\beta$ T cells, significant expansion $\gamma\delta$ T cells can occur. Furthermore, these cells appear capable of inducing colitis, albeit less efficiently than CD4$^+$ $\alpha\beta$ T cells, and it is possible that the pathogenic effects of these cells are mediated via IFN$\gamma$ production.

## C. Cytokines and Inflammation

The results discussed so far strongly suggest that the key effector in all of the IBD models as well as in human IBD is IFN$\gamma$ (MacDonald et al., 1990; Sartor, 1994). With this in mind, we will consider briefly what effects excessive IFN$\gamma$ production would have to explain its pathogenic effects in IBD. IFN$\gamma$ has long been known to have a downregulatory effect on Th2-mediated responses, acting to inhibit proliferation of Th2-differentiated cells (Kaufman, 1995; Kelso, 1995). At the same time, IFN$\gamma$ has a profound effect on promoting the differentiation of Th1 CD4$^+$ T cells (Kaufman, 1995; Kelso, 1995). The importance of IFN$\gamma$ in promoting aberrant Th1 responses in murine IBD was clearly demonstrated by the inhibition of colitis in SCID recipients of CD45RB$^{hi}$ CD4$^+$ T cells, by in vivo blockade using an anti-IFN$\gamma$ antibody (Powrie et al., 1994b).

Another principal role of IFN$\gamma$ is to activate macrophages, which leads in turn to the production of proinflammatory mediators such as TNF, IL-1, IL-12, reactive oxygen species, and nitric oxide (Kaufman, 1995). Acting either directly or indirectly, these substances, in excessive quantities, can cause significant damage to intestinal mucosa (Madara and Stafford, 1989; MacDonald et al., 1990). Indeed, elevated levels of these proinflammatory cytokines have been measured in human IBD (MacDonald et al., 1990; Sartor, 1994; Ligumski et al., 1990; Mihada et al., 1989). As expected, substantial levels of TNF$\alpha$ were found in a number of different IBD models, including IL-10$^{null}$ mice, transplanted tg$\epsilon$26 mice, and SCID mice reconstituted with CD45RB$^{hi}$, CD4$^+$ T cells. In the latter two cases, treatment with anti-TNF antibodies significantly, but not completely, attenuated the progression of disease, emphasizing the important role of this cytokine in murine IBD (Powrie et al., 1994b; our unpublished observations).

INF$\gamma$ is also known to upregulate MHC class I and class II expression on a variety of cell types, and in several of the IBD models class II expression was dramatically elevated on the epithelial cells of the colon (Sadlack et al., 1993; Mombaerts et al., 1993; Kühn et al. 1993; Holländer et al., 1995b). Similarly, increased class II expression on colonic epithelium is a consistent feature of human IBD (Mayer et al., 1991). Damage caused to the colonic epithelium, by the direct activity of IFN$\gamma$ (Madara and Stafford, 1989) or indirect actions via other proinflammatory cytokines, could profoundly alter the antigenic balance within the colon. In synergy with elevated class II expression, these effects could greatly exacerbate inappropriate immune responses caused by dysregulation of mucosal T-cell responses.

## D. CD8$^+$ T Cells and Cytotoxicity

Evident in a number of the rodent colitis models was that the inflammatory infiltrate in the colon comprised a high number of CD8$^+$ $\alpha\beta$ T cells as well as CD4$^+$ T cells. CD8$^+$ cells could be involved in the immunopathology of colitis via cytotoxic activity, possibly stimulated by excessive local levels of IFN$\gamma$. This is supported by findings in some cases of human IBD (Stevens *et al.*, 1995). We observed that colonic CD8$^+$ $\alpha\beta$ T cells from IL-2$^{null}$ mice were strongly cytotoxic compared with *wt* colonocytes, which showed poor constitutive cytotoxicity *ex vivo* (Simpson *et al.*, 1995a; Camarini *et al.*, 1993). Although these $\alpha\beta$ TCR$^+$, CD8$^+$ CTL could have been involved in the pathology observed in the colitis in the IL-2$^{null}$ mouse, they were not critical for disease, since IL-2$^{null}$ animals crossed with class I-deficient $\beta_2$m$^{null}$ mice [which lack CD8$^+$ $\alpha\beta$ T cells (Koller *et al.*, 1990)] still developed colitis (Simpson *et al.*, 1995a). In fact, the accelerated appearance of colitis in $\beta_2$m$^{null}$ × IL-2$^{null}$ mice suggests that CD8$^+$ T cells may be more important in a regulatory or counterinflammatory capacity. For example, CD8$^+$ CTLs could be recruited to the colon kill-damaged epithelial cells in an effort to restore disruption to the luminal epithelial interface caused by inflammatory mediators (Klein and Mosely, 1993).

We also observed a strong constitutive T-cell-mediated cytotoxic activity in IEL and LPL preparations from colons of transplanted tg$\epsilon$26 mice. In light of the predominance of CD4$^+$ T cells in these fractions, we considered it likely that a substantial proportion of this activity was due to CD4$^+$ T cells and that this may have contributed to the pathogenesis of colitis in transplanted tg$\epsilon$26 mice. Previous studies have shown that CD4$^+$ CTLs are predominantly Th1-like and mediate killing via expression of FAS-ligand (FAS-L) that induces apoptosis in the target cell via FAS-receptor signaling (Ju *et al.*, 1994; Nagata and Goldstein, 1995; Berke, 1995a,b). Other studies have also implicated an important role for excessive FAS-L expression by activated CD4$^+$ T cells in the development of a GVHD-like wasting syndrome in *wt* mice transplanted with syngeneic FAS-deficient *(lpr)* bone marrow (Chu *et al.*, 1995). To test whether FAS-L expression was important in mediating pathogenic effects seen in tg$\epsilon$26 colitis, we engrafted tg$\epsilon$26 mice with bone marrow from *gld/gld* mice, which have a defect in FAS-L expression (Takahashi *et al.*, 1994). Onset of colitis in these animals was not affected, demonstrating that FAS-L expression was not critical in the progression of colitis (unpublished observations). Consistent with this, we found that the short-term CTL activity observed in transplanted tg$\epsilon$26 mice was principally mediated by a Ca$^{2+}$ dependent (perforin/serine protease) mechanism (Berk 1995a,b) and showed only moderate FAS/FAS-ligand-dependent killing. The importance of perforin-mediated cytotoxic activity in the pathogenesis of colitis in bone marrow-transplanted tg$\epsilon$26 mice could be tested by transplantation of tg$\epsilon$26 mice with bone marrow from perforin-deficient mice (reviewed by Berke 1995a,b).

## V. Regulation and Dysregulation within the Intestine

Although much evidence has now accumulated to demonstrate the importance of regulatory T cells in the prevention of colitis, many questions are outstanding concerning the development and mode of action of these cells. Clues to some of these questions may be provided by the studies of the bone marrow transplanted tgϵ26 mice, in which the importance of thymic selection in the development regulatory T cells was made apparent (Holländer *et al.,* 1995b). In related experiments, the role of the thymus in selecting pathogenic and nonpathogenic T cells was also demonstrated in mice which had been thymectomized at 3 days postpartum (3dTx mice). In later life, these animals developed a number of organ-specific autoimmune conditions, including some gastrointestinal pathology that was driven by T cells that emerged prior to thymectomy (Bonomo *et al.,* 1995).

A common interpretation that could be applied to both of the above experiments and the CD45RB/SCID transfer model is that in the absence of regulatory T cells, naive T cells could mediate their pathogenic effects unabaited. In the case of 3dTx mice, this would imply that the development-regulatory T cells may ensue at a later point in thymic development. Similarly, thymocyte development in transplanted tgϵ26 mice is supported for only a window of time post-transplantation (3–4 weeks) after which double-positive ($CD4^+$, $CD8^+$) thymocytes disappear, presumably stemming the emergence of new (regulatory?) T cells (Holländer *et al.,* 1995b). Another (not mutually exclusive) explanation for these findings is that the general T-cell lymphopenia found in transplanted tgϵ26 mice and 3dTx mice may limit the normal regulatory interactions required for T-cell homeostasis (Powrie, 1995). However, the absence of IBD in SCID mice reconstituted with even very small numbers of unseparated ($CD45RB^{hi/lo}$) T cells argues against this explanation (Powrie *et al.,* 1994b).

Regulatory T cells have been characterized previously by the repertoire of cytokines they produce. As already discussed, Th2 cells, known to be responsible for controlling B-cell activity, produce at least two cytokines that have distinct effects on generation of Th1 cells, namely IL-4 and IL-10 (Kelso, 1995). IL-4 can effectively counter the polarization of Th0 cells into Th1 cells. However, the finding that $IL-4^{null}$ mice do not develop colitis suggests that this pathway of cytokine regulation may not be very important in controlling pathogenic Th-1 responses in murine IBD (Kühn *et al.,* 1991). Experiments in which administration to colitic CD45RB-transferred SCID mice with recombinant IL-4 had no effect on development of colitis also support this conclusion (Powrie *et al.,* 1994b).

IL-10 is an efficient anti-inflammatory cytokine that acts primarily to shut down macrophages, which could have an indirect, yet profound, impact on the generation of Th1 responses by attenuating IL-12 and INFγ production (Kelso, 1995). Indeed, the development of colitis in IL-10-deficient mice and the effective abrogation of disease in CD45RB-transferred mice treated with recombinant IL-10 strongly illustrate the important role of this cytokine in protecting against aberrant Th1 responses (Powrie *et al.,* 1994b). Similarly, TGFβ1, part of a family of proteins produced primarily by activated macrophages, is important in regulating inflammatory responses. The central role of this cytokine in T-cell regulation was demonstrated in TGFβ1-deficient mice, which developed a variety of inflammatory lesions in different organs, including the colon and the stomach, depending on the genetic background on which the null mutation was carried. The direct role of $TGF_\beta$ in restraining T-cell responses in murine IBD was also demonstrated by *in vivo* administration of anti-$TGF_\beta$ antibody to SCID mice that received $CD45RB^{hi}$ T cells. In treated mice, the protective capacity of $CD45RB^{lo}$ cells was efficiently abrogated (Powrie *et al.*, 1995b).

The accumulation of memory-like T cells that accompanies pathology in many forms of murine IBD may reflect a failure to shut down immune responses. In normal circumstances this is achieved by activation-induced cell death (AICD) which occurs, via apoptosis, as a default pathway to ensure the clearance of activated T cells after their useful participation in an immune response. Remaining T cells that fail to undergo AICD become long-lived (memory) T cells. IL-2, known to be pivotal in the activation of T cells, also appears to be important in programming T cells to undergo AICD, at least *in vitro* (Lenardo, 1991). Thus, the appearance of large numbers of mucosal-homing, memory-like T cells in IL-2$^{null}$ mice would suggest that AICD may occur less efficiently in these animals.

$TNF\alpha$ and $INF\gamma$, unlike IL-2, have been shown to attenuate the ability of $CD4^+$ T cells to undergo AICD, at least in response to chronic superantigen activation (Vella *et al.*, 1995). It is possible therefore that either in the absence of a factor required for priming cells for AICD (e.g., IL-2) or in the presence of excessive levels of factors that antagonize this process (e.g., $TNF\alpha$ and $INF\gamma$), the accumulation of memory-like (AICD "resistant") T cells results. In large numbers, such cells, which also acquire a mucosal-homing phenotype (characterized by low L-selectin expression), could place a considerable burden on the intestinal immune system. Although the large numbers of activated/memory T cells found in many forms of murine IBD could support this hypothesis, the importance of compromised AICD as a mechanism in perpetuating T-cell pathogenesis in IBD requires further investigation.

The question of antigen specificity of the immune responses in each of the murine IBD models remains a complex puzzle. However, a significant clue to the etiology of animal and possibly human IBD comes from the finding that in some cases IBD does not develop, or is significantly attenuated, in animals reared under gnotobiotic or specific pathogen-free environments (Sadlack *et al.*, 1993; Taurog *et al.*, 1994; Sartor, 1995). (See chapter by Sartor in this volume). Clearly, these findings implicate a central role for intestinal bacterial flora in the development of IBD. The absence of pathogenic microorganisms in the different immunodeficient mouse strains kept under standard conditions further suggests that normal, non-pathogenic enteric flora are the most likely candidates.

Together, the presence of Th1-like cytokines and the apparent correlation of bacterial flora with development of colitis point toward aberrant cell-mediated responses to normal bacterial antigens as central to the disease. However, at a more fundamental level, the development of IBD in these animals reflects a failure of systemic immunoregulation that is most likely not confined to the intestinal mucosa. For this reason it is intriguing that each of the mouse lines so far studied does not reveal more evidence of systemic autoimmunity. Although immunopathology was noted in other organs in some animals (e.g., in IL-2$^{null}$ mice, TGF-$\beta^{null}$ mice, and HLA$\beta_{27}$ rat) the colon was the most frequently and, often, the most severely affected organ. This may be explained simply by the substantial load of bacterial antigens found within the colon. By comparison the relative paucity of other organ-specific self-antigens may constrain potentially autoaggressive responses. The mechanism of antigenic stimulation of T cells may also be considerably different within the colonic mucosa. For example, polyclonal activation by bacterial superantigens may occur at a high frequency in the colon and initiate abnormally aggressive inflammatory responses. The antigenic specificities of intestinal T-cell responses in normal as well as in diseased states will obviously be an important issue to address.

## VI. Lessons for Human IBD

It is apparent that a common picture is emerging from the collective studies of the rodent IBD models, namely, that interruption of normal T-cell homeostasis is pivotal in the development of colitis. The effects of TNF$\alpha$ and INF$\gamma$ are clearly central to pathogenesis in most forms rodent IBD, not just as mediators of inflammation but also as powerful modulators of T-cell regulation. Studies in human patients of Crohn's disease have linked high levels of INF$\gamma$ and TNF$\alpha$ to the disease, and preliminary studies have shown encouraging responses by patients to treatment with anti-TNF antibody administration (Van Dullman et al., 1995). The pivotal roles of regulatory T cells and their cytokines, including IL-10 and TGF$\beta$, in moderating the activity pathogenic T cells have also been illustrated clearly in the rodent IBD models.

It is likely that IBD in each of the rodent models discussed results from fundamental defects of systemic immunoregulation, and in this regard, questions concerning how regulatory T cells operate and how they are selected are most pertinent. Although many of the lessons from studies of rodent models of IBD have yet to be learned, the rapid progress made so far in understanding the mechanisms underlying these diseases sheds an optimistic light on the potential design of more effective strategies for treatment of human IBD.

### Acknowledgments

We thank Dr. Samir Shah for critical reading of the manuscript and useful discussion. Work described here was supported by grants from the Crohn's and Colitis Foundation of America, the Elanor Dana Naylor Foundation, and the NIH (P30DK 433–51, RO1 DK 47677, A.K.B.). S. J. S. is a recipient of a Research Fellowship from the Crohn's and Colitis Foundation of America.

### References

Berke, G. (1995a). Unlocking the secrets of CTL and NK cells. (1995). Immunol. Today **16**, 343–346.
Berke, G. (1995b). The CTL's kiss of death. Cell. (Cambridge, Mass.) **81**, 9–12.

Bonomo, A., Kehn, P. J., and Shevach, E. M. (1995). Post-thymectomy autoimmunity: Abnormal T cell homeostasis. *Immunol. Today* **16**, 61–67.

Bottomly, K., Luqman, M., Greenbaum, L., Carding, S., West, J., Pasqualini, T., and Murphy, D. B. (1989). A monoclonal antibody to CD45R distinguishes CD4 T cell populations that produce different cytokines. *Eur. J. Immunol.* **16**, 617–623.

Bradley, L. M., Atkins, G. G., and Swain, S. L. (1992). Long term CD4$^+$ memory T cells from the spleen lack MEL-14, the lymph node homing receptor. *J. Immunol.* **148**, 324–331.

Camarini, V., Panawala, C., and Kronenberg, M. (1993). Regional specialization of the mucosal immune system. Intra-epithelial lymphocytes of the large intestine have a different phenotype and function from those of the small intestine. *J. Immunol.* **151**, 1765–1776.

Chu, J. L., Ramos, P., Rosendorff, A., Nikolic-Zugic, J., Lacy, E., Matsuzawa, A., and Elkon, K. B. (1995). Massive up-regulation of the Fas-ligand in *lpr* and *gld* mice: Implications for Fas regulation and the graft-versus-host disease-like wasting syndrome. *J. Exp. Med.* **181**, 393–398.

Hammer, R. E., Maika, S. D., Richardson, J. A., Tang, J., and Taurog, J. D. (1990). Spontaneous inflammatory disease in transgenic rats expressing HLA-$\beta_{27}$ and human $\beta_2$m: An animal model of HLA$\beta_{27}$-associated disorders. *Cell (Cambridge, Mass.)* **63**, 1099–1112.

Holländer, G. A., Wang, B., Nichogiannopoulou, A., Platenberg, P.-P., van Ewijk, W., Burakoff, S. J., Gutierrez-Ramos, J.-C., and Terhorst, C. (1995a). A development control point in the induction of the thymic cortex regulated by a sub-population of pro-thymocytes. *Nature (London)* **373** 350–353.

Holländer, G. A., Simpson, S. J., Mizoguchi, E., Nickogiannopoulo, A., She, S., Gutierrez-Ramos, J.-C., Bhan, A., Burakoff, S. J., Wang, B., and Terhorst, C. (1995b). Severe colitis resulting from aberrant thymic selection. *Immunity* **3**, 27–38.

Ju, S. T., Cui, H., Panka, D. J., Ettinger, R., and Marshak-Rothstein, A. (1994). Participation of target FAS protein in apoptosis pathway induced by CD4$^+$ Th1 and CD8$^+$ cytotoxic T cells. *Proc. Natl. Acad. Sci. U.S.A.* **91**, 4185–4189.

Kaufman, S. H. E. (1995). Immunity to intracellular microbial pathogens. *Immunol. Today* **16**, 338–342.

Kelso, A. (1995). Th1 and Th2 subsets: Paradigms lost? *Immunol. Today* **16**, 374–379.

Klein, J. R., and Mosley, R. L. (1993). Phenotypic and cytotoxic characteristics of intraepithelial lymphocytes. In "Mucosal Immunology: Intraepithelial Lymphocytes" (H. Kiyono and J. R. McGhee, eds.), pp. 33–60. Raven, New York.

Koller, B. H., Marrack, P., Kappler, J., and Smithies, O. (1990). Normal development of mice deficient in $\beta_2$m MHC class I proteins, and CD8$^+$ T cells. *Science* **248**, 1227–1230.

Kühn, R., Rajewsky, K., and Müller, W. (1991). Generation and analysis of interleukin-4 deficient mice. *Science* **254**, 707–710.

Kühn, R., Lohler, J., Rennick, D., Rajewski, K., and Muller, W. (1993). Interleukin-10 deficient mice develop chronic enterocolitis. *Cell (Cambridge, Mass.)* **75**, 263–274.

Kulkarni, A. B., Huh, C. G., Becker, D., Geiser, A., Lyght, M., Flanders, K. C., Roberts, A. B., Sporn, M. B., Ward, J. M., and Karlsson, S. (1993). Transforming growth factor $\beta_1$ null mutation in mice causes excessive inflammatory response and early death. *Proc. Natl. Acad. Sci. U.S.A.* **90**, 770–774.

Lee, W. T., Yin, X. M., and Vitetta, E. S. (1990). Functional and ontogenetic analysis of murine CD45R$^{hi}$ and CD45R$^{lo}$ CD4+ T cells. *J. Immunol.* **144**, 3288–3295.

Lenardo, M. J. (1991). IL-2 programs mouse $\alpha\beta$ T lymphocytes for apoptosis. *Nature (London)* **353**, 858–861.

Ligumski, M., Simon, P. L., Karmeli, F., and Rachmilewitz, D. (1990). Role of interleukin-1 in inflammatory bowel disease: Enhanced production during active disease. *Gut* **31**, 686–689.

Ma, A., Datta, M., Chen, J., Margosian, and Horak, I. (1995). T cells, but not B cells, are required for bowel inflammation in interleukin 2-deficient mice. *J. Exp. Med.* **182**, 1567–1572.

MacDermott, R. P., and Stenson, W. F. (1988). Alterations of the immune system in ulcerative colitis and Crohn's disease. *Adv. Immunol.* **42**, 285–328.

MacDonald, T. T., Hutchings, P., Choy, M. Y., Murch, S., and Cooke, A. (1990). Tumour necrosis factor-alpha and interferon-gamma production measured at the single cell level in normal and inflammed human intestine. *Clin. Exp. Immunol.* **81**, 301–305.

Madara, J. L., and Stafford, J. (1989). Interferon-gamma directly affects the barrier function of cultured intestinal epithelial monolayers. *J. Clin. Invest.* **83**, 724–727.

Mayer, L., Eisenhardt, D., Salomon, P., Bauer, W., Pluos, R., and Piccinini, L. (1991). Expression of class II molecules on intestinal epithelial cells in humans. Differences between normal and inflammatory bowel disease. *Gastroenterology* **100**, 3–12.

Mihada, Y. R., Wu, K., and Jewell, D. P. (1989). Enhanced production of interleukin-1β by mononuclear cells isolated from mucosa with active ulcerative colitis or Crohn's disease. *Gut* **30**, 835–838.

Mombaerts, P., Iacomini, J., Johnson, R. S., Herrup, K., Tonegawa, S. and Pappaionnou, V. E. (1992). RAC-1-deficient mice have no mature B and T lymphocytes. *Cell* **68**, 869–877.

Mombaerts, P., Mizoguchi, E., Grusby, M. J., Glimcher, L. H., Bhan, A. K., and Tonegawa, S. (1993). Spontaneous development of inflammatory bowel disease in T cell receptor mutant mice. *Cell (Cambridge, Mass.)* **75**, 275–282.

Morrissey, P. J., Charrier, K., Braddy, S., Liggitt, D., and Watson, J. D. (1993). CD4$^+$ T cells that express high levels of CD45RB induce wasting disease when transferred into congenic severe combined immunodeficient mice. Disease development is prevented by co-transfer of purified CD4$^+$ T cells. *J. Exp. Med.* **178**, 237–244.

Nagata, S., and Goldstein, P. (1995). The fas death factor. *Science* **267**, 1449–1456.

Podolsky, D. (1991a). Inflammatory bowel disease (1). *N. Engl. J. Med.* **325**, 928–937.

Podolsky, D. (1991b). Inflammatory bowel disease II. *N. Engl. J. Med.* **325**, 1008–1016.

Powrie, F., Leach, M. W., Mauze, S., Caddle, L. B., and Coffman, R. B. (1993). Phenotypically distinct subsets of CD4$^+$ T cell induce or protect from chronic intestinal inflammation in C.B-17 SCID mice. *Int. Immunol.* **5**, 1461–1471.

Powrie, F., Correa-Oliveira, R., Mauze, S., and Coffman, R. L. (1994a). Regulatory interactions between CD45RB$^{high}$ and CD45RB$^{low}$ CD4$^+$ T cells are important for the balance between protective and pathogenic cell-mediated immunity. *J. Exp. Med.* **179**, 589–600.

Powrie, F., Leach, M. W., Mauze, S., Menon, S., Barcomb Caddle, L., and Coffman, R. L. (1994b). Inhibition of TH1 responses prevents inflammatory bowel disease in SCID mice reconstituted with CD45RB$^{hi}$ CD4$^+$ T cells. *Immunity* **1**, 553–562.

Powrie, F. (1995a). T cells in inflammatory bowel disease: Protective and pathogenic roles. *Immunity* **3**, 171–174.

Powrie, F., Carlino, J., Leach, M. W., Mauze, S., and Coffman, R. L. (1995b). A critical role for TGF$_β$ but not IL-4 in the suppression of Th-1 mediated colitis by CD4-5Rb$^{lo}$ CD4$^+$ T cells. *J. Exp. Med.* (in press).

Rudolph, U., Finegold, M. J., Rich, S. S., Harriman, G. H., Srinivasan, Y., Boulay, G., and Birnbaumer, L. (1995). Ulcerative colitis and adenocarcinoma of the colon in β alphai z-deficient mice. *Nat. Genet.* **10**, 143–150.

Rudolphi, A., Boll, G., Poulsen, S. S., Claesson, M. H., and Reimann, J. (1994). Gut homing CD4$^+$ T cell receptor αβ$^+$ T cells in the pathogenesis of murine inflammatory bowel disease. *Eur. J. Immunol.* **24**, 2803–2812.

Sadlack, B., Merz, H., Schorle, H., Schimpl, A. C., and Horak, I. (1993). Ulcerative colitis-like disease in mice with a disrupted interleukin-2 gene. *Cell (Cambridge, Mass.)* **75**, 253–261.

Sartor, R. B. (1990). Role of intestinal microflaora in initiation and perpetuation of inflammatory bowel disease. *Can. J. Gastroenterol.* **4**, 271–277.

Sartor, R. B. (1994). Cytokines in intestinal inflammation: Patho-physiological and clinical considerations. *Gastroenterology* **106**, 533–539.

Sartor, B. (1995). Insights into the pathogenesis of inflammatory bowel diseases provided by new rodent models of spontaneous colitis. *Inflammatory Bowel Diseases* **1**, 64–75.

Shull, M. M., Ormsby, I., Kier, A. B., Pawlowski, S., Diebold, R. J., Yin, M. Y., Allen, R., Sidman,

C., Proetzel, G., Calvin, D., Annuziata, N., and Doetschman, T. (1992). Targeted disruption of the mouse growth factor $\beta 1$ gene results in multi-focal inflammatory disease. *Nature (London)* **359**, 693–699.

Simpson, S. J., Mizoguchi, E., Allen, D., Bhan, A. K., and Terhorst, C. (1995a). Evidence that CD4[+], but not CD8[+] T cells are responsible for murine interleukin-2-deficient colitis. *Eur. J. Immunol.* **25**, 2618–2625.

Simpson, S. J., Hollander, G. A., Mizoguchi, E., Bhan, A. K., Wang, B., and Terhorst, C. (1995b). A novel form of murine colitis mediated by Th-1 CD4[+] T cells and TCR$\gamma\delta$+ T cells: A common role for INF-$\gamma$. Manuscript in preparation.

Stevens, A. C., Lipman, M. P., Spivack, J. E., Roddey, G., Bitton, A. M., Peppercorn, M., and Strom, T. B. (1995). Enhanced intramucosal cytotoxic lymphocyte gene expression in ulcerative colitis. *Inflammatory Bowel Diseases* **1**, 101–107.

Strober, W., and Ehrhardt, R. O. (1993). Chronic intestinal inflammation: An unexpected outcome in cytokine and T cell receptor mutant mice. *Cell (Cambridge, Mass.)* **75**, 203–205.

Sundberg, J. P., Elso, C. O., Bedigian, H. *et al.* (1994). Spontaneous heritable colitis in a new substrain of C3H/Hej mice. *Gastroenetrology* **107**, 1726–1735.

Takahashi, T., Tanaka, M., Brannan, C. I., Jenkins, N. A., Copeland, N. G., T., Suda, T., and Nagata, S. (1994). Generalized lymphoproliferative disease in mice, caused by a point mutation in the fas ligand. *Cell (Cambridge, Mass.)* **76**, 969–976.

Taurog, J. D., Richardson, J. A., Croft, J. T., Simmons, W. A.,. Zhou, M., Fernandez-Sueiro, J. L., Balish, E., and Hammer, R. E. (1994). The germ free state prevents development of gut and joint inflammatory disease in J HLA-B27 transgenic rats. *J. Exp. Med.* **180**, 2359–2364.

Van Dullman, H. M., van Deventer, S. J. H., Hommes, D. W., Bijl, H. A., Jansen, J., Tytgat, G. N. Y., and Woody, J. (1995). Treatment of Crohn's disease with anti-tumor necrosis factor chimeric monoclonal antibody (cA2). *Gastroentrology* **109**, 129–135.

Vella, A. T., McCormack, J. E., Linsley, P. S., Kappler, J. W., and Marrack, P. M. (1995). Lipopolysaccharide interferes with the induction of peripheral cell death. *Immunity* **2**, 261–270.

Wang, B., Biron, C., She, J., Higgins, K., Sunshine, M.-C., Lacy, L., Lonberg, N., and Terhorst, C. (1994). A block in both early T lymphocyte and natural killer cell development in transgenic mice with high copy numbers of the CD3-$\epsilon$ gene. *Proc. Natl. Acad. Sci. U.S.A.* **91**, 9402–9406.

Wang, B., Levelt, C., Salio, M., Zheng, D., Sancho, J., Liu, C.-P., Huang, M., Higgins, K., Sunsine, M.-J., Eichman, K., Lacy, E., Lonberg, N., and Terhorst, C. (1995). Abrogation of early T cell development by excessive signal transduction through CD3-$\epsilon$. *Int. Immunol.* **7**, 435–448.

## part
# IV

# MUCOSAL INFLAMMATION

# Chapter 23

# The Role of Endogenous Luminal Bacteria and Bacterial Products in the Pathogenesis of Experimental Enterocolitis and Systemic Inflammation

R. Balfour Sartor

*Division of Digestive Diseases, University of North Carolina at Chapel Hill, Chapel Hill, North Carolina 27599*

## I. INTRODUCTION

Although ulcerative colitis and Crohn's disease appear to be the result of an unrestrained inflammatory response, the antigen(s) which initiate and perpetuate these chronic, relapsing disorders remain uncertain (Sartor, 1995a). Clinicians have a longstanding belief that the normal enteric microbial flora were somehow involved in the pathogenesis of these diseases because inflammation occurs in the distal ileum and colon (the sites of the highest luminal bacterial concentrations), antibiotics and bowel rest benefit patients with Crohn's disease, and inflammatory bowel disease (IBD) patients have increased immune responses to ubiquitous luminal bacteria (Sartor, 1995b). Recent investigations using the older induced models of intestinal inflammation and new genetically engineered rodent models that develop spontaneous enterocolitis (Sartor, 1995c; Elson *et al.*, 1995) provide compelling evidence (Table I) to support the hypothesis that normal luminal bacteria and their products can induce and perpetuate chronic intestinal and systemic inflammation in genetically susceptible hosts (Sartor, 1995d). This hypothesis is rational, given the high concentrations of predominantly anaerobic bacteria and bacterial components in the distal ileum (approximately $10^8$ viable bacteria/g luminal contents) and colon ($10^{11-12}$ bacteria/g) (Donaldson, 1981; Simon and Gorbach, 1984). Mucosal inflammation enhances mucosal uptake and systemic transport of luminal bacterial components (Chadwick and Anderson, 1992; Sartor, 1995b) and promotes secondary invasion of mucosal ulcers and fistulae by enteric bacteria (Cartun *et al.*, 1993) (Fig. 1). These phlogistic bacterial constituents activate mucosal phagocytic cells and lymphocytes to secrete proinflammatory cytokines and solu-

*Essentials of Mucosal Immunology* Copyright © 1996 by Academic Press, Inc. All rights of reproduction in any form reserved.

TABLE *I*

EVIDENCE THAT UBIQUITOUS ENTERIC BACTERIA MEDIATE EXPERIMENTAL INTESTINAL
AND SYSTEMIC INFLAMMATION

1. Germ-free (sterile) environment attenuates acute injury and prevents chronic inflammation.

2. Antibiotics prevent and treat intestinal and systemic inflammation.

3. Small-bowel bacterial overgrowth induces and reactivates extraintestinal lesions.

4. Induction and perpetuation of inflammation by purified bacterial products.

5. Development of humoral and cellular immune responses to luminal bacteria.

*Note.* Modified from Sartor (1995d).

ble inflammatory mediators and stimulate specific immune responses which perpetuate the inflammatory process (Schwab, 1993; Sartor, 1995b). This chapter will summarize evidence generated in animal models of enterocolitis which supports this hypothesis.

## II. ABSENCE OF ENTEROCOLITIS IN GERM-FREE RODENTS

The most compelling evidence that ubiquitous luminal bacteria are involved in the pathogenesis of intestinal inflammation is provided by the consistent finding that

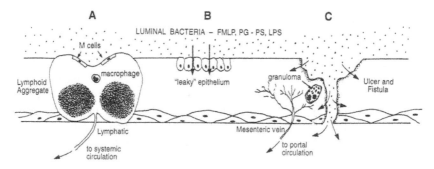

**FIGURE 1.** Mechanisms of mucosal uptake of normal bacterial flora and bacterial products in intestinal inflammation. Luminal bacteria and bacterial products such as chemotactic f-Met oligopeptides (FMLP), peptidoglycan–polysaccharide polymers (PG–PS), and lipopolysaccharide (LPS, endotoxin) are present in the distal ileum and colon. (A) Specialized epithelial cells (M cells) over Peyer's patches and organized lymphoid follicles preferentially transport luminal macromolecules in the normal state, initiating a tightly regulated, controlled mucosal immune response. (B) Normally the intact epithelium provides a relatively impenetrable barrier, but with nonulcerative inflammation, NSAID exposure, or perhaps subclinical Crohn's disease, the epithelium is "leaky," permitting enhanced uptake of luminal bacterial products. (C) With intestinal ulceration there is secondary invasion of viable bacteria and unrestricted uptake of bacterial products and antigens, further intensifying inflammation. Systemic uptake of bacterial products through the lymphatic and portal circulations leads to extraintestinal inflammation. Reprinted from Sartor and Powell (1991), with permission of Appleton and Lange Publishing Co.

"germ-free" rodents raised under completely sterile conditions fail to develop chronic enterocolitis (Table II).

## A. Induced Enterocolitis Models

Lewis rats populated with enteric bacteria devoid of all recognizable pathogens [specific pathogen-free (SPF)] develop chronic, mid-small-bowel ulceration with hepatobiliary inflammation, anemia, leukocytosis, and transient colonic ulcers when subcutaneously injected with indomethacin (Sartor *et al.,* 1992; Yamada *et al.,* 1993b). One to three days after indomethacin injection, germfree rats exhibit attenuated small-bowel ulcers and no evidence of colonic ulcers, compared with littermates conventionalized with SPF flora (Robert and Asano, 1977; Davis *et al.,* 1990). Germ-free Lewis rats have no evidence of intestinal or extraintestinal inflammation 14 days after indomethacin injection, in striking contrast to active enteritis, hepatobiliary inflammation, anemia, and leukocytosis in SPF littermates (Sartor *et al.,* 1994). Of considerable interest to the concept that bacterial polymers can potentiate intestinal inflammation, Davis *et al.* (1990) demonstrated that feeding purified, sterile peptidoglycan–polysaccharide (PG–PS) complexes to germfree rats increased small-bowel ulceration almost to levels seen in littermates populated with SPF bacteria, but had no such potentiating effect on colonic inflammation.

Similar results have been obtained with several other induced colitis models, suggesting a near universal requirement for ubiquitous bacteria in intestinal inflammation. Some studies have also explored which bacterial species have a dominant role in inducing intestinal inflammation. Onderdonk and colleagues (1981) showed that germ-free guinea pigs fed carrageenan, a red seaweed extract, failed to display any evidence of colitis, in marked contrast to animals populated with conventional bacteria. In a series of elegant experiments, these investigators found that *Bacteroides vulgatus* was the bacterial species which had the greatest ability to induce colitis in this model (Onderdonk *et al.,* 1981). Similarly, Phillips and

TABLE II

EFFECT OF BACTERIAL COLONIZATION ON EXPERIMENTAL ENTEROCOLITIS

| Model | Conventional or SPF flora | Sterile |
|---|---|---|
| Indomethacin (rat) | Enterocolitis | Attenuated acute, absent chronic |
| Carrageenan (guinea pig) | Colitis | Normal |
| Ameba (guinea pig) | Colitis | Normal |
| Dextran sodium sulfate (mouse) | Colitis | Colitis, ↑ mortality |
| IL-2 knockout (mouse) | Colitis | Normal |
| IL-10 knockout (mouse) | Enterocolitis | Normal |
| HLA-B27 transgenic (rat) | Gastroduodenitis, colitis | Normal |

*Note.* SPF, specific pathogen-free.

Gorstein (1966) demonstrated that bacteria-free guinea pigs do not develop cecal lesions following colonization with ameba. Guinea pigs monoassociated with *Clostridium perfringens, Lactobacillus acidophilus,* A-2 microccocus, and *Bacillus subtilis* before infection with ameba had more aggressive lesions than those colonized with *Streptococcus faecalis. Escherichia coli* monoassociation produced the lowest incidence of colitis following amebic infection, suggesting that anaerobic bacteria have a dominant role in experimental colitis. In contrast, germ-free mice fed dextran sodium sulfate (DSS) have a higher mortality rate than conventional mice (A. Onderdonk, unpublished data), raising the possibility that bacterial metabolism of this epithelial toxin is partially protective. It should be noted that this model has only been investigated in the acute phase, and that enteric bacteria may be capable of perpetuating chronic DSS-induced colitis.

## B. Genetically Engineered Rodents

Similar results have been observed in the newer models of deletion or overexpression of regulatory genes in mice or rats. The HLA-$B_{27}/\beta_2$ microglobulin transgenic rat model has been investigated most thoroughly. Taurog and colleagues (1994) showed that $B_{27}$ transgenic rats raised in a sterile environment had no evidence of colitis or arthritis, but continued to develop hair loss, epididymitis, and seizures. Rath and colleagues (1995a) confirmed these observations and also demonstrated an absence of gastritis and duodenitis in germ-free $B_{27}$ transgenic rats. Furthermore, these investigators found that colitis progressively developed during a 4-week period after colonization of gnotobiotic rats with SPF flora. Cytokine profiles of inflamed cecal tissues document activation of both macrophages and T lymphocytes following bacterial colonization (Rath *et al.,* 1995a), which is consistent with the ability of lymphocytes to transfer disease to nude rats (J. Taurog, unpublished results).

Similar results have been observed in preliminary studies of IL-2 and IL-10 knockout mice and SCID mice populated with CD45RB$^{hi}$ lymphocytes. IL-2-deficient (IL-2$^{-/-}$) mice housed in conventional rodent quarters develop aggressive colitis with bloody diarrhea and crypt abscesses (Sadlack *et al.,* 1993). However, in an SPF environment, these mice have subclinical colitis with only mild histologic inflammation and, when sterile, have neither clinical nor histologic evidence of colitis. Similarly, IL-10$^{-/-}$ mice, which have jejunal and colonic inflammation when conventionally housed, have isolated colitis under SPF conditions (Kuhn *et al.,* 1993). In preliminary studies, germ-free IL-10 knockout mice have no clinical evidence of intestinal inflammation (E. Balish, unpublished observations).

## III. PREVENTION OF INFLAMMATION BY ANTIBIOTICS

Diminishing luminal bacterial concentrations can attenuate or even entirely prevent experimental intestinal and systemic inflammation in a number of different models (Table III). These results are consistent with the absence of inflammation

***TABLE III***

ATTENUATION OF EXPERIMENTAL INTESTINAL AND SYSTEMIC INFLAMMATION BY ANTIBIOTICS

| Inducing event | Inflamed organ | Antibiotic therapy | Reference |
|---|---|---|---|
| Indomethacin | Small bowel | Metronidazole, tetracycline | Robert and Asano (1977) Yamada et al. (1993b) |
| Carrageenan | Colon | Metronidazole, clindamycin | Onderdonk et al. (1978) |
| TNB-SA | Colon | Imipeneum and vancomycin, Amoxicillin/clavulonic acid | Videla et al. (1994) |
| HLA-B27 TG | Colon, stomach, joints | Metronidazole | Rath et al. (1995b) |
| Jejunal SFBL | Liver, joints | Metronidazole | Lichtman et al. (1991a) Lichtman et al. (1995) |

*Note.* DSS, dextran sodium sulfate; TNB-SA, trinitrobenzene sulfonic acid; SFBL, self-filling blind loop; TG, transgenic.

in germ-free rodents and suggest that enteric bacteria have an essential role in the pathogenesis of intestinal inflammation. Broad-spectrum antibiotics, especially metronidazole and others with an anaerobic spectrum, are particularly active, implying a dominant role for anaerobic bacteria.

## IV. SYSTEMIC INFLAMMATION INDUCED BY SMALL-BOWEL BACTERIAL OVERGROWTH

Lichtman and colleagues (1990, 1991a,b, 1992, 1995) have demonstrated that surgical creation of experimental small-bowel bacterial overgrowth in genetically susceptible rats induces chronic hepatobiliary inflammation and reactivates arthritis.

### A. Hepatobiliary Inflammation

Surgical creation of a self-filling blind loop (SFBL) in the jejunum of rats leads to stasis and rapid proliferation of predominantly anaerobic bacteria, enhanced mucosal permeability, and intra- and extrahepatic biliary inflammation that resembles certain features of sclerosing cholangitis (Lichtman *et al.,* 1990). The inflammatory response is centered around bile ducts and is manifested by infiltration of mononuclear cells and occasional neutrophils, epithelial damage, ductal proliferation, and periportal fibrosis. Focal parenchymal inflammation, elevated serum AST concentrations, and increased numbers of Kupffer cells provide evidence of hepatic inflammation. Anaerobic luminal bacteria mediate the hepatobiliary injury, since inflammation is prevented by metronidazole and tetracycline, but not gentamicin (Lichtman *et al.,* 1991a). PG–PS from anaerobic bacteria are implicated, since mutanolysin, which selectively degrades peptidoglycan by splitting the $\beta_{1-4}$ linkage between *N*-acetyl muramic acid and *N*-acetyl glucosamine, prevents and treats injury in this model (Lichtman *et al.,* 1992). Furthermore, PG–PS polymers are absorbed to a greater degree from the blind loop than from the normal intestine, circulating PG–PS complexes are excreted in the bile, and serum anti-pepti-doglycan antibodies are increased following bacterial overgrowth (Lichtman *et al.*, 1991b). Although there is evidence of enhanced translocation of viable enteric bacteria to mesenteric lymph nodes, cultures of the liver, bile, blood, and perito-neal cavity are reproducibly negative (Lichtman *et al.*, 1990).

The ability of sterile bacterial products to cause systemic inflammation is fur-ther supported by the demonstration that repeated injections of heat-killed *E. coli* into the portal or systemic veins of rabbits causes hepatobiliary inflammation (Kono *et al.*, 1990). Although LPS absorption and endotoxemia are increased in this model (Brand *et al.*, 1994), complexing LPS with polymyxin B does not attenuate inflammation, and serum anti-LPS antibodies are not increased (Licht-man *et al.*, 1991b). Periportal inflammation accompanying chronic indomethacin-induced small intestinal ulceration (Sartor *et al.*, 1992) may share similar patho-genic mechanisms, since luminal bacteria proliferate in the inflamed small intes-tine, there is increased translocation of enteric bacteria to mesenteric lymph nodes, and metronidazole almost completely inhibits intestinal and systemic inflammation in the both models (Yamada *et al.*, 1993b). Like the PG–PS model, host genetic susceptibility is an important factor in the SFBL model, since Lewis rats develop inflammation 2–4 weeks after bacterial overgrowth and Wistar rats within 8–12 weeks, but Fischer and Buffalo rats fail to develop hepatobiliary injury even though they have identical concentrations of bacteria in the blind loop (Lichtman *et al.*, 1990).

## B. Arthritis

Using the same SFBL model in Lewis rats, Lichtman and associates (1995) showed that PG–PS polymers from ubiquitous luminal bacteria are capable of reactivating inflammation in previously injured ankles. Creation of experimental small-intestinal bacterial overgrowth caused arthritis in joints which had been in-jected intraarticularly with PG–PS 11 days previously, but there was no inflamma-tion in contralateral saline-injected joints. Reactivation of inflammation could be prevented by metronidazole, but not gentamicin or polymyxin B, by metronida-zole, IL-1 receptor antagonist, anti-tumor necrosis factor α (TNFα) antibody, and cyclosporine. This study implicates PG–PS from luminal anaerobic bacteria, T lymphocytes, IL-1, and TNFα in the pathogenesis of arthritis in this model.

## V. Inflammation Induced by Purified Bacterial Products

### A. Proinflammatory Properties of Bacterial Components

Several components of normal enteric bacteria, including chemotactic-formylated oligopeptides such as f-met–leu–phe (FMLP) and cell-wall polymers such as LPS (endotoxin) and PG–PS complexes are capable of activating phagocytic cells, lymphocytes, and proteolytic cascades (Table IV) (Chadwick and Anderson, 1992; Schwab, 1993; Sartor, 1995b). Many cytokines and soluble inflammatory mediators stimulated by FMLP, LPS, and PG–PS are increased in experimental intestinal inflammation (Herfarth and Sartor, 1994; Sartor, 1994, 1995a; Elson *et al.*, 1995). Because these bacterial components coexist in the lumen of the distal intestine and mucosal uptake of FMLP, LPS, and PG–PS is increased with intestinal inflammation, it is likely that mucosal inflammatory cells are simultaneously exposed to these phlogistic agents, which have overlapping properties and synergistic activities. For example, inflammation induced by PG–PS can be reactivated by LPS (Stimpson *et al.*, 1987) and LPS can prime a macrophage so that FMLP triggers greater production of reactive oxygen radicals (Baldassano *et al.*, 1993).

## B. Experimental Enterocolitis and Systemic Inflammation

The ability of purified bacterial products to initiate and perpetuate intestinal and systemic inflammation suggests that these sterile components may mediate many of the inflammatory effects of enteric bacteria and that invasion of the mucosa by viable bacteria is not essential (Sartor, 1995b). Experimentally, LPS and FMLP can induce acute, self-limited inflammation, whereas poorly biodegradable PG–PS from certain bacterial species causes spontaneously relapsing enterocolitis and extraintestinal inflammation. Acute colitis is induced by high luminal concentrations of FMLP (Chester *et al.*, 1985); more physiologic amounts increase mucosal permeability in the distal ileum (von Ritter *et al.*, 1988). LPS, when intravenously injected, causes mid-small-bowel hemorrhage, which is mediated by platelet-activating factor (Hseuh *et al.*, 1987), and stimulates chloride secretion, resulting in diarrhea (Ciancio *et al.*, 1993). Subcutaneous administration of LPS induces intes-

TABLE IV

PROINFLAMMATORY EFFECTS OF BACTERIAL PRODUCTS (FMLP, PG-PS, AND LPS)

---

*Macrophage and neutrophil activation*
Cytokines (IL-1, IL-6, IL-8, TNF$\alpha$, etc.)
Arachidonic acid metabolites (prostaglandins, leukotrienes, thromboxanes, platelet-activating factor)
Reactive oxygen metabolites
Nitric oxide
Proteases
*Proteolytic cascades*
Complement pathway
Kallikrein-kinin system
*Lymphocyte activation*
T-lymphocyte activation, mitogenic stimulation, adjuvant effect
B-cell mitogenic and antigenic activation

---

*Note.* Modified from Sartor (1995d).

tinal microvascular lesions (Mathan *et al.,* 1988), and intraperitoneal injection of endotoxin enhances bacterial translocation (Deitch *et al.,* 1989).

In contrast to the self-limited inflammation induced by LPS and FMLP, intramural (subserosal) injection of poorly biodegradable PG–PS induces chronic, spontaneously relapsing, granulomatous enterocolitis and associated arthritis, hepatic granulomas, anemia of chronic disease, and leukocytosis (Sartor *et al.,* 1985; Yamada *et al.,* 1993a; McCall *et al.,* 1994). This model exhibits a biphasic pattern of inflammation. Acute injury at the site of injection peaks at 1–3 days and is mediated, in part, by interleukin-1 (IL-1) and kallikrein (McCall *et al.,* 1994; Stadnicki *et al.,* 1994). After resolution of acute inflammation over 5–7 days, granulomatous, fibrotic enterocolitis spontaneously reactivates in Lewis rats approximately 14 days after PG–PS injection and is accompanied by erosive arthritis, hepatic granulomas, anemia, and leukocytosis (McCall *et al.,* 1994). The chronic granulomatous phase is T lymphocyte-mediated, as determined by the absence of chronic inflammation in nude (athymic) Lewis rats, complete inhibition by cyclosporine, and upregulation of cecal interferon-$\gamma$ (Sartor *et al.,* 1993). In addition to T-cell activation, monokines, including IL-1$_{\alpha \text{ and } -\beta}$, IL-6, gro, and IL-1 receptor antagonist are upregulated (McCall *et al.,* 1993, 1994). Recombinant IL-1 receptor antagonist and IL-10 significantly attenuate chronic enterocolitis and arthritis (McCall *et al.,* 1994; Herfarth and Sartor, unpublished results).

Chronicity of inflammation in this model depends on host genetic susceptibility and biodegradability of the PG–PS polymers. Inbred Lewis rats develop aggressive granulomatous enterocolitis with fibrosis and extraintestinal manifestations that persist for at least 4 months, whereas Buffalo and Fischer F$_{344}$ rats, the latter MHC-matched with Lewis rats, exhibit only transient, self-limited intestinal inflammation with no fibrosis or systemic responses (McCall *et al.,* 1994). Poorly biodegradable PG–PS polymers derived from group A streptococci, enterococci, group D streptococci, and certain *Eubacterial* strains induce chronic granulomatous inflammation, whereas easily biodegradable PG–PS from *Peptostreptococcus* incites only transient inflammation (Schwab, 1993). Of potential therapeutic importance, degradation of PG–PS by a muralytic enzyme, mutanolysin, can prevent and treat chronic granulomatous enterocolitis and systemic inflammation (Sartor *et al.,* 1991; Schwab, 1995). In addition to its ability to induce inflammation after intramural injection, luminal PG–PS has been shown to potentiate acetic acid-induced colitis (Sartor *et al.,* 1988) and indomethacin-induced enteritis (Davis *et al.,* 1990) and has been implicated in the pathogenesis of hepatobiliary inflammation in the SFBL model (Lichtman *et al.,* 1992). Furthermore, mucosal uptake and systemic transport of luminal PG–PS is increased following acetic acid injury of the colon (Sartor *et al.,* 1988) and experimental small-bowel bacterial overgrowth (Lichtman *et al.,* 1991b). Portal and systemic venous endotoxemia is also increased in the SFBL model (Brand *et al.,* 1994).

Complexing LPS with luminal adsorbents such as kaolin or tarra fullonica reduced endotoxemia, but had no effect on intestinal inflammation in the trinitrobenzene sulfonic acid model (Gardiner *et al.,* 1993). These results are consistent with the lack of benefit complexing LPS with polymyxin B in hepatobiliary and joint inflammation in the SFBL model (Lichtman *et al.,* 1991a, 1995).

## VI. IMMUNE RESPONSES TO UBIQUITOUS BACTERIA AND BACTERIAL COMPONENTS

Evidence emerging from newer rodent models strongly suggests that chronic intestinal inflammation is immunologically mediated, with a role for $CD4^+$ T lymphocytes (Sartor, 1995a,e). However, the antigens driving this chronic immune response are just beginning to be investigated. Elson and associates have demonstrated T- and B-lymphocyte responses to ubiquitous enteric bacteria in $C_3H/HeJ$ Bir substrain mice which spontaneously develop colitis (Sundberg *et al.,* 1994). By Western blot analysis, serum from these mice recognizes multiple epitopes in homogenates of normal enteric bacteria (Brandwein *et al.,* 1995). More antigens were recognized from homogenates of aerobic gram-negative rods, such as *E. coli,* than from intestinal anaerobes, such as *Bacteroides* or *Eubacterium* sp., and outer membrane components seemed to be the dominant antigens. However, maximum serologic responses occurred in older mice ($>6$ months of age), which is long after colitis in this model spontaneously resolves (inflammation peaks between 3 and 6 weeks of age). This kinetic pattern suggests that the serum antibody response may be more a reflection of mucosal absorption of bacterial antigens rather than an integral pathogenic process. Recently, this same group showed a Th1-dominant response to ubiquitous luminal bacteria, including *E. coli,* which occurred during active inflammation (Cong, 1995), suggesting a more pathogenic role for cell-mediated than for humoral immune responses. Of interest, the apparently spontaneous mutation which confers susceptibility to colitis occurs on a genetic background of resistance to LPS stimulation (McCabe *et al.,* 1993). LPS-nonresponding C3H/HeJ mice are high responders to several types of induced colitis (Sartor, 1995c). Consistent with the observations of an immune response to bacterial membrane proteins, outer membrane proteins of *B. vulgatus* are capable of enhancing carrageenan-induced colitis in guinea pigs (Breeling *et al.,* 1988). In preliminary studies, our group has demonstrated T lymphocyte responses to PG–PS in the chronic phase of indomethacin-induced enteritis in rats (S. Tonkonogy, unpublished results).

## VII. CONCLUSIONS

Results in a large number of disparate models consistently demonstrate that normal luminal bacteria and their products can induce and perpetuate chronic intestinal and systemic inflammation in genetically susceptible hosts. This conclusion is consistent with clinical observations, which suggest that anaerobic bacteria have a dominant role in Crohn's disease and that aerobes influence ulcerative colitis (Sartor, 1995b). Ongoing studies in rodent models will determine whether a single bacterial species, or groups of bacteria, can preferentially influence chronic intestinal inflammation.

A conceptual paradigm is presented in Fig. 2, illustrating the dynamic interaction between proinflammatory luminal bacterial constituents and mucosal protective forces. Because phlogistic bacterial products are present in the lumen of the distal ileum and colon of all rodents and humans, host susceptibility factors must determine the course of the inflammatory response. Critical protective mechanisms include the ability of the normal mucosal barrier to exclude proinflammatory bacterial products and active downregulation of the inflammatory response by immunosuppressive T lymphocytes, cytokines, prostaglandins, and neuropeptides. Genetic alterations of immunoregulation or barrier function could alter the delicate balance between protective and aggressive factors to favor chronic inflammation. Similarly, environmental agents which derange barrier function, inhibit protective cytokines or prostaglandins, or alter luminal bacterial constituents could preturb mucosal homeostasis, thereby favoring acute or chronic inflammation. It is apparent from rodent studies that host genetic background is an essential determinant of chronicity of inflammation (Sartor, 1995f). However, an essential role for ubiquitous luminal bacteria is equally evident from the studies discussed in this chapter; thus, chronic intestinal inflammation is the result of an interaction between environmental and genetic factors.

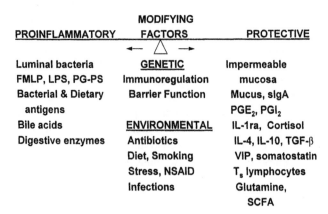

**FIGURE 2.** The balance between luminal proinflammatory factors and mucosal protective mechanisms. The genetically determined immune response to bacterial products or epithelial barrier function can influence host susceptibility to chronic inflammation while environmental factors can influence initial onset and spontaneous reactivation of inflammation. FMLP, $n$-formyl-methionyl-leucyl-phenylalanine; IL, interleukin; TGF$_\beta$, transforming growth factor-$\beta$; NSAID, nonsteroidal anti-inflammatory drug; T$_s$, T suppressor lymphocytes; SCFA, short-chain fatty acids. Adapted from Sartor, R.B. (1990). *Can. J. Gastroenterol.* **4**, 271–277, and used with permission of Pulsus Group, Inc.

Future studies are necessary to determine which bacterial species and bacterial products exert a dominant driving force and to develop novel approaches to selectively eliminate key proinflammatory luminal constituents. Although it is impossible to chronically sterilize the mammalian gut, it may be possible to eliminate targeted bacterial strains by selective antibiotics, blockade of epithelial attachment, immunization, or competition for ecologic niches by noninflammatory bacteria. Similarly, novel approaches to complexing, degrading, or inactivating bacterial products such as PG–PS, LPS, and FMLP, or blocking membrane receptors for these molecules on immune effector cells, may prove to be effective. Therapeutic approaches which target factors that initiate and perpetuate inflammation are conceptually superior to those that attempt to block ongoing advanced inflammatory reactions. However, the development of therapeutic strategies that selectively target specific bacteria and bacteria constituents is dependent on identifying which bacterial components preferentially stimulate chronic intestinal inflammation in genetically susceptible hosts.

## ACKNOWLEDGMENTS

The author gratefully acknowledges the expert secretarial and editorial assistance of Brian C. Springer and constructive review by Rance Sellon, DVM, Ph.D. Original research in this review was supported by NIH Grants DK 40249 and DK 34987, the Crohn's and Colitis Foundation of America, and the Deutsche Forschungsgemeinschaft (DFG).

## REFERENCES

Baldassano, R. N., Schreiber, S., Johnston, R. B., Jr., Fu, R. D., Muraki, T., and MacDermott, R. P. (1993). Crohn's disease monocytes are primed for accentuated release of toxic oxygen metabolites. *Gastroenterology* **105,** 60.

Brand, H. S., Maas, M. A. W., Bosma, A., Van Ketel, R. J., Speelman, P., and Chamuleau, R. A. F. M. (1994). Experimental colitis in rats induces low-grade endotoxinemia without hepatobiliary abnormalities *Dig. Dis. Sci.* **39,** 1210–1215.

Brandwein, S., McCabe, R. P., Dadrat, A., Ridwan, K. B. Waites, B. U., Birkenmeier, E. H., Sundberg, J. P., and Elson, C. O. (1995). Spontaneously colitic C₃H/HeJ Bir mice demonstrate antibody reactivity to isolated colonies of enteric bacteria. *Gastroenterology* **108,** A787.

Breeling, J. L., Onderdonk, A. B., Cisneros, R. L., and Kasper, D. L. (1988). *Bacteroides vulgatus* outer membrane antigens associated with carrageenan-induced colitis in guinea pigs. *Infect. Immun.* **56,** 1754–1759.

Cartun, R. W., Van Kruiningen, H. J., Pedersen, C. A., and Berman, M. M. (1993). An immunocytochemical search for infectious agents in Crohn's disease. *Mod. Pathol.* **6,** 212–219.

Chadwick, V. S., and Anderson, R. P. (1992). Microorganisms and their products in inflammatory bowel disease. *In* "Inflammatory Bowel Disease" (R. P. MacDermott and W. F. Stenson, eds.), pp. 241–258. Elsevier, New York.

Chester, J. F., Ross, J. S., Malt, R. A., and Weitzman, S. A. (1985). Acute colitis produced by chemotactic peptides in rats and mice. *Am. J. Pathol.* **121,** 284.

Ciancio, M. J., Vittiritti, L., Dhar, A., and Chang, E. B. (1993). Endotoxin-induced alterations in rat colonic water and electrolyte transport. *Gastroenterology* **103,** 1437–1443.

Cong, Y., Brandwein, S. L., McCabe, R. P., Ridwan, B. U., Birkenmeier, E. H., Sundberg, J. P., and Elson, C. O. (1995). Th1 response to enteric bacteria in colitis C3H/HeJ Bir mice. *Clin. Immunol. Immunopathol.* **76,** S44.

Davis, S. W., Holt, L. C., and Sartor, R. B. (1990). Luminal bacteria and bacterial polymers potentiate indomethacin-induced intestinal injury in the rat. *Gastroenterology* **98,** 455A.

Deitch, E. A., Ma, L., Ma, W. J., Grisham, M. B., Granger, D. N., Specian, R. D., and Berg, R. D. (1989). Inhibition of endotoxin-induced bacterial translocation in mice. *J. Clin. Invest.* **84,** 36.

Donaldson, R. M., Jr. (1981). Normal bacterial population of the intestine and their relation to intestinal function. *N. Engl. J. Med.* **270,** 938–943.

Elson, C. O., Sartor R. B., Tennyson, G., and Riddel, R. (1995). Experimental models of IBD. *Gastroenterology* **109,** 1344–1367.

Gardiner, K. R., Anderson, N. H., McCaigue, M. D., Erwin, P. J., Halliday, M. I., and Rowlands, B. J. (1993). Adsorbents as antiendotoxin agents in experimental colitis. *Gut* **34,** 51.

Herfarth, H., and Sartor, R. B. (1994). Cytokine regulation of experimental intestinal inflammation. *Curr. Opin. Gastroenterol.* **10,** 625–632.

Hsueh, W., Gonzalez-Crussi, F., and Arroyave, J. L. (1987). Platelet-activating factor: An endogenous mediator for bowel necrosis in endotoxemia. *FASEB J.* **1,** 403.

Kono, K., *et al.* (1990). Experimental portal fibrosis produced by intraportal injection of killed non-pathogenic *Escherichia coli* in rabbits. *Gastroenterology* **98,** 414.

Kuhn, R., Lohler, J., Rennick, D., Rajewsky, K., and Muller, W. (1993). Interleukin-10-deficient mice develop chronic enterocolitis. *Cell (Cambridge, Mass.)* **75,** 263–274.

Lichtman, S. N., Sartor, R. B., Schwab, J. H., and Keku, J. (1990). Hepatic inflammation in rats with experimental small intestinal bacterial overgrowth. *Gastroenterology* **98,** 414–423.

Lichtman, S. N., Keku, J. Schwab, J. H., and Sartor, R. B. (1991a). Hepatic injury associated with small bowel bacterial overgrowth in rats is prevented by metronidazole and tetracycline. *Gastroenterology* **100,** 513–519.

Lichtman, S. N., Keku, J., Schwab, H. J., and Sartor, R. B. (1991b). Evidence for peptidoglycan absorption in rats with experimental small bowel bacterial overgrowth. *Infect. Immun.* **59,** 555–562.

Lichtman, S. N., Okoruwa, E. E., Keku, J., Schwab, J. H., and Sartor, R. B. (1992). Degradation of endogenous bacterial cell wall polymers by the muralytic enzyme mutanolysin prevents hepatobiliary injury in genetically susceptible rats with experimental intestinal bacterial overgrowth. *J. Clin. Invest.* **90,** 1313–1322.

Lichtman, S. N., Wang, J., Sartor, R. B., Zhang, C., Bender, D. E., Dalldorf, F. G., and Schwab, J. H. (1995). Reactivation of arthritis induced by small bowel bacterial overgrowth in rats: Role of cytokines luminal bacteria and bacterial polymers. *Infect. Immun.* **63,** 2295–2301.

Mathan, V. I., Penney, G. R., Mathan, M. M., and Rowley, D. (1988). Bacterial lipopolysaccharide-induced intestinal microvascular lesions leading to acute diarrhea. *J. Clin. Invest.* **82,** 1714.

McCabe, R. P., Mills, T., Ridwan, B., Dadrat, A., Thaggard, G., Beagley, K. Birkenmeier, E., Sundberg, J., and Elson, C. O. (1993). Immune reactivity of C3H/HeJ mice with spontaneous colitis. *Gastroenterology* **104,** A656.

McCall, R. D., Haskill, J. S., and Sartor, R. B. (1993). Constitutive expression of TNFα and of an IL-8-like gene is associated with genetic susceptibility to chronic granulomatous enterocolitis in inbred rats. *Gastroenterology* **104,** 740A.

McCall, R. D., Haskill, S., Zimmermann, E. M., Lund, P. K., Thompson, R. C., and Sartor, R. B. (1994). Tissue interleukin-a and interleukin-2 receptor antagonist expression in enterocolitis in resistant and susceptible rats. *Gastroenterology* **106,** 960–972.

Onderdonk, A. B., Hermos, J. A., Dzink, J. L., and Bartlett, J. G. (1978). Protective effect of metronidazole in experimental ulcerative colitis. *Gastroenterology* **74,** 521–526.

Onderdonk, A. B., Franklin, M. L., and Cisneros, R. L. (1981). Production of experimental ulcerative colitis in gnotobiotic guinea pigs with simplified microflora. *Infect. Immun.* **32,** 325–331.

Phillips, B. P., and Gorstein, F. (1966). Effects of different species of bacteria on the pathology of enteric amebiasis in monocontaminated guinea pigs. *Am. J. Trop. Med. Hyg.* **15**, 863.

Rath, H. C., Bender, D. E., Grenther, T., Holt, L. C., Herfarth, H. H., Mohanty, S., Taurog, J. D., Hammer, R. E., and Sartor, R. B. (1995a). Normal bacteria stimulate colonic, gastric, and systemic inflammation in HLA-B$_{27}$/$\beta_2\mu$ microglobulin transgenic rats. *Gastroenterology* **108**, A899.

Rath, H. C., Bender, D. E., Holt, L. C., Grenther, T., Taurog, J. D., Hammer, R. E., and Sartor, R. B. (1995b). Metronidazole attenuates colitis in HLA-B$_{27}$/$\beta_2\mu$ transgenic (TG) rats: A pathogenic role for anaerobic bacteria. *Clin. Immunol. Immunopathol.* **76**, S45.

Robert, A., and Asano, T. (1977). Resistance of germfree rats to indomethacin-induced intestinal lesions. *Prostaglandins* **14**, 333–341.

Sadlack, B., Merz, H., Schorle, H., Schimpl, A., Feller, A. C., and Horak, I. (1993). Ulcerative colitis-like disease in mice with a disrupted interleukin-2 gene. *Cell (Cambridge, Mass.)* **75**, 253–261.

Sartor, R. B. (1990). Role of intestinal microflora in initiation and perpetuation of inflammatory bowel disease. *Can. J. Gastroenterol.* **4**, 271–277.

Sartor, R. B. (1994). Cytokines in intestinal inflammation: Pathophysiologic and clinical considerations. *Gastroenterology* **106**, 533–539.

Sartor, R. B. (1995a). Current concepts of the etiology and pathogenesis of Crohn's disease and ulcerative colitis. *Gastroenterol. Clin. North Am.* **24**, 475–508.

Sartor, R. B. (1995b). Microbial factors in the pathogenesis of Crohn's disease, ulcerative colitis and experimental intestinal inflammation. *In* "Inflammatory Bowel Disease" (J. B. Kirsner and R. J. Shorter, Eds.), 4th ed., pp. 96–124. Williams & Wilkins, Baltimore, MD.

Sartor, R. B. (1995c). Insights into the pathogenesis of inflammatory bowel disease provided by new rodent models of spontaneous colitis. *Inflammatory Bowel Diseases* **1**, 64–75.

Sartor, R. B. (1995d). The role of normal enteric bacteria and bacterial products in chronic intestinal inflammation. *In* "Inflammatory Bowel Disease" (G. N. J. Tytgat and S. N. J. van Deventer, eds.), in press. Kluwer, Dordrecht, The Netherlands.

Sartor, R. B. (1995e). The use of transgenic and knockout rodents as models of inflammatory bowel disease. *Mucosal Immunology Update* **3**, 9–12.

Sartor, R. B. (1995f). Genetic factors in animal models of intestinal inflammation. *Can. J. Gastroenterol.* **9**, 147–152.

Sartor, R. B., and Powell, D. W. (1991). Mechanisms of diarrhea in intestinal inflammation and hypersensitivity. *In* "Controversies in Gastroenterology, Diarrheal Diseases" (M. Field, Ed.), pp. 75–114. Appleton and Lange, Norwalk, CT.

Sartor, R. B., Cromartie, W. J., Powell, D. W., and Schwab, H. J. (1985). Granulomatous enterocolitis induced in rats by purified bacterial cell wall fragments. *Gastroenterology* **89**, 587–595.

Sartor, R. B., Bond, T. M., and Schwab, J. H. (1988). Systemic uptake and intestinal inflammatory effects of luminal bacterial cell wall polymers in rats with acute colonic injury. *Infect. Immun.* **56**, 2101–2108.

Sartor, R. B., Holt, L. C., Bender, D. E., and Schwab, J. H. (1991). Prevention and treatment of chronic relapsing enterocolitis in rats by *in vivo* degradation of bacterial cell wall polymers. *Gastroenterology* **100**, 613A.

Sartor, R. B., Bender, D. E., and Holt, L. C. (1992). Susceptibility of inbred rat strains to intestinal and extraintestinal inflammation induced by indomethacin. *Gastroenterology* **102**, A690.

Sartor, R. B., Bender, D. E., Allen, J. B., Zimmermann, E. M., Holt, L. C., Pardo, M. S., Lund, P. K., and Wahl, S. M. (1993). Chronic experimental enterocolitis and extraintestinal inflammation are T lymphocyte dependent. *Gastroenterology* **104**, 775A.

Sartor, R. B., Bender, D. E., Grenther, T., and Holt, L. C. (1994). Absolute requirement for ubiquitous luminal bacteria in the pathogenesis of chronic intestinal inflammation. *Gastroenterology* **106**, A767.

Schwab, J. H. (1993). Phlogistic properties of peptidoglycan–polysaccharide polymers from cell walls of pathogenic and normal-flora bacteria which colonize humans. *Infect. Immun.* **61**, 4535–4539.

Schwab, J. H. (1995). Bacterial cell-wall induced arthritis: Models of chronic recurrent polyarthritis and reactivation of monoarticular arthritis. *In* "Mechanisms and Models in Rheumatoid Arthritis" (B. Henderson, R. Pettifer, and J. Edwards, eds.), pp. 439–454. Academic Press, London.

Simon, G. I., and Gorbach, S. L. (1984). Intestinal flora in health and disease: A review. *Gastroenterology* **86,** 174.

Stadnicki, A., dela Cadena, R. A., Kettner, C., Sartor, R. B., Adam, A., and Colman, R. W. (1994). A selective plasma kallikrein inhibitor modulates the development of peptidoglycan-induced acute intestinal inflammation. *Clin. Res.* **42,** A243.

Stimpson, S. A., Esser, R. E., Carter, P. B., Sartor, R. B., Cromartie, W. J., and Schwab, H. J. (1987). Lipopolysaccharide induces recurrence of arthritis in rat joints previously injured by peptidoglycan–polysaccharide. *J. Exp. Med.* **165,** 1688–1702.

Sundberg, J. P., Elson, C. O., Bedigian, H., and Birkenmeier, E. H. (1994). Spontaneous, heritable colitis in a new substrain of $C_3H/HeJ$ mice. *Gastroenterology* **107,** 1726–1735.

Taurog, J. D., Richardson, J. A., Croft, J. T., Simmons, W. A., Zhou, M., Fernandez-Sueiro, J. L., Balish, E., and Hammer, R. E. (1994). The germfree state prevents development of gut and joint inflammatory disease in HLA-$B_{27}$ transgenic rats. *J. Exp. Med.* **180,** 2359–2364.

von Ritter, C., Sekizuka, E. Grisham, M. B., and Granger, D. N. (1988). The chemotactic peptide *N*-formyl methionyl-leucyl-phenylalanine increases mucosal permeability in the distal ileum of the rat. *Gastroenterology* **95,** 651.

Videla, S., Vilaseca, J., Guarner, F., Salas, A., Treserra, F., Crespo, E., Antolin, M., and Malagelada, J. R. (1994). Role of intestinal microflora in chronic inflammation and ulceration of the rat colon. *Gut* **35,** 1090–1097.

Yamada, T., Sartor, R. B., Marshall, S., Specian, R. D., and Grisham, M. B. (1993a). Mucosal injury and inflammation in a model of chronic granulomatous colitis. *Gastroenterology* **104,** 759–771.

Yamada, T., Deitch, E., Specian, R. D., Perry, M. A., Sartor, R. B., and Grisham, M. B. (1993b). Mechanisms of acute and chronic intestinal inflammation induced by indomethacin. *Inflammation* **17,** 641–662.

*Chapter 24*

# The Role of the Mucosal Immune System in Inflammatory Bowel Disease

Richard P. MacDermott

*Section of Gastroenterology, Lahey Hitchcock Medical Center,
Burlington, Massachusetts 01805; Department of Immunology, Massachusetts General Hospital,
Boston, Massachusetts 02115; and Harvard Medical School,
Boston, Massachusetts 02115*

## I. INTRODUCTION

The normal human intestinal mucosal immune system has important protective functions, which should not lead to damage of the intestine. In healthy individuals, nutrients cross the interface from the external environment (the gut lumen) into the intestinal mucosa, while the translocation of potentially injurious agents must be prevented efficiently and completely (Mestecky, 1987; Mestecky and McGhee, 1987). A critical function, therefore, of the normal intestinal immune system is the ability to specifically recognize and neutralize infectious agents as well as potentially injurious toxins (Mestecky, 1987; Mestecky and McGhee, 1987). Discrimination between self and nonself is also critical so that host tissues are not damaged during the time that host protective defense mechanisms are being employed.

Cytokines, produced by macrophages (Dinarello, 1988) and T cells, induce B cells to mature into plasma cells and to secrete immunoglobulins, including IgA (Mestecky, 1987; Mestecky and McGhee, 1987). Presentation of antigens to B cells initiates an orderly and precise sequence of activation steps during which genes that code for variable regions are joined with genes that code for constant regions of heavy and light chains of immunoglobulins (Mestecky, 1987; Mestecky and McGhee, 1987). This sequence of events results in the formation of specific DNA, which produces a specific messenger RNA that, in turn, allows a B cell to secrete an isotype and subclass-defined antibody specific for the initiating antigen (Mestecky, 1987; Mestecky and McGhee, 1987). The mucosal immune system has unique mechanisms that allow mucosal B cells to "switch" from predominantly IgM production to IgA production (Kawanishi *et al.*, 1983a,b). A series of cell-mediated and cytokine-mediated regulatory events are involved in the production of IgA, which is the major intestinal mucosal protective immunoglobulin (Mestecky, 1987; Mestecky and McGhee, 1987). Within normal human mucosal lymphoid follicles, T-cell subsets produce specific B-cell switch, differentiation, and growth factors, which regulate IgA production by B cells (Coffman et al., 1987).

In ulcerative colitis (UC) and Crohn's disease (CD), the normally protective mucosal immune response is not appropriately downregulated, and highly activated effector cells produce prolonged, severe inflammation. Chronic inflammatory processes within the intestine thus exacerbate and perpetuate intestinal injury in inflammatory bowel disease (IBD). Advances in the understanding of normal immune and inflammatory processes in the intestinal mucosa have continued to provide new insights into the immunopathogenic mechanisms involved in the idiopathic, chronic inflammatory intestinal diseases UC and CD (MacDermott and Stenson, 1988; MacDermott, 1994). In this chapter, a brief overview of current concepts regarding the role of the mucosal immune system in IBD will be presented.

## II. ALTERATIONS IN IMMUNOGLOBULIN SYNTHESIS AND SECRETION

Long-standing IBD is characterized by a mixed cellular infiltrate composed predominantly of B cells and T cells. In the normal intestine, IgA-positive B cells predominate. In IBD, however, IgG-containing cells are increased more than IgA-containing cells and are present in deeper tissue layers (Brandtzaeg et al., 1988). The intestinal lumen contains numerous immunogenic molecules that physiologically stimulate the normal mucosal immune system, which, in turn, reacts by mounting a protective response. In IBD, the mucosal immune system exhibits a markedly heightened IgG immune response. Our studies have provided evidence for the presence of highly activated T cells and B cells, as evidenced by the heightened spontaneous immunoglobulin secretion observed from intestinal and peripheral blood mononuclear cells, particularly with regard to IgG and the IgG subclasses (MacDermott, 1988, 1994; MacDermott and Nahm, 1987; MacDermott and Stenson, 1988; MacDermott et al., 1989).

Both phenotypic and functional parameters indicate an increased state of activation of normal lamina propria T and B cells, which may be induced through continuous antigenic stimulation by lumenal antigens (Peters et al., 1989). The enhanced in vivo activation of normal intestinal B lymphocytes in comparison to peripheral blood mononuclear cells (MNC) may lead to heightened spontaneous in vitro immunoglobulin secretion (Schreiber et al., 1991a,b, 1992). IBD intestinal MNC exhibit markedly increased IgG secretion compared with control intestinal MNC (Scott et al., 1986). When compared with normal control intestinal MNC, we observed that a marked increase in spontaneous secretion of IgG is observed from IBD intestinal MNC (Scott et al., 1986). The greatest increase in spontaneous IgG secretion is seen with UC intestinal MNC, owing to the secretion of large amounts of IgG1 with a concomitant increase in IgG3 secretion. CD intestinal MNC exhibit increased IgG secretion primarily consisting of IgG1 and IgG2 (Scott *et al.*, 1986). We have observed similar alterations in IgG subclass concentrations in the sera of active, untreated IBD patients, thus underscoring the *in vivo* relevance of our *in vitro* findings (MacDermott *et al.*, 1989).

Increased total IgG and IgG subclass secretion by isolated IBD intestinal MNC *in vitro* is most likely due to increased numbers and altered ratios of intestinal plasma cell populations in IBD. The total lymphocyte number has been observed to be 4 times greater than normal in intestinal specimens from patients with both UC and CD (Brandtzaeg *et al.*, 1988; Van Spreeuwel *et al.*, 1985) with the major increase occurring in IgG-containing cells. Compared with control specimens, the number of IgG-containing cells was 30 times greater, whereas the number of IgA-containing cells were 2 times greater than normal (Brandtzaeg *et al.*, 1988; Van Spreeuwel *et al.*, 1985). The increased *in vitro* secretion of total IgG and IgG subclasses from IBD intestinal MNC is most likely related to the increased percentage of IgG-containing cells present *in vivo* in inflamed mucosa. Both IgG1 and IgG3 are better complement pathway activators and opsonins than IgG2 and IgG4 (Heiner, 1984, Oxelius, 1984).

It is now apparent that within the intestine involved with disease itself, major alterations in antibody secretion occur, particularly with regard to spontaneous IgG subclass secretion. Delineation of the stimuli and antigens that induce increased secretion of IgG subclasses in intestinal mucosa may, thus, provide valuable insights into possible etiologic and immunopathogenic aspects of IBD (MacDermott and Nahm, 1987; MacDermott and Stenson, 1988; MacDermott, 1994). Recent studies have demonstrated that perinuclear anti-neutrophil cytoplasmic antibodies (pANCA) are found in 70% of culture supernatants from UC lamina propria lymphocytes, indicating the existence of pANCA-producing B-cell clones in active UC intestinal mucosa (Targan *et al.*, 1995).

## III. THE ROLE OF COMPLEMENT IN IBD

The possible role of complement activation in tissue destruction in IBD (Halstensen *et al.*, 1989a,b) has been studied using monoclonal antibodies that recognized a neoepitope only expressed by activated $C_3b$ and the cytolytically active terminal complement complex. This approach was used to identify potential complement-induced damage in tissue sections from inflamed IBD intestine. Nine of 11 patients with UC showed activated $C_3b$ deposited apically on the surface epithelium of involved mucosa, whereas no deposits were seen in 31 matched noninflamed specimens or in 16 of 17 healthy controls. Moreover, a striking colocalization of IgG1, activated $C_3b$, and terminal complement complex was observed in 4 of the 11 UC patients. Thus, IgG1, secreted into the lumen during active UC, immune processes may provide a mechanism for contiguous bowel destruction via complement activation.

An increased vascular deposition of terminal complement complex in both UC and CD (Halstensen *et al.,* 1989a) has also been demonstrated. Interestingly, 5 out of 10 UC specimens and 1 out of 5 CD samples contained terminal complement complex located outside of the blood vessels in the mucosa or submucosa. In IBD, significantly more $C_3c$ reactivity was associated with terminal complement complex deposition, thus indicating continuous complement activation and deposition within the blood vessel wall (Halstensen *et al.,* 1989a). These findings are consistent with the *in vivo* studies by Ahrenstedt *et al.* (1990) who found that both $C_3$ and $C_4$ levels in jejunal perfusates of CD patients were increased when compared with healthy controls. Complement activation in IBD may lead to the initiation of both acute and chronic tissue destruction. In addition, complement as a component of immune activation may result in enhanced recruitment of granulocytes and macrophages, which can lead in turn to the increased *in vitro* release of potent chemotactic mediators such as $LTB_4$ and IL-8 by the newly recruited macrophages and neutrophils.

## IV. GRANULOCYTE AND MACROPHAGE FUNCTION

During active IBD, large numbers of neutrophils and monocytes leave the bloodstream and migrate into the inflamed mucosa and submucosa. These cells carry out a series of destructive inflammatory events and then continue to migrate on through the bowel wall into the intestinal lumen. The biological events that occur during intestinal inflammation are the result of a multiplicity of interacting inflammatory mediators, cytokines, and chemokines.

Saverymuttu *et al.* (1985a,b) carried out functional studies that demonstrated the movement of inflammatory cells in IBD. Patients' peripheral blood phagocytes (granulocytes and monocytes) were isolated, labeled *in vitro* with [111]indium tropolonate, and reinjected. The migration of the [111]indium-labeled phagocytes was then assessed with time, using a whole-body gamma camera. In 20 of 22 patients with CD, over 90% of radiolabeled phagocytes accumulated rapidly in the inflamed intestine (Saverymuttu *et al.,* 1985a,b). A similar study conducted in 15 UC patients showed enhanced migration into areas of inflamed bowel (Saverymuttu *et al.,* 1985b). These studies demonstrated the greatly increased migration of monocytes, macrophages, and polymorphonuclear neutrophils (PMNs) into the intestine that occurs in IBD and in addition showed that monitoring phagocytic cell movement could be of potential value in the clinical assessment of IBD patients (Saverymuttu *et al.,* 1985a,b).The introduction of [99m]technetium-hexamethyl propylene amine oxine as a leukocyte label in CD has further refined techniques for assessing phagocytic cell migration in IBD (Schoelmerich, 1988). The selective labeling of mononuclear phagocytes (monocytes) by [99m]technetium stannous colloid has allowed focus on better understanding of macrophage migration in IBD (Pullman *et al.,* 1988).

## V. PROINFLAMMATORY CYTOKINES

Both lymphocytes and macrophages in inflamed intestinal mucosa synthesize and secrete large numbers of potent proinflammatory mediators. Inflammatory destructive processes are mediated in part by IL-1 (IL-1$_\alpha$ and IL-1$_\beta$), IL-6, and TNF$\alpha$ (cachectin). When the two forms of IL-1 ($\alpha$ and $\beta$) are compared, they exert very similar functions despite their different sources and their structural dissimilarities. The best known activities of IL-1 include the induction of fever *(endogenous pyrogen)*, the stimulation of acute-phase protein synthesis, and the initiation of lymphocyte activation events. TNF, which shares only 3% homology with IL-1, is identical with cachectin, which causes hemodynamic shock and cachexia associated with various disease states. Human T-cell activation requires both a cross-linking mechanism for the T-cell antigen receptor complex and the presence of IL-1, which, under physiologic conditions, are both provided by the macrophage. In addition to macrophages, it should be noted that B cells, astrocytes, mesangial cells, keratinocytes, and endothelial cells can also act as accessory cells by producing or expressing membrane-bound IL-1.

Isaacs *et al.* (1992) as well as Stevens *et al.* (1990) demonstrated that IL-1 mRNA was present in the inflamed mucosa of a majority of IBD patients. Increasing interest has, therefore, focused on the role of proinflammatory cytokines in the initiation and enhancement of intestinal inflammatory processes. Mahida *et al.* (1989) studied IL-1$\beta$ release from isolated intestinal lamina propria mononuclear cells and observed enhanced spontaneous secretion by monocytes from IBD patients when compared with normal controls. Lipopolysaccharide further enhanced IL-1$_\beta$ production by IBD lamina propria mononuclear cells but not by those from normal controls (Mahida *et al.*, 1989). Moreover, depletion of macrophages abolished IL-1$_\beta$ secretion (Mahida *et al.*, 1989). Cominelli and Dinarello (1989) and Cominelli *et al.* (1990) demonstrated that increased IL-1 concentrations play a key role in the pathogenesis of rabbit immune complex colitis and that tissue levels of IL-1 correlate with the severity of inflammation. IL-1 mRNA was detectable as early as 4 hr after induction of colitis, thus indicating that IL-1 gene expression occurs as an early event in experimental immune complex colitis (Cominelli *et al.*, 1990). The rise in IL-1 preceded the increase of PGE$_2$ and LTB$_4$. Moreover, treatment with IL-1 receptor antagonist (IL-1Ra) reduced the extent and severity of the inflammatory response associated with immune complex colitis (Cominelli *et al.*, 1990).

Studies by Isaacs *et al.* (1992) using the polymerase chain reaction to detect cytokines in intestinal lamina propria showed a more frequent occurrence of IL-1, IL-6, and TNF$\alpha$ in CD and UC patients when compared to normal patients. We have observed that lamina propria mononuclear cells (LPMNC) isolated from endoscopic biopsy specimens from patients with active IBD secreted high amounts of IL-1$_\beta$, TNF$\alpha$, and IL-6 (Reinecker *et al.*, 1993). MacDonald *et al.* (1990a,b) investigated the secretion of TNF$\alpha$ in IBD by using a spot enzyme-linked immunosorbent assay (ELISA) technique. In both CD and a subgroup of UC patients, TNFα-secreting intestinal mononuclear cells were increased in frequency in comparison with normal controls (MacDonald *et al.*, 1990a,b). We have found that there is very low spontaneous *in vitro* release of TNFα by LPMNC isolated from endoscopic biopsy specimens from normal donors and IBD patients (Reinecker *et al.*, 1993). Stimulation of LPMNC with pokeweed mitogen (PWM), interestingly, induced an enhancement of TNFα release, which was significantly higher in IBD than normal controls (Reinecker *et al.*, 1993). TNFα activates endothelial cells and can induce IL-1 and IL-6. Both IL-2 and TNFα stimulate $PGI_2$, $PGE_2$ and PAF secretion by cultured endothelial cells. Sustained inflammation leading to tissue destruction in IBD could potentially be mediated to a significant degree by the potent biologic activities of the proinflammatory cytokines IL-1 and TNFα.

## VI. Leukotrienes

The 5-lipoxygenase pathway is found primarily in cells of bone marrow origin involved in inflammatory processes (i.e., mast cells, neutrophils, monocytes, and macrophages) (Borgeat and Samuelsson, 1979; Stenson and Parker, 1984). The major products of the 5-lipoxygenase pathway are 5-hydroxy-6,8,11,14-eicosatetraenoic acid (5-HETE) and leukotrienes $B_4$, $C_4$, $D_4$, and $E_4$ ($LTB_4$, $LTC_4$, $LTD_4$, and $LTE_4$). $LTB_4$ and, to a lesser extent, 5-HETE exert potent chemotactic activities for neutrophils. $LTB_4$, in the presence of neutrophils, also induces enhanced vascular permeability. The sulfidoleukotrienes induce smooth muscle contraction in the lung, blood vessels, and gastrointestinal tract (Stenson and Parker, 1984).

Incubation of IBD mucosa with radiolabeled arachidonic acid results in the synthesis of large quantities of $LTB_4$ and 5-HETE and smaller quantities of $PGE_2$ and thromboxane $B_2$ (Sharon and Stenson, 1984). IBD mucosa produces larger quantities of leukotrienes than normal mucosa (Sharon and Stenson, 1984). Levels of both $PGE_2$ and $LTB_4$ were markedly higher in rectal dialysates from UC patients and declined to normal levels after treatment with a short course of prednisolone (Lauritsen *et al.*, 1985). The presence of large numbers of neutrophils and mononuclear phagocytes in IBD mucosa suggests that there is a chemotactic factor (or factors) present in IBD mucosa that induces neutrophils to migrate out of the circulation and into the tissue. $LTB_4$ is a potent chemoattractant for human neutrophils (Ford-Hutchinson *et al.*, 1984); there are, however, other potent chemotactic molecules, such as chemokines, that we now believe are likely to be critical and central to the perpetuation of IBD.

## VII. Chemokines (Chemotactic Cytokines)

The migration of immune competent cells is specifically regulated by a recently described family of chemotactic cytokines termed chemokines (Yoshimura *et al.*,

1987; Oppenheim *et al.*, 1991; Baggiolini *et al.*, 1989, 1994; Matsushima *et al.*, 1988; Standiford *et al.*, 1990a; Miller and Krangel, 1992; Yoshimura and Leonard, 1991). Chemokines are chemotactic cytokines induced by proinflammatory stimuli that, when secreted, are involved in activating and regulating the multistep process of selective adhesion, cell activation, and migration of leukocytes (Yoshimura *et al.*, 1987; Oppenheim *et al.*, 1991; Baggiolini *et al.*, 1989, 1994; Matsushima *et al.*, 1988; Standiford *et al.*, 1990a; Miller and Krangel, 1992; Yoshimura and Leonard, 1991). Chemokines have the ability to initiate, upregulate, and perpetuate inflammation. In contrast to most previously recognized chemoattractants, chemokines direct the migration of specific leukocyte subpopulations, and thus chemokines may lead to processes that either increase or inhibit mucosal inflammation by discrete cell types. Our recent studies have demonstrated the expression of several chemokines within the intestinal mucosa, and have established the involvement of chemokines in mucosal inflammation in IBD. Our studies have also demonstrated that, in addition to lamina propria leukocytes and endothelial cells, intestinal epithelial cells synthesize and secrete chemokines. Intestinal epithelial cells may therefore participate in the processes leading to the attraction of leukocytes into the intestinal mucosa, and may regulate the composition of different leukocyte subsets in the intestinal lamina propria. The interaction of intestinal epithelial cells and intestinal leukocytes in the regulation of the recruitment of immune competent cells into the intestinal mucosa may be pivotal for the function of the mucosal immune system in both health and disease.

Chemokines are a family of low-molecular-weight (8–10 kDa), basic, heparin-binding proteins that are related by both the primary structure and the position of four cysteines in their amino acid sequence (Yoshimura *et al.*, 1987; Oppenheim *et al.*, 1991; Baggiolini *et al.*, 1989, 1994; Matsushima *et al.*, 1988; Standiford *et al.*, 1990a; Miller and Krangel, 1992; Yoshimura and Leonard, 1991). At least 20 different chemokines have been described to date. The chemokine family has been divided into two subfamilies based on the arrangement of the first two cysteines (Oppenheim *et al.*, 1991; Baggiolini *et al.*, 1994; Miller and Krangel, 1992). The members of the two subfamilies can be distinguished based upon structural characteristics and the chromosomal location of their genes (Oppenheim *et al.*, 1991; Baggiolini *et al.*, 1994). In the C–X–C, or $\alpha$-chemokine, subfamily, the first two cysteines are separated by one amino acid. Members of this branch include interleukin-8, platelet factor 4 (PF4), melanocyte growth stimulatory activity (MGSA, also termed GRO$\alpha$), GRO$\beta$, GRO$\gamma$, NAP-2, ENA-78 (epithelial cell-derived neutrophil activator with 78 residues), $\gamma$IP-10 ($\gamma$-interferon inducible protein of 10 kDa). The genes for the $\alpha$-chemokines are clustered together on human chromosome 4, q12-21. In the C–C branch or $\beta$-chemokine subfamily the first two cysteines are adjacent. Members of the C–C branch include: monocyte chemoattractant protein-1, -2, and -3 (MCP-1, MCP-2, and MCP-3), RANTES (regulated on activation, normal T cell expressed and secreted), and macrophage inflammatory proteins 1$\alpha$ and 1$\beta$ (MIP-1$\alpha$ and MIP-1$\beta$), I-309, and Eotaxin. The genes for the β-chemokines are colocalized on chromosome 17, q11-21. The location of the two different subfamilies on two entirely different genes may prove of importance in the future in that cell activation pathways and regulatory mechanisms may prove to be different for the α- as opposed to the β-chemokines.

In general, α-chemokines, such as IL-8, GROα, and ENA-78, are potent chemo-attractants and activators of neutrophils but not monocytes, while β-chemokines, including MCP-1, RANTES, MIP-1α, and MIP-1β, are potent chemoattractants and activators of monocytes but not neutrophils. Some chemokines are also able to specifically attract lymphocytes: RANTES is a chemoattractant for memory T cells; IL-8 attracts T cells *in vitro* and *in vivo* (Baggiolini *et al.*, 1994), and MCP-1, MCP-2, and MCP-3 are able to direct the migration of stimulated human CD4$^+$ and CD8$^+$ T lymphocytes (Loetscher *et al.*, 1994). Chemokines also have effects on other blood leukocytes. Both MCP-1 and RANTES are direct mediators of the release of histamine by human basophils, while RANTES and MIP-1α are chemoattractants and activators of eosinophils (Baggiolini *et al.*, 1994). Proin-flammatory cytokines are potent upregulators and stimulators of chemokine synthesis and secretion (Barker *et al.*, 1990). Dexamethasone inhibits chemokine synthesis and secretion (Tobler *et al.*, 1992); therefore, one possible anti-inflammatory mechanism of steroids in IBD may be downregulation of chemokine production. Monocytes and macrophages synthesize and secrete most of α-chemokines. Autocrine feedback mechanisms could further stimulate the recruitment of leukocytes by chemokines. Many diverse cell types, when stimulated by proinflammatory cytokines, produce chemokines, including endothelial cells, epithelial cells, and fibroblasts (Oppenheim *et al.*, 1991; Baggiolini *et al.*, 1994; Standiford *et al.*, 1990b; Yoshimura and Leonard, 1990a). Therefore, in the intestine there are a large number of different cell types that have the potential of producing chemo-kines.

## VIII. Chemokine Actions

Chemokines are potent chemoattractants and activators of granulocytes and macro-phages. As part of the chemoattractant process, granulocytes and macrophages undergo a shape change, termed diapedesis, which is the development of long cytoplasmic outpouchings that reach ahead from the cell in the direction of move-ment (Baggiolini *et al.*, 1994). Diapedesis is one of the earliest processes triggered by chemokines. In order for leukocytes to attach and adhere to capillary wall endothelial cells, they first must slow, marginate, and then roll along the endothe-lial lining cells. Migration of leukocytes between the endothelial cells and on into the intestinal mucosa is mediated by families of cell-surface molecules including selectins and integrins (Albelda *et al.*, 1994; Springer, 1994). Selectin and integrin molecule expression is upregulated by chemokine activation of endothelial cells (Albelda and Buck, 1990; Butcher, 1991; Bevilacqua and Nelson, 1993; Lasky, 1992). Chemokine activation of endothelial cells, as well as circulating granulocytes and macrophages, leads to increased expression of selectins and integrins so that attachment, rolling, adhesion, and subsequent migration events can occur (Albeda *et al.,* 1994; Springer, 1994; Albeda and Buck, 1990; Butcher, 1991; Bevilacqua and Nelson, 1993; Lasky, 1992). The adherent leukocytes transmigrate between the endothelial cells, and continue to move into areas of mucosal inflammation, a process which requires a chemotactic gradient. Potent, long-lived chemokines, such as IL-8, are capable of providing upregulatory activation and chemotactic stimuli that are central to both the adherence and transmigration of granulocytes and monocytes (Oppenheim *et al.,* 1991; Baggiolini *et al.,* 1994). Therefore, adhesion molecules, selectins, and integrins, which are upregulated by chemokines, promote the increased flux of leukocytes into areas of inflammation.

After migration of granulocytes and monocytes into the internal mucosa, chemokines can then activate the respiratory burst during which oxygen radicals are formed by leukocytes. Reactive oxygen metabolites are highly toxic and can both protect against infectious agents and damage nearby "innocent bystander" cells. Chemokines very effectively stimulate the respiratory burst and oxygen radical production by neutrophils and macrophages (Oppenheim *et al.,* 1991; Baggiolini *et al.,* 1994; Rollins *et al.,* 1991), which is one of the major destructive processes in the pathogenesis of inflammatory bowel disease. A second destructive process, which chemokines activate in leukocytes, is the process of exocytosis, in which a wide variety of potent enzymes are released from granules within granulocytes and macrophages (Oppenheim *et al.,* 1991; Baggiolini *et al.,* 1994). By stimulating intracellular storage granules to release preformed destructive enzymes, chemokines convert macrophages and granulocytes into potent "rapid strike force" effector cells that are able to quickly destroy a large number of substrates, including proteins, sugars, and major components of cell membranes as well as the extracellular matrix. Third, in leukocytes that are triggered by chemokines another important group of proinflammatory molecules is the increased formation of all arachidonic acid metabolism pathway products. Chemokines stimulate cells to increase their production of arachidonic acid metabolism pathway products (Baggiolini *et al.,* 1994) including the potent chemotactic molecule $LTB_4$, which then contributes to increasing the nonspecific migration of inflammatory cells into the mucosa.

## IX. Chemokine (Serpentine) Receptors

The chemokine receptors, like their ligands, consist of a large family of structurally and functionally related cell-surface membrane proteins. They are members of a superfamily of seven transmembrane domain rhodopsin-like, G-protein-coupled receptors that can be defined by amino acid homologies, and that belong to the serpentine family of transmembrane receptors (Kelvin *et al.,* 1993; Grob *et al.,* 1990; Samanta *et al.,* 1990; Holmes *et al.,* 1991; Murphy and Tiffany, 1991; Yoshimura and Leonard, 1990b). Each receptor has seven sequential hydrophobic membrane-spanning regions with an extracellular N-terminus and an intracellular C-terminus. The intracellular loops that connect the seven membrane-spanning regions interact with G-proteins (Kelvin *et al.*, 1993), which then trigger a sequence of intracellular enzymes leading to activation of the cell. The chemokine receptor family includes receptors specific for $\alpha$-chemokines (IL-8 receptor A and B), receptors specific for $\beta$-chemokines (MIP-1$\alpha$/RANTES receptor, MCP-1 receptor A and B), and receptors that are able to bind both $\alpha$-chemokines and $\beta$-chemokines (Duffy antigen/erythrocyte chemokine receptor).

Classically, $\alpha$-chemokine and $\beta$-chemokine receptors selectively bind different proteins of the corresponding chemokine families. Each chemokine receptor, however, exhibits different affinities and specificities for certain chemokines. For example, the two major receptors for IL-8 are IL-8 receptor A (Holmes *et al.*, 1991) and IL-8 receptor B (Murphy and Tiffany, 1991). IL-8 receptor A is highly specific for IL-8, to which it binds with high affinity. In contrast, IL-8 receptor B binds not only IL-8, but also two other $\alpha$-chemokines: monocyte growth-stimulating activity (GRO/MGSA) and neutrophil-activating peptide (NAP-2) (Lee *et al.*, 1992; Gayle *et al.*, 1993). Thus, IL-8 receptor B is "promiscuous" in its binding when compared to IL-8 receptor A. In addition, IL-8 receptor A, which is the receptor with higher IL-8-specificity, is found almost exclusively on neutrophils, while IL-8 receptor B is found not only on neutrophils but also on monocytes and T cells (Kelvin *et al.*, 1993; Holmes *et al.*, 1991; Murphy and Tiffany, 1991; Lee *et al.*, 1992; Gayle *et al.*, 1993).

Similar observations have been made for the serpentine receptors that interact with the $\beta$-chemokine subfamily members (Ahuja *et al.*, 1994; Wang *et al.*, 1993b). Monocyte chemotactic and activating factor (MCAF)/MCP-1 binds with very high affinity to the MCAF/MCP-1 receptor found predominantly on monocytes (Yoshimura and Leonard, 1990b). Monocytes also express a second MCP-1 receptor that is able to bind two other $\beta$-chemokines: macrophage inflammatory protein-1$\alpha$ (MIP-1$\alpha$) and macrophage inflammatory protein-1$\beta$ (MIP-1$\beta$) (Oh *et al.*, 1991). Finally, a third receptor on monocytes exhibits binding "promiscuity" because it exhibits low affinity, binding with MCAF/MCP-1, as well as with both MIP-1$\alpha$ and MIP-1$\beta$ (Wang *et al.*, 1993b) and also with RANTES (Wang *et al.*, 1993a).

Different chemokines may therefore be able to selectively direct a discrete, focused cellular response by activating certain cell types through high-affinity receptors. The promiscuous receptor sharing among chemokines, on the other hand, may be an important regulatory mechanism to allow the increased attraction of a mixed leukocyte population. The final composition of the inflammatory cell population in response to chemokine stimulation and activation may depend on both the composition of the secreted chemokines and the relative expression of different chemokine cell-surface receptors. Because related receptors with different affinities and cross-reactive binding capabilities are present on each type of cell, relative differences in receptor distribution and receptor affinity for specific chemokines may significantly influence which cells are actually attracted to and activated by each individual chemokine.

The current model of signal transduction in leukocytes by chemokines involves a receptor whose binding ability is increased by conformational changes induced by association with the GDP bound state of a pertussis toxin-sensitive heterotrimeric G protein. The short, third, intracellular loop of the serpentine receptor family of molecules may serve as the G-protein recognition site based on similarities to the well-characterized intracellular regions involved in rhodopsin-induced cellular activation (Baggiolini et al., 1994). After ligand binding, the activated receptor catalyzes the exchange of GDP for GTP by the G-protein $\alpha$ subunit, resulting in dissociation of $\alpha$ from $\beta\gamma$ subunits. In turn, $\beta\gamma$ activates a phosphoinositide-specific phospholipase C (PLC), leading to the accumulation of inositol triphosphate and diacylglycerol in the cytoplasm. Inositol triphosphate results in the increased release of calcium from within the cell, while diacylglycerol activates protein kinase C, leading to the delayed activation of phospholipase D (PLD). Early PLC-mediated and late PLD-mediated biochemical events have been temporally correlated with the highly sensitive migratory response and relatively insensitive cytotoxic responses of phagocytes to chemoattractants. Chemokine activation through serpentine family receptors therefore leads to signal transduction and intracellular activation processes. This in turn causes the granulocyte or macrophage to change shape, move between endothelial cells into sites of inflammation, and then exhibit increased respiratory burst activity with the production of oxygen radicals as well as granule exocytosis with the release of potent destructive enzymes.

## X. INTERLEUKIN-8 AND MONOCYTE CHEMOATTRACTANT PROTEIN-1 IN ULCERATIVE COLITIS AND CROHN'S DISEASE

The role of chemokines in the pathophysiology of UC and CD has just begun to be examined. Chemokines could play a central role in IBD because the chemokines are relatively resistant to inactivation in vivo, in contrast to other chemoattractants such as $LTB_4$, FMLP, and PAF, which have shorter half-lives (Oppenheim et al., 1991; Baggiolini et al., 1994). Furthermore, chemokines are produced by a number of different cell types after stimulation by proinflammatory cytokines; therefore, similar chemotactic signals could be produced quickly in response to the stimulation of intestinal cells by a variety of different stimulatory processes (Oppenheim et al., 1991; Baggiolini et al., 1994).

The potential involvement of chemokines in the pathophysiology of various diseases has centered to date on the measurement of chemokine levels in involved sites of disease activity. Inflammatory skin diseases were among the first to be examined, with psoriatic lesions being shown to contain markedly increased concentrations of IL-8. IL-8 has been thought to be involved in mediating the formation of neutrophilic skin microabscesses that are commonly found in psoriatic skin lesions (Schröder, 1992). The second chronic inflammatory condition that has been extensively examined for elevated levels of chemokines is arthritis (Seitz *et al.*, 1991). Very high levels of IL-8 have been found in the synovial fluid of patients with rheumatoid arthritis (Rampart *et al.*, 1992). In addition, the concentration of MCAF/MCP-1 has also been found to be elevated in the synovial fluid of patients with arthritis (Koch *et al.*, 1992). Inflammatory pulmonary diseases that are known to be associated with a marked increase in neutrophils have also been examined for elevated chemokine levels. Increased expression of IL-8 mRNA has been observed in alveolar macrophages, coupled with increased IL-8 levels in bronchoalveolar lavage fluid from idiopathic pulmonary fibrosis patients (Carre *et al.*, 1991). Studies carried out by Mahida and co-workers (1992), Izzo and co-workers (1992), and Hommes and co-workers (1992) have demonstrated increased synthesis and production of IL-8 in UC.

We developed a quantitative polymerase chain reaction (RT-PCR) assay (Izutani *et al.*, 1994) to determine the amount of IL-8 mRNA and MCP-1 mRNA in mucosal sections obtained from resected specimens from patients with CD and UC (Izutani *et al.*, 1995; Reinecker *et al.*, 1995). The quantitative PCR is based on the use of an internal standard RNA that differs in size from the original RNA (Izutani *et al.*, 1994). The standard RNA (sRNA) is then reverse transcribed together with the sample RNA, and amplified by PCR using the same set of primers (Izutani *et al.*, 1994). The size difference between the two PCR products allows electrophoretic separation and quantification of the radioactively labeled PCR products (Izutani *et al.*, 1994). Templates for the generation of synthetic RNA specific for human IL-8 and MCP-1 were constructed (Izutani *et al.*, 1995; Reinecker *et al.*, 1995). The amount of IL-8 mRNA or MCP-1 mRNA was then determined (Izutani *et al.*, 1995; Reinecker *et al.*, 1995).

We observed very high levels of IL-8 mRNA in involved UC mucosa and significantly increased IL-8 mRNA levels in involved CD mucosa (Izutani *et al.*, 1995). Much higher levels of IL-8 mRNA expression were observed in involved, as opposed to noninvolved, intestinal mucosal sections obtained from UC and CD patients (Izutani *et al.*, 1995). Mucosa from diverticulitis patients used as disease specificity control specimens showed moderately increased IL-8 mRNA. Similar patterns of IL-8 mRNA expression were observed in isolated epithelial cells obtained from the same mucosal sections (Izutani *et al.*, 1995). Our studies (Izutani *et al.*, 1995) have demonstrated that IL-8 mRNA levels are markedly increased to extraordinarily high amounts in inflamed mucosa and isolated epithelial cells from UC patients.

In normal intestinal mucosa, analysis by immunohistochemistry demonstrated MCP-1 predominantly in the surface epithelium (Reinecker *et al.*, 1995). In contrast, inflamed mucosa from patients with UC or CD contained multiple cells immunoreactive for MCP-1, including spindle cells, mononuclear cells, and endothelial cells (Reinecker *et al.*, 1995). MCP-1 mRNA expression (Reinecker *et al.*, 1995) was equally and markedly increased in inflamed intestinal biopsies from patients with UC, CD, and diverticulitis. MCP-1 expression within freshly isolated intestinal epithelial cells was able to be upregulated by IL-1$_\beta$ and PMA (Reinecker *et al.*, 1995). Immunoprecipation detected MCP-1 in conditioned media from Caco-2 cells (Reinecker *et al.*, 1995). Caco-2 cell-conditioned media stimulated monocyte chemotaxis activity that was inhibited by anti-MCP-1 antibodies (Reinecker *et al.*, 1995). Constitutive MCP-1 mRNA levels in Caco-2 cells were upregulated by interleukin-1$\beta$ and downregulated by dexamethasone (Reinecker *et al.*, 1995).

Chemokines have been characterized, and have begun to be implicated as important components in promoting chronic inflammation in a variety of different diseases. Chemokines are relatively resistant to inactivation, have long half-lives *in vivo,* are produced by many different cell types, interact with a wide variety of specific serpentine family chemokine receptors on leukocyte cell surfaces, and have selective chemotactic activities with regard to defined subtypes of leukocytes. Therefore, chemokines have become prime candidates as molecules that may play pivotal roles in the perpetuation and upregulation of the chronic inflammatory process in UC and CD patients (Izutani *et al.*, 1995; Reinecker *et al.*, 1995).

Because of the different target cell specificities that characterize the $\alpha$-chemokine versus $\beta$-chemokine subfamilies, a wide range of leukocyte chemotactic and activation responses may be seen. Thus, different types of inflammatory cell infiltrates could be seen pathologically in IBD tissue, depending on variations in the repertoire of serpentine family receptor distribution on the surface of circulating leukocytes. Furthermore, because a large number of different chemokine molecules can be stimulated and produced, differences in disease activity and tissue pathology may ultimately be able to be explained in part by differences in the relative production of different types of chemokines.

The mRNA levels in isolated and purified intestinal epithelial cells from involved versus noninvolved UC mucosa showed a correlation with IL-8 mRNA levels in the mucosal sections, suggesting a potentially pivotal and important contribution by epithelial cells themselves in the establishment of chemotactic gradients for granulocytes within the lamina propria of UC patients (Izutani *et al.*, 1995). In further support of this hypothesis, human intestinal epithelial tumor cell line cells (Caco-2) express mRNA for IL-8 and respond to stimulation due to IL-1 with an increase in IL-8 mRNA (Izutani *et al.*, 1995). Cytokines such as IL-1 and TNF could thus act to stimulate the increased production of IL-8 from surrounding immune and nonimmune cells, thereby further amplifying the migration of additional granulocytes from the vascular compartment into the intestinal mucosa. IL-8 secretion by intestinal epithelial cells may be of particular importance in UC and may in part account for the dominant role of granulocytes in UC mucosa.

Our data also strongly suggest that MCP-1 may play a particularly significant role in CD (Reinecker *et al.*, 1995). Production of MCP-1 by endothelial cells, LPMNC, and epithelial cells could establish a chemotactic gradient capable of influencing the increased migration of monocytes/macrophages from the blood stream through the endothelium into both the mucosa and submucosa during chronic active CD. The ability of MCP-1 to induce monocyte activation, macrophage exocytosis, increased release of destructive enzymes, and upregulation of respiratory burst activity indicates that there may be a variety of different processes in which MCP-1 may markedly increase monocyte/macrophage function in CD.

Therefore, the most intriguing and provocative aspect of our studies to date is that the relative patterns of IL-8 mRNA and MCP-1 mRNA differ, depending upon the nature of the IBD process (Izutani *et al.*, 1995; Reinecker *et al.*, 1995). The most striking finding is the enormous elevation in IL-8 mRNA seen in actively involved UC mucosa and epithelial cells (Izutani *et al.*, 1995). Although it is unclear as to whether this marked increase in IL-8 mRNA is primary or secondary, there may be a close relationship between increased IL-8 and the predominantly granulocytic infiltrate seen in UC.

At a clinical level, the measurement of chemokine mRNA levels in tissue or secreted chemokines into the intestinal lumen could prove helpful in the future as a measurement of the amount of ongoing mucosal inflammation in UC and/or CD. Measurement of chemokines could possibly provide ways of determining the level of disease activity and/or of following the response to therapy in IBD patients. Based upon our observations (Izutani *et al.*, 1995; Reinecker *et al.*, 1995), IL-8 mRNA and/or IL-8 levels may prove to be of particular interest in objectively assessing mucosal inflammation and/or disease activity in UC. Conversely, MCP-1 mRNA and/or MCP-1 levels may prove to be closely related to the state of disease activity and tissue destruction in CD.

Our observations (Izutani *et al.*, 1995; Reinecker *et al.*, 1995) suggest that the development of selective inhibitors for chemokines will be of great interest as potential novel therapeutic strategies in UC and CD. Compounds that inhibit chemokine synthesis, or that block chemokine binding to serpentine family receptors on granulocytes and monocytes, may have the potential of inhibiting the process of granulocyte and monocyte migration into the mucosa and submucosa of involved intestine in IBD patients, which could diminish the severity of the inflammatory response and, thus, clinical disease activity. A more complete understanding of the role of chemokines in UC and CD will follow studies that investigate in detail the intracellular and molecular mechanisms by which chemokines activate and attract inflammatory cells into the intestinal mucosa, upregulate the expression of adhesion molecules on both submucosal capillary endothelial cells and circulating leukocytes, and activate the production of proinflammatory cytokines by cells within the intestine.

### Acknowledgment

This work was supported in part by National Institutes of Health Grant DK21474.

# REFERENCES

Ahrenstedt, O., Knutson, L., Nilsson, B., Nilsson-Ekdahl, K., Odlind, B., and Hallgren, R. (1990). Enhanced local production of complement components in the small intestines of patient with Crohn's disease. *N. Engl. J. Med.* **322,** 1345–1349.

Ahuja, S. K., Gao, J. L., and Murphy, P. M. (1994). Chemokine receptors and molecular mimicry. *Immunol. Today* **15,** 281–287.

Albelda, S. M., and Buck, C. A (1990). Integrins and other cell adhesion molecules. *FASEB J.* **4,** 2868–2880.

Albelda, S M., Smith, C. W., and Ward, P. A. (1994). Adhesion molecules and inflammatory injury. *FASEB J.* **8,** 504–512.

Baggiolini, M., Walz, A., and Kunkel, S. L. (1989). Neutrophil-activating peptide-1/interleukin-8 a novel cytokine that activates neutrophils. *J. Clin. Invest.* **84,** 1045–1049.

Baggiolini, M., Dewald, B., and Moser, B. (1994). Interleukin-8 and related chemotactic cytokines—CXC and CC chemokines. *Adv. Immunol.* **55,** 97–179.

Barker, J. N., Sarma, V., Mitra, R. S., Dixit, V. M., and Nickoloff, B. J. (1990). Marked synergism between tumor necrosis factor-alpha and interferon-gamma in regulation of keratinocyte-derived adhesion molecules and chemotactic factors. *J. Clin. Invest.* **85,** 605–608.

Bevilacqua, M., and Nelson, R. M. (1993). Selectins. *J. Clin. Invest.* **91,** 379–387.

Borgeat, P., and Samuelsson, B. (1979). Transformation of arachidonic acid by rabbit polymorphonuclear leukocytes. *J. Biol. Chem.* **254,** 2643–2646.

Brandtzaeg, P., Sollid, L. M., Thrane, P. S., Kvale, D., Bjerke, K., Scott, H., Kett, K., and Rognum, T. O. (1988). Lymphoepithelial interactions in the human mucosal immune system. *Gut* **29,** 1116–1130.

Butcher, E. C. (1991). Leukocyte–endothelial cell recognition: Three (or more) steps to specificity and diversity. *Cell (Cambridge, Mass.)* **67,** 1033–1036.

Carre, P. C., Mortenson, R. L., King, T. E., Jr., Noble, P. W., Sable, C. L., and Riches, D. W. (1991). Increased expression of the interleukin-8 gene by alveolar macrophages in idiopathic pulmonary fibrosis. A potential mechanism for the recruitment and activation of neutrophils in lung fibrosis. *J. Clin. Invest.* **88,** 1802–1810.

Coffman, R. L., Shrader, B., Carty, J., Mosmann, T. R., and Bond, M. W. (1987). A mouse T cell product that preferentially enhances IgA production. I. Biologic characterization. *J. Immunol.* **139,** 3685–3690.

Cominelli, F., and Dinarello, C. A. (1989). Interleukin-1 in the pathogenesis of and protection from inflammatory bowel disease. *Biotherapy* **1,** 369–375.

Cominelli, F., Nast, C. C., Clark, B. D., Schindler, R., Lierena, R., Eysselein, V. E., Thompson, R. C., and Dinarello, C. A. (1990). Interleukin-1 (IL-1) gene expression, synthesis, and effect of specific IL-1 receptor blockade in rabbit immune complex colitis. *J. Clin. Invest.* **86,** 972–980.

Dinarello, C. A. (1988). Biology of interleukin-1. *FASEB J.* **2,** 108–115.

Ford-Hutchinson, W. W., Bray, M. A., and Doig, M. V. (1984). Leukotriene B, a potent chemotactic and aggregating substance released from polymorphonuclear leukocytes. *Nature (London)* **266,** 264–265.

Gayle III, R. B., Sleath, P. R., Srinivason, S., Birks, C. W., Weerawarna, K. S., Cerretti, D. P., Kozlosky, C. J., Nelson, N., Vanden Bos, T., and Beckmann, M. P. (1993). Importance of the amino terminus of the interleukin-8 receptor in ligand interactions. *J. Biol. Chem.* **268,** 7283–7289.

Grob, P. M., David, E., Warren, T. C., DeLeon, R. P., Farina, P. R., and Homon, C. A. (1990). Characterization of a receptor for human monocyte-derived neutrophil chemotactic factor/interleukin-8. *J. Biol. Chem.* **265,** 8311–8316.

Halstensen, T. S., Mollnes, T. E., and Brandtzaeg, P. (1989a). Persistent complement activation in submucosal blood vessels of active inflammatory bowel disease: Immunohistochemical evidence. *Gastroenterology* **97,** 10–19.

Halstensen, T. S., Mollnes, T. E., Fausa, O., and Brandtzaeg, P. (1989b). Deposits of terminal complement complex (TCC) in muscular mucosa and submucosal vessels in ulcerative colitis and Crohn's
disease of the colon. *Gut* **30,** 361–366.

Heiner, D. C. (1984). Significance of immunoglobulin G (IgG) subclasses. *Am. J. Med.* **76,** 1.

Holmes, W. E., Lee, J., Kuang, W. J., Rice, G. C., and Wood, W. I. (1991). Structure and functional
expression of a human interleukin-8 receptor. *Science* **253,** 1278–1280.

Hommes, D. W., Jansen, J., Smit, F., Fockens, P., Zhao, Y., Tytgat, G. N. J., Ceska, M., and van
Deventer, S. J. H. (1992). Enhanced production of interleukin-8 in ulcerative colitis. *Gastroenterology* **102,** A927.

Isaacs, K. L., Sartor, R. B., and Haeskil, J. S. (1992). Cytokine messenger RNA profiles in inflammatory bowel disease mucosa detected by polymerase chain reaction amplification. *Gastroenterology*
**103,** 1587–1595.

Izutani, R., Ohyanagi, H., and MacDermott, R. P. (1994). Quantitative PCR for detection of femtogram
quantities of interleukin-8 mRNA expression. *Microbiol. Immunol.* **38,** 233–237.

Izutani, R., Loh, E. Y., Reinecker, H.-C., Ohno, Y., Fusunyan, R. D., Lichtenstein, G. R., Rombeau,
J. L., and MacDermott, R. P. (1995). Increased expression of interleukin-8 mRNA in ulcerative
colitis and Crohn's disease mucosa and epithelial cells. *Inflammatory Bowel Diseases,* **1,**
37–47.

Izzo, R. S., Witkon, K., Chen, A. I., Hadjiyane, C., Weinstein, M. I., and Pellechia, C. (1992). Interleu-
kin-8 and neutrophil markers in colonic mucosa from patients with UC. *Am. J. Gastroenterol.* **87,**
1447–1452.

Kawanishi, H., Saltzman, L. E., and Strober, W. (1983a). Mechanisms regulating IgA class-specific
immunoglobulin production in murine gut-associated lymphoid tissues. I. T cells derived from
Peyer's patches that switch sIgM B cells *in vitro. J. Exp. Med.* **157,** 433–450.

Kawanishi, H., Saltzman, L., and Strober, W. (1983b). Mechanisms regulating IgA class-specific immunoglobulin production in murine gut-associated lymphoid tissues. II. Terminal differentiation of
postswitch sIgA-bearing Peyer's patch B cells. *J. Exp. Med.* **158,** 649–669.

Kelvin, D. J., Michiel, D. F., Johnston, J. A., Lloyd, A. R., Sprenger, H., Oppenheim, J. J., and Wang,
J. M. (1993). Chemokines and serpentines: The molecular biology of chemokine receptors. *J. Leukocyte Biol.* **54,** 604–612.

Koch, A. E., Kunkel, S. L., Harlow, L. A., Johnson, B., Evanoff, H. L., Haines, G. K., Burdick,
M. D., Pope, R. M., and Streiter, R. M. (1992). Enhanced production of monocyte chemoattractant
protein-1 in rheumatoid arthritis. *J. Clin. Invest.* **90,** 772–779.

Lasky, L. A. (1992). Selectins: interpreters of cell-specific carbohydrate information during inflammation. *Science* **258,** 964–969.

Lauritsen, K., Laursen, L. S., Bukhave, K., and Rask-Madsen, J. (1985). Effects of systemic prednisolone on arachidonic acid metabolites determined by equilibrium *in vivo* dialysis of rectum in severe
relapsing ulcerative colitis. *Gastroenterology* **88,** A1466.

Lee, J., Horuk, R., Rice, G. C., Bennett, G. L., Camerato, T., and Wood, W. I. (1992). Characterization
of two high affinity human interleukin-8 receptors. *J. Biol. Chem.* **267,** 16283–16287.

Loetscher, P., Seitz, M., Clark-Lewis, I., Baggiolini, M., and Moser, B. (1994). Monocyte chemotactic
proteins MCP-1, MCP-2, and MCP-3 are major attractants for human CD4+ and CD8+ T lymphocytes. *FASEB J.* **8,** 1055–1060.

MacDermott, R. P. (1988). Altered secretion patterns of IgA and IgG subclasses by IBD intestinal
mononuclear cells. *In* "Inflammatory Bowel Diseases—Basic Research and Clinical Implications"
(H. Geobell, B. M. Peskar, and H. Malchow, eds.), pp. 105–111. MTP Press, Flacon House, Lancas-
ter, U.K.

MacDermott, R. P. (1994). Alterations in the mucosal immune system in ulcerative colitis and Crohn's
disease. *Med. Clin. North Am.* **78,** 1207–1231.

MacDermott, R. P., and Nahm, M. H. (1987). Expression of human immunoglobulin G subclassed in
inflammatory bowel disease. *Gastroenterology* **93,** 1127–1129.

MacDermott, R. P., and Stenson, W. F. (1988). Alterations in the mucosal immune system in ulcerative colitis and Crohn's disease. *Adv. Immunol.* **42,** 285–323.

MacDermott, R. P., Nash, G. S., Auer, I. O., Shlien, R., Lewis, B. S., Madassery, J., and Nahm, M. H. (1989). Alterations in serum IgG subclasses in patients with ulcerative colitis and Crohn's disease. *Gastroenterology* **94,** A275.

MacDonald, T. T., Choy, M. Y., Hutchings, P., and Cooke, A. (1990a). Activated T cells and macrophages in the intestinal mucosa of children with inflammatory bowel disease. *In* "Advances in Mucosal Immunology" (T. T. MacDonald, S. J. Chalacombe, P. W. Bland, C. R. Stokes, R. V. Heatley, and A. M. Mowat, Eds.), pp. 683–699. Kluwer, Boston.

MacDonald, T. T., Hutchings, P., Choy, M. Y., Murch, S., and Cooke, A. (1990b). Tumor necrosis factor-alpha and interferon-gamma production measured at the single-cell level in normal and inflamed human intestine. *Clin. Exp. Immunol.* **81,** 301–305.

Mahida, Y. R., Wu, K., and Jewell, D. P. (1989). Enhanced production of interleukin-1-beta by mononuclear cells isolated from mucosa with active ulcerative colitis or Crohn's disease. *Gut* **30,** 835–838.

Mahida, Y. R., Ceska, M., Effenberger, F., Kurlak, L., Lindley, I., and Hawkey, C. J. (1992). Enhanced synthesis of neutrophil-activating peptide-1/interleukin-8 in active ulcerative colitis. *Clin. Sci.* **82,** 273–275.

Matsushima, K., Morishita, K., Yoshimura, T., Lavu, S., Kobayashi, Y., Lew, W., Appella, E., Kung, H. F., Leonard, E. J., and Oppenheim, J. J. (1988). Molecular cloning of human monocyte-derived neutrophil chemotactic factor (MDNCF) and induction of MDNCF mRNA by interleukin-1 and tumor necrosis factor. *J. Exp. Med.* **167,** 1883–1893.

Mestecky, J. (1987). The common mucosal immune system and current strategies for induction of immune responses in external secretions. *J. Clin. Immunol.* **7,** 265–276.

Mestecky, J., and McGhee, J. R. (1987). Immunoglobulin A (IgA): Molecular and cellular interactions involved in IgA biosynthesis and immune response. *Adv. Immunol.* **40,** 153–245.

Miller, M. D., and Krangel, M. S. (1992). Biology and chemistry of the chemokines: A family of chemotactic and inflammatory cytokines. *Crit. Rev. Immunol.* **12,** 17–46.

Murphy, P. M., and Tiffany, H. L. (1991). Cloning of complementary DNA encoding a functional human interleukin-8 receptor. *Science* **253,** 1280–1283.

Oh, K. O., Zhou, Z., Kim, K. K., Samanta, H., Fraser, M., Kim, Y. J., Broxmeyer, H. E., and Kwon, B. S. (1991). Identification of cell surface receptors for murine macrophage inflammatory protein-1 alpha. *J. Immunol.* **147,** 2978–2983.

Oppenheim, J. J., Zachariae, C. O., Mukaida, N., and Matsushima, K. (1991). Properties of the novel proinflammatory supergene intercrine cytokine family. *Annu. Rev. Immunol.* **9,** 617–648.

Oxelius, V. A. (1984). Immunoglobulin G (IgG) subclasses and human disease. *Am. J. Med.* **76,** 7–18.

Peters, M. G., Secrist, H., Anders, K. R., Nash, G. S., Rich, S. R., and MacDermott, R. P. (1989). Normal human intestinal B lymphocytes: Increased activation compared to peripheral blood. *J. Clin. Invest.* **83,** 1827–1833.

Pullman, W. E., Sullivan, P. J., Barrett, P. J., Lising, J., Booth, J. A., and Doe, W. F. (1988). Assessment of inflammatory bowel disease activity by technetium 99m phagocyte scanning. *Gastroenterology* **95,** 989–996.

Rampart, M., Herman, A. G., Grillet, B., Opdenakker, G., and Van Damme, J. (1992). Development and application of a radioimmunoassay for interleukin-8: Detection of interleukin-8 in synovial fluids from patients with inflammatory joint disease. *Lab. Invest.* **66,** 512–518.

Reinecker, H.-C., Steffen, M., Witthoeft, T., Pfleuger, I., Schreiber, S., MacDermott, R. P., and Raedler, A. (1993). Enhanced secretion of TNF-alpha, IL-6, and IL-1-beta by isolated lamina propria mononuclear cells from patients with ulcerative colitis and Crohn's disease. *Clin. Exp. Immunol.* **94,** 174–181.

Reinecker, H. D., Loh, E. Y., Ringler, D. J., Mehta, A., Rombeau, J. L., and MacDermott, R. P. (1995). Monocyte-chemoattractant protein 1 gene expression in intestinal epithelial cells and inflammatory bowel disease mucosa. *Gastroenterology* **108,** 40–50.

Rollins, B. J., Walz, A., and Baggiolini, M. (1991). Recombinant human MCP-1/JE induces chemo-taxis, calcium flux, and the respiratory burst in human monocytes. *Blood* **78,** 1112–1116.

Samanta, A. K., Oppenheim, J. J., and Matsushima, K. (1990). Interleukin-8 (monocyte-derived neutro-phil chemotactic factor) dynamically regulates its own receptor expression on human neutrophils. *J. Biol. Chem.* **265,** 183–189.

Saverymuttu, S. H., Chadwick, V. S., and Hodgson, H. J. (1985a). Granulocyte migration in ulcerative colitis. *Eur. J. Clin. Invest.* **15,** 60–68.

Saverymuttu, S. H., Peters, A. M., Lavender, J. P., Chadwick, V. S., and Hodgson, H. J. (1985b). *In vivo* assessment of granulocyte migration to diseased bowel in Crohn's disease. *Gut* **26,** 378–383.

Scholmerich, J., Schmidt, E., Schumichen, C., Billmann, P., Schmidt, H., and Gerok, W. (1988). Scinti-graphic assessment of bowel involvement and disease activity in Crohn's disease using technetium 99m hexamethyl propylene amine oxine as leukocyte label. *Gastroenterology* **95,** 1287–1293.

Schreiber, S., MacDermott, R. P., Raedler, A., Pinnau, R., Bertovich, M. J., and Nash, G. S. (1991a). Increased activation of isolated intestinal lamina propria mononuclear cells in inflammatory bowel disease. *Gastroenterology* **101,** 1020–1030.

Schreiber, S., Nash, G. S., Raedler, A., Pinnau, R., Bertovich, M. J., and MacDermott, R P. (1991b). Human lamina propria mononuclear cells are activated in inflammatory bowel disease. *In* "Frontiers of Mucosal Immunology" (M. Tsuchiya, Ed.), pp. 749–753. Elsevier, Amsterdam.

Schreiber, S., Raedler, A., Conn, . R., Rombeau, J. L., and MacDermott, R. P. (1992). Increased *in vitro* release of soluble interleukin-2 receptor by colonic lamina propria mononuclear cells in in-flammatory bowel disease. *Gut* **33,** 236–241.

Schröder, J. M. (1992). Generation of NAP-1 and related peptides in psoriasis and other inflammatory skin diseases. *Cytokines* **4,** 54–76.

Scott, M. G., Nahm, M. H., Macke, K., Nash, G. S., Bertovich, M. J., and MacDermott, R. P. (1986). Spontaneous secretion of IgG subclasses by intestinal mononuclear cells: Differences between ul-cerative colitis, Crohn's disease and controls. *Clin. Exp. Immunol.* **66,** 209–215.

Seitz, M., Dewald, B., Gerber, N., and Baggiolini, M. (1991). Enhanced production of neutrophil-activating peptide-1/interleukin-8 rheumatoid arthritis. *J. Clin. Invest.* **87,** 463–469.

Sharon, P., and Stenson, W. F. (1984). Enhanced synthesis of leukotriene B4 by colonic mucosa in inflammatory bowel disease. *Gastroenterology* **86,** 453–460.

Springer, T. A. (1994). Traffic signals for lymphocyte recirculation and leukocyte emigration: The multistep paradigm. *Cell (Cambridge, Mass.)* **76,** 301–314.

Standiford, T. J., Kunkel, S. L., Basha, M. A., Chensue, S. W., Lynch III, J. P., Toews, G. B., Westwick, J., and Strieter, R. M. (1990a). Interleukin-8 gene expression by a pulmonary epithelial cell line. A model for cytokine network in the lung. *J. Clin. Invest.* **86,** 1945–1953.

Standiford, T. J., Strieter, R. M., Kasahara, K., and Kunkel, S. L. (1990b). Disparate regulation of interleukin 8 gene expression from blood monocytes, endothelial cells, and fibroblasts by interleu-kin 4. *Biochem. Biophys. Res. Commun.* **171,** 531–536.

Stenson, W. F., and Parker, C. W. (1984). Leukotrienes. *Adv. Intern. Med.* **30,** 175–199.

Stevens, C., Walz, G., and Zanker, B. (1990). Interleukin-6, interleukin-1-beta and tumor necrosis factor: Expression in inflammatory bowel disease. *Gastroenterology* **98,** A475.

Targan, S. R., Landers, C. J., Cobb, L., MacDermott, R. P., and Vidrich, A. (1995). Perinuclear antineu-trophil cytoplasmic antibodies are spontaneously produced by mucosal B cells of ulcerative colitis patients. *J. Immunol.* **155,** 3262–3267.

Tobler, A., Meier, R., Seitz, M., Dewald, B., Baggiolini, M., and Fey, M. F. (1992). Glucocorticoids downregulate gene expression of GM-CSF, NAP-1/IL-8, and IL-6, but not of M-CSF in human fibroblasts. *Blood* **79,** 45–51.

Van Spreeuwel, J. P., Lindeman, J., and Meijer, A. C. J. L. M. (1985). A quantitative study of immuno-globulin-containing cells in the differential diagnosis of acute colitis. *J. Clin. Pathol.* **38,** 774–777.

Wang, J. M., McVicar, D. W., Oppenheim, J. J., and Kelvin, D. J. (1993a). Identification of RANTES receptors on human monocytic cells: Competition for binding and desensitization by homologous chemotactic cytokines. *J. Exp. Med.* **177,** 699–705.

Wang, J. M., Sherry, B., Fivash, M. J., Kelvin, D. J., and Oppenheim, J. J. (1993b). Human recombinant macrophage inflammatory protein-1 alpha and -beta and monocyte chemotactic and activating factor utilize common and unique receptors on human monocytes. *J. Immunol.* **150,** 3022–3029.

Yoshimura, T., Matsushima, K., Oppenheim, J. J., and Leonard, E. J. (1987). Neutrophil chemotactic factor produced by lipopolysaccharide (LPS)-stimulated human blood mononuclear leukocytes: Partial characterization and separation from interleukin-1 (IL-1). *J. Immunol.* **139,** 788–793.

Yoshimura, T., and Leonard, E. J. (1990a). Secretion by human fibroblasts of monocyte chemoattractant protein-1, the product of gene JE. *J. Immunol.* **144,** 2377–2383.

Yoshimura, T., and Leonard, E. J. (1990b). Identification of high affinity receptors for human monocyte chemoattractant protein-1 on human monocytes. *J. Immunol.* **145,** 292–297.

Yoshimura, T., and Leonard, E. J. (1991). Human monocyte chemoattractant protein-1 (MCP-1). *Adv. Exp. Med. Biol.* **305,** 47–56.

# Chapter 25

## Mast Cell Heterogeneity and Functions in Mucosal Defenses and Pathogenesis

A. Dean Befus

*Pulmonary Research Group, Department of Medicine, University of Alberta, Edmonton, Alberta, Canada T6G 2S2*

### I. INTRODUCTION

Mast cells are most often thought of as the major effector cells of allergic reactions. They are almost ubiquitous in their distribution throughout the body and exhibit site-specific adaptations to their microenvironments which undoubtedly have important functional implications. They bear thousands of high-affinity receptors for IgE which become occupied by specific IgE antibodies, and upon reexposure to the sensitizing allergens they undergo anaphylactic degranulation. This activation leads to the rapid release of several potent mediators stored in the cytoplasmic granules or newly synthesized from membrane phospholipids or other constituents. Classical allergic reactions ensue with their cascades of inflammatory events and sequelae of symptoms. At mucosal surfaces, food allergy, allergic asthma, conjunctivitis, or rhinitis are well-known expressions of these reactions.

However, mast cells have other functions that are less well known and are believed to be independent of IgE antibodies. In delayed type hypersensitivity reactions in mice, mast cell activation and, particularly serotonin release, is an important initiating factor of vascular changes and cellular infiltration (Askenase *et al.*, 1980). The numbers of mast cells increase and they become activated in sites of tissue injury and remodeling such as bone fractures, keloid scars, and fibrosis. Mast cell hyperplasia is evident in some tumors and in sites of chronic inflammation throughout the body. The mechanisms that control these changes, the nature of the signals that activate the mast cells, and the functions of the mast cells under these conditions are poorly known.

In this brief review of the properties of mast cells and their functions, some recent advances will be highlighted and some of the more novel associations between mast cell numbers, activation, and physiologic or pathophysiologic events will be discussed. Such information helps provide insight into the complex biology of the cell and encourages a broad view of its physiological roles. There are many other recent reviews of mast cell biology to assist the reader with this intriguing and rapidly evolving subject (e.g., Galli, 1990; Schulman, 1993; Schwartz and Huff, 1993; Befus, 1995; Razin *et al.*, 1995).

## II. Mast Cell Activation and Mediator Release

### A. Activation

As indicated above, mast cells can be activated in several ways, not all of which involve IgE-mediated mechanisms (Fig. 1).

### 1. IgE-Dependent Mechanisms

Both high- and low-affinity receptors for IgE are present on mast cells and when these are occupied by IgE and cross-linked by antigen, activation and mediator secretion occurs. The structure of the high-affinity receptor is well known and components of its kinase-dependent signaling have been defined (Beaven and Metzger, 1993). Low-affinity receptors for IgE on mast cells are less well understood, but include FcγRII/III (Takizawa *et al.*, 1992) and perhaps also CD23 (Frandji *et al.*, 1993). Interestingly, both high- and low-affinity IgE receptors are glycosylated, and in populations of mast cells derived from the rat body cavity or intestinal mucosa significant molecular weight heterogeneity of the receptors exists (Swieter *et al.*, 1989). The relevance of this heterogeneity is unknown, but presumably it plays some role in IgE receptor function.

### 2. Antigen-Specific T-Cell Factor

In addition to the IgE ligand–receptor-mediated pathway, a distinct antigen-specific T-cell-mediated pathway exists that induces the release of serotonin in murine delayed-type hypersensitivity reactions (Askenase *et al.*, 1980). This pathway, despite its potential significance, has not been investigated by many laboratories.

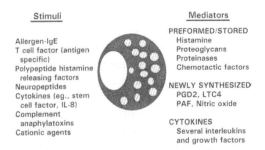

| Stimuli | Mediators |
| --- | --- |
| | PREFORMED/STORED |
| Allergen-IgE | Histamine |
| T cell factor (antigen | Proteoglycans |
| specific) | Proteinases |
| Polypeptide histamine | Chemotactic factors |
| releasing factors | |
| Neuropeptides | NEWLY SYNTHESIZED |
| Cytokines (eg., stem | PGD2, LTC4 |
| cell factor, IL-8) | PAF, Nitric oxide |
| Complement | |
| anaphylatoxins | CYTOKINES |
| Cationic agents | Several interleukins |
| | and growth factors |

*FIGURE 1.* Stimuli that activate mast cells and the spectrum of mediators produced by these cells.

Accordingly, its characteristics are poorly known and its molecular components have not been defined. Whether mast cells in all tissue sites possess this pathway, or whether it is restricted to cutaneous mast cells in mice remains to be established. Its biological and clinical relevance must be determined; perhaps the pathophysiology of several poorly understood inflammatory conditions are initiated or perpetuated by this pathway.

### 3. Histamine-Releasing Factors (HRF)

Another mechanism for the activation of mast cells and basophils involves a series of HRF derived from mononuclear cells, eosinophils, neutrophils, platelets, etc. (Kaplan *et al.*, 1991). For example, activated mononuclear cells produce at least three types of HRF, one 8 to 10 kDa, one 15 to 17 kDa, and one 35 to 41 kDa. The 8- to 10-kDa form is homologous with connective tissue activating peptide II (CTAP-II) and its cleavage product, neutrophil activating peptide (NAP-2). Other authors have shown that NAP-1, now recognized as IL-8, also acts as a low-molecular-weight HRF. The molecular identity of the 15 to 17 factor appears to be monocyte chemotactic and activating factor (Kuna *et al.*, 1992), whereas that of the 35- to 41-kDa HRF remains to be determined.

Neutrophils produce cationic peptides that have HRF activity (White *et al.*, 1988). This activity is constitutively produced, heat stable, and <5 kDa. Of the cationic peptides produced by neutrophils, defensins or corticostatins have been extensively studied because of their antimicrobial activities (Lehrer *et al.*, 1993). Interestingly, we have established that these cysteine-rich peptides are potent histamine secretagogues for peritoneal mast cells from rats, but are without effect on intestinal mucosal mast cells from the same species. It will be intriguing to determine if the close relatives of defensins, namely the cryptdins found selectively in Paneth cells at the base of the intestinal crypts (Eisenhauer *et al.*, 1992), will activate the intestinal mucosal mast cells, but be without effects on histamine secretion from peritoneal mast cells. Such an observation would be consistent with the evolving model of mast cell heterogeneity which suggests that site-specific pathways of activation exist.

### 4. Neuropeptides, Microbial Toxins

Other cationic moieties that induce histamine secretion from at least some mast cell populations include neuropeptides such as substance P, somatostatin, vasoactive intestinal polypeptide, and endorphins (e.g., Shanahan *et al.*, 1985). Until recently the amounts of neuropeptide used to study mast cell activation were considered by many to be nonphysiological ($\mu M$ levels needed to induce histamine secretion). However, work by Janiszewski *et al.* (1994) studying ion channels in mast cells showed significant effects at $nM$ levels of the neuropeptide substance P. The biological significance of this mode of mast cell activation is incompletely known, but the close anatomical association of mast cells and nerves (Stead *et al.*, 1987), exciting examples of classical Pavlovian conditioning of mast cell secretion

(MacQueen *et al.*, 1989), and *in vivo* models of wheal and flare reactions (Kiernan, 1975) or enteritis induced by *Clostridium difficile* toxin A (Castagliuolo *et al.*, 1994; Kurose *et al.*, 1994; Pothoulakis *et al.*, 1994; see below) suggest that this may be a prominent pathway of mast cell activation.

Until recently mast cell activation was not often considered to be important in bacterial, or even viral, infections, because elevations in mast cell numbers or in IgE levels were not associated with these infections. This emphasizes the disservice that the focus on IgE has given the field of mast cell biology. However, one can be optimistic that the recent literature will diversify the approaches taken to elucidate the functional roles of mast cells.

## 5. Other Cationic Agents

The list of other cationic agents that activate some mast cell populations is extensive, including: compound 48/80, bee venom peptides 401 and mastoparan, polylysine, polymyxin, and complement cleavage products such as C3a (Befus, 1995). Even proteolytic breakdown of food proteins such as albumin can release peptides with mast cell secretagogue activity apparently independent of IgE antibodies (Carraway *et al.*, 1989). Thus, it is evident that the activation of mast cells can be initiated by several factors of diverse origin. Unravelling the biological significance of these modes of activation will make major contributions to our understanding of mast cell biology.

## B. Mediators

Mast cells construct and secrete a plethora of mediators that fall into categories of being preformed and stored in the granules, or being newly synthesized following activation (Fig. 1). Only a select few of these mediators will be discussed here; other reviews have a comprehensive coverage of the full spectrum of mediators (e.g., Schwartz and Huff, 1993).

## 1. Histamine

Histamine is a well-known mediator stored in mast cell granules. When mast cells are activated it is secreted into the surrounding environment, but has a short half-life in the circulation. Histamine stores in the mast cell are replenished, most probably by regranulation of existing mast cells and/or development of mast cells from their progenitors (Miller, 1971; Dvorak *et al.*, 1986).

## 2. Proteinases

Although they have not had as high a profile in the literature as biogenic amines, several different proteinases are stored in granules and released following mast cell activation (Schwartz, 1990; Caughey, 1995). These proteinases are abundant, in some mast cells representing at least 50% of the cellular protein (Abe *et al.*, 1990). Both chymase- and tryptase-like serine proteinases, as well as carboxypeptidase-like metalloproteinases, are widespread in mast cells from the body cavity, skin, and lungs of mice, rats, and humans. However, marked heterogeneity in proteinase expression in mast cells has been identified in each of these species. In rodents mast cells from the peritoneum express multiple differentially glycosylated forms of the chymases, rat proteinase 1 (analogous to mouse proteinase 4) and 5, and carboxypeptidase A and small amounts of tryptase (Befus *et al.*, 1995). By contrast, intestinal mucosal mast cells express only the chymase, rat proteinase 2 (Befus *et al.*, 1995). In mice a similar pattern appears to exist (Newlands *et al.*, 1993; Caughey, 1995), although at least five distinct types of chymase have been described, all closely linked to T-cell granzyme genes on murine chromosome 14 (Gurish *et al.*, 1993). Two of these are selectively expressed in mucosal mast cells (mouse proteinases 1 and 2). In addition, two mast cell tryptases have been described in mice (Caughey, 1995). The expression of these distinct chymases in murine mast cells is regulated by several cytokines, including IL-3, IL-4, IL-10, and stem cell factor (e.g., Eklund *et al.*, 1993).

Mast cells from humans also express chymases, tryptases, and carboxypeptidase (Caughey, 1995). A single chymase gene has been identified in humans, but four tryptase genes have been found. Interestingly, mast cells found in greatest abundance at mucosal sites in humans express tryptase, but not chymase, a marked contrast to observations in rodents (Schwartz, 1990). The functions of these various mast-cell-specific enzymes is incompletely known, but reports include: fibroblast activation (Ruoss *et al.*, 1991), smooth muscle contraction (Sekizawa *et al.*, 1989), submucosal gland secretion in the respiratory tract (Sommerhoff *et al.*, 1989), neuropeptide degradation (Tam and Caughey, 1990), protein processing (Mizutani *et al.*, 1991), and extracellular matrix degradation (Banovac *et al.*, 1993). As selective inhibitors of the expression or functions of these proteinases are developed, important new knowledge of mast cell function will be uncovered.

### 3. Cytokines

In the late 1980s it first was recognized that mast cells produce several cytokines such as tumor necrosis factor-$\alpha$ (TNF$\alpha$) (e.g., Young *et al.*, 1987). Since these initial observations, the number of cytokines that have been identified in mast cells, at the level of either functional protein or mRNA, has grown rapidly. There are few cytokines that have not been identified in *in vivo*-derived mast cells or at least in mast cell lines in rodents or humans (Fig. 2). A critical question is whether mast cells are an important source of these cytokines *in vivo* or whether many of the observations merely reflect cultural artifact or mRNA without protein production. Some cytokines are constitutively produced in some mast cell populations and stored in the granules, whereas the expression of other cytokines must be induced by selected stimuli. For example, TNF$\alpha$ is abundant in rat and mouse peritoneal mast cells (e.g., 404 pg/$10^6$ rat mast cells), but rat intestinal mucosal mast cells store about 17% of this amount (68 pg/$10^6$ mast cells) (Bissonnette *et al.*, 1995a). However, activated intestinal mucosal mast cells are induced to pro-

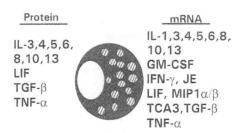

Protein                                              mRNA

IL-3,4,5,6,                                        IL-1,3,4,5,6,8,
8,10,13                                            10,13
LIF                                                GM-CSF
TGF-β                                              IFN-γ, JE
TNF-α                                              LIF, MIP1α/β
                                                   TCA3,TGF-β
                                                   TNF-α

**FIGURE 2.** Cytokines identified in mast cells, either as the protein or biological activity or as mRNA. Abbreviations: IL, interleukins; LIF, leukemia inhibitory factor; TGF, transforming growth factor; TNF, tumor necrosis factor; GM-CSF, granulocyte monocyte colony-stimulating factor; IFN, interferon; MIP, monocyte inhibitory peptide; TCA, T-cell activation gene.

duce up to 90% of the TNFα cytotoxicity of peritoneal mast cells. Similarly, human skin mast cells store little TNFα, but can rapidly synthesize it once activated (Benyon *et al.,* 1991). Bradding *et al.* (1995) have provided additional evidence that mast cells are heterogeneous in their cytokine content. Their investigations demonstrated that mast cells from human skin that express both chymase and tryptase are largely positive for IL-4, IL-5, and IL-6, whereas only a low proportion (15%) of mast cells that express tryptase only express IL-4. Williams and Coleman (1995) recently showed that activation of rat peritoneal mast cells with anti-IgE antibodies for 4 hr induced expression of IL-5, IL-6, TNFα, MIP-2, and IFNγ. Cyclosporine A and dexamethasone inhibited this gene expression.

One of the intriguing observations from this rapidly evolving work is that mast cells are capable of expressing cytokines that fall into both the so-called Th1 and Th2 patterns associated in the extreme with distinct types of immune and inflammatory responses (Mosmann and Coffman, 1989). This is perhaps not surprising as the Th1/Th2 distinction is often unclear in T cells as well (Kelso, 1995). However, it will be important to determine if the same mast cell can express several cytokines and if these cytokines fall into the extreme categories associated with both Th1 and Th2 immune responses (e.g., IL-4 and IFNγ), or with only one of these types of responses (e.g., Th2, IL-4, and IL-5). If the same mast cell expresses both IL-4 and IFNγ, are these stored in the same compartment in the cell and capable of being released together, or is their release differentially controlled through distinct storage compartments or secretion mechanisms? There is certainly precedent for differential control of mediator secretion, e.g., histamine and TNFα release (e.g., Bissonnette *et al.,* 1995a) and TNFα and IL-6 release (Leal-Berumen *et al.,* 1995).

Perhaps the most important question about mast cell cytokines relates to their role in health and disease. When is mast-cell-derived IL-4 or TNFα the most abundant source of these cytokines, and when is it the most relevant source? Double-labeling approaches have shown that in bronchial biopsies from individuals with asthma, mast cells are a major source of IL-4, IL-5, IL-6, and TNFα (Bradding *et al.*, 1994). Additional studies are required to establish that mast-cell-derived cytokines are highly relevant sources in several settings. Indeed, it has been postulated that sources of cytokines such as the mast cell may produce the initial pulse of a cytokine during a natural immune response that subsequently directs the acquired immune response (Romagnani, 1992; e.g., IL-4 directs Th2-type allergic responses). This may be especially true where the mast cell expresses a cytokine constitutively. Lastly, it is important to recognize that these types of questions are not restricted to considerations of mast cell biology, but apply equally to other cell types as well. For example, eosinophils produce a similar plethora of cytokines and are undoubtedly an important source in several settings (Moqbel, 1996).

## III. REGULATION OF CYTOKINE PRODUCTION AND SECRETION

There is a wealth of literature about the inhibition of histamine secretion and production of arachidonic acid metabolites by mast cells. Much of this involves anti-allergic and anti-inflammatory drugs. However, until recently there has been little information about the regulation of cytokine production in mast cells and about the role of cytokines in regulating mast cell secretion and functions.

### A. Cytokines

Stem cell factor is an important growth and differentiation factor for mast cells (Galli *et al.*, 1994). In addition, it is a powerful secretagogue for human mast cells and potentiates antigen-induced histamine secretion and arachidonic acid production from mast cells of several species. Interestingly, we have recently shown that with rat peritoneal mast cells stem cell factor does not alter the antigen-induced release of TNFα (Lin *et al.*, 1996). The pathways involved in this differential regulation of mast cell mediators by stem cell factor are unknown, but given increasing evidence that stem cell factor is involved in allergic reactions such as asthma (Undem *et al.*, 1994), understanding of these pathways will be important. Whether or not the lack of effect of stem cell factor on TNFα release is true also for all mast cell cytokines must be determined.

By contrast to stem cell factor, other cytokines inhibit the release of cytokines by mast cells or the steady state levels of cytokine mRNA in mast cells (Fig. 3). For example, interferons (IFN) α, β, and γ inhibit both histamine and TNFα secretion from rat peritoneal mast cells (Bissonnette *et al.*, 1995a). IL-10 behaves differently, inhibiting antigen-induced TNFα production, but stimulating antigen-induced histamine release (Lin *et al.*, 1996). Marshall and co-workers showed that LPS stimulates IL-6 production by mast cells, but inhibits TNFα production (Leal-Berumen *et al.*, 1995). The complexity of the regulatory relationships among cytokines and mast cell mediators worsens when other mast cell populations, even

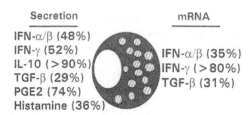

**FIGURE 3.** Inhibition of tumor necrosis factor-α production and secretion, and its steady-state mRNA levels in mast cells, by cytokines. Abbreviations: legend to see Fig. 2; PGE$_2$, prostaglandin E$_2$.

in the rat, are considered. For example, although interferons inhibit TNFα by both rat peritoneal and mucosal mast cells, and inhibit histamine release from peritoneal mast cells, they do not inhibit histamine release from intestinal mucosal mast cells (Bissonnette et al., 1995a). This emphasizes the distinctions between mast cell types and the differential regulation of their mediators.

## B. Anti-allergic and Anti-inflammatory Drugs

Several drugs used to treat allergic and other inflammatory conditions inhibit the release of TNFα from mast cells or its steady state levels of mRNA (Fig. 4). Disodium cromoglycate (SCG) and nedocromil sodium (NED) are widely used anti-allergic drugs, but whether their principle mode of action is through inhibition of histamine release or of cytokine release is unclear. Moreover, these drugs act in an analogous fashion to IFNγ on histamine and TNFα release from rat peritoneal and mucosal mast cells, inhibiting both from peritoneal cells, but inhibiting only TNFα and not histamine from mucosal mast cells (Bissonnette et al., 1995b). In contrast to SCG and NED, which only partially inhibit TNFα release, sulfasalazine and its metabolites, as well as β$_2$ agonists, can almost completely inhibit TNFα release from mast cells (Bissonnette et al., 1996; E. Y. Bissonnette and A. D. Befus, unpublished). One of the important actions of corticosteroids in the treatment of allergic disease is thought to be regulation of cytokine production in mast cells (Wershil et al., 1995; Williams and Coleman, 1995).

## IV. MAST CELL HETEROGENEITY

It has been well known for many years that mast cells exhibit marked heterogeneity both within and between species. Two principal subtypes have been identified, namely connective tissue and mucosal mast cells. However, mast cell heterogeneity is more complex than just two subtypes, as each cell is unique in both time and space as compared to any other cell; the reasons for distinctions within and between mast cell populations may relate to many factors such as phases of ontogeny, activation, and recovery. Although space restrictions prohibit a comprehensive

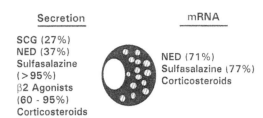

**Secretion**

SCG (27%)
NED (37%)
Sulfasalazine
(>95%)
β2 Agonists
(60 - 95%)
Corticosteroids

**mRNA**

NED (71%)
Sulfasalazine (77%)
Corticosteroids

*FIGURE 4.* Inhibition of tumor necrosis factor-α production and secretion, and its steady state mRNA levels in mast cells, by anti-allergic and anti-inflammatory drugs. Abbreviations: NED, nedocromil sodium; SCG, sodium cromoglycate.

review of this intriguing subject, several examples of such heterogeneity have been provided above.

For example, IgE receptors in rat peritoneal and mucosal mast cells exhibit heterogeneity in their size, presumably as a result of glycosylation differences (Swieter *et al.*, 1989). Some secretagogues activate peritoneal mast cells, but not mucosal mast cells (e.g., defensins, neuropeptides, and other cationic moieties). Proteinase composition differs markedly between rodent connective tissue (peritoneal) and mucosal mast cells, and chymase and tryptase content is used to distinguish human mast cell types (e.g., Caughey, 1995). Cytokine content varies among mast cell populations and in humans it may correlate with the proteinase phenotype (Bradding *et al.*, 1995). Lastly, the regulation of cytokine production in rat mast cells correlates with the mast cell subtypes involved (e.g., Bissonnette *et al.*, 1995a,b). Further information about mast cell heterogeneity is essential before we will fully appreciate its functional significance and the underlying cellular and molecular mechanisms.

## V. ONTOGENY

Mast cells develop from multipotent stem cells in the bone marrow. Through a series of incompletely understood processes mast cell progenitors arise from the stem cells and ultimately differentiate into phenotypically distinct mast cell subtypes (Schwartz and Huff, 1993; Befus, 1995). A current model of the developmental regulation of mast cell heterogeneity is that a widely distributed common progenitor is instructed by microenvironmental signals to express selected components of its mast cell potential. Moreover, the mast cell phenotype initially expressed is not irreversibly fixed, and given a different set of microenvironmental signals, clonal populations of mast cells can transdifferentiate from one phenotype to another (see Galli, 1990; Befus, 1995). Stem cell factor, IL-3, IL-4, IL-9, IL-10, IFNγ, and transforming growth factor-β are among the factors involved in the developmental regulation of mast cell subtypes.

The extent to which programmed cell death or apoptosis regulates the numbers or types of mast cell populations in tissues is unknown. However, IL-3 and stem cell factor enhance survival of mast cells (Mekori *et al.*, 1993), whereas treatment with systemic corticosteroids leads to the selective depletion of mucosal mast cells in rats (King *et al.*, 1985), apparently by a process of apoptosis and macrophage engulfment (Soda *et al.*, 1991). Further understanding of these processes may uncover novel therapeutic strategies for the treatment of mast-cell-dependent inflammatory responses.

## VI. Functions

Given the cornucopia of mediators and their respective target cells, together with the diversity of activation signals, it is not surprising that mast cells exhibit a wealth of functional activities. Not all of these are obviously linked to IgE-mediated allergic or inflammatory reactions. Nevertheless, IgE-mediated reactions are a pivotal component of mast cell activation and function. Both immediate and late-phase reactions involve mast cell mediators, although the precise roles of mast cells in the late reaction are unclear. It may be that TNF$\alpha$ released from mast cells is a critical component in the generation of the late reaction in asthma. Similarly, although there is strong evidence in the mouse that mast cells are an integral part of a classical delayed-type hypersensitivity response (Askenase *et al.* 1980), the roles of mediators other than serotonin in this response are unknown.

The work of Gauchet *et al.* (1993) uncovered a novel aspect of the relationship between mast cells and IgE, namely that mast cells may be able to replace T cells in the induction of IgE synthesis by B lymphocytes. Because both mast cells and basophils bear CD40 ligand on their surface and contain IL-4, they can induce IgE synthesis by ligation of CD40 on the B cells and the provision of IL-4 for IgE production. Interestingly, mast cells have also been shown recently to produce IL-13 (Burd *et al.* 1995; Lin *et al.*, 1996), a cytokine that can mimic IL-4 function in IgE synthesis. The relationship between these observations about mast cells and IgE synthesis and earlier observations by Mayrhofer *et al.* (1976) that mast cells store IgE in their cytoplasm is unclear. However, it might be productive to further investigate the role of mast cells in IgE synthesis, storage, and catabolism.

A curious observation made in recent years is the close association between mast cell activation, as evidenced by mast cell proteinase 2 in the serum, and weaning in newborn rats. Serum levels of proteinase 2 peak Day 22 after birth and are thus temporally associated with weaning and intestinal closure (Cummins *et al.*, 1989). Cyclosporine A inhibits this rise, an observation interpreted by some as suggesting T-cell involvement in mast cell activation (Cummins *et al.*, 1989). Substance P does not appear to be involved, as its depletion with capsaicin has no effect on the changes in the proteinase levels (Cummins *et al.*, 1994). The role of mast cell activation in weaning and the nature of the stimulus responsible are unknown. It could be that there is an inflammatory component in weaning, or that the high serum levels of proteinase 2 reflect an immaturity in the regulatory control of mucosal mast cells at this early phase in their development and has no physiologic consequence. Toxin A of *C. difficile* induces intestinal inflammation in a mast-cell-dependent manner that appears to be independent of IgE (Castagliuolo *et al.*, 1994; Kurose *et al.*, 1994). Histamine is an important mediator in this inflammation, and it appears that neuronal mechanisms are central to the activation of the mast cell (Castagliuolo *et al.*, 1994; Pothoulakis *et al.*, 1994). This is perhaps the most clear example of mast cell activation at a mucosal surface by a neurogenic mechanism. The extent to which this pathway is relevant in human disease is unknown, but it serves as an important example of non-IgE activation of mast cells.

The mast-cell-deficient mouse strains W/W$^v$ (mutation in the receptor for stem cell factor, c-kit) and Sl/Sl$^d$ (mutation in stem cell factor) have proven to be excellent tools with which to study mast cell functions (Galli, 1990). The former can be reconstituted systemically with normal bone marrow, or locally by injection of mast cells. These models have been used to show the mast cell dependency of peritonitis (Zhang *et al.*, 1992), the role of substance P in mast-cell-dependent neutrophil accumulation in skin (Yano *et al.*, 1989), and the dependency of anaphylaxis on mast cells (Galli, 1990; Zhang *et al.*, 1992). Several other studies using these models have suggested that mast cells have diverse functions.

These murine models will continue to provide valuable information about mast cell functions and, when combined with transgenic or knockout manipulations of murine genotype, promise to be increasingly powerful experimental tools. In addition, human studies which employ *in situ* assessments of mast cell contents, activation, and function will be essential to unravel the mysteries of the roles of the mast cell in health and disease.

## REFERENCES

Abe, T., Swieter, M., Imai, T., denHollander, N., and Befus, A. D. (1990). Mast cell heterogeneity: Two-dimensional gel electrophoretic analysis of rat peritoneal and intestinal mucosal mast cells. *Eur. J. Immunol.* **20,** 1941–1947.

Askenase, P. W., Bursztajn, S., Gershon, M. D., and Gershon, R. K. (1980). T cell-dependent mast cell degranulation and release of serotonin in murine delayed-type hypersensitivity. *J. Exp. Med.* **152,** 1358–1374.

Banovac, K., Banovac, F., Yang, J., and Koren, E. (1993). Interaction of osteoblasts with extracellular matrix: Effect of mast cell chymase. *Proc. Soc. Exp. Biol. Med.* **203,** 221–235.

Beaven, M. A., and Metzger, H. (1993). Signal transduction by Fc receptors: The FcεRI case. *Immunol. Today* **14,** 222–226.

Befus, A. D. (1995). The immunophysiology of mast cells in intestinal immunity and symbiosis. *In* "Infections of the Gastrointestinal Tract" (M. J. Blaser, P. D. Smith, J. I. Ravdin, H. B. Greenberg, and R. L. Guerrant, eds.), pp. 227–236. Raven, New York.

Befus, A. D., Chin, B., Pick, J., Evans, S., Osborn, S., and Forstrom, J. (1995). Proteinase of rat mast cells: Peritoneal but not intestinal mucosal mast cells express mast cell proteinase 5 and carboxypeptidase A. *J. Immunol.* **155,** 4406–4411.

Benyon, R. C., Bissonnette, E. Y., and Befus, A. D. (1991). Tumor necrosis factor-α dependent cytotoxicity of human skin mast cells is enhanced by anti-IgE antibodies. *J. Immunol.* **147,** 2253–2258.

Bissonnette, E. Y., Chin, B., and Befus, A. D. (1995a). Interferons differentially regulate histamine and TNF-$\alpha$ in rat intestinal mucosal mast cells. *Immunology* **86,** 12–17.

Bissonnette, E. Y., Enciso, J. A., and Befus, A. D. (1995b). Inhibition of tumour necrosis factor-alpha (TNF-$\alpha$) release from mast cells by the anti-inflammatory drugs, sodium cromoglycate and nedocromil sodium. *Clin. Exp. Immunol.* **102,** 78–84.

Bissonnette, E. Y., Enciso, J. A., and Befus, A. D. (1996). Inhibitory effects of sulfasalazine and its metabolites on mediator release from mast cells. *J. Immunol.* **156,** 218–223.

Bradding, P., Roberts, J. A., Britten, M., Montefort, S., Djukanovic, R., Mueller, R., Heusser, C. H., Howarth, P. H., and Holgate, S. T. (1994). Interleukin-4, -5, and -6 and tumor necrosis factor-$\alpha$ in normal and asthmatic airways: Evidence for the human mast cell as a source of these cytokines. *Am. J. Respir. Cell Mol. Biol.* **10,** 471–480.

Bradding P., Okayama, Y., Howarth, P. H., Church, M. K., and Holgate, S. T. (1995). Heterogeneity of human mast cells based on cytokine content. *J. Immunol.* **155,** 297–307.

Burd, P. R., Thompson, W. C., Max, E. E., and Mills, F. C. (1995). Activated mast cells produce interleukin 13. *J. Exp. Med.* **181,** 1373–1380.

Carraway, R. E., Cochrane, D. E., Boucher, W., and Mitra, S. P. (1989). Structures of histamine-releasing peptides formed by the action of acid proteases on mammalian albumin(s). *J. Immunol.* **143,** 1680–1684.

Castagliuolo, I., LaMont, J. T., Letourneau, R., Kelly, C., O'Keane, J. C., Jaffer, A., Theoharides, T. C., and Pothoulakis, C. (1994). Neuronal involvement in the intestinal effects of *Clostridium difficile* toxin A and *Vibrio cholerae* enterotoxin in rat ileum. *Gastroenterology* **107,** 657–665.

Caughey, G. H. (1995). "Mast Cell Proteases in Immunology and Biology." Dekker, New York.

Cummins, A. G., Labrooy, J. T., and Shearman, D. J. C. (1989). The effect of cyclosporin A in delaying maturation of the small intestine during weaning in the rat. *Clin. Exp. Immunol.* **75,** 451–456.

Cummins, A. G., Antoniou, D., and Thompson, F. M. (1994). Neuropeptide depletion by capsaicin does not prevent mucosal mast cell activation in the rat at weaning. *Immunol. Cell Biol.* **72,** 230–233.

Dvorak, A. M., Schleimer, R. P., Schulman, E. S., and Lichtenstein, L. M. (1986). Human mast cells use conservation and condensation mechanisms during recovery from degranulation. *Lab. Invest.* **54,** 663–678.

Eisenhauer, P. B., Harwig, S. S. S. L., and Lehrer, R. I. (1992). Cryptdins: Antimicrobial defensins of the murine small intestine. *Infect. Immun.* **60,** 3556–3565.

Eklund, K. K., Ghildyal, N., Austen, K. F., and Stevens, R. L. (1993). Induction by IL-9 and suppression by IL-3 and IL-4 of the levels of chromosome-derived transcripts that encode late-expressed mouse mast cell proteases. *J. Immunol.* **151,** 4266–4273.

Frandji, P., Oskéritzian, C., Cacaraci, F., Lapeyre, J., Peronet, R., David, B., Guillet, J.-G., and Mécheri, S. (1993). Antigen-dependent stimulation by bone marrow-derived mast cells of MHC class II-restricted T cell hybridoma. *J. Immunol.* **151,** 6318–6328.

Galli, S. J. (1990). Biology of disease. New insights into "the riddle of the mast cells": microenvironmental regulation of mast cell development and phenotypic heterogeneity. *Lab. Invest.* **13,** 35–70.

Galli, S. J., Zsebo, K. M., and Geissler, E. N. (1994). The kit ligand, stem cell factor. *Adv. Immunol.* **55,** 1–96.

Gauchat, J.-F., Henchoz, S., Mazzel, G., Aubry, J.-P., Brunner, T., Blasey, H., Life, P., Talabot, D., Flores-Romo, L., Thompson, J., Kishi, K., Butterfield, J., Dahinden, C., and Bonnefoy, J.-Y. (1993). Induction of human IgE synthesis in B cells by mast cells and basophils. *Nature (London)* **365,** 340–342.

Gurish, M. F., Nadeau, J. H., Johnson, K. R., McNeil, H. P., Grattan, K. M., Austen, K. F., and Stevens, R. L. (1993). A closely linked complex of mouse mast cell-specific chymase genes on chromosome 14. *J. Biol. Chem.* **268,** 11372–11379.

Janiszewski, J., Bienenstock, J. and Blennerhassett, M. G. (1994). Picomolar doses of substance P trigger electrical responses in mast cells without degranulation. *Am. J. Physiol.* **267,** C138–145.

Kaplan, A. P., Reddigari, S., Baeza, M., and Kuna, P. (1991). Histamine releasing factors and cytokine-dependent activation of basophils and mast cells. *Adv. Immunol.* **50,** 237–254.

Kelso, A. (1995). Th1 and Th2 subsets: Paradigms lost? *Immunol. Today* **16,** 374–379.

Kiernan, J. A. (1975). A pharmacological and histological investigation of the involvement of mast cells in cutaneous axon reflex vasodilation. *Q. J. Exp. Physiol.* **60,** 123–130.

King, S. J., Miller, H. R. P., Newlands, G. F. J., and Woodbury, R. G. (1985). Depletion of mucosal mast cell protease by corticosteroids: Effect on intestinal anaphylaxis is the rat. *Proc. Natl. Acad. Sci. U.S.A.* **82,** 1214–1218.

Kuna, P., Reddigari, S. R., Rucinski, D., Oppenheim, J. J., and Kaplan, A. P. (1992). Monocyte chemotactic and activating factor is a potent histamine-releasing factor for human basophils. *J. Exp. Med.* **175,** 489–493.

Kurose, I., Pothoulakis, C., LaMont, J. T., Anderson, D. C., Paulson, J. C., Miyasaka, M., Wolf, R., and Granger, D. N. (1994). *Clostridium difficile* toxin A-induced microvascular dysfunction. Role of histamine. *J. Clin. Invest.* **94,** 1919–1926.

Leal-Berumen, I., O'Byrne, P., Gupta, A., Richards, C. D., and Marshall, J. S. (1995). Prostanoid enhancement of interleukin-6 production by rat peritoneal mast cells. *J. Immunol.* **154,** 4759–4767.

Lehrer, R. I., Lichtenstein, A. K., and Ganz, T. (1993). Defensins': Antimicrobial and cytotoxic peptides of mammalian cells. *Annu. Rev. Immunol.* **11,** 105–128.

Lin, T.-J., Enciso, J. A., Bissonnette, E. Y., Szczepek, A., and Befus, A. D. (1996). Cytokine and drug modulation of TNF-$\alpha$ in mast cells. *In* "Proceedings International Symposium on Molecular Biology of Allergens and the Atopic Immune Response" (A. Sehon and D. Kraft, Eds.), Plenum, New York (in press).

MacQueen, G., Marshall, J., Perdue, M., Siegel, S., and Bienenstock, J. (1989). Pavlovian conditioning of rat mucosal mast cells to secrete rat mast cell proteinase II. *Science* **243,** 83–85.

Mayrhofer, G., Bazin, H., and Gowans, J. L. (1976). Nature of cells binding anti-IgE in rats immunized with *Nippostrongylus brasiliensis:* IgE synthesis in regional lymph nodes and concentration in mucosal mast cells. *Eur. J. Immunol.* **6,** 537–545.

Mekori, Y. A., Oh, C. K., and Metcalfe, D. D. (1993). IL-3 dependent murine mast cells undergo apoptosis on removal of IL-3. *J. Immunol.* **151,** 3775–3784.

Miller, H. R. P. (1971). Immune reactions in mucous membranes. *Lab. Invest.* **24,** 339–347.

Mizutani, H., Schechter, N., Lazarus, G., Black, R. A., and Kupper, T. S. (1991). Rapid and specific conversion of precursor interleukin 1$\beta$ (IL-1$_\beta$) to an active IL-1 species by human mast cell chymase. *J. Exp. Med.* **174,** 821–825.

Moqbel, R. (1996). Synthesis and storage of regulatory cytokines in human eosinophils. *In* "Proceedings International Symposium on Molecular Biology of Allergens and the Atopic Immune Response" (A. Sehon and D. Kraft, Eds.), Plenum, New York (in press).

Mosmann, T. R., and Coffman, R. L. (1989). TH$_1$ and TH$_2$ cells: Different patterns of lymphokine secretion lead to different functional properties. *Annu. Rev. Immunol.* **7,** 145–173.

Newlands, G. F. J., Knox, D. P., Pirie-Shepherd, S. R., and Miller, H. R. P. (1993). Biochemical and immunological characterization of multiple glycoforms of mouse mast cell protease 1: Comparison with an isolated murine serosal mast cell protease (MMCP-4). *Biochem. J.* **294,** 127–135.

Pothoulakis, C., Castagliuolo, I., LaMont, J. T., Jaffer, A., O'Keane, J. C., Snider, R. M., and Leeman, S. E. (1994). CP-96, 345, a substance P antagonist, inhibits rat intestinal responses to *Clostridium difficile* toxin A but not cholera toxin. *Proc. Natl. Acad. Sci. U.S.A.* **91,** 947–951.

Razin, E., Pecht, I., and Rivera, J. (1995). Signal transduction in the activation of mast cells and basophils. *Immunol. Today* **16,** 370–373.

Romagnani, S. (1992). Induction of TH$_1$ and TH$_2$ responses: A key role for the "natural" immune response? *Immunol. Today* **13,** 379–381.

Ruoss, S. J., Hartmann, T., and Caughey, G. H. (1991). Mast cell tryptase is a mitogen for cultured fibroblasts. *J. Clin. Invest.* **88,** 493–499.

Schulman, E. S. (1993). The role of mast cells in inflammatory responses in the lung. *Crit. Rev. Immunol.* **13,** 35–70.

Schwartz, L., and Huff, T. (1993). Biology of mast cells and basophils. *In* "Allergy Principles and Practice" (S. Manning, Ed.), Vol. 1, pp. 135–168. Mosby-Year Book, St. Louis, Missouri.

Schwartz, L. B. (1990). "Neutral Proteases of Mast Cells." Karger, Basel.

Sekizawa, K., Caughey, G. H. Lazarus, S. C., Gold, W. M., and Nadel, J. A. (1989). Mast cell tryptase causes airway smooth muscle hyperresponsiveness in dogs. *J. Clin. Invest.* **83,** 175–179.

Shanahan, F., Denburg, J. A., Fox, J., Bienenstock, J., and Befus, D. (1985). Mast cell heterogeneity: Effects of neuroenteric peptides on histamine release. *J. Immunol.* **135,** 1331–1337.

Soda, K., Kawabori, S., Perdue, M. H., and Bienenstock, J. (1991). Macrophage engulfment of mucosal mast cells in rats treated with dexamethasone. *Gastroenterology* **100,** 929–937.

Sommerhoff, C. P., Caughey, G. H., Finkbeiner, W. E., Lazarus, S. C., Basbaum, C. B., and Nadel, J. A. (1989). Mast cell chymase. A potent secretagogue for airway gland serous cells. *J. Immunol.* **142,** 2450–2456.

Stead, R. H., Tomioka, M., Quinonez, G., Simon, G. T., Felten, S. Y., and Bienenstock, J. (1987). Intestinal mucosal mast cells in normal and nematode-infected rat intestines are in intimate contact with peptidergic nerves. *Proc. Natl. Acad. Sci. U.S.A.* **84,** 2975–2979.

Swieter, M., Chan, B. M. C., Rimmer, C., McNeill, K., Froese, A., and Befus, D. (1989). Isolation and characterization of IgE receptors from rat intestinal mucosal mast cells. *Eur. J. Immunol.* **19,** 1879–1885.

Takizawa, F., Adamczewski, M., and Kinet, J.-P. (1992). Identification of the low affinity receptor for immunoglobulin E on mouse mast cells and macrophages as FcγRII and FcγRIII. *J. Exp. Med.* **176,** 469–476.

Tam, E. K., and Caughey, G. H. (1990). Degradation of airway neuropeptides by human lung tryptase. *Am. J. Resp. Cell Mol. Biol.* **3,** 32–37.

Undem, B. J., Lichtenstein, L. M., Hubbard, W. C., Meeker, S., and Ellis, J. L. (1994). Recombinant stem cell factor-induced mast cell activation and smooth muscle contraction in human bronchi. *Am. J. Respir. Cell Mol. Biol.* **11,** 646–650.

Wershil, B. K., Furuta, G. T., Lavigne, J. A., Roy-Choudhury, A., Wang, Z.-S., and Galli, S. J. (1995). Dexamethasone or cyclosporin A suppress mast cell-leukocyte cytokine cascades. *J. Immunol.* **154,** 1391–1398.

White, M. V., Kaplan, A. P., Haak-Frendscho, M., and Kaliner, M. (1988). Neutrophils and mast cells: Comparison of neutrophil-derived, histamine-releasing activity (HRA-N) with other histamine releasing factors. *J. Immunol.* **141,** 3575–3583.

Williams, C. M. M., and Coleman, J. W. (1995). Induced expression of mRNA for IL-5, IL-6, TNF-$\alpha$, MIP-2 and IFN-$\gamma$ in immunologically activated rat peritoneal mast cells: Inhibition by dexamethasone and cyclosporin A. *Immunology* **86,** 244–249.

Yano, H., Wershil, B. K., Arizono, N., and Galli, S. J. (1989). Substance P-induced augmentation of cutaneous vascular permeability and granulocyte infiltration in mice is mast cell dependent. *J. Clin. Invest.* **84,** 1276–1286.

Young, J. D.-E., Liu, C.-C., Butler, G., Cohn, Z. A., and Galli, S. J. (1987). Identification, purification, and characterization of a mast cell-associated cytolytic factor related to tumor necrosis factor. *Proc. Natl. Acad. Sci. U.S.A.* **84,** 9175–9179.

Zhang, Y., Ramos, B. F., and Jakschik, B. A. (1992). Neutrophil recruitment by tumor necrosis factor from mast cells in immune peritonitis. *Science* **258,** 1957–1959.

# Chapter 26

# Hepatocellular Autoantigens

Michael Peter Manns, Christian Straßburg, Maria Gracia Clemente, and
Petra Obermayer-Straub

*Division of Gastroenterology and Hepatology,
Medizinische Hochschule Hannover,
D-30623 Hannover, Germany*

## I. INTRODUCTION

Rapid progress has been made concerning the etiology and pathogenesis of chronic hepatitis. Three major hepatitis viruses have been identified as agents responsible for the induction of chronic hepatitis, i.e., hepatitis B, C, and D virus (Table I) (1). Furthermore the "syndrome" of autoimmune hepatitis which usually runs a chronic course has been defined more precisely (2), partly because of a molecular definition and analysis of hepatocellular autoantigens. Numerous autoantibodies have been described in liver diseases. This chapter summarizes the present knowledge of hepatocellular autoantigens as far as they are recognized by circulating autoantibodies and may be relevant as diagnostic markers, scientific tools, or candidates to be involved in pathogenesis. Some autoantibodies have clinical relevance since they are useful markers to differentiate subgroups of chronic hepatitis of presumed different etiology (1–5). Since we now not only diagnose but also treat some forms of chronic hepatitis according to specific etiological diagnoses, some of these autoantibodies are useful to distinguish autoimmune hepatitis from chronic viral hepatitis. This is important since autoimmune hepatitis benefits from immunosuppression while interferons which are given to patients with chronic viral hepatitis may cause deterioration (6).

## II. METHODOLOGICAL APPROACH TO IDENTIFY HEPATOCELLULAR AUTOANTIGENS

The first hint that immune mechanisms may play a significant role in liver diseases comes from the observation that a particular group of young women with hypergammaglobulinemia responds well to corticosteroids. This syndrome was later found to be associated with autoantibodies to nuclear antigens (ANA) (7). In viral

*Essentials of Mucosal Immunology*   Copyright © 1996 by Academic Press, Inc. All rights of reproduction in any form reserved.

TABLE I

CLASSIFICATION OF CHRONIC HEPATITIS ON THE BASIS OF ETIOLOGY

| Hepatitis type | HBsAg | HBV DNA | HDV antibody (HDV RNA) | HCV antibody (HCV RNA) | Autoantibodies |
|---|---|---|---|---|---|
| B | + | ± | − | − | — |
| D | + | − | + | − | 10–20% anti-LKM-3 |
| C | − | − | − | + | 2–10% anti-LKM-1 (*) |
| Autoimmune | | | | | |
|   Type 1 | − | − | − | − | ANA |
|   Type 2 | − | − | − | − | LKM-1 |
|   Type 3 | − | − | − | − | SLA/LP |
| Drug-induced | − | − | − | − | Some: ANA, LKM, LM |
| Cryptogenic | − | − | − | − | — |

hepatitis clinicians observed that patients with a deficient immune system produce high amounts of virus in their liver although biochemical and histological liver tissue damage was often marginal. This led to the assumption that the immune system and not the hepatitis B virus is mediating hepatocellular injury. Reactions against the patient's own liver had already been discussed at a very early stage, and tissue-infiltrating T lymphocytes viewed as primary candidates in liver cell destruction. However, the targets of autoimmunity remained unknown. Interest has focused on the characterization of autoantibodies circulating in the patients' blood. Of particular interest are autoantibodies that are specifically associated with liver diseases or that are directed against liver membrane constituents. However, most autoantibodies recognize intracellular antigens; as in other autoimmune diseases an important question is whether these intacellular antigens or parts of them (i.e., autoepitopes) are expressed on the cell surface and thus become targets for T-lymphocyte- or autoantibody-mediated cytotoxicity.

As in all fields of biological science, progress depends on methodological developments. Tools of molecular biology facilitated an identification and molecular analysis of hepatocellular autoantigens. First autoantibodies were determined by indirect techniques such as the LE (lupus erythematosus) cell phenomenon, then by complement fixation test to detect ANA. In the 1960s indirect immunofluorescence became a great advantage since this technique enabled investigators to localize the antigen to subcompartments of the cell, such as the nucleus, mitochondria, and cytoplasm. Further significant progress resulted from the advent of immunoblotting techniques in the mid 1980s. Mitochondrial and microsomal autoantigens became identified according to their appropriate molecular weight. The most recent development has been the application of molecular cloning. An increasing number of hepatocellular autoantigens have been identified after screening human liver cDNA libraries with human serum. These sera used for library screening have to be well characterized in terms of their monospecific reactivity to protein bands in immunoblotting (Western blotting). Isolation and sequencing of the cDNAs encoding these proteins facilitated the production of recombinant human autoantigens which are useful for epitope mapping and developing assays for auto-antibody testing. Furthermore recombinant antigens may be used to evaluate the antigen specificity of liver-derived T lymphocytes. Finally, isolated cDNAs facilitate investigations of the antigen's role in cell biology.

In principal there are two different approaches to identify hepatocellular autoantigens. In one approach, a particular antigen, already identified in another autoimmune disease or previously identified in an animal model, is purified biochemically and used in an assay for circulating autoantibody reactivity in patient sera. A different approach starts with the patients' serum, which is tested for reactivity toward autologous liver tissue. This second approach permits recognition of significant autoantibody reactivity, characterization of antibody titer and avidity, and identification of tissue autoantigens.

## III. AUTOANTIGENS OF THE HEPATOCELLULAR MEMBRANE

Antibodies against the liver plasma cell membrane are primary candidates to identify pathogenetically relevant autoantibodies. They may mediate liver cell damage by immunological mechanisms such as antibody-dependent cell-mediated cytotoxicity (ADCC). Another possibility would be that these antibodies identify structures expressed on the liver cell membrane that may be targets of cell-mediated immunity, in particular by cytotoxic T lymphocytes. In 1972, Meyer zum Büschenfelde and Miescher (8) prepared a crude antigen fraction from liver homogenate and identified a liver-specific component by heterologous antisera. McFarlane et al. (9) further purified this fraction and called it "liver specific lipoprotein (LSP)." The term "LSP" was misleading for such a crude fraction containing numerous proteins. McFarlane et al. (10) empirically identified the asialoglycoprotein receptor (ASGPR) as a liver-specific membrane-derived constituent of LSP. McFarlane et al. described increased titers for the anti ASGPR antibodies in patients with liver diseases. The occurrence of anti ASGPR antibodies is closely associated with autoimmune liver diseases although they may also be found in viral hepatitis (11). Results differ slightly depending on whether rodent or human tissue is used for antigen preparation. However, one has to consider that affinity-purified receptor protein is nonspecifically bound to ELISA plates. One would like to see other purified liver plasma cell membrane as constituents for control. The accumulated data on antiASGPR autoantibodies may be summarized as follows: anti-ASGPR occur in inflammatory liver diseases, and antibodies to human ASGPR seem to be rather specific for autoimmune hepatitis and primary biliary cirrhosis. Their titers decline if immunosuppressive therapy is effective. If they occur in viral hepatitis they decline in titer if interferon is effective. T lymphocytes of the CD4-positive T helper cell phenotype have been cloned from liver tissue that specifically proliferate in the presence of purified ASGPR. It was shown that these CD4-positive cells give help to peripheral blood lymphocytes to produce anti-ASGPR antibodies *in vitro*. ASGPR receptors are predominantly expressed on periportal hepatocytes, i.e., where the histological lesion of piecemeal necrosis is found. Recombinant ASGPR could not be used to map B-cell epitopes. However, the major epitope could be localized close to glycosylated areas of the ASGPR molecule (11). The roles of other membrane receptors remain to be analyzed as targets of autoimmunity.

## IV. NUCLEAR AUTOANTIGENS

Antinuclear antibodies (ANA) have been known for almost three decades to occur in chronic hepatitis. However, compared to the tremendous progress that has been achieved in the molecular analysis of ANA and their antigens in rheumatological diseases, basic data on ANA in liver disease are very limited. It is known that ANA in liver diseases are heterogeneous and that most of the specificities found in rheumatological disorders are also found in autoimmune hepatitis. This includes anti-DNA antibodies. Basic work is still necessary and modern molecular biological tools must be applied to determine whether a liver-specific nuclear antigen or an ANA associated with a particular liver disease exists. Recently, antibodies to a nuclear transcription factor, SP100, gained some attention (12). These antibodies were first identified by Western blotting using sera from patients with Sjögren's syndrome. Later it became obvious that the anti-SP100 antibodies have a particularly high association with primary biliary cirrhosis. Preliminary data also demonstrate close association with autoimmune hepatitis (12, 13).

Recently, our laboratory identified cyclin A as a major nuclear autoantigen in autoimmune liver diseases (14). We addressed this question since a nuclear antigen in systemic lupus erythematosus, i.e., proliferating cell nuclear antigen (PCNA) was previously called cyclin (15). It is now known to be an auxilliary protein for DNA polymerase delta. It is used as a marker for cell proliferation and it is highly expressed in regenerating liver tissue and in hepatocellular carcinoma. Furthermore, hepatitis B virus sequences were shown to be integrated into the cyclin A gene in a patient with hepatitis B-associated hepatocellular carcinoma (16).

Our data show that recombinant cyclin A is a major nuclear antigen in autoimmune liver diseases, i.e., autoimmune hepatitis and primary biliary cirrhosis. Future experiments are needed to investigate the membrane expression of cyclin A epitopes, the effect of anti-cyclin A antibodies on the antigen's function, the mapping of the B-cell epitope, and the evaluation of a potential T-cell response. It is also necessary to search for liver-specific nuclear antigens or ANA specificity associated with liver disease. Western blot experiments with nuclear cell extracts have to be performed to identify major nuclear autoantigens in liver diseases. Sera with high titers to these antigens should be used for screening human liver cDNA libraries.

## V. MICROSOMAL AUTOANTIGENS

In 1973 Rizzetto *et al.* (17) described autoantibodies by indirect immunofluorescence that stained the cytoplasma of liver and kidney tissue. Since the staining pattern was different from that of antimitochondrial antibodies and since in a complement fixation assay highest reactivity was seen with the microsomal fraction, these autoantibodies were termed "liver–kidney–microsomal antibodies." These antibodies were found to be associated with a particular subgroup of chronic hepatitis, also called autoimmune hepatitis type 2 (4) (Table II). These LKM-1 antibodies associated with autoimmune hepatitis type 2 had to be distinguished from LKM-2 antibodies which are associated with a particular drug-induced hepatitis caused by the diuretic drug tienilic acid (or ticrynafen) (18) (Table I). Ticrynafen was used in France and the United States and has now been withdrawn from the market. LKM-3 antibodies were identified by indirect immunofluorescence in a proportion of patients with chronic hepatitis D (19) (Table II). Further differentiation of autoantibody reactivity toward microsomal antigens was achieved with molecular techniques which will be described below. Recently a rare antimicrosomal autoantibody was observed in a dihydralazine-induced hepatitis and autoimmune hepatitis of children that predominantly stains the perivenous hepatocytes. Since the antibodies exclusively stain liver tissue they were termed liver–microsomal (LM) antibodies. Untill now the application of molecular biological techniques has permitted molecular characterization of most but not all of these microsomal antigens (Table II).

*TABLE II*

HETEROGENEITY OF MICROSOMAL AUTOANTIGENS

| Antibody | kDa | Target antigen | Disease association |
|---|---|---|---|
| LKM-1 | 50 | Cytochrome P450 2D6 | Autoimmune hepatitis type 2 (hepatitis C) |
| LKM-2 | 50 | Cytochrome P450 2C9 | Ticrynafen-induced hepatitis |
| LKM-3 | 55 | Family 1 UGT Family 2 UGT | Chronic hepatitis D (Autoimmune hepatitis type 2) |
| LM | 52 | Cytochrome P450 1A2 | Dihydralazine-induced hepatitis, autoimmune hepatitis, APS-1 |
| | 57 | Disulfide isomerase | Halothane-hepatitis |
| | 59 | Carboxylesterase | Halothane-hepatitis |
| | 59 | ? | Chronic hepatitis C |
| | 64 | ? | Autoimmune hepatitis |
| | 70 | ? | Chronic hepatitis C |

## VI. Cytochrome P450 IID6: Antigen of Liver–Kidney–Microsomal Antibodies Type 1 (LKM-1)

LKM-1 antibodies were identified and characterized by indirect immunofluorescence and complement fixation assay (17). Immunoblotting techniques showed that the major antigen was a protein of 50 kDa (20, 21). However, additional minor antigen bands were recognized by Western blot using human microsomes and sera from patients with chronic hepatitis (22, 23). Screening of human liver cDNA libraries and immunopurification led to the identification of human cytochrome P450 IID6 as the major 50-kDa microsomal LKM-1 antigen (22, 24, 25). This was confirmed by inhibition of enzyme function and affinity purification of human LKM-1 autoantibodies from recombinant cytochrome P450 IID6. Cytochrome P450 IID6 is a drug-metabolizing enzyme responsible for the metabolism of several classes of agents in man, including $\beta$-blockers, antiarhythmic drugs, and antidepressent drugs. Endogenous substrates are unknown. This enzyme is known for its profound genetic polymorphism. At least eight deficient alleles have been described (26). Up to 10% of the normal white population is deficient for drug metabolism mediated by P450 IID6, due to deficient alleles and consequent lack of expression of P450 IID6 protein in the liver. The molecular basis of this genetic polymorphism has been elucidated (26).

## VII. LKM-1 Autoantibodies Inhibit Cytochrome P450 IID6 Function *In Vitro* but Not *In Vivo*

Zanger *et al.* (24) have shown that sera from patients with LKM-1 autoantibodies inhibit the hydroxylation of bufuralol in isolated human liver microsomes. Later this was shown for sparteine metabolism (27). It can be concluded from these experiments that LKM-1 autoantibodies react with the active site of the enzyme and that obviously an expression of the P450 protein in the liver is a prerequisite for the induction of LKM-1 autoantibodies. The capacity of cytochrome P450 IID6-mediated drug metabolism in isolated microsomes correlates with the amount of P450 IID6 protein in these microsomes, as evidenced by Western blot analysis (24, 26). While bufuralol is an experimental $\beta$-blocker, the antiarhythmic drug sparteine can be used to measure the patients' phenotype for P450 IID6-mediated drug metabolism *in vivo*. This means that for the first time the function of an autoantigen could be measured *in vivo* (27). In their study the *in vivo* phenotype was evaluated at the time of a liver biopsy which had been obtained for diagnostic purposes. The P450 IID6 content was measured semiquantiatively by Western blotting (27). All of the more than 50 patients tested so far are extensive metabolizers for drug metabolism mediated by P450 IID6, and a poor metabolizer has not been found (unpublished data). Molecular studies have confirmed that poor metabolizers carry two of the defective alleles, resulting in a lack of P450 IID6 protein expression in the patients' liver, whereas the patients studied so far usually carry one defective and one wild-type allele (unpublished data). Because P450 II D6 activity remains in patients with anti-LKM-1 autoantibodies, it can be concluded that antibodies do not penetrate the intact liver cell membrane sufficiently to inhibit enzyme function *in vivo*. Similar studies, which evaluate the effect of an autoantibody on its autoantigen's function *in vivo* have not been performed for any other autoantigen to date.

## VIII. CYTOCHROME P450 IID6 MAY BE EXPRESSED ON THE HEPATOCELLULAR MEMBRANE

For many years expression on the plasma membrane was postulated to be crucial for an antigen's involvement in immunopathogenesis. Several years ago Lenzi *et al.* (28) demonstrated staining of LKM positive serum from patients with chronic hepatitis on the surface of rabbit hepatotcytes. After the identification of cytochrome P450 enzymes as targets of LKM-antibodies, this question was addressed again by Loeper *et al.* (29, 30). This group of investigators has presented data that support a plasma membrane expression of cytochrome P450 enzymes, among them cytochrome P450 IID6. These authors used isolated rat and human hepatocytes as well as isolated plasma membrane fractions. Indirect immunofluorescence, Western blotting, and immunoelectron microscopy with either patient serum or murine monoclonal antibodies were employed. Others, including our own group, were unable to demonstrate surface expression of cytochrome P450 IID6 on isolated viable hepatocytes using fluorescence-activated cell sorting (FACS) analysis or indirect immunofluorescence on hepatocytes (31, 32). Possibly the membrane expression of cytochrome P450 enzymes or fragments of them occur during the disease process mediated by inflammatory cytokines. These questions still need to be addressed experimentally, despite the difficulties involved.

## IX. CELLULAR IMMUNE RESPONSE TO CYTOCHROME P450 IID6

Since LKM-1 autoantibodies do not penetrate through the intact liver cell membrane sufficiently to inhibit enzyme function *in vivo,* and since tissue-infiltrating T lymphocytes are major components of piecemeal necrosis, it was logical to search for antigen-specific T lymphocytes in liver tissue. Löhr *et al.* (33) prepared 189 T-cell clones isolated from liver biopsies of four different patients with autoimmune hepatitis type 2. These T-cell clones were isolated by limiting dilution and propagated *in vitro* by recombinant IL-2. Four of these clones proliferated specifically in response to human recombinant cytochrome P450 IID6. These T lymphocytes expressed the helper T-cell phenotype and antigen-specific proliferation was inhibited by MHC class II monoclonal antibodies. In order to evaluate the pathogenetic significance of cellular immune reactions against cytochrome P450 IID6 it will be necessary to develop an autologous cytotoxicity system. It may also be necessary to express the P450 IID6 gene in cultured autologous cells such as fibroblasts.

## X. Cytochrome P450 IID6 Is Regulated Like a Negative Acute-Phase Protein

Little is known about how the expression of hepatocellular autoantigens is regulated. Since cytochrome P450 enzymes are markers of highly differentiated cells, it is understandable that P450 gene expression is absent in many hepatoma cell lines. Primary hepatocyte cultures often lose expression of cytochrome P450 enzymes early during cultivation. Specific entracellular matrix components, e.g., laminin, may help to maintain the expression of P450 proteins in isolated cultured hepatocytes (C. Trautwein et al., unpublished). Furthermore it seems necessary to evaluate whether cytokines, many of them synthesized locally by cells of the inflammatory infiltrate, modulate the expression of antigens. Initially we had choosen acute-phase mediators IL-1, IL-6, and TNFα (34). Administration of these recombinant cytokines to mice led to the pretranslational suppression of cytochrome P450 IID6 expression by up to 75% at 6 hr. Very recently this observation was confirmed by a different experimental approach, in which recombinant cytokines administered in vivo to mice diminished the metabolic ratio, i.e., the capacity to metabolize P450 IID6-dependent drugs (35) in vivo. In the meantime it became evident that several cytochrome P450 enzymes are regulated like negative acute phase reactants (36). Until now no cytokine has been identified that upregulates the expression of P450 proteins.

## XI. Genetics of LKM-1 Antibody-Associated Liver Disease

The data on genetics in liver diseases are still very limited. Progress has been made mainly in ANA-positive autoimmune hepatitis type 1 as summarized in a recent review (37). In whites there is a dual association of autoimmune hepatitis with HLA antigens, either with HLA DR3 or HLA DR4. Patients associated with HLA A1-B8-DR3 haplotype are younger, have a lower age at onset, relapse after treatment more frequently, and require liver transplatation more often compared to the HLA DR4-positive individuals with this disease. In Japan autoimmune hepatitis type 1 is predominantly associated with HLA DR4. However, serological markers associated with this genetic background have not been identified. Furthermore C4A gene deletions responsible for an increase in C4A-Q0 alleles was found in ANA positive autoimmune hepatitis type 1 (38, 39). C4A gene deletion seems to be in linkage disequilibrium with the HLA A1-B8-DR3 haplotype. An increased frequency of C4A-Q0 alleles was found in several other diseases with a presumed autoimmune background (37). In some of them, an infectious etiology is either discussed or already proven, such as in measle virus-induced subacute sclerosing panencephalitis (SSPE). Since C4 is involved in immune complex clearence and virus elimination this phenomenon may be involved in pathogenesis.

The preliminary analysis by others (4, 40) and our group (41) suggests that in LKM-1 antibody-associated liver disease there is an association with HLA DR3 and C4A-Q0. It is of interest whether the analysis of the genetic polymorphism of the autoantigen locus itself reveals an additional genetic predisposition. A PCR technology applying allele specific amplification enables us to address this question. Our own data and those of others (41,42) indicate that patients with LKM-1 autoantibodies are all extensive metabolizers, and suggest that these patients carry one defective and in addition one wild-type allele (41) possibly associated with HLA DR3 or another gene at the HLA locus. It may be hypothesized that a particular drug is metabolized by wild-type. P450 IID6 into a reactive metabolite or that an infection with a particular virus leads to a loss of tolerance against a mutant P450 IID6 through presentation of this autoantigen by a specific HLA allele expressed on the hepatocyte surface. Our future studies will examine this hypothesis.

## XII. RELATIONSHIP BETWEEN HEPATOTROPIC VIRUSES AND CYTOCHROME P450 IID6

Depending on the geographical origin, a variable proportion of patients with LKM-1 antibody-associated liver disease have signs of HCV infection. More than 90% of the patients in Japan (43) and Italy (44), about 50% in France (45) and Germany (46), and less than 10% in England (44) are hepatitis C antibody (anti-HCV) positive and the majority of them are also HCV RNA-positive. The involvement of HCV in immunopathogenesis is also supported by the observation that anti-GOR, an antibody to a HCV-associated nuclear antigen, is found only in patients with markers of hepatitis C virus infection. Interestingly the two LKM-1 antibody-associated patient populations differ clinically (45, 46). The HCV-negative patients are young, female predominance is striking, inflammatory activity is high, and response to immunosuppression is good. They represent genuine autoimmune hepatitis type 2. In contrast, the HCV-positive patients resemble chronic hepatitis C. Age at onset is above 40 years, inflammatory activity is low, response to corticosteroids is not convincing, and a majority of these patients do not require treatment since disease activity is low (46).

Recently there has been a debate whether anti-LKM-1 antibodies in HCV-positive autoimmune hepatitis type 2 recognize the 50-kDa cytochrome P450 IID6 antigen (47, 48) Manns et al. reported that the antigen is different from the 50-kDa antigen (49). In a previous publication we reported that some HCV-positive sera do not react with the recombinant human cytochrome P450 IID6 antigen, while the majority of anti-HCV and anti-LKM-1 positive sera from patients with chronic hepatitis recognize a larger epitope sequence of cytochrome P450 IID6

(49). Yamamoto *et al.* (50) confirmed and extended this observation. We reported that apart from the 50-kDa P450 IID6 antigen other proteins at 59 and 70 kDa are recognized by Western analysis (51). These proteins remain to be characterized at the molecular level. Patients who react with the 50- and 70-kDa antigens seem to have the best response to interferon-$\alpha$ treatment (51). We have investigated the possible association of a specific HCV strain or viral sequence with the induction of autoimmunity to microsomal antigens, among them cytochrome P450 IID6 (52). We found that HCV genotype II, according to the Okamoto classification (53), is the dominant strain in Italian and German patients with chronic hepatitis C and autoimmunity to LKM antigens (52). Since some sequence homology exists between the core, envelope, and NS5 region of the HCV and cytochrome P 450 IID6, we amplified and sequenced the appropriate regions of the HCV genome. The analysis of the viral genome isolated from anti-LKM-1- and anti-HCV-positive patients revealed no closer sequence homology. However, deletions in the envelope region of hepatitis C virus adjacent to the homology region were detected only in anti-LKM-1-positive patients and not in patients with chronic hepatitis C without autoimmunity.

Because it is still unknown what triggers autoimmune hepatitis type 2, i.e., anti-LKM-1-positive, HCV-negative young females with high disease activity and good response to immunosuppression, we investigated possible sequence homologies between cytochrome P450 IID6 and hepatotropic viruses. We found that the major B-cell epitope on cytochrome P450 IID6 (49), an eight-amino acid peptide, has a high sequence homology with the immediate early protein of the herpes simplex virus type I (Fig. 1). LKM-1 antibodies affinity-purified from a synthetic peptide with the sequence of this epitope react with the cellular cytochrome P450 IID6 and the viral protein. Indirect clinical evidence supports this hypothesis: We observed a family with identical female twins, 13 years old (54). Only the child suffering from autoimmune hepatitis type 2 and in addition from ulcerative colitis had signs of herpes simplex virus type I (HSV-1) infection. No other family member including the healthy twin sister had serological evidence of HSV or HCV infection. However, the twins both carried the autoimmune haplotype A1-B8-DR3-C4A-Q0. Furthermore, we observed a child with fulminant hepatic failure and LKM antibodies that was high titer positive for IgM herpes simplex virus antibodies (Tillmann *et al.*, unpublished). Therefore herpes simplex virus could be a candidate in triggering this autoimmune liver disease.

### XIII. CYTOCHROME P450 IIC9—THE MAJOR ANTIGEN OF LIVER–KIDNEY–MICROSOMAL ANTIBODIES TYPE 2 (LKM-2)

Another type of LKM antibody was observed in a drug-induced hepatitis caused by the diuretic drug tienilic acid. This autoantibody was termed LKM-2 (55). It was never seen in Germany since the drug had only been prescribed in France and

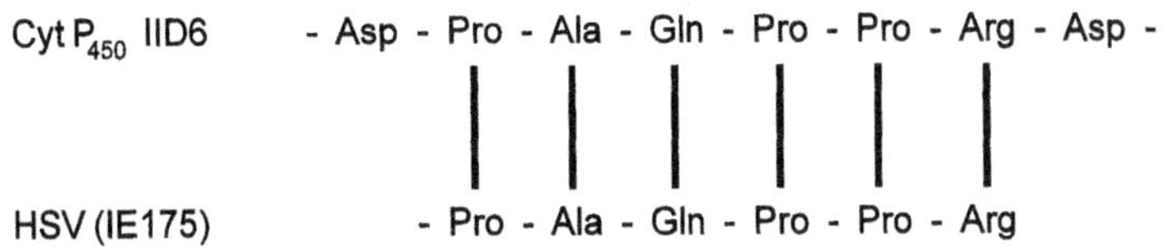

Cyt P$_{450}$ IID6     - Asp - Pro - Ala - Gln - Pro - Pro - Arg - Asp -

HSV (IE175)     - Pro - Ala - Gln - Pro - Pro - Arg

FIGURE 1. Sequence homology between the major B-cell epitope of cytochrome P450 IID6 (LKM-1 – antigen) and the immediate early protein 175 (IE 175) of herpes simplex virus type 1 (HSV). Modified according to Ref. (49).

the United States. Once the drug is withdrawn liver disease subsides and LKM-2 antibody titers decline and finally become negative. LKM-2 antigen became the first cytochrome P450 enzyme to be identified as an autoantigen (56), i.e., cytochrome P450 IIC9. This drug-induced liver disease may become a model for immune-mediated drug-induced liver disease (Fig. 2).

Thus, a drug, e.g., tienilic acid, is metabolized by the cytochrome P450 enzyme (P450 IIC9). The reactive metabolite binds covalently to the metabolizing enzyme (P450 IIC9). Now cytochrome P450 IIC9 acts as an autoantigen and induces anti LKM-2 antibodies. However, there are still questions left to be answered, such as whether LKM-2 autoantibodies themselves mediate liver cell necrosis. A membrane expression has already been postulated for P450 IIC9 (29,30).

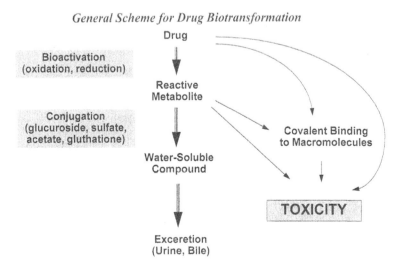

General Scheme for Drug Biotransformation

Drug

Bioactivation (oxidation, reduction)

Reactive Metabolite

Conjugation (glucuroside, sulfate, acetate, gluthatione)

Covalent Binding to Macromolecules

Water-Soluble Compound

TOXICITY

Exceretion (Urine, Bile)

FIGURE 2. Hypothesis for autoimmunity against cytochrome P450 enzymes in drug-induced hepatitis. Modified according to Refs. (71,74).

## XIV. CYTOCHROME P450 IA2: TARGET OF LIVER MICROSOMAL ANTIBODIES (LM)

The antihypertensive drug dihydralazine may lead to an immune-mediated drug-induced hepatitis associated with autoantibodies directed against periportal hepatocytes but not reacting with other tissue including the kidney. This antigen was identified as cytochrome P450 IA2 (57). At the same time autoantibodies against P450IA2 were found in a child with idiopathic autoimmune hepatitis (58,59). Cytochrome P450 IA2 is highly inducible by dioxin. In man it is responsible for the metabolism of phenacetin. It is unknown whether this enzyme is genetically polymorphic. Anti-P450 IA2 antibodies also inhibit enzyme function *in vitro*. The B-cell epitope has not been identified yet. Recently cytochrome P450 IA2 was identified as a major hepatocellular autoantigen in autoimmune polyendocrine syndrome type 1 (APS 1) (60). This genetically determined multiorgan autoimmune process mainly affects endocrine organs including the adrenal, thyroid, parathyroid, and skin. However, in 10% of these patients the liver is involved. If the syndrome is associated with adrenal insufficiency the patient's serum usually contains autoantibodies that react with adrenal P450 enzymes that are crucial for corticosteroid synthesis. Thus autoantibodies are associated with this syndrome that specifically react with the enzymes that are involved in the metabolism of hormones whose deficiency is responsible for the clinical manifestations. In this context it is of particular interest that a liver-specific P450 is recognized by autoantibodies occurring in this syndrome once the liver is involved (60). Retrospectively, the child described in 1990 (58, 59) with anti-P450 IA2 antibodies presumably had APS-1 syndrome, or at least suffered from multiple skin lesions; his brother had died at the age of 8 from Addison's disease. Studies are in progress that further elucidate this relationship (P. Obermayer-Straub *et al.*, unpublished).

## XV. UDP-GLUCURONOSYLTRANSFERASES: A NEW FAMILY OF HEPATOCELLULAR AUTOANTIGENS AND TARGET OF LKM-3 AUTOANTIBODIES

In their original report Crivelli *et al.* (19) observed in 11 of their 81 (13%) chronic hepatitis D carriers serum antibodies to the cytoplasms of hepatocytes and proximal renal tubules. The strongest reaction was seen with human and primate tissue. In tissue from other animal species (ox, pig, rabbit, and rat) the fluorescence intensity declined progressively. In addition to liver and kidney, weak reactivity was seen with pancreas, adrenal gland, thyroid, and stomach, whereas reactivity of LKM-1 and LKM-2 is restricted to liver and kidney tissue (17). These antibodies are now called LKM-1, characterize autoimmune hepatitis type 2 (4) and mainly recognize cytochrome P450 IID6 (22, 24, 25). These LKM-1 antibodies may also occur in some cases with hepatitis C, i.e., around 2%, and rarely in immune-mediated halothane hepatitis.

Recently our laboratory identified and characterized the microsomal antigens in hepatitis D. Immunochemical characterization with one- and two-dimensonal immunoblotting revealed that the sera react with an antigen around 55 kDa which is weakly expressed in neonatal liver and which is inducible by various agents such as dioxin, phenobarbital, and rifampicin (61). The isoelectric point of the antigen is around 8. When testing purified cytochrome P450s the highest reactivity was seen with cytochrome P450 IIIA6. However, when testing the LKM-3 sera against recombinant P450 IIIA6 a negative result was obtained.

Finally, cloning of a human liver cDNA library revealed a cDNA that encodes the major LKM-3 antigen associated with hepatitis D (61). The derived fusion protein reacted specifically with LKM-3 sera. The sequence of this cDNA was highly homologous to a family one UDP-glucuronosyltransferase. Testing several recombinant family one and two recombinant proteins revealed that the major autoepitope is expressed on exon 2–5 of family one UDP-glucuronosyltransferases (UGT). These exons (2 to 5) are common for all family one UGTs while exon one is unique and determines specific function and inducibility (Fig. 3). Some sera react in addition with a minor epitope on family two UDP-glucuronosyltransferases.

To evaluate the clinical relevance of recombinant UGT proteins as diagnostic reagents for the detection of LKM-3 antibodies we applied an immunoblotting technique with rabbit recombinant UGT 1.6. All sera obtained from patients with hepatitis D that were positive for LKM-3 antibodies by immunofluorescence also reacted positive for anti-UGT. Only 1 out of 11 LKM-1 sera from patients with

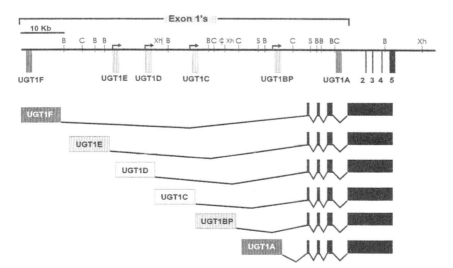

FIGURE 3. Gene locus for family one UDP-glucuronosyltransferases according to Ritter *et al.* (72).

autoimmune hepatitis type 2 was positive for anti-UGT reactivity while all the other sera from many hepatic and nonhepatic diseases were negative. These sera included material from patients with hepatitis D that were negative for LKM antibodies, hepatitis C (either LKM-positive or -negative), hepatitis B, autoimmune hepatitis type 1 and 3, primary biliary cirrhosis, primary sclerosing cholangitis, and lupus erythematosus.

Thus the major LKM-3 autoepitope is expressed on exon 2–5 of family one UDP-glucuronosyltransferases, and a minor epitope is localized on family two UDP-glucuronosyltransferase. UDP-glucuronosyltransferases become the first enzymes of phase II drug metabolism to be identified as human autoantigens (Fig. 3). Autoimmunity against UDP-glucuronosyltransferases may be another good model for the study of virus-induced autoimmunity in man. In this context the membrane expression of UGT proteins has to be evaluated, as does the inhibitory activity of these autoantibodies on UGT function. Finally, the T-cell response to these proteins has to be elucidated.

Concerning the diagnostic relevance of anti-UGT antibodies, their occurrence will need to be correlated with disease activity, level of HDV replication, treatment response, and prognosis. Even if anti-UGT are only secondary phenomena and are not related to pathogenesis, they may become useful diagnostic tools for the diagnosis and management of patients with chronic hepatitis D. It is of particular interest that autoimmunity is a common phenomenon in hepatitis D while autoimmunity only rarely occurs in hepatitis B virus infection alone. The relationship between autoimmunity to UDP-glucuronosyltransferases and the phase I enzymes of drug metabolism, i.e., cytochrome P450 enzymes, needs to be investigated in detail. Preliminary evidence indicates a molecular relationship between autoimmunities to phase I and phase II enzymes of drug metabolism (Fig. 4). Several other autoantibodies occur in chronic hepatitis D. Autoantibodies against forestomach basal layer cells and stellate epithelial cells of the thymus seem to react against an identical antigen of 46 kDa which is expressed in both tissues (62). This 46-kDa antigen awaits molecular identification. Conceivably, it is another enzyme involved in the metabolism of environmental and endogenous substrates (63,64).

## XVI. Cytosolic Autoantigens

In 1987 antibodies to a soluble liver antigen (SLA) were described as a constituent of the cytosol (3). They could be identified by enzyme-linked immunosorbent assay or radioimmunoassay but not by immunofluorescence. They seem to recognize cytokeratins (65). These cytosolic antibodies may help to identify patients with autoimmune hepatitis that are negative for other autoantibodies which are detectable by immunofluorescence (3,5,66,67). Therefore they were used to identify another subgroup of autoimmune hepatitis. Antibodies with similar diagnostic significance directed against a cytosolic component of liver and pancreas tissue

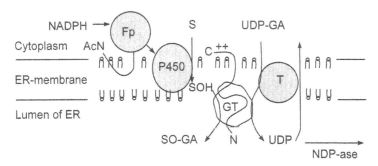

***FIGURE 4.*** Molecular relationship between cytochrome P450 enzymes (P450) (autoantigens LKM-1 = P450IID6, LKM2 = P450 IIC9, LM = P450IA2) and UDP-glucuronosyltransferases (T) (autoantigen LKM-3 = UGT-family 1) within the membranes of the endoplasmatic reticulum of hepatocytes. Modified according to Ref. (73).

were also described (68). The molecular identification still has to be achieved for LC1 and LC2 antigen (69,70), antibodies which are also directed against cytosolic components, and detected by imunofluorescence. Their identity is unknown. However, they frequently occur together with LKM-1 antibodies (69,70).

## XVII. Discussion

Significant progress was made in recent years concerning the molecular identification of hepatocellular autoantigens. This was facilitated by technical developments such as molecular cloning. Several liver diseases are associated with a significant number of autoantibodies. Among these diseases are autoimmune hepatitis, primary biliary cirrhosis, and primary sclerosing cholangitis. The etiology of all these diseases of presumed autoimmune background is unknown. It remains to be determined whether autoantibodies specifically associated with these diseases can give us any clues toward an etiology, e.g., via molecular mimicry between the sequence of B- and T-cell epitopes of these autoantigens and infectious agents. Furthermore, it needs to be determined whether a T-cell response against such constituents of the liver cell is pathogentically relevant. In addition, these autoantibodies may help to identify subsets of these syndromes which share a common response to specific treatment, e.g., immunosuppressive agents, interferons, or bile acids. Furthermore particular autoantibodies such as LKM-1 and LKM-3 occur in association with a proportion of patients with either hepatitis C or D. It has to be investigated whether autoimmunity against these self antigens contributes to tissue damage in these viral infections of the liver or whether these autoantibodies again identify subsets of liver diseases with a particular response to treatment, e.g., interferons versus corticosteroids. Finally, hepatitis C and hepatitis D may provide clinical models useful for the study of virus-induced autoimmunity in man.

Like many other autoantigens which have already been identified, hepatocellular autoantigens are intracellular enzymes that are inhibited by their autoantibodies *in vitro*. These autoantibodies react with conserved regions of their molecules which are usually active sites. In view of the fact that most of the major hepatocellular autoantigens are not organ-specific, it is not clear why the disease is usually restricted to the liver. Possibly these antigens or parts of them are exclusively expressed on the surface of hepatocytes. Alternatively, a specific activation of the immune system via specific HLA molecules only occurs in the liver.

Nevertheless, naturally occuring autoantibodies in the serum of patients with chronic hepatitis may be used as scientific tools to study the nature and biology of these antigens. Autoantibodies, in contrast to murine monoclonal antibodies, usually react with conserved regions of these molecules and often inhibit the function of their antigen *in vitro*. As has been shown for the LKM-1 antigen, cytochrome P450 IID6, these autoantibodies do not sufficiently penetrate the intact liver cell membrane to inhibit the functions of these cytoplasmic antigens *in vivo*. These antibodies—as scientific tools—may help us to analyze the relationship between structure and function of these proteins. This may be of particular interest in the newly discovered hepatocellular autoantigens of hepatitis D, e.g., the UDP-glucuronosyltranserases. The UGT supergene family is still poorly characterized, presumably due to the lack of good monoclonal antibodies. Hopefully, anti-UGT (anti-LKM-3) antibodies in hepatitis D may be as useful as some antinuclear antibodies in lupus erythematosus to study these aspects of cell biology. It seems to be a matter of time until such autoantibodies help to identify as yet unknown proteins which significantly contribute to liver cell function

## ACKNOWLEDGMENT

Our work was supported by the Deutsche Forschungsgemeinschaft SFB 244.

## REFERENCES

1. Desmet, V., Gerber, M. A., Hoofnagle, J. H., Manns, M., and Scheuer, P. (1994). Classification of chronic hepatitis: Diagnosis, grading and staging. *Hepatology (Baltimore)* **19**, 1513–1520.
2. Johnson, P. J., McFarlane, I. G., Alvarez, F., *et al.* (1987). Meeting report of the international autoimmune hepatitis group. *Hepatology* **7**, 1372–1375.
3. Manns, M., Gerken, G., Kyriatsoulis, A., Staritz, M., and Meyer zum Büschenfelde, K.-H. (1987). Characterization of a new subgroup of autoimmune chronic active hepatitis by autoantibodies against a soluble liver antigen, *Lancet* **1**, 292–294.
4. Homberg, J. C., Abuaf, N., Bernard, O., Islam, S., Alvarez, F., Khalil, S. H., Poupon, R., Darnis, F., Levy, V.-G., Grippon, P., Opolon, P., Bernuau, J., Benhamou, J.-P., and Alagille, D. (1987). Chronic active hepatitis associated with anti-liver/kidney microsomes antibody type I: A second type of "autoimmune hepatitis". *Hepatology (Baltimore)* **197**, 1333–1339.
5. Czaja, A. J., and Manns, M. P. (1995). The validity and importance of subtypes in autoimmune hepatitis: a point of view. *Am. J. Gastroenterol.* **90**, 1206–1211.
6. Ruiz-Moreno, M., Rua, M. J., Carreno, V., Quiroga, J. A., Manns, M., and Meyer zum Büschen-

felde, K.-H. (1991). Autoimmune chronic active hepatitis type 2 manifested during interferon therapy in children. *J. Hepatol.* **12,** 265–266.

7. Mackay, I.R., Taft, C. O., and Cowling, D. S. (1956). Lupoid hepatitis. *Lancet* **2,** 1323–1326.

8. Meyer zum Büschenfelde, K.-H., and Miescher, P. A. (1972). Liver specific antigens, purification and characterization. *Clin. Exp. Immunol.* **10,** 89–102.

9. McFarlane, I. G., Wojcika, M. B., Zucker, G. M., and Eddlestone, A.L. W. F. (1977). Purification and characterization of human liver-specific membrane lipoprotein (LSP). *Clin. Exp. Immunol.* **27,** 381.

10. McFarlane, I. G., McFarlane, B. M., Major, G. N., Tolley, P., and Willams, R. (1985). Identification of the hepatic asialoglycoprotein receptor (hepatic lectin) as a component of liver specific membrane lipoprotein (LSP). *Clin. Exp. Immunol.* **55,** 347–354.

11. Poralla, T., Treichel, V., Löhr, H., and Fleischer, B. (1991). The asialoglycoprotein receptor as target structure in autoimmune liver disease. *Semin. Liver Dis.* **11,** 215–222.

12. Szoztecki, C., Krippner, H., Penner, E., and Bautz, F. A. (1987). Autoimmune sera recognize a 100 kDa nuclear protein antigen (SP-100). *Clin. Exp. Immunol.* **68,** 108–116.

13. Szostecki, C., Guldner, H. H., Netter, H. J., and Will, H. (1990). Isolation and characterization of a cDNA encoding a human nuclear antigen predominantly recognized by autoantibodies from patients with primary biliary cirrhosis. *J. Immunol.* **145,** 4338–4347.

14. Strassburg, C. P., Alex, B., Zindy, F., Gerken, G., Lüttig, B., Meyer zum Büschenfelde, K.-H., Bréchot, C., and Manns, M. P. (1995). Identification of cyclin A as a molecular target of antinuclear antibodies (ANA) in autoimmune liver diseases. *J. Hepatol.* **23**(Suppl.1), 127.

15. Bravo, R., Rainer, F., Blundell, R. A., and Macdonald Bravo, H. (1987). Cyclin/PCNA is the auxiliary protein of DNA polymerase delta. *Nature (London)* **326,** 515–517.

16. Wang, J., Chenivesse, X., Henglein, B., and Brechot, C. (1990). Hepatitis B virus integration in a cyclin A gene in hepatocellular carcinoma. *Nature (London)* **343,** 555–557.

17. Rizzetto, M., Swana, G., and Doniach, D. (1973). Microsomal antibodies in active chronic hepatitis and other disorders. *Clin. Exp. Immunol.* **15,** 331–344.

18. Homberg, J. C., Andre, C., and Abuaf, N. (1984). A new anti-liver/kidney microsome antibody (anti.LKM2) in tienilic acid-induced hepatitis. *Clin. Exp. Immunol.* **55,** 561–570.

19. Crivelli, O., Lavarini, C., Chiaberge, E., Amoroso, A., Farci, P., Negro, F., and Rizzetto, M. (1983). Microsomal autoantibodies in chronic infection with the HBsAg associated delta (d) agent. *Clin. Exp. Immunol.* **54,** 232–238.

20. Alvarez, F., Bernard, O., Homberg, J. C., and Kreibich, G. (1985). Anti-liver kidney microsomes antibody recognizes a 50,000 molecular weight protein of the endoplasmic reticulum. *J. Exp. Med.* **161,** 1231–1236.

21. Kyriatsoulis, A., Manns, M., Gerken, G., Lohse, A. W., Ballhausen, W., Reske, K., and Meyer zum Büschenfelde, K.-H. (1987). Distinction between natural and pathological autoantibodies by immunoblotting and densitometric subtraction: Liver-kidney-microsomal antibody (LKM) positive sera identify multiple antigens in human liver tissue. *Clin. Exp. Immunol.* **79,** 53–60.

22. Manns, M., Johnson, E. F., Griffin, K. J., Tan, E. M., and Sullivan, K. F. (1989). The major target antigen of liver kidney microsomal autoantibodies in idiopathic autoimmune hepatitis is cytochrome P450 db1. *J. Clin. Invest.* **83,** 1066–1072.

23. Codoner-Franch, P., Paradis, K., Gueguen, M., Bernard, O., Amar-Costesec, A., and Alvarez, F. (1989). A new antigen recognized by anti-liver-kidney-microsome antibody (LKMA). *Clin. Exp. Immunol.* **75,** 354–358.

24. Zanger, U. M., Hauri, H. P., Loeper, J., Homberg, J. C., and Meyer, U. A. (1988). Antibodies against human cytochrome P-450db1 in autoimmune hepatitis type II. *Proc. Natl. Acad. Sci. U.S.A.* **85,** 8256–8260.

25. Gueguen, M., Yamamoto, A. M., Bernard, O., and Alvarez, F. (1989). Anti-liver kidney microsome antibody type 1 recognizes human cytochrome P450 db 1. *Biochem. Biophys. Res. Commun.* **159,** 542–547.

26. Gonzales, F. J., Skoda, R. C., Kimura, S., *et al.* (1988). Characterization of the common genetic defect in humans deficient in debrisoquine metabolism. *Nature (London)* **331**, 442–446.

27. Manns, M., Zanger, U., Gerken, G., Sullivan, K. F., Meyer zum Büschenfelde, K.-H., Meyer, U. A., and Eichelbaum, M. (1990). Patients with type II autoimmune hepatitis express functionally intact cytochrome P450db1 that is inhibited by LKM-1 autoantibodies *in vitro* but not *in vivo*. *Hepatology (Baltimore)* **12**, 127–132.

28. Lenzi, M., Bianchi, F. B., Cassani, F., and Pisi, E. (1984). Liver cell surface expression of the antigen reacting with liver kidney microsomal antibody (LKM). *Clin. Exp. Immunol.* **55**, 36–40.

29. Loeper, J., Descatoire, V., Maurice, M., Beaune, P., Houssin, D., Belghiti, J., Feldmann, G., and Pessayre, D. (1990). Presence of cytochrome P450 on human hepatocyte plama membrane. Recognition by several autoantibodies. *Hepatology (Baltimore)* **12**, 909 (Abstract).

30. Loeper, J., Descatoire, V., Maurice, M., Beaune, A., Belghiti, J., Houssin, D., Ballet, F., Feldmann, G., Guengerich, F. P., and Pessayre, D. (1993). Cytochrome P-450 in human hepatocyte plasma membrane: Recognition by several autoantibodies. *Gastroenterology* **104**, 203–216.

31. Yamamoto, A. M., Mura, C., De Lemos-Chirandini, C., Krishnamoorthy, R., and Alvarez, F. (1993). Cytochrome P450IID6 recognized by LKM1 antibody is not exposed on the surface of hepatocytes. *Clin. Exp. Immunol.* **92**, 381–390.

32. Trautwein, C., Gerken, G., Löhr, H., Meyer zum Büschenfelde, K.-H., and Manns, M. (1993). Lack of surface expression for the B-cell autoepitope of cytochrome P450 IID6: Evidence by flow cytometry. *Z. Gastroenterol.* **31**, 225–230.

33. Löhr, H., Manns, M., Kyriatsoulis, A., Lohse, A. W., Trautwein, C., Meyer zum Büschenfelde, K.-H., and Fleischer, B., (1991). Clonal analysis of liver infiltrating T cells in patients with chronic active hepatitis (AI-CAH). *Clin. Exp. Immunol.* **84**, 297–302.

34. Trautwein, C., Ramadori, G., Gerken, G., Meyer zum Büschenfelde, K.-H., and Manns, M. (1992). Regulation of cytochrome P450 IID by acute phase mediators in C3H/HeJ mice. *Biochem. Biophys. Res. Commun.* **182**, 617–623.

35. Orishiki, M., Nishioka, M., Tsuneoka, Y., Matsuo, Y., and Ichikawa, Y. (1992). Human CYP2D6 gene in chronic liver disease. Symposium: "Immunology and the Liver" Basel, October 18–20, 1992, Abstract No. 161.

36. Razzak, Z. A., Loyer, P., Corcos, L., Fautrel, A., Gautier, A., Turlin, B., Beaune, P., and Guillouzo, A. (1993). Cytokines down-regulated expression of various cytochromes P-450 in human hepatocytes cultures. *Hepatology* **18**, 130A.

37. Manns, M., and Krüger, M. (1994). Genetics in liver diseases. *Gastroenterology* **106**, 1676–1697.

38. Vergani, D., Wells, L., Larcher, V. F. *et al.* (1985). Genetically determined low C4: A predisposing factor to autoimmune chronic active hepatitis. *Lancet* **2**, 294–298.

39. Scully, L. J., Toze, C., Sengar, D. P. S., and Goldstein, R. (1993). Early-onset autoimmune hepatitis is associated with a C4A gene deletion. *Gastroenterology* **104**, 1478–1484.

40. Lenzi, M., Mantovani, W., Cataleta, M., Basllardini, G., Cassani, F., Giostra, F., Muratori, L., and Bianchi, F. B. (1992). HLA typing in autoimmune hepatitis (AI-CAH) type 2. *J. Hepatol.* **16**, 59.

41. Manns, M. P., Jentzsch, M., Mergener, K., Gerken, G., Thiers, V., Brechot, C., Meyer zum Büschenfelde, K.-H., and Eichelbaum, M. (1990). Discordant manifestation of LKM-1 antibody positive autoimmune hepatitis in identical twins. *Hepatology (Baltimore)* **12**, 840.

42. Yamamoto, A. M., Mura, C., Morales, M. G., Bernard, O., Krishnamoorthy, R., and Alvarez, F. (1992). Study of CYP2D6 gene with autoimmune hepatitis and P450 IID6 autoantibodies. *Clin. Exp. Immunol.* **87**, 251–255.

43. Miyachi, K. (1992). Personal communication.

44. Lenzi, M. Johnson, P. J., McFarlane, I. G., Ballardini, G., Smith, H. M., McFarlane, B. M., Bridger, C., Vergani, D., Bianchi, F. B., and Williams, R. (1991). Antibodies to hepatitis C virus in autoimmune liver disease; evidence for geographical heterogenity. *Lancet* **338**, 277–280.

45. Lunel, F., Abuaf, N., Frangeul, L., Grippon, P., Perrin, M., Le Coz, Y., Valla, D., Borotto, E.,

Yamamoto, A.-M., Huraux, L.-M., Opolon, P., and Homberg, J.-C. (1992). Liver/kidney microsomes antibody type 1 and hepatitis C virus infection. *Hepatology (Baltimore)* **16**, 630–636.

46. Michel, G., Ritter, A., Gerken, G., Meyer zum Büschenfelde, K.-H., Decker, R., and Manns, M. (1992). Anti-GOR and hepatitis C virus in autoimmune liver disease. *Lancet* **339**, 267–269.

47. Vergani, D., and Mieli-Vergani, G. (1993). Type II autoimmune hepatitis. What is the role of the hepatitis C virus? *Gastroenterology* **104**, 1870–1873.

48. Ma, Y., Lenzi, M., Gäken, J., Thomas, M. G., Farzaneh, F., Ballardini, G., Cassani, F., Mieli-Vergani, G., Bianchi, F. B., and Vergani, D. (1992). The target antigen of liver kidney microsomal antibody is different in type II autoimmune chronic active hepatitis and chronic hepatitis C virus infection. *J. Hepatol.* **16**, 4.

49. Manns, M. P., Griffin, K. J., Sullivan, K. F., and Johnson, E. F. (1991). LKM-1 autoantibodies recognize a short linear sequence in P450 IID6. *J. Clin. Invest.* **88**, 1370–1378.

50. Yamamoto, A. M., Cresteil, D., Homberg, J. C., and Alvarez, F. (1993). Characterization of anti-liver-kidney microsome antibody (anti-LKM1) from hepatitis C virus-positive and -negative sera. *Gastroenterology* **104**, 1762–1767.

51. Durazzo, M., Philipp, T., van Pelt, F. N. A. M., Lüttig, B., Borgesio, E., Michel, G., Schmidt, E., Loges, S., Rizzetto, M., and Manns, M. P. (1995). Heterogeneity of microsomal autoantibodies (LKM) in chronic hepatitis C and D virus infection. *Gastroenterology* **108**, 455–462.

52. Michitaka, K., Durazzo, M., Tillmann, H. L., Walker, D., Philipp, T., and Manns, M. P. (1994). Analysis of hepatitis C virus genome in patients with autoimmune hepatitis type 2. *Gastroenterology* **106**, 1603–1610.

53. Okamoto, H., Sugiyama, Y., Okada, S., *et al.* (1992). Typing hepatitis C virus by polymerase chain reaction with type-specific primers: Application to clinical survays and tracing infectious sources. *J. Gen. Virol.* **73**, 673–679.

54. Manns, M. P., Kaletzko, S., Löhr, H., Borchard, F., Rittner, C., Meyer zum Büschenfelde, K.-H., and Eichelbaum, M. (1990). Discordant manifestation of LKM-1 antibody positive autoimmune hepatitis in identical twins. *Hepatology* **12**, 840.

55. Homberg, J. C., Andre, C., and Abuaf, N. (1984). A new anti-liver-kidney microsome antibody (anti-LKM2) in tienilic acid-induced hepatitis. *Clin. Exp. Immunol.* **55**, 561–570.

56. Beaune, P., Dansette, P. M., Mansuy, D., Kiffel, L., Finck, M., Amar, C., and Leroux, J. P. (1987). Human antiendoplasmatic reticulum autoantibodies appearing in a drug-induced hepatitis are directed against a human liver cytochrome P-450 that hydroxylates the drug. *Proc. Natl. Acad. Sci. U.S.A.* **84**, 551–555.

57. Bourdi, M., Larrey, D., Nataf, J., Bernuau, J., Pessayre, D., Iwasaki, M., Guengerich, F. P., and Beaune, P. (1990). Anti-liver endoplasmatic reticulum autoantibodies are directed against human cytochrome P450 IA2. *J. Clin. Invest.* **85**, 1967–1973.

58. Sacher, M., Blümel, P., Thaler, H., and Manns, M. (1990). Chronic active hepatitis associated with vitiligo, nail dystrophy, alopecia, and a new variant of LKM antibodies. *J. Hepatol.* **10**, 364–369.

59. Manns, M. P., Griffin, K. J., Quattrochi, L. C., Sacher, M., Thaler, H., Tukey, R. H., and Johnson, E. F. (1990). Identification of cytochrome P450 IA2 as a human autoantigen. *Arch. Biochem. Biophys.* **280**, 229–232.

60. Clemente, M. G., Obermayer-Straub, P., Meloni, A., Tukey, R. H., Cao, A., DeVirgiliis, S., and Manns, M. P. (1995). Cytochrome P450 1A2 as the hepatocellular autoantigen in autoimmune polyendocrine syndrome type 1. *J. Hepatol.* **23**(Suppl. 1), 126.

61. Philipp, T., Durazzo, M., Trautwein, C., Alex, B., Straub, P., Lamb, G., Johnson, E. F., Tukey, R. H., and Manns, M. P. (1994). LKM-3 autoantibodies in chronic hepatitis D recognize the UDP-glucuronosyltransferases. *Lancet* **344**, 578–581.

62. Philipp, T., Straub, P., Durazzo, M., Tukey, R. H., and Manns, M. P. (1995). Molecular analysis of autoantigens in hepatitis D. *J. Hepatol.* **22**(Suppl. 2), 132–135.

63. Buti, M., Amengual, M. J., Esteban, R., Pujol, A., Jardi, R., Allende, H., Roget, M., Casacoberta,

J. M., Guardia, J., and Rodriguez, J. L. (1989). Serological profile of tissue autoantibodies during acute and chronic delta hepatitis. *J. Hepatol.* **9**, 345–350.

64. Amengual, M. J., Catalfamo, M., Pujol, A., Juarez, C., Gelpi, C., and Rodriguez, J. L. (1989). Autoantibodies in chronic delta virus infection recognize a common protein of 46 kD in rat forestomach basal cell layer and stellate thymic epithelial cells. *Clin. Exp. Immunol.* **78**, 80–84.

65. Wächter, B., Kyriatsoulis, A., Lohse, A. W., Gerken, W., Meyer zum Büschenfelde, K.-H., and Manns, M. (1990). Characterization of liver cytokeratin as a major target antigen of anti-SLA antibodies. *J. Hepatol.* **11**, 232–239.

66. Czaja, A., Manns, M. P., and Homburger, H. (1992). Frequency and significance of antibodies to liver/kidney microsome type 1 in adults with chronic active hepatitis. *Gastroenterology* **103**, 1290–1295.

67. Czaja, A. J., Carpenter, H. A., and Manns, M. P. (1993). Antibodies to soluble liver antigen, P450IID6, and mitochondrial complexes in chronic hepatitis. *Gastroenterology* **105**, 1522–1528.

68. Berg, P. A., and Stachemessar, E. (1981). Hypergammaglobulinamische chronisch aktive Hepatitis mit Nachweis komplement-bindender partiell leberspezifischer Antikörper. *Verg. Dtsch. Ges. Inn. Med.* **87**, 921.

69. Martini, E., Abuaf, N., Cavalli, F., Durand, V., Johanet, C., and Homberg, J. C. (1988). Antibody to liver cytosol (anti-LC1) in patients with autoimmune chronic active hepatitis type 2. *Hepatology (Baltimore)* **8**, 1662–1666.

70. Abuaf, N., Hohanet, C., Soulie, E., Loeper, J., and Homberg, J.-C. (1992). Anti-liver cytosol antibodies in hepatology: Autoimmune hepatitis, viral hepatitis C and graft-versus-host disease. *In* "Immunology and Liver" Kluwer, Dordrecht, London, and Boston. (K.-H. Meyer zum Büschenfelde, J. Hoofnagle, and M. Manns, eds.), pp. 215–226.

71. van Pelt, F.N.A.M., Straub, P., and Manns, M. P. (1995). Molecular basis of drug-induced immunological liver injury. *Semin. Liver Dis.*

72. Ritter, J. K., Chen, F., Sheen, Y. Y., Tran, H. M., Kimurai, S., Yeatman, M. T., and Owens, I. S. (1992). A novel complex locus UGT1 encodes human bilirubin, phenol, and other UDP-glucuronsyltransferase isozymes with identical carboxyl termini. *J. Biol. Chem.* **267**, 3257–3261.

73. Iyanagi, T., Haniu, M., Sogawa, K., Fujii-Kuriyama, Y., Watanabe, S., Shively, J. E., and Anan, K. F. (1986). Cloning and characterization of cDNA endcoding methylcholantrene inducible rat mRNA for UDP-glucuronosyltransferase. *J. Biol. Chem.* **261**, 15607–15614.

74. Beaune, P., Bourdi, M., Lecoeur, S., Lopez-Garcia, P., Dansette, P., Mansuy, D., Belloc, C., Gautier, J-C., Larrey, D., Pessayre, D., Catinot, R., and Ballet, F. (1992). Mechanism of adverse drug reactions directed against cytochromes P450. *In:* "Immunology and Liver" (Meyer zum Büschenfelde, K-H., Hoofnagle, J., and Manns, M., Eds.), pp. 277–283. Kluwer Academic Publishers, Dordrecht, London/Boston.

*part*
# V

# MUCOSAL INFECTION

# Chapter 27

# Helicobacter pylori: Lessons of "Slow" Bacteria for the Host–Parasite Interaction

Martin J. Blaser

*Department of Medicine and Department of Microbiology and Immunology, Division of Infectious Diseases, Vanderbilt University School of Medicine, Nashville, Tennessee 37232*

## I. INTRODUCTION

In 1982, a spiral Gram-negative bacteria, now called *Helicobacter pylori,* was discovered in the human stomach (1). This was a surprising finding since most doctors and scientists considered the stomach to be essentially sterile. However, we now know that about one-half of the world's population is infected with *H. pylori* (2), and that it is the most important cause of both peptic ulcer disease and gastric adenocarcinoma, especially involving the distal stomach (3–6).

The hallmark of *H. pylori* infection is the presence of inflammation in the gastric mucosa. *Helicobacter pylori*-infected gastric tissue shows an inflammatory infiltrate in the lamina propria including both T and B lymphocytes, macrophages, mast cells, eosinophils, and neutrophils. In addition, there is disturbance of epithelial gland struction and function, with infiltration by inflammatory cells and diminished mucus production (4). This lesion is called chronic superficial gastritis (CSG), it is present in essentially all *H. pylori*-infected persons, and it now is clear that *H. pylori* causes this tissue injury (5).

In essence, *H. pylori* can be considered the first of a new class of pathogens, which I have called "slow" bacteria (6). The characteristics of *H. pylori* that in total differentiate it from other described bacteria include the following. It persists for decades (probably for life) in most infected persons. Unlike other persistent bacterial agents that spend most of their tenure in the human host in dormancy (e.g., *Mycobacterium tuberculosis*), *H. pylori* is undergoing active replication. As evidenced by its near universality in human populations in developing countries, and its persistence, it is superbly adapted for the human host. In conjunction with the near universality of closely related strains in other primates, and the tremendous diversity among strains (7,8), these data suggest that it has long been a parasite of humans, possibly since before we differentiated from other mammals.

Infection with *H. pylori* may lead to disease (such as cancer or ulceration) years or decades after its introduction; however, disease is not an inevitable consequence of infection. In that specific sense *H. pylori* resembles other chronic infectious agents of humans such as *M. tuberculosis* and *Shistosoma* species, but in total its characteristics as listed above differentiate it from other known human pathogens. It is likely that other slow bacterial pathogens will be recognized in the future as causing one or more of a variety of chronic inflammatory diseases of unknown cause (9).

Unlike other host–microbial interactions in which the result is an all-or-none phenomenon (elimination of the microbe or death of the host), *H. pylori* infection represents a dynamic equilibrium in which neither host nor microbe can eliminate the other, so they coexist for long periods. The presumed long history of *H. pylori* infections in humans suggests that there has in fact been a coevolution of host and microbe in response to selective pressures.

## II. PATHOGENESIS OF INFLAMMATION

In such circumstances, not unexpectedly, the pathogenesis of *H. pylori* infection is complex. In the first case, most (>90%) organisms are free-living within the secreted mucus in the stomach. In a sense, these lumenal bacteria may be considered as living outside the human host. However, a minority of *H. pylori* cells adhere to gastric epithelial cells, after producing apparent adherence pedestals, and some evidence suggests that a small number of organisms may locally invade the epithelial cells, although this latter point is controversial. What is clear, however, is that *H. pylori* cells are not present in the lamina propria, which is the site for the bulk of the inflammatory reaction. However, *H. pylori* antigens may be visualized in the lamina propria (10). As evidenced by the strong B-cell responses to *H. pylori* infection, there is clear recognition of *H. pylori* antigens and production of a sustained humoral immune response (11). With eradication of infection, the antibody response gradually wanes, but it may revive with new or recrudescent infection; this indicates that the response requires the continued presence of the antigen, and thus may be modulated (12).

There now is substantial evidence from both *in vitro* and *in vivo* studies that *H. pylori* antigens may both attract and activate inflammatory cells (10,13). Similarly, *H. pylori* stimulates epithelial cells to produce proinflammatory cytokines including IL-6 and IL-8. Thus, a model can be created in which *H. pylori* infection leads to a long and complex cascade of proinflammatory events involving epithelial cells, inflammatory cells, and cytokines.

## III. ECONOMY OF THE INFLAMMATORY
## RESPONSE: DOWNREGULATION

Nature is economical, and for well-adapted pathogens like *H. pylori* it is likely that much, if not all, that occurs is adaptive rather than accidental. It is likely that unrestricted inflammation is bad for both host and microbe. For the host, mounting a strong inflammatory response against a microbe that can not be eliminated is maladaptive, one cost of which is the elimination of normal gastric structure and function. For the microbe, intense inflammation hastens the development of atrophic gastritis, a condition in which bacterial numbers fall toward zero. Maintenance of a long-term niche requires that inflammation be minimized to the lowest levels consistent with the health of the microbial population.

I have previously proposed a model of this interaction (Fig. 1), in which *H. pylori* deliberately (adaptively) releases proinflammatory effectors that stimulate the host to respond. This response has as a consequence: the release of nutrients allowing the "offshore" *H. pylori* population to be fed. On its own, this is a positive feedback cycle, which we know cannot persist. I have proposed that evolution has selected for those hosts in which the mucosal immune system downregulates this inflammation. Parenthetically, such downregulation would be adaptive in relation to other chronic pathogens that cannot be eliminated such as the *Plasmodium* species. In addition, I have proposed that evolution has selected for *H. pylori* strains that can finely modulate its proinflammatory activities to the level required both to sustain the microbial population and to ensure transmission to a new host. Thus, the positive-feedback system has two brakes, and in total this proposal represents an autoregulation model. Mathematical analysis in fact indicates that a regulated model is the only way *H. pylori* can remain in steady state for long periods (14).

Is this model correct? A number of observations are consistent with the hypothesis raised, but I will highlight two. First, the lipopolysaccharide (endotoxin) of *H. pylori* has remarkably little biological activity. Our experiments have shown that approximately 10,000-times more LPS from *H. pylori* compared with *Esche-*

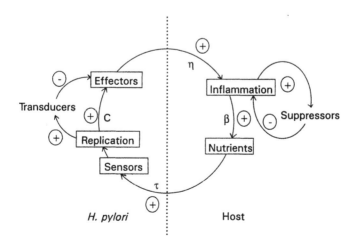

FIGURE 1. Model of *H. pylori* persistence. Reprinted from Ref. (6), with permission.

*richia coli* is required to activate macrophages (15). This bespeaks an extremely strong selection for bacteria that the host can tolerate. Conversely, despite much evidence for an extremely strong B-cell response to *H. pylori,* most studies suggest that the T-cell response is blunted or essentially absent (16). Although the definitive experiments to examine the model of downregulation have not yet been performed, the hypotheses are testable and can be addressed in the future.

## IV. VARIATION IN CLINICAL OUTCOME OF *H. PYLORI* INFECTION

Regardless of the mechanism by which *H. pylori* induces inflammation, the natural history of this infection has gradually been established (Fig. 2). Within weeks to a month of its acquisition, the host develops chronic superficial gastritis, and this lesion persists for decades. Most infected persons have chronic superficial gastritis or mild atrophic gastritis when they die, never having had any clinical consequences of infection. As such, for most infected persons, *H. pylori* has been a harmless commensal, and the possibility that the infection may be beneficial (a symbiont with humans) has not been ruled out. In a minority of persons (less than 10%) there is the development of peptic ulceration; in others, severe atrophic gastritis increases risk for development of gastric adenocarcinoma, and in a few

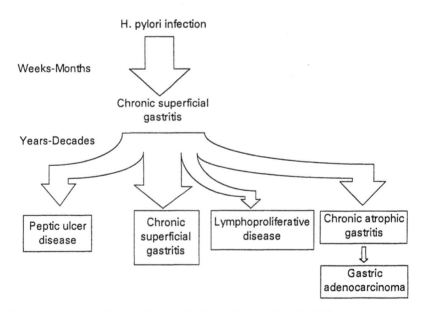

**FIGURE 2.** Natural history of *H. pylori* infection. Reprinted from Ref. (6), with permission.

others there may be lymphoproliferative disorders, such as MALT-type lymphomas (17).

The paradigm that a persistent pathogen that has coevolved with humans only causes disease in a small fraction of infected hosts is a common theme (i.e., schistosomiasis, *M. tuberculosis* infection). The determinants of risk of clinical consequences may be divided into four major categories. Different outcomes may reflect differences in: (i) virulence of infecting organisms, (ii) genetic background of infected hosts, (iii) exposure of hosts to other environmental agents, and (iv) the age at which infection was acquired. Although there has been evidence that each of these factors may play a role in explaining the complexity of the responses to *H. pylori* infection, the remainder of this chapter will focus on two differences among *H. pylori* strains that are associated with clinical differences.

## V. THE VACUOLATING CYTOTOXIN

In 1988, Dr. Robert Leunk found that culture supernatants from a subset of *H. pylori* strains could induce vacuole formation in a variety of eukaryotic cells (18). This activity was unlike that due to most known bacterial toxins, and could not be neutralized by several anti-toxins (18). Leunk found that about 50% of *H. pylori* strains express this activity in culture supernatants, an observation that has been confirmed (19,20). At first, there was doubt as to whether a cytotoxin actually existed, since ammonia released by the strong urease activity of *H. pylori* also can induce vacuoles to form (21); however, careful analyses showed that there existed a vacuolating activity independent of that related to ammonia (22). In 1992, Cover and Blaser reported on the purification of the toxin; the mature toxin migrated at about 90 kDa on SDS–PAGE (23). Furthermore, they and others showed that *H. pylori*-infected persons could possess neutralizing antibodies in their serum, confirming that the toxin was being produced *in vivo* (24,25). These observations put to rest any doubts that the toxin existed. The toxin induces formation of numerous vacuoles in affected cells (26), a process that requires vacuolar-type ATPase activity in the target cell (27,28). The vacuoles are products of the endocytic pathway (29), but certain molecules inhibit or augment activity (30).

Since cytotoxicity represented a phenotype that could be detected *in vitro*, numerous investigators began to study *H. pylori* isolates from patients with different clinical manifestations to determine whether the *in vitro* phenotypes correlated with clinical outcome (19,31–33). Although the exact methods used by the investigators varied, the results all were in the same direction; cytotoxigenic strains were significantly more frequently isolated from patients with peptic ulceration than from patients with gastritis alone (Table I). Thus, cytotoxicity was a marker for more virulent strains. Similar studies were conducted to examine the association of cytotoxicity with atrophic gastritis or gastric cancer (34,35) but results were more equivocal.

TABLE I

TABLE I
ISOLATION OF CYTOTOXIGENIC *H. PYLORI* STRAINS FROM PATIENTS WITH PEPTIC ULCERATION
OR GASTRITIS ALONE

| Study | Reference | Peptic ulcer disease | | Gastritis alone | | P value |
| | | Number of patients | % positive | Number of patients | % positive | |
|---|---|---|---|---|---|---|
| Figura *et al.* | 19 | 24 | 67 | 53 | 30 | 0.007 |
| Cover *et al.* | 31 | 5 | 100 | 19 | 32 | 0.02 |
| Tee *et al.* | 32 | 93 | 66 | 53 | 36 | <0.001 |
| Goosens *et al.* | 33 | 41 | 49 | 89 | 25 | 0.007 |

## VI. CHARACTERISTICS OF *vacA*

Cloning of the gene encoding the toxin was accomplished essentially simultaneously by four research groups (36–39). Fortunately, by agreement, each group named the gene *vacA,* since it encoded the vacuolating cytotoxin, and mutation of *vacA* ablated the cytotoxic activity (36). Analysis of the gene suggested that it encoded a short N-terminal cleaved signal sequence and a more substantial (about 50 kDa) carboxyl terminal (36–39). Structural analysis and homology searches suggested that the cleaved N-terminus permits passage of the toxin through the cytoplasmic membrane of the bacterium, whereas the C-terminal portion serves as a pore, allowing transit of the toxin molecule through the outer membrane before it is cleaved (38). Sequence analysis of the mature toxin shows no obvious homologies to other known genes (36–39).

Importantly, although not all *H. pylori* strains express vacuolating cytotoxin activity *in vitro,* essentially all strains possess *vacA* (36–39). However, in certain regions of the gene, *vacA* is well-conserved from strain to strain whereas in other regions there is substantial diversity (35,40,41). In the highly diverse middle region, sequences from strains that are toxigenic form a family in which the sequences are highly related to one another (>90%). The nontoxigenic strains form a second highly related family (>90% identity in the middle region) (36,40). This is highly unusual for a region within a conserved gene, as *vacA* is in *H. pylori,* and in contrast, the upstream gene *cysS* is highly conserved across all strains (41). Telford and colleagues found that supernatants from tox[+] strains but not tox[−] strains could cause severe mucosal injury when inoculated into the mouse stomach (37). To better assess the active agent, culture supernatants were compared from a wild-type tox[+] strain (84-183) and an isogenic strain in which *vacA* was mutated and in which no toxin production was observed (84-183V) (42). Whereas supernatants from both strains induced inflammation of the mucosa to a similar extent, mutation of *vacA* markedly reduced the degree of gastric epithelial mucosal injury.

These findings indicate that the *vacA* product is an aggressive factor involved in mucosal damage.

## VII. *vacA* DIVERSITY

Recent studies by Atherton *et al.* have further characterized *vacA* diversity, and found important clinical correlates (40). They defined two alleles of the middle region, called m1 and m2, and found three alleles of the signal sequence s1a, s1b, and s2. Alleles s1a and s1b are closely related but distinct. In total, any *H. pylori* strain could have one of six possible genotypes, but in a study of 62 isolates, no strain of the s2m1 *vacA* type was identified. vacA genotype correlated well with toxin phenotype. In general, s2m2 strains were not toxin producers, s1/m1 strains were high toxin producers, and s1/m2 strains had a bimodal distribution in the middle (40). In 57 (92%) of 62 strains, *cagA* status was concordent with *vacA* genotype: all s2 strains were *cagA*⁻ and all *cagA*⁺ strains were s1. There also were 5 *cagA*⁻ strains that were s1.

When the clinical status of the patients from whom these strains were obtained was ascertained, important clinical information emerged. Of 23 persons who had past or present peptic ulcer disease, 21 (91%) were infected with an s1 strain whereas this genotype was observed in 16 (48%) of the 33 patients with gastritis alone. Further studies are on-going but these investigations indicate a strong association between vacA genotype and the liklihood of having peptic ulceration. If confirmed, this observation may have substantial clinical utility. In any event, the mechanism for the association of particular s-types and peptic ulcer disease is not at all understood. Subanalyses suggest that the effects of s-types on gastric inflammation are independent of *cagA* status or m-type.

## VIII. THE CagA PROTEIN

In the late 1980s, investigators were examining *H. pylori* strains to determine the extent of antigenic diversity (20,43,44). Several groups noted that a subset of strains (from 60 to 80% depending on the study population) expressed a protein migrating between 120 and 130 kDa, and that this band was absent in other strains. In 1990, Cover *et al.* first reported that 100% of persons with duodenal ulceration had serum IgG antibodies that recognized a 128-kDa band, versus only about 60% in patients with gastritis alone (20). The next year, Crabtree *et al.* found almost identical gastric IgA responses to a 120-kDa band (which we now know is identical to Cover's 128-kDa band) (45). These proteins have been called the CagA protein and on careful examination have been found to range in size from 120 to 140 kDa (46,47). Several other investigators have confirmed a strong association between the presence of serum antibodies to the CagA protein and duodenal ulceration. It now appears that 40–60% of patients with gastritis alone are infected with *cagA*⁺ strains compared to 80 to 100% of patients with duodenal ulceration (20,45,48). For patients with gastric ulceration, results are intermediate (20,48). Recent studies also have shown an association between infection with a CagA⁺ strain and the development of both atrophic gastritis (49), as well as adenocarcinoma of the stomach (50,51). Thus, strains expressing the CagA protein appear more virulent than CagA⁻ strains.

## IX. THE *cagA* LOCUS

Two research groups cloned the gene encoding CagA, and by agreement called it *cagA* (46,47). In contrast to *vacA, cagA* is not present in every *H. pylori* strain; strains that do not express the CagA protein lack *cagA*. In total, in developed countries about 60% of strains are *cagA*⁺ and the remainder are *cagA*⁻, but in developing countries the *cagA*⁺ proportion appears higher. An interesting feature of the *cagA* sequence is the presence of multiple repeating patterns. A variable number of repeats explains the size range of CagA proteins, from about 120 to 140 kDa (46). We have recently identified two new genes upstream of *cagA,* but oriented in the opposite direction, that we have called *picA* and *picB* (52). These genes appear to be cotranscribed, and all strains that carry *cagA* carry *picA* and *picB,* whereas strains lacking one of the genes lack all three, and thus they appear completely linked at the genetic level (52). We now have created isogenic mutant strains in which we have ablated CagA, PicA, or PicB protein production by insertion of an antibiotic (kanamycin) resistance cassette into each of these genes (52,53). Mutation of *picA* also knocks out the downstream *picB* which is cotranscribed.

## X. *cagA* AND INFLAMMATION

Because *cagA*⁺ strains are more virulent (more highly associated with duodenal ulceration, atrophic gastritis, and adenocarcinoma of the stomach), we investigated whether these strains induced more profound inflammation than did *cagA*⁻ strains. The results were remarkably consistent. *cagA*⁺ strains have an average sixfold higher density of bacterial cells in the gastric antrum than do *cagA*⁻ strains (54); *cagA*⁺ strains are associated with substantially higher levels of gastric inflammation and injury than are *cagA*⁻ strains (45,55). *In vitro, cagA*⁺ strains induce substantially greater IL-8 production by AGS gastric epithelial cells than do *cagA*⁻ wild-type strains (56). In total, these data suggest that *cagA*⁺ stains have a more inflammatory life-style than do *cagA*⁻ cells, and that this process turns up the "gain," resulting in higher levels of gastric injury (Fig. 3).

## XI. ROLE OF picAB

To answer the question of whether the *cagA* product itself causes more inflammation or is merely a marker for this phenomenon, we compared wild type *cagA*⁺

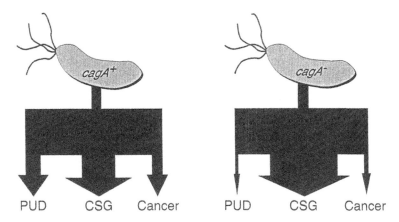

**FIGURE 3.** Comparison of *cagA*⁺ and *cagA*⁻ strains. Epidemiological studies indicate that persons infected with *cagA*⁻ strains are most likely to continue to have chronic superficial gastritis (CSG) with no other sequelae during life. Peptic ulcer diseaser (PUD) and gastric cancer (GC) are uncommon outcomes of infection. Persons infected with *cagA*⁺ strain also are most likely to develop only CSG; however, the likelihood of developing PUD or GC is much increased. The reason for this difference between *cagA*⁺ and *cagA*⁻ strains is unknown but the author hypothesizes that the former strains have a more proinflammatory lifestyle, and that the clinical sequelae are consequences of this phenomenon.

strains with isogenic mutants that differed only in that *cagA* was knocked out by insertion mutagenesis (53). When we examined ability of the wild type and the isogenic *cagA*⁻ mutant strains to possess vacuolating cytotoxin activity or to induce IL-8 production by AGS cells, there were no differences. These data suggested that the presence of *cagA* was merely a marker for strains that induced enhanced inflammation. We then compared the *picA* and the *picB* mutants with their respective wild-type cells. All strains showed essentially equal levels of cytotoxin activity. However, ablation of *picA* or *picB* sharply diminished the ability of the mutant strains to induce AGS cells to produce IL-8 (52). These data suggest that *picA* and/or *picB* are essential for the proinflammatory activity induced by wild-type cells that are *cagA*⁺. Whether the products of *picA* or *picB* themselves are the proinflammatory substances or merely facilitate such activity is not yet known. However, the strong homology of *picB* with *Bordetella pertussis* PtlC and *Agrobacterium tumefaciens* VirB4 suggest a role in a secretory pathway (52). Further work is on-going.

## XII. CONCLUSIONS

*Heliobacter pylori* appear to have conserved mechanisms permitting persistance in the human host. Current evidence indicates that *H. pylori* has been a pathogen of humans since time immemorial. Prolonged coevolution helps explain the relative innocuity of these slow bacteria. In addition, at least two different markers, the genotype of the vacuolating cytotoxin and the presence or absence of *picA* or *picB*, are characteristics that differentiate among strains. Such characteristics reflect differences in virulence, and may reflect genetic elements that have been acquired more recently.

## ACKNOWLEDGMENTS

The author acknowledges the hard work and imagination of the following individuals who performed much of the work covered in this review: Timothy Cover, John Atherton, Paolo Ghiari, Uwe Mai, Geraldine Miller, Richard Peek, Guillermo Pérez-Pérez, Rino Rappuoli, Smita Sharma, Phillip Smith, and Murali Tummuru. The work presented in this review was supported in part by the Medical Research Service of the Departments of Veterans Affairs and by the National Cancer Institute (RO1 CA58834).

## REFERENCES

1. Marshall, B. J., and Warren, J. R. (1984). Unidentified curved bacilli in the stomach of patients with gastritis and peptic ulceration. *Lancet* **1,** 1311–1315.
2. Pounder, R. E., and Ng, D. (1995). The prevalence of *Helicobacter pylori* infection in different countries. *Aliment Pharmacol. Ther.* **9,** S33–S39.
3. Hentschel, E., Brandstatter, G., Dragoisics, B., *et al.* (1993). Effect of ranitidine and amoxicillin plus metronidazole on the eradication of *Helicobacter pylori* and the recurrence of duodenal ulcer. *N. Engl. J. Med.* **328,** 308–312.
4. Dixon, M. F. (1991). *Helicobacter pylori* and peptic ulceration: Histopathological aspects. *J. Gastroenterol. Hepatol.* **6,** 125–130.
5. Blaser, M. J. (1990). *Helicobacter pylori* and the pathogenesis of gastroduodenal inflammation. *J. Infect. Dis.* **161,** 626–633.
6. Blaser, M. J., and Parsonnet, J. (1994). Parasitism by the "slow" bacterium *Helicobacter pylori* leads to altered gastric homeostasis and neoplasia. *J. Clin. Invest.* **94,** 4–8.
7. Fujimoto, S., Marshall, B., and Blaser, M. J. (1994). PCR-based restriction fragment length polymorphism typing of *Helicobacter pylori*. *J. Clin. Microbiol.* **32,** 331–334.
8. Akopyanz, N., Bukanov, N. O., Westblom, T. U., Kresovich, S., and Berg, D. E. (1992). DNA diversity among clinical isolates of *Helicobacter pylori* detected by PCR-based RAPD fingerprinting. *Nucleic Acids Res.* **20,** 5137–5142.
9. Blaser, M. J. (1994). Bacteria and diseases of unknown cause. *Ann. Intern. Med.* **121,** 144–145.
10. Mai, U. E., Pérez-Pérez, G. I., Allen, J. B., Wahl, S. M., Blaser, M. J., and Smith, P. D. (1992). Surface proteins from *Helicobacter pylori* exhibit chemotactic activity for human leukocytes and are present in gastric mucosa. *J. Exp. Med.* **175,** 517–525.
11. Pérez-Pérez, G. I., Dworkin, B. M., Chodos, J. E., and Blaser, M. J. (1988). *Campylobacter pylori* antibodies in humans. *Ann. Intern. Med.* **109,** 11–17.
12. Kosunen, T. U., Seppala, K., Sarna, S., and Sipponen, P. (1992). Diagnostic value of decreasing IgG, IgA, and IgM antibody titres after eradication of *Helicobacter pylori*. *Lancet* **339,** 893–895.
13. Mai, U. E. H., Pérez-Pérez, G. I., Wahl, L. M., Wahl, S. M., Blaser, M. J., and Smith, P. D. (1991). Soluble surface proteins from *Helicobacter pylori* activate monocytes/macrophages by lipopolysaccharide-independent mechanism. *J. Clin. Invest.* **87,** 894–900.
14. Kirschner, D. E., and Blaser, M. J. (1995). The dynamics of *Helicobacter pylori* infection of the human stomach. *J. Theor. Biol.* **176,** 281–290.
15. Pérez-Pérez, G. I., Shepherd, V. L., Morrow, J. D., and Blaser, M. J. (1995). Activation of human THP-1 and rat bone marrow-derived macrophages by *Helicobacter pylori* lipopolysaccharide. *Infect. Immun.* **63,** 1183–1187.

16. Sharma, S. A., Miller, G. G., Pérez-Pérez, G. I., and Gupta, R. S. (1994). Humoral and cellular immune recognition of *Helicobacter pylori* proteins are not concordant. *Clin. Exp. Immunol.* **97**, 126–132.

17. Wotherspoon, A. C., Doglioni, C., Diss, T. C., *et al.* (1993). Regression of primary low-grade B-cell lymphoma of mucosa-associated lymphoid tissue type after eradication of *Helicobacter pylori*. *Lancet* **342**, 575–577.

18. Leunk, R. D., Johnson, P. T., David, B. C., Kraft, W. G., and Morgan, D. R. (1988). Cytotoxic activity in broth-culture filtrates of *Campylobacter pylori*. *J. Med. Microbiol.* **26**, 93–99.

19. Figura, N., Guglielmetti, P., Rossolini, A., *et al.* (1989). Cytotoxin production by *Campylobacter pylori* strains isolated from patients with peptic ulcers and from patients with chronic gastritis only. *J. Clin. Microbiol.* **27**, 225–226.

20. Cover, T. L., Dooley, C. P., and Blaser, M. J. (1990). Characterization of and human serologic response to proteins in *Helicobacter pylori* broth culture supernatants with vacuolizing cytotoxin activity. *Infect. Immun.* **58**, 603–610.

21. Xu, J. K., Goodwin, C. S., Cooper, M., and Robinson, J. (1990). Intracellular vacuolization caused by the urease of *Helicobacter pylori*. *J. Infect. Dis.* **161**, 1302–1304.

22. Cover, T. L., Puryear, W., Pérez-Pérez, G. I., and Blaser, M. J. (1991). Effect of urease on HeLa cell vacuolation induced by *Helicobacter pylori* cytotoxin. *Infect. Immun.* **59**, 1264–1270.

23. Cover, T. L., and Blaser, M. J. (1992). Purification and characterization of the vacuolating toxin from *Helicobacter pylori*. *J. Biol. Chem.* **267**, 10570–10575.

24. Cover, T. L., Cao, P., Murthy, U. K., Sipple, M. S., and Blaser, M. J. (1992). Serum neutralizing antibody response to the vacuolating cytotoxin of *Helicobacter pylori*. *J. Clin. Invest.* **90**, 913–918.

25. Leunk, R. D., Ferguson, M. A., Morgan, D. R., Low, D. E., and Simor, A. E. (1990). Antibody to cytotoxin in infection by *Helicobacter pylori*. *J. Clin. Microbiol.* **28**, 1181–1184.

26. Cover, T. L., Halter, S. A., and Blaser, M. J. (1992). Characterization of HeLa cell vacuoles induced by *Helicobacter pylori* broth culture supernatant. *Hum. Pathol.* **23**, 1004–1010.

27. Papini, E., Bugnoli, M., Debernard, M., Figura, N., Rappuoli, R., and Montecucco, C. (1993). Bafilomycin-A1 inhibits *Helicobacter pylori*-induced vacuolization of HeLa cells. *Mol. Microbiol.* **7**, 323–327.

28. Cover, T. L., Reddy, L. Y., and Blaser, M. J. (1993). Effects of ATPase inhibitors on the response of HeLa cells to *Helicobacter pylori* vacuolating toxin. *Infect. Immun.* **61**, 1427–1431.

29. Papini, E., De Bernard, M., Milia, E., *et al.* (1994). Cellular vacuoles induced by *Helicobacter pylori* originate from late endosomal compartments. *Proc. Natl. Acad. Sci. U.S.A.* **91**, 9720–9724.

30. Cover, T. L., Vaughn, S. G., and Blaser, M. J. (1992). Potentiation of *Helicobacter pylori* vacuolating toxin activity by nicotine and other weak bases. *J. Infect. Dis.* **166**, 1073–1078.

31. Cover, T. L., Cao, P., Lind, C. D., Tham, K. T., and Blaser, M. J. (1993). Correlation between vacuolating cytotoxin production by *Helicobacter pylori* isolates *in vitro* and *in vivo*. *Infect. Immun.* **61**, 5008–5012.

32. Tee, W., Lambert, J. R., Pegorer, M., and Dwyer, B. (1993). Cytotoxin production by *Helicobacter pylori* more common in peptic ulcer disease. *Gastroenterology* **104**, A789.

33. Goossens, H., Glupczynski, Y., Burette, A., Lambert, J., Vlaes, L., and Butzler, J. (1992). Role of the vacuolating toxin from *Helicobacter pylori* in the pathogenesis of duodenal and gastric ulcer. *Med. Microbiol. Lett.* **1**, 153–159.

34. Hirai, M., Azuma, T., Ito, S., Kato, T., Kohli, Y., and Fujiki, N. (1994). High prevalence of neutralizing activity to *Helicobacter pylori* cytotoxin in serum of gastric-carcinoma patients. *Int. J. Cancer* **56**, 56–60.

35. Blaser, M. J., Kobayashi, K., Cover, T. L., Cao, P., Feurer, I. D., and Pérez-Pérez, G. I. (1993). *Helicobacter pylori* in Japanese patients with adenocarcinoma of the stomach. *Int. J. Cancer* **55**, 799–802.

36. Cover, T. L., Tummuru, M. K. R., Cao, P., Thompson, S. A., and Blaser, M. J. (1994). Divergence

of genetic sequences for the vacuolating cytotoxin among *Helicobacter pylori* strains. *J. Biol. Chem.* **269**, 10566–10573.

37. Telford, J. L., Ghiara, P., Dell'Orco, M., *et al.* (1994). Gene structure of the *Helicobacter pylori* cytotoxin and evidence of its key role in gastric disease. *J. Exp. Med.* **179**, 1653–1658.

38. Schmitt, W., and Haas, R. (1994). Genetic analysis of the *Helicobacter pylori* vacuolating cytotoxin: Structural similarities with the IgA protease type of exported protein. *Mol. Microbiol.* **12**, 307–319.

39. Phadnis, S. H., Ilver, D., Janzon, L., Normark, S., and Westblom, T. U. (1994). Pathological significance and molecular characterization of the vacuolating toxin gene of *Helicobacter pylori*. *Infect. Immun.* **62**, 1557–1565.

40. Atherton, J. C., Cao, P., Peek, R. M., Jr., Tummuru, M. K. R., Blaser, M. J., and Cover, T. L. (1995). Mosaicism in vacuolating cytotoxin alleles of *Helicobacter pylori:* Association of specific *vacA* types with cytotoxin production and peptic ulceration. *J. Biol. Chem.* **270**, 17771–17777.

41. Garner, J. A., and Cover, T. L. (1995). Analysis of genetic diversity in cytotoxin-producing and non-cytotoxin-producing *Helicobacter pylori* strains. *J. Infect. Dis.* **172**, 290–293.

42. Ghiari, P., Marchetti, M., Blaser, M. J., *et al.* (1995). Role of the *Helicobacter pylori* virulence factors vacuolating cytotoxin, CagA, and urease in a mouse model of disease. *Infect. Immun.* **63**, 4154–4160.

43. Apel, I., Jacobs, E., Kist, M., and Bredt, W. (1988). Antibody response of patients against a 120 kDa surface protein of *Campylobacter pylori. Zentralbl. Bakteriol. Mikrobiol. Hyg. A.* **268**, 271–276.

44. Pérez-Pérez, G. I., and Blaser, M. J. (1987). Conservation and diversity of *Campylobacter pyloridis* major antigens. *Infect. Immun.* **55**, 1256–1263.

45. Crabtree, J. E., Taylor, J. D., Wyatt, J. I., *et al.* (1991). Mucosal IgA recognition of *Helicobacter pylori* 120 kDa protein, peptic ulceration, and gastric pathology. *Lancet* **338**, 332–335.

46. Covacci, A., Censini, S., Bugnoli, M., *et al.* (1993). Molecular characterization of the 128-kDa immunodominant antigen of *Helicobacter pylori* associated with cytotoxicity and duodenal ulcer. *Proc. Natl. Acad. Sci. U.S.A.* **90**, 5791–5795.

47. Tummuru, M. K. R., Cover, T. L., and Blaser, M. J. (1993). Cloning and expression of a high molecular weight major antigen of *Helicobacter pylori:* Evidence of linkage to cytotoxin production. *Infect. Immun.* **61**, 1799–1809.

48. Cover, T. L., Glupczynski, Y., Lage, A. P., *et al.* (1995). Serologic detection of infection with *cagA*⁺ *Helicobacter pylori* strains. *J. Clin. Microbiol.* **33**, 1496–1500.

49. Kuipers, E. J., Pérez-Pérez, G. I., Meuwissen, S. G. M., and Blaser, M. J. (1995). *Helicobacter pylori* and atrophic gastritis: importance of the *cagA* status. *J.N.C.I.* **87**, 1777–1780.

50. Crabtree, J. E., Wyatt, J. I., Sobala, G. M. *et al.* (1993). Systemic and mucosal humoral responses to *Helicobacter pylori* in gastric cancer. *Gut* **34**, 1339–1343.

51. Blaser, M. J., Pérez-Pérez, G. I., Kleanthous, H., *et al.* (1995). Infection with *Helicobacter pylori* strains possessing *cagA* associated with an increased risk of developing adenocarcinoma of the stomach. *Cancer Res.* **55**, 2111–2115.

52. Tummuru, M. K., Sharma, S. A., and Blaser, M. J. (1995). *Helicobacter pylori picB*, a homologue of the *Bordetella pertussis* toxin secretion protein, is required for induction of IL-8 in gastric epithelial cells. *Mol. Microbiol.* **18**, 867–876.

53. Tummuru, M. K. R., Cover, T. L., and Blaser, M. J. (1994). Mutation of the cytotoxin-associated *cagA* gene does not affect the vacuolating cytotoxin activity of *Helicobacter pylori. Infect. Immun.* **62**, 2609–2613.

54. Atherton, J. C., Peek, R. M., Tham, K. T., Pérez-Pérez, G. I., and Blaser, M. J. (1994). Quantitative culture of *Helicobacter pylori* in the gastric antrum: Association of bacterial density with duodenal ulcer status and infection with *cagA* positive bacterial strains, and negative association with serum IgG levels. *Am. J. Gastroenterol* **89**, 1322.

55. Peek, R. M., Blaser, M. J., and Miller, G. G. (1994). *cagA*-positive *Helicobacter pylori* strain induce preferential cytokine expression in gastric mucosa. *Am. J. Gastroenterol.* **89,** 1344.
56. Sharma, S. A., Tummuru, M. K. R., Miller, G. G., and Blaser, M. J. (1995). Interleukin-8 response of gastric epithelial cell lines to *Helicobacter pylori* stimulation *in vitro*. *Infect. Immun.* **63,** 1681–1687.

# Chapter 28

# *Helicobacter pylori:* Infection, Inflammation and the Host Immune Response

Steven J. Czinn and John G. Nedrud

*Division of Pediatric Gastroenterology and Nutrition, Rainbow Babies and Childrens Hospital, and Institute of Pathology, Case Western Reserve University, Cleveland, Ohio 44106*

Gastric diseases ranging from gastritis and ulcers to adenocarcinoma have historically been major health concerns which afflict millions of people worldwide. Until recently, the causes of such diseases have been attributed to dietary factors, medications, or physiologic abnormalities of the patient. However, recent work involving a novel bacterial pathogen, *Helicobacter pylori,* suggests that this microorganism plays an etiologic role in the development of gastric disease.

The concept of spiral organisms within the stomach is not a new one. Investigators in the 19th century described spiral organisms in the gastric mucosa of several animal species. Similar organisms were subsequently identified on the surface of human gastric mucosa. These observations were confirmed by Freedberg and Barron (1940), who identified spiral-shaped organisms in approximately 50% of adults with gastric and/or peptic ulcer disease. Despite early enthusiasm, skepticism regarding the bacterial etiology of peptic ulcer disease was promoted by Palmer in a study involving an excess of 1000 gastric biopsy specimens, which failed to demonstrate these organisms (Palmer, 1954). Fitzgerald and Murphy (1950) discussed the role of gastric urease and peptic ulcer disease, and other investigators concluded that the gastric urease present in patients with peptic ulcer disease was of bacterial origin. It was not until the early 1980s, when Marshall and Warren successfully cultured this unique bacteria from a human gastric biopsy (Marshall and Warren, 1983), that evidence began to mount to support an etiologic role for this bacteria in the development of gastroduodenal disease and cancer.

Morphologically, *H. pylori* is a gram-negative, s-shaped rod, $0.5 \times 3.0$ $\mu$m in length. It has polar flagella, and produces a series of enzymes, such as urease, catalase, and oxidase. *Helicobacter pylori* requires a microaerophilic environment for culture, and is associated with the gastric epithelium of man. Despite a number of reports confirming spiral organisms associated with the presence of gastritis and ulcers, the medical community remained skeptical regarding the etiologic role this

*Essentials of Mucosal Immunology* Copyright © 1996 by Academic Press, Inc. All rights of reproduction in any form reserved.

microorganism played in the development of gastroduodenal disease. It is estimated that between 50 and 80% of adult humans are infected worldwide and it is now clear that virtually 100% of patients with duodenal ulcers and 80–90% of gastric ulcer patients have this infection in the stomach (NIH Consensus Conference, 1994; Peterson, 1991). It also appears that *Helicobacter*-infected individuals have a significantly increased rate of gastric cancer (Eurogast Study Group, 1993; World Health Organization, 1994; Parsonnet, 1993). Although it is possible to use multidrug antibiotic therapy to eradicate this infection, there are a number of adverse effects of antibiotic treatment including poor patient compliance, antimicrobial resistance, abdominal pain, and diarrhea (Bell *et al.,* 1992; Chiba *et al.,* 1992). Therefore, if one could develop a way to immunologically prevent or treat infection, it would be extremely beneficial, and as early as 1991 studies in animals suggested the feasibility of an *H. pylori* vaccine (Czinn and Nedrud, 1991).

The evidence that implicates *H. pylori* in the pathogenesis of gastroduodenal disease comes from a series of studies. The first are volunteer studies. In the early 1980s, when Barry Marshall first rediscovered *H. pylori,* there was tremendous skepticism in the medical community. Support for the relationship between *H. pylori* and human illness was derived from novel experiments performed by Barry Marshall and Arthur Morris (Marshall *et al.,* 1985; Morris and Nicholson, 1987), who satisfied Koch's postulates by creating histologically confirmed gastritis following consumption of viable organisms with subsequent recovery of bacteria. Antimicrobial studies now show very convincingly that eradication of the infection induces rapid, complete remission of ulcers. Although recurrence rates after antimicrobial therapy have been reported to be low, this may have more to do with exposure rates and opportunity for reinfection than the existence of effective immunity after antimicrobial cure. Indeed, animal studies have shown that in contrast to vaccination, triple-therapy cure of *Helicobacter* infections does not lead to immunity to reinfection (Chen *et al.,* 1993; Fox *et al.,* 1994; S. J. Czinn, *et al.,* 1996). In addition, the widely accepted cohort theory for *H. pylori* infection suggests that *H. pylori* infection is primarily acquired in childhood and that as the population ages, new infections of adults are relatively rare (Banatvala *et al.,* 1993). Thus, eradication of infection in adults could yield low reinfection rates because adults have low exposure rates rather than because of immunity. If this hypothesis were true, then in a situation where adults do have high exposure rates, as might be expected in a developing country, one might expect a relatively high rate of reinfection after triple-therapy cure. In fact, one recent study from Brazil showed exactly this result (Coelho *et al.,* 1992).

A series of animal models has been developed which has provided the opportunity to study host responses to this infection. When one begins to study the immune response to this infection, a paradox becomes apparent. We and others have shown that vaccination can prevent, and may even cure, *Helicobacter* infections (Chen *et al.,* 1993; Corthesy-Theulaz *et al.,* 1995; Czinn *et al.,* 1993; Ferrero *et al.,* 1994, 1995; Marchetti *et al.,* 1995; Michetti *et al.,* 1994). However, humans and animals infected with *Helicobacter* species develop anti-*Helicobacter* immune responses, but do not clear the infection. There are a number of possible resolutions to this paradox. This microorganism is not invasive, and in some ways is not really within the body. It lives on the surface of the gastric epithelium, in an area where neither cell-mediated nor humoral immune mechanisms may be able to clear the infection. A second possible resolution of the paradox may be that preexisting immunity such as induced by vaccination may be able to block the infection, whereas postinfection immune responses may be unable to clear an existing infection. The issue of local/mucosal immune responses as opposed to systemic immunity may also be important. Finally, there may be quantitative and/or qualitative differences in the antibody response when an individual is immunized as compared to naturally infected. Accumulating evidence suggests that the latter explanation may be the most plausible (see below).

A number of laboratories have begun to study the feasibility of prophylactic and therapeutic vaccination for the prevention and treatment of *H. pylori* infection. The animal models that most investigators have used to investigate *H. pylori* vaccination is an adaptation of the germ-free/*H. felis* mouse model. Originally, this model employed 6-week-old germ-free outbred Swiss–Webster mice and has since been adapted for conventional inbred strains of mice (Lee *et al.,* 1990; Michetti *et al.,* 1994; Mohammadi *et al.,* 1996). Once mice are infected with *H. felis,* they develop chronic inflammation which appears to be lifelong (Fox *et al.,* 1993; Lee *et al.,* 1993) Similar to humans, treatment of murine *H. felis* infection requires triple-antimicrobial therapy; a single antimicrobial agent is unable to cure the disease (Dick-Hegedus and Lee, 1991). There are, however, a number of significant differences between *H. felis* and *H. pylori.* Specifically, *H. felis* does not appear to have cagA or vacA, which are markers of virulence in *H. pylori,* and finally, this is a nonadherent microorganism.

Using this model, the generally accepted oral immunization protocol employs three to five weekly oral immunizations consisting of inactivated *H. felis,* inactivated *H. pylori,* or purified *Helicobacter* proteins plus cholera toxin. One week after the final immunization, the animals are challenged with viable *H. felis* and sacrificed at various time intervals. Gastric biopsies are then obtained for rapid urease testing and/or visualizing organisms on histologic sections for determination of infection. The results of such studies indicate that a significant IgA and IgG anti-*Helicobacter* response was generated in serum, gastric, and intestinal secretions in immunized mice as compared to nonimmunized controls. Additionally, significant protection was observed when the mice were immunized prior to challenge with live *H. felis* (Fig. 1). As can be seen in Fig. 1, oral immunization prevents *Helicobacter* infection in 82% of immunized animals, whereas 90% of control animals become infected following challenge.

In an effort to resolve the paradox regarding why oral immunization is able to prevent *Helicobacter* infection although the immune response following natural infection is unable to clear the organisms, we began to study the antibody response

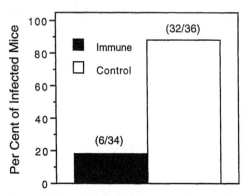

**FIGURE 1.** Groups of Swiss–Webster germ-free mice were orally immunized four or five times over a 1-month period with 2–4 mg of sonicated *H. felis* lysate plus 10 µg of cholera toxin and were then challenged orally with approximately $10^6$ viable *H. felis* bacteria. One to two weeks after challenge, mice were sacrificed and gastric biopsies were collected. The biopsies were scored for the presence of *H. felis* by rapid urease test and/or culture positivity. Pooled data from four experiments, the numbers in parentheses represent the number of protected animals/total number of mice per group. Adapted from Czinn *et al.* (1993).

following oral immunization and infection (Fig. 2). In this experiment, we took a series of naive and immunized animals and challenged them with *H. felis*. As expected, the immunized animals had preexisting antibodies. At 1 and 3 weeks following challenge, immunized animals were protected, and had significant titers of serum IgA and serum IgG antibody. However, the more interesting point is that by 6 weeks following infection, there was virtually no difference between the two groups. Therefore, oral immunization could induce antibodies prior to infectious challenge, but did not appear to enhance the magnitude of the antibody response relative to infection of nonimmunized mice. Similar results were seen in the intestinal washes (Fig. 2). Once again, there were preexisting intestinal IgA and intestinal IgG antibodies after immunization, but after about 6 weeks there was virtually no difference between the preimmunized/infected mice and the infected mice. Similar results were also observed in gastric washes of immunized versus infected mice but the anti-*H. felis* titers were lower. Collectively, these results are consistent with the hypothesis that preexisting antibodies can block infection, and this may resolve the paradox noted earlier. At about this time, however, several laboratories began to report successful therapeutic immunization against *Helicobacter* infection. In these studies, mice which had been chronically infected with *H. felis* were successfully cured of *H. felis* infection following oral immunization with *H. felis* antigens and cholera toxin (Corthesy-Theulaz *et al.*, 1995; Doidge *et al.*, 1994).

Our laboratory has also investigated therapeutic immunization using the ferret model. We believe the ferret model has specific advantages over the murine model

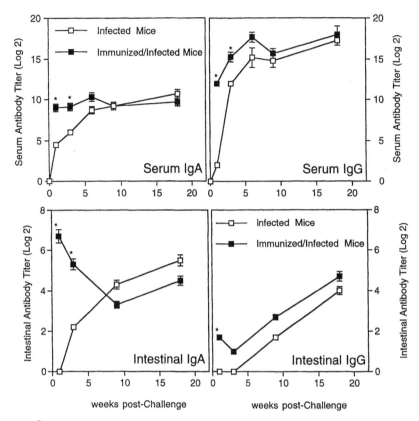

**FIGURE 2.** Serum and intestinal antibody titers in germ-free mice after oral immunization with *H. felis* lysate plus cholera toxin. Naive mice had undetectable levels of anti-*H. felis* antibody (data not shown). Titers in the immunized/infected group that were significantly greater ($P < 0.05$) than titers in the infected only group are indicated by an asterisk (*). Adapted from Sellman *et al.* (1995).

when performing therapeutic immunization studies. Specifically, *H. mustelae* is indigenous to ferrets, and, for the most part, only infects ferrets. Consistent with humans, natural infection occurs early in life. There is also serologic conversion with the development of histologic gastritis. It is also very difficult to eradicate this infection with antimicrobial agents; similar to humans, it requires triple therapy for a minimum of 2 weeks. Finally, eradication of *H. mustelae* in ferrets results in resolution of gastritis.

Chronically infected ferrets were immunized five times with purified *H. pylori* urease plus cholera toxin. Animals that were treated with *H. pylori* urease plus cholera toxin had a 30% rate of cure while all animals receiving cholera toxin alone or sham immunization remained infected. Despite the fact that we only cured 30% of the animals, we saw a reduction in inflammation in all immunized animals (Cuenca *et al.*, 1996). If these experiments in mice and ferrets continue to yield consistent results, it could lead to immunotherapy therapy for *H. pylori* infection of humans. Finally, based on these intriguing results, it appears that we have not yet resolved the paradox regarding the immune responses and *Helicobacter* infections; the immunity which results in clearance of infection after therapeutic immunization is clearly not due to preexisting antibodies.

Since therapeutic immunization rules out the notion that preexisting antibodies are the sole reason that immunization works and since there were no differences in the magnitude of antibody responses between infected and immunized (protected) animals (Fig. 2), we have begun to examine qualitative differences in antibody responses among immunized vs infected animals. Western blots were performed to examine the humoral immune response against *H. felis* in the immunized only mice, immunized-challenged (protected) mice, and nonimmunized infected mice. Immunization alone, or immunization followed by challenge and ultimate protection, resulted in the presence of an additional band of 60–70 kDa, consistent with antibody to ureB (data not shown). Additional bands in immunized or immunized and challenged animals in the range of 16–20 kDa were also seen. We have recently observed a similar set of circumstances in a pediatric patient. In this case report, a 10-year-old boy with a documented duodenal bulb ulcer, as well as chronic gastric inflammation and the presence of *H. pylori*, spontaneously cleared his *Helicobacter* infection. The Western blot analysis from this patient, shown in Fig. 3, demonstrates numerous bands during chronic infection but only one prominent band with a molecular weight of 76 kDa following spontaneous clearance of infection. Subsequent Western blot analysis using purified recombinant *H. pylori* ureB showed that this convalescent serum did, in fact, react with urease (not shown). Although these results reflect serum rather that secretory antibodies, another recent animal study has shown that secretory IgA antibodies reactive with ureB correlated with protection of *H. felis*-immunized mice (Lee *et al.*, 1995). Additional evidence for the potential role of anti-urease antibodies in prevention or cure of *Helicobacter* infections comes from passive immunization studies where anti-urease monoclonal antibodies blocked *H. felis* infection of mice (Blanchard *et al.*, 1995a). The striking inverse correlation between antibodies reacting with urease and the absence of colonization or disease in both animal and human studies suggests that qualitative differences in antibody responses between infected as opposed to immunized individuals may be a critical element which allows immunized animals (and hopefully humans) to either prevent or clear *Helicobacter* infections.

Why should there be a qualitative difference in the antibody responses of infected versus immunized subjects? One important fact regarding successful immunization versus *Helicobacter* spp. to date is that they have all included cholera toxin or the biologically similar heat labile toxin of *Escherichia coli*, or derivatives of these toxins as a mucosal adjuvant (Chen *et al.*, 1993; Corthesy-Theulaz *et al.*, 1995; Czinn *et al.*, 1993; Ferrero *et al.*, 1994, 1995; Lee and Chen, 1994; Lee *et*

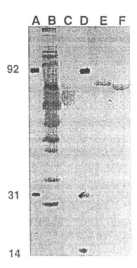

**FIGURE 3.** Western blot of serum anti-*H. pylori* antibodies from a patient who spontaneously cleared his infection. Lanes A and D, molecular weight standards. Western blot of serum against *H. pylori* lysate (lane B) and *H. pylori* outer membranes (lane C) during phase of chronic infection. Western blot of serum against *H. pylori* lysate (lane E) and *H. pylori* outer membranes (lane F). Following spontaneous clearance of *H. pylori* infection.

*al.*, 1995; Marchetti *et al.*, 1995; Michetti *et al.*, 1994). Immunizations which have not used one of these adjuvants have not been successful at preventing infection and in some cases have actually exacerbated the disease which results when animals are challenged (Chen *et al.*, 1993; Eaton and Krakowa, 1992; Lee *et al.*, 1995; Palley *et al.*, 1993). Perhaps it is the addition of cholera toxin which is responsible for the qualitative differences in the antibody response which we have observed, or for other undefined qualitative aspects of the immune response which are responsible for protective immunization. The mechanism(s) by which cholera toxin alters immune responses after oral immunization are complex and probably multifactorial. (See Holmgren *et al.*, 1993, for a review of this subject.) One things seems certain: their inherent toxicity makes it unlikely that unmodified cholera toxin or heat-labile toxin will be acceptable adjuvants for use in humans, although a clinical trial is currently underway in humans evaluating heat labile toxin as a potential mucosal adjuvant. Cholera toxin and heat-labile toxin consist of 5 B subunits which bind the toxin to cellular ganglioside $GM_1$, and one A subunit with ADP ribosylation activity which activates adenylate cyclase, thus raising intracellular cyclic AMP levels and mediating the toxicity. Although there has been some controversy regarding the requirement for active A subunit for adjuvant activity, in nearly all cases at least a small amount of pharmacologic activity contributed by the A subunit has been present when adjuvant activity is observed. Early studies using a murine Sendai virus experimental system suggested that only a small amount of A subunit activity may be required for the adjuvant effects (Liang *et al.*, 1989), and additional studies have suggested that a small amount of active A subunit may synergize with larger amounts of B subunit in promoting enhanced immune responses (Tamura *et al.*, 1994; Wilson *et al.*, 1990). Numerous studies have suggested that purified B subunit might act as an oral adjuvant (Holmgren *et al.*, 1993) but in most cases the B subunit preparations have been contaminated with small amounts of holotoxin. Indeed, it has been possible to successfully immunize mice against *H. felis* using commercially prepared, cholera toxin B subunit as an oral adjuvant (Lee and Chen 1994; Nedrud *et al.*, 1995). However, in these cases contaminating A subunit probably played a critical role since when recombinant cholera toxin B subunit devoid of any detectable ADP ribosylation activity was used, neither enhanced antibody responses nor protection from infection was observed (Nedrud *et al.*, 1995). We can conclude from these studies that although toxin B subunits alone will probably not be successful oral adjuvants for a *Helicobacter* vaccine, very small amounts of added holotoxin such as might be present in B subunit purified from holotoxin may be enough to ensure a successful *H. pylori* vaccine. Such "purified" B subunit has minimal to no toxicity and has been safely administered to tens of thousands human volunteers (Clemens *et al.*, 1988). Another approach for a safe version of a cholera toxin/heat-labile toxin mucosal adjuvant is to genetically detoxify the molecule by introducing point mutations at critical amino acid residues (Burnette, *et al.*, 1991; Dickinson and Clements, 1995; Douce *et al.*, 1995; Grant *et al.*, 1994). With one exception, which involved intranasal rather than oral immunization (Douce *et al.*, 1995), a small amount of ADP ribosyl transferase activity was retained by mutants with adjuvant activity, although all mutants tested were devoid of overt toxicity. In preliminary experiments, we have used several of these genetically detoxified molecules as adjuvants to immunize and protect mice against *H. felis* infection (Nedrud and Cieplak, unpublished observations).

In addition to vaccination, another area where immune and inflammatory responses may play an important role in *Helicobacter* infections is in disease pathogenesis. Many more people are infected with *H. pylori* than progress to overt, severe disease requiring medical intervention. What are the factors which determine whether an infected individual will progress to severe disease? One possible factor is duration of infection. Virtually all infected individuals possess so-called active chronic inflammation (NIH Consensus Conference, 1994) which if given enough time might progress to atrophy, ulceration, or even gastric cancer. Another hypothesis suggests that phenotypic differences among bacterial isolates may be important in disease. Indeed, there is accumulating evidence that individuals infected with strains of *H. pylori* which express the vacuolating toxin vacA and/or the cytotoxin associated gene product cagA are more likely to develop peptic ulcers or gastric cancer than are individuals who are infected with vacA/cagA negative strains (Covacci *et al.*, 1993; Cover and Blaser, 1995; Crabtree *et al.*, 1991; Xiang *et al.*, 1995). A third hypothesis to explain the varied clinical outcomes of

*Helicobacter* infection is that variation in the host response is important. We and others have been using the *H. felis* model described above to examine this possibility (Mohammadi *et al.,* 1996; Sakagami *et al.,* 1994). We looked at a series of inbred strains of mice (BALB/c, C3H, C57BL/6, and MHC congenic partners on the BALB/c and C57BL/6 backgrounds) infected with a single strain of *H. felis.* We observed that mice with a BALB/c background had minimal inflammatory responses after *Helicobacter* infection but that mice with a C57BL/6 background had much more severe inflammation (Table I). C3H mice also had more severe inflammation after infection with *H. felis,* which was partially ameliorated in mice which are nonresponsive to bacterial endotoxin (Sakagami *et al.,* 1994). These results suggest that the nature of the host immune or inflammatory responses are also important in disease outcome after *H. pylori* infection of humans. It is probable that duration of infection, bacterial strain, and the host response all play a role in disease outcome after *Helicobacter* infection.

To further investigate the role of the immune response in *Helicobacter*-associated disease, we have also begun to characterize cellular immune responses in the *H. felis* model. Initially, we did some studies in severe combined immunodeficient (SCID) mice on the BALB/c background. These animals have a minimal inflammatory response to *Helicobacter.* Of interest, however, is that in SCIDs or non-SCIDs, the inflammation was, for the most part, the same (Blanchard *et al.,* 1995b). This suggested that perhaps the inflammation associated with *Helicobacter* infection is T- and B-cell independent, and that perhaps the cellular immune response does not play a significant role in disease pathogenesis. However, when the cellular immune response was examined in C57BL/6 mice, which exhibit severe inflammation after infection, the magnitude of the cellular response was found to correlate with the degree of inflammation. In addition, adoptive transfer of sensitized lymphocytes from *H. felis*-infected mice enhanced the inflammatory process when recipient mice were challenged with *H. felis* (Mohammadi *et al.,* 1995). In

*TABLE I*

SEVERITY OF INFLAMMATION AFTER
*HELICOBACTER* INFECTION VARIES
WITH THE MOUSE STRAIN

| Mouse strain | Inflammation score |
| --- | --- |
| BALB/c | $0.8 \pm 0.6$ |
| C3H | $1.3 \pm 0.9$ |
| C57BL/6 | $2.5 \pm 0.5$ |

*Note.* Inbred mice were infected with a single isolate of *H. felis* and were sacrificed 11 weeks later. The intensity of inflammation was graded on a semiquantitative score of 0–3.

BALB/c mice where inflammation was minimal, the magnitude of the *Helico-bacter*-specific lymphocyte stimulation was also lower. This mouse strain variation in the magnitude of the *Helicobacter*-specific cellular immune response may be analogous to the human situation where the results are quite divergent. When one looks at the human response, there are some groups that identify a specific cellular response in positive patients, other groups suggest that there is a cellular response in both seropositive and seronegative patients, and a third group of investigators reports reduced cellular response in seropositive patients (Karttunen *et al.,* 1990; Sharma *et al.,* 1994; Tosi *et al.,* 1992).

A number of conclusions can be drawn from from these studies on the host immune response to *Helicobacter* infection. Natural infection or immunization results in a systemic and mucosal immune response of equivalent magnitude. However, there appears to be a qualitative difference in the immune response following immunization which results in protection. Specifically, antibodies against urease and perhaps other antigens appear to be prominent following immunization and may play a key role in prevention or protection from *Helicobacter* infection. Finally, the cellular immune response following infection and immunization requires further study to determine its role in protection and/or pathogenesis of *Helicbacter* infection.

## REFERENCES

Banatvala, N., Mayo, K., Megraud, F., Jennings, R., Deeks, J. J., and Feldman, R. A. (1993). The cohort effect and *Helicobacter pylori. J. Infect. Dis.* **168,** 219–221.

Bell, G. D., Powell, K., Burridge, S. M., Pallecaros, A., Jones, P. H., Gant, P. W., Harrison, G., and Trowell, J. E. (1992). Experience with 'triple' anti-Helicobacter eradication therapy: Side effects and the importance of testing the pre-treatment bacterial isolate for metronidazole resistance. *Alimentary Pharmacology and Therapy* **6,** 427–435.

Blanchard, T. G., Czinn, S. J., Maurer, R., Thomas, W. D., Soman, G., and Nedrud, J. G. (1995a). Urease-specific monoclonal antibodies prevent *Helicobacter felis* infection in mice. *Infect. Immun.* **63,** 1394–1399.

Blanchard, T. G., Czinn, S. J., Nedrud, J. G., and Redline, R. W. (1995b). Helicobacter-associated gastritis in SCID mice. *Infect. Immun.* **63,** 1113–1115.

Burnette, W. N., Mar, V. L., Platler, B. W., Schlotterbeck, J. D., McGinley, M. D., Stoney, K. S., Rohde, M. F., and Kaslow, H. R. (1991). Site-specific mutagenesis of the catalytic subunit of cholera toxin: Substituting lysine forarginine 7 causes loss of activity. *Infect. Immun.* **59,** 4266–4270.

Chen, M., Lee, A., Hazell, S., Hu, P., and Li, Y. (1993). Immunisation against gastric infection with *Helicobacter* species: First step in the prophylaxis of gastric cancer? *Zentralbl. Bakteriol.* **280,** 155–165.

Chiba, N., Babu, V. R., Rademaker, J. W., and Hunt, R. F. (1992). Meta-analysis of the efficiency of antibiotic therapy in eradicating *Helicobacter pylori. Am. J. Gastroenterol.* **87,** 1716–1727.

Clemens, J. D., Harris, J. R., Khan, M. R., Ali, M., Yunus, M., Khan, M. U., Svennerholm, A. M., Sack, D. A., Chakraborty, J., Stanton, B. F., Ahmed, F., Kay, B. A., Rao, M. R., and Holmgren, J. (1988). Impact of B subunit killed whole-cell and killed whole-cell-only oral vaccines against cholera upon treated diarrhoeal illness and mortality in an area endemic for cholera. *Lancet* **1,** 1375–1379.

Coelho, L. G. V., Passos, M. C. F., Chausson, Y., Costa, E. L., Maia, A. F., Brandao, M. J. C., Rodrigues, D. C., and Castro, L. P. (1992). Duodenal ulcer and eradication of *Helicobacter pylori* in a developing country. An 18 month follow up study. *Scand. J. Gastroenterol.* **27**, 362–366.

Corthesy-Theulaz, I., Porta, N., Glauser, M., Saraga, E., Vaney, A.-C., Haas, R., Kraehenbuhl, J. P., Blum, A. L., and Michetti, P. (1995). Oral immunization with *Helicobacter pylori* urease B subunit as a treatment against Helicobacter infection in mice. *Gastroenterology* **109**, 115–121.

Covacci, A., Censini, S., Bugnoli, M., Petracca, R., Burroni, D., Macchia, G., Massone, A., Papini, E., Xiang, Z., Figura, N., and Rappuoli, R. (1993). Molecular characterization of the 120 kDa immunodominant antigen of *Helicobacter pylori* associated with cytotoxicity and duodenal ulcer. *Proc. Natl. Acad. Sci. U.S.A.* **90**, 5791–5795.

Cover, T. L., and Blaser, M. J. (1995). *Helicobacter pylori:* A bacterial cause of gastritis, peptic ulcer disease, and gastric cancer. *ASM News* **61**, 21–26.

Crabtree, J. E., Taylor, J. D., Wyatt, J. I., Heatley, R. V., Shallcross, T. M., Tompkins, D. S., and Rathbone, B. J. (1991). Mucosal IgA recognition of *Helicobacter pylori* 120 kDa protein, peptic ulceration, and gastric pathology. *Lancet* **338**, 332–335.

Cuenca, R., Blanchard, T. G., Czinn, S. J., Nedrud, J. G., Monath, T. P., Lee, C. K., and Redline, R. W. (1996). Therapeutic immunization against *Helicobacter mustelae* infection in naturally infected ferrets. *Gastroenterology* (in press).

Czinn, S. J., and Nedrud, J. G. (1991). Oral immunization against *Helicobacter pylori*. *Infect. Immun.* **59**, 2359–2363.

Czinn, S. J., Cai, A., and Nedrud, J. G. (1993). Protection of germfree mice from infection by *Helicobacter felis* after active oral or passive IgA immunization. *Vaccine* **11**, 637–642.

Czinn, S. J., Bierman, J. C., Diters, R. W., Blanchard, T. G., and Leunk, R. D. (1996). Characterization and therapy for experimental infection by *Helicobacter mustelae* in ferrets. *Helicobacter* **1**, 43–51.

Dick-Hegedus, E., and Lee, A. (1991). Use of a mouse model to examine anti-*Helicobacter pylori* agents. *Scand. J. Gastroenterol.* **26**, 909–915.

Dickinson, B. L., and Clements, J. D. (1995). Dissociation of *Escherichia coli* heat-labile enterotoxin adjuvanticity from ADP-ribosyltransferase activity. *Infect. Immun.* **63**, 1617–1623.

Doidge, C., Gust, I., Lee, A., Buck, F., Hazell, S., and Manne, U. (1994). Therapeutic immunization against Helicobacter infection. *Lancet* **343**, 913–914.

Douce, G., Trucotte, C., Cropley, I., Roberts, M., Pizza, M., Domenighini, M., Rappuoli, R., and Dougan, G. (1995). Mutants of *Escherichia coli* heat labile toxin lacking ADP-ribosyltransferase activity act as nontoxic, mucosal adjuvants. *Proc. Natl. Acad. Sci. U.S.A.* **92**, 1644–1648.

Eaton, K. A., and Krakowa, S. (1992). Chronic active gastritis due to *Helicobacter pylori* in immunized Gnotobiotic piglets. *Gastroenterology* **103**, 1580–1586.

Eurogast Study Group (1993). An international association between *Helicobacter pylori* infection and gastric cancer. *Lancet* **341**, 1359–1362.

Ferrero, R. L., Thiberge, J.-M., Huerre, M., and Labigne, A. (1994). Recombinant antigens prepared from the urease subunits of *Helicobacter* spp.: Evidence of protection in a mouse model of gastric infection. *Infect. Immun.* **62**, 4981–4989.

Ferrero, R. L., Thiberge, J.-M., Kansau, I., Wuscher, N., Huerre, M., and Labigne, A. (1995). The GroES homolog of *Helicobacter pylori* confers protective immunity against mucosal infection in mice. *Proc. Natl. Acad. Sci. U.S.A.* **92**, 6499–6503.

Fitzgerald, O., and Murphy, P. (1950). Studies on the physiological chemistry and clinical significance of urease and urea with special reference to the human stomach. *Irish J. Med. Sci.* **292**, 97–159.

Fox, J. G., Blanco, M., Murphy, J. C., Taylor, N. S., Lee, A., Kabok, Z., and Pappo, J. (1993). Local and systemic immune responses in murine *Helicobacter felis* active chronic gastritis. *Infect. Immun.* **61**, 2309–2315.

Fox, J. G., Batchelder, M., Hayward, A., Yan, L., Palley, L., Murphy, J. C., and Shames, B. (1994). Prior *Helicobacter mustelae* infection does not confer protective immunity against experimental reinfection in ferrets. *Am. J. Gastroenterol.* **89**, 1318.

Freedberg, A. S., and Barron, L. E. (1940). The presence of spirochaetes in human gastric mucosa. *Am. J. Dig. Dis.* **38,** 443–445.

Grant, C. C. R., Messer, R. J., and Cieplak, W. J. (1994). Role of trypsin-like cleavage at arginine 192 in the enzymatic and cytotonic activities of *Escherichia coli* heat-labile enterotoxin. *Infect. Immun.* **62,** 4270–4278.

Holmgren, J., Lycke, N., and Czerkinsky, C. (1993). Cholera toxin and cholera B subunit as oral–mucosal adjuvant and antigen vector systems. *Vaccine* **11,** 1179–1184.

Karttunen, R., Andersson, G., Poiikonen, K., Kosunen, T. U., Karttunen, T., Juutinen, K., and Niemela, S. (1990). *Helicobacter pylori* induces lymphocyte activation in peripheral blood cultures. *Clin. Exp. Immunol.* **82,** 485–488.

Lee, A., and Chen, M. (1994). Successful immunization against gastric infection with *Helicobacter* species: Use of a cholera toxin B-subunit-whole-cell vaccine. *Infect. Immun.* **62,** 3594–3597.

Lee, A., Fox, J. G., Otto, G., and Murphy, J. (1990). A small animal model of human *Helicobacter pylori* active chronic gastritis. *Gastroenterology* **99,** 1315–1323.

Lee, A., Chen, M., Coltro, N., O'Rourke, J., Hazell, S., Hu, P., and Li, Y. (1993). Long term infection of the gastric mucosa with *Helicobacter* species does induce atrophic gastritis in an animal model of *Helicobacter pylori* infection. *Zentralbl. Bakteriol.* **280,** 38–50.

Lee, C. K., Weltzin, R., Thomas, W. D. J., Kleanthous, H., Ermak, T. H., Soman, G., Hill, J. E., Ackerman, S. K., and Monath, T. P. (1995). Oral Immunization with recombinant *Helicobacter pylori* urease Induces secretory IgA antibodies and protects mice from challenge with *Helicobacter felis. J. Infect. Dis.* **172,** 161–172.

Liang, X., Lamm, M. E., and Nedrud, J. G. (1989). Cholera toxin as a mucosal adjuvant: Glutaraldehyde treatment dissociates adjuvanticity from toxicity. *J. Immunol.* **143,** 484–490.

Marchetti, M., Arico, B., Burroni, D., Figura, N., Rappuoli, R., and Ghiara, P. (1995). Development of a mouse model of *Helicobacter pylori* infection that mimics human disease. *Science* **267,** 1655–1658.

Marshall, B. J., Armstrong, J. A., and McGechie, D. B. (1985). Attempt to fulfill Koch's postulate for pyloric Campylobacter. *Med. J. Aust.* **142,** 436–439.

Marshall, M. J., and Warren, R. J. (1983). Unidentified curved bacilli on gastric epithelium in active chronic gastritis. *Lancet* **1,** 1273–1275.

Michetti, P., Corthesy-Thelaz, I., Davin, C., Haas, R., Vaney, A.-C., Heitz, M., Bille, J., Kraehenbuhl, J. P., Saraga, E., and L., B. A. (1994). Immunization of Balb/c mice against *Helicobacter felis* infection with *Helicobacter pylori* urease. *Gastroenterology* **107,** 1002–1011.

Mohammadi, M., Nedrud, J. R. R., and Czinn, S. (1995). Adoptive transfer of Helicobacter-specific lymphocytes enhances inflammation in mice. *Clin. Immuno. Immunopathol.* **76,** S8.

Mohammadi, M., Redline, R., Nedrud, J., and Czinn, S. (1996). Role of the host in pathogenesis of Helicobacter associated gastritis: *H. felis* infection of inbred and congenic mouse strains. *Infect. Immunol.* **64,** 238–245.

Morris, A., and Nicholson, G. (1987). Ingestion of *Campylobacter pyloridis* causes gastritis and raised fasting gastric pH. *Am. J. Gastroenterol.* **82,** 192–199.

Nedrud, J., Blanchard, T., Czinn, S., and Lycke, N. (1995). Recombinant cholera toxin B subunit is not an adjuvant for oral immunization against *Helicobacter felis* in mice. *J. Cell. Biochem. Suppl.* **19A,** 261.

NIH Consensus Conference, N. C. (1994). *Helicobacter pylori* in peptic ulcer disease. *JAMA, J. Am. Med. Assoc.* **272,** 65–69.

Palley, L. S., Murphy, J., Yan, Y., Taylor, N., Polidoro, D., and Fox, J. (1993). The effects of an oral immunization scheme using muramyl dipeptide as an adjuvant to prevent gastric *Helicobacter mustelae* infection of ferrets. *Acta Gastroenterol. Belg.* **56**(Suppl.), 54.

Palmer, E. D. (1954). Investigation of the gastric *spirchaetes* of the human. *Gastroenterology* **27,** 218–220.

Parsonnet, J. (1993). *Helicobacter pylori* as a risk factor for gastric cancer. *Eur. J. Gastroenterol. Hepatol.* **5** (Suppl. 1), S103–S107.

Peterson, W. L. (1991). *Helicobacter pylori* and peptic ulcer disease. *N. Engl. J. Med.* **324**, 1043–1048.

Sakagami, T., Shimoyama, T., O'Rourke, J., and Lee, A. (1994). Back to the host: Severity of inflammation induced by *Helicobacter felis* in different strains of mice. *Am. J. Gastroenterol.* **89**, 1345 (Abstract 241).

Sellman, S., Blanchard, T. G., Nedrud, J. G., and Czinn, S. J. (1995). Vaccine strategies for prevention of *Helicobacter pylori* infections. *Eur. J. Gastroenterol. Hepatol.* **7**, S1–S6.

Sharma, S. A., Miller, G. G., Perez-Perez, G. I., Gupta, R. S., and Blaser, M. J. (1994). Humoral and cellular immune recognition of *Helicobacter pylori* proteins are not concordant. *Clin. Exp. Immunol.* **97**, 126–132.

Tamura, S.-I., Yamanaka, A., Shimohara, M., Tomita, T., Komase, K., Tsuda, Y., Suzuki, Y., Nagamine, T., Kawahara, K., Danbara, H., Aizawa, C., Oya, A., and Kurata, T. (1994). Synergistic action of cholera toxin B subunit (and *Escherichia coli* heat-labile toxin B subunit) and a trace amount of cholera whole toxin as an adjuvant for nasal influenza vaccine. *Vaccine* **12**, 419–426.

Tosi, M. F., Sorensen, R. U., and Czinn, S. J. (1992). Cell-mediated immune responsiveness to Helicobacter pylori in healthy seropositive and seronegative adults. *Immunol. Infect. Dis.* **2**, 133–136.

Wilson, A. D., Clarke, C. J., and Stokes, C. R. (1990). Whole cholera toxin and B subunit act synergistically as an adjuvant for the mucosal immune response of mice to keyhole limpet haemocyanin. *Scand. J. Immunol.* **31**, 443–451.

World Health Organization (1994). Infection with *Helicobacter pylori*. *IARC Monographs on the Evaluation of Carcinogenic Risks to Humans* **61**(Schistosomes, Liver Flukes and *Helicobacter pylori*), 218–220.

Xiang, Z., Censini, S., Bayeli, P. F., Telford, J. H., Figura, N., Rappuoli, R., and Covacci, A. (1995). Analysis of expression of CagA and VacA virulence factors in 43 strains of *Helicobacter pylori* reveals that clinical isolates can be divided into two major types and that CagA is not necessary for expression of the vacuolating cytotoxin. *Infect. Immun.* **63**, 94–98.

# Chapter 29

# Mechanisms of Mucosal Immunopathology in Respiratory Syncytial Virus Infection

Roberto Garofalo and Pearay L. Ogra

*Department of Pediatrics, University of Texas Medical Branch, Galveston, Texas 77555*

Respiratory syncytial virus (RSV) is the most important cause of viral lower-respiratory tract disease in infants and young children. It is estimated that 1 out of 100 primary infections leads to hospital admission (Holberg *et al.*, 1991) and substantial mortality occurs in infants with underlying heart and lung disease (MacDonald *et al.*, 1982; Groothuis *et al.*, 1988). In addition to acute morbidity, there are long-term consequences of RSV infection in infancy. RSV has been shown to predispose to the development of hyperreactive airway disease (Hall *et al.*, 1984), and recurrent episodes of wheezing in asthmatic children are often precipitated by RSV infection (Sly *et al.*, 1989). The association between viral respiratory infections and asthma has been acknowledged for several decades. Viruses provoke wheezing in some asthma patients, and viral respiratory infections may also promote the development and intensity of airway hyperresponsiveness (Horn *et al.*, 1975, 1979). Common pathogenetic mechanisms link viral bronchiolitis in infancy and asthma in later life, both airway disorders associated with mucosal inflammation.

Despite the large number of studies on the pathogenesis of RSV infection in humans and experimental animals, the mechanisms of the disease and the delicate balance between immunopathology and immunoprotection are not well understood.

## I. INFLAMMATORY RESPONSE IN RSV DISEASE

Postmortem studies in children have demonstrated that RSV bronchiolitis is characterized by a peribronchiolar mononuclear infiltration with edema of the walls and surrounding tissue, necrosis of the epithelium of the small airways, and plugging of the lumens by the necrotic material and mucus (reviewed in Hall, 1992). Several observations have suggested that immunologic mechanisms may play a key role in the severity of RSV lower respiratory tract disease. Children with RSV infection have been shown to develop an RSV-specific IgE response in the airway

*Essentials of Mucosal Immunology*   Copyright © 1996 by Academic Press, Inc. All rights of reproduction in any form reserved.

mucosa (Welliver *et al.*, 1981). Virus-specific IgE appeared more frequently and in higher concentrations in patients with wheezing due to RSV infection than in patients infected with RSV who did not have wheezing. The degree of RSV-IgE responsiveness was highly correlated with severity of illness, as determined by the degree of hypoxia. In addition, the development of virus-specific IgE response correlated with increased concentrations of histamine in nasopharyngeal secretions (NPS) of patients with bronchiolitis. The fact that the RSV-IgE response was more strongly correlated with the degree of hypoxia than was the concentrations of histamine suggested that the release of other soluble mediators may play an equally important part in determining the severity of illness due to RSV infection. Indeed, leukotriene (LT)$C_4$, a potent bronchoconstrictor metabolite of the arachidonic acid cascade in eosinophils, has been detected in samples of NPS obtained in the acute phase of RSV infection (Volovitz *et al.*, 1988). Two-third of infants with bronchiolitis had detectable levels of $LTC_4$ in NPS. Concentrations of $LTC_4$ in children with bronchiolitis were fivefold higher than those measured in children with upper respiratory illness. Moreover, $LTC_4$ was found in 83% of the children developing an RSV-IgE response and quantities of $LTC_4$ were correlated directly with the magnitude of the RSV-IgE response in secretions. $LTE_4$, recently recognized as a selective eosinophil chemotactic factor (Laitinen *et al.*, 1993), and $LTB_4$ were also present in the respiratory tract at the time of RSV bronchiolitis (Garofalo *et al.*, 1991). Infants who developed an $LTB_4$ response had lower arterial $pO_2$ concentrations and individual concentrations of $LTB_4$ significantly correlated with the degree of hypoxia. Since $LTB_4$ has little or no bronchoconstrictor activity but is a potent inflammatory and immunomodulatory substance, the correlation of $LTB_4$ concentrations with hypoxia may reflect the migration and activation of inflammatory cells, such as neutrophils and eosinophils, to the airway mucosa. In this regard, a massive infiltration of eosinophils has been described in postmortem lung specimens of children who were previously vaccinated with a formalin-inactivated RSV vaccine (Kim *et al.*, 1969). Recipients of this RSV vaccine preparation also had an increase in peripheral blood eosinophil counts at the time of subsequent naturally acquired RSV infection (Chin *et al.*, 1969). In other studies, samples of NPS obtained from a group of children with various forms of illness related to RSV or bacterial pneumonia were tested for the presence of eosinophil cationic protein (ECP), a specific eosinophil granule-associated protein which plays an important role in the pathogenesis of asthma. Concentrations of ECP in children with bronchiolitis were significantly higher (169 ng/ml) than those in children with upper respiratory infection (43 pg/ml) or with lower respiratory disease but without wheezing (29 ng/ml). Negligible concentrations of ECP were found in children with bacterial pneumonia. Among those individuals with detectable concentrations of ECP, the degree of hypoxia was significantly correlated with the amount of ECP present in the respiratory tract, suggesting that eosinophil activation occurs in the respiratory tract during RSV bronchiolitis and may play a significant role in the development of virus-induced airway obstruction (Garofalo *et al.*, 1992).

## II. INTERACTION OF RSV WITH BASOPHILS AND EOSINOPHILS

Common respiratory viruses such as influenza, rhinovirus, and RSV are capable of enhancing *in vitro* IgE-mediated histamine release from basophils in the presence (Ida *et al.*, 1977) or absence (Chonmaitree *et al.*, 1988) of interferon (IFN). Sendai virus-induced IFN can also augment the *in vitro* chemotactic response of basophils (Lett-Brown *et al.*, 1981). Evidence suggesting that factors other than IFN may also play a role in virus-induced enhancement of histamine release has been reported (Busse *et al.*, 1983). Furthermore, the observation that heat-, UV-, or ether-inactivated viruses were also able to enhance the IgE-mediated histamine release (Ida *et al.*, 1977; Busse *et al.*, 1983) raised the possibility that basophils could have been activated or primed by soluble factors released by epithelial cells in which viruses were grown and contaminating virus preparations used in those studies. To determine the nature of the interaction between viruses and eosinophils, we investigated *in vitro* whether eosinophils were activated with respect to oxidative and nonoxidative metabolism after incubation with RSV (Kimpen *et al.*, 1992). Activation of normodense blood eosinophils obtained from healthy subjects was evident from the release of superoxide and $LTC_4$. Using a cytochrome c reduction assay, superoxide could be detected in the cell supernatant 30 min after exposure to RSV. The magnitude of superoxide production due to RSV stimulation varied among the subjects but was clearly detectable in 63% of those tested. Furthermore, the virus primed eosinophils to release significantly more superoxide on subsequent challenge with phorbol esters (PMA) and also sensitized eosinophils to release higher amounts of $LTC_4$ in response to calcium ionophore A23187. Although we have demonstrated by immunofluorescence a direct interaction between RSV and eosinophils, the possibility that eosinophils, as previously mentioned for basophils, were indirectly activated by factors released by epithelial cells (Hep-2) employed for the preparation of the virus pools could not be ruled out at the time of those studies.

## III. RSV MODULATION OF EPITHELIAL BARRIER FUNCTION

Several studies suggest an association between respiratory infections and appearance of allergic disease, especially in atopic individuals. Possible explanations for these observations include that viral agents induce an inflammatory response in the airway mucosa, or may alter the immune defense and act as adjuvants or as allergens (reviewed in Björkstén, 1994). In addition, alteration of the permeability of the respiratory epithelial barrier during viral infections may have an important role in the enhanced uptake of environmental antigens, thus facilitating access of antigens to local immunocompetent cells.

We have shown that serum igG and IgE antibody response to ragweed antigen following primary exposure developed at significantly higher levels in mice infected with RSV, compared to sham-infected controls (Leibovitz *et al.*, 1988). In another study (Freihorst *et al.*, 1988), mice that were exposed intranasally to OVA 4–8 days after RSV infection attained significantly higher peak concentrations of OVA antigen in serum samples compared to uninfected animals. Furthermore, serum IgG anti-OVA antibody titer was higher in RSV-infected animals 9, 16, and 24 days after the last administration of OVA. IgE anti-OVA activity was determined in serum samples collected before RSV infection or sham infection and 17 and 32 days postinfection. No anti-OVA-specific IgE activity was observed in RSV-infected or uninfected animals before and up to 9 days after administration of OVA with an adjuvant (aluminum hydroxide). However, half of the adjuvant-treated, RSV-infected animals exhibited a detectable OVA-specific IgE response 2 weeks later.

Although our data clearly showed enhancement of systemic antigen uptake during acute RSV infection, the histopathological findings of the lungs of RSV-infected mice did not exhibit marked damage of the bronchioalveolar epithelium. The mechanisms underlying the increased antigen uptake observed could not be defined based on these data. However, several possible explanations may exist. These include suppression of phagocytic or mucociliary clearance of antigens, increased permeability of the respiratory epithelium to concurrently available antigens for local and systemic uptake and processing, or possible alterations of mucosal transportation mechanisms secondary to the release of pharmacologic mediators and cytokines during acute RSV infection (Ogra *et al.*, 1984). The role of mucosal damage in the uptake of antigens has been investigated in a number of experimental models demonstrating that the macromolecular absorption across the alveolar capillary barrier may be controlled by inflammatory as well as immunologic mechanisms (Gordon *et al.*, 1983; Braley *et al.*, 1979; Tenner-Raez *et al.*, 1979). Recently it has been shown that IFN$\gamma$ can significantly alter the barrier function of human intestinal epithelial monolayers, as evidenced by a dose-dependent reduction in the transepithelial electrical resistance (Adams *et al.*, 1993). This effect is not associated with epithelial cell death. Other proinflammatory cytokines which are produced in the mucosa (IL-1, IL-6, TNF, TGF$\beta$) have not been investigated to elucidate their effect on epithelial barrier function.

## IV. ROLE OF RESPIRATORY EPITHELIUM

Respiratory epithelial cells are the primary target of viruses which enter the airway. RSV infection results from inhalation or self-inoculation of the virus into the nasal mucosa followed by infection of the local respiratory epithelium. Spreading along the respiratory tract occurs mainly by cell-to-cell transfer of the virus along the intracytoplasmic bridges (Hall *et al.,* 1981). The insult to the respiratory epithelium which is induced by viruses and by a variety of environmental stimuli may be the initial "trigger" of airway inflammation. Several investigators have indeed demonstrated that airway epithelium can generate proinflammatory and immunomodulatory cytokines such as GM-CSF, IL-1, and IL-6, and the chemokines IL-8 and monocyte chemotactic protein (MCP)-1 in response to a number of stimuli including inflammatory agents, injury, and microbial infection (Otsuka *et al.,* 1987; Ohtoshi *et al.,* 1991; Marini *et al.,* 1992; Churchill *et al.,* 1992; Heis *et al.,* 1993; Arnold *et al.,* 1993; Bromander *et al.,* 1993; Cromwell *et al.,* 1992; Standiford *et al.,* 1990, 1991). These studies suggest that respiratory epithelium is in a key position to induce and sustain inflammatory and immunological events in lung diseases such as asthma through the production of cytokines. GM-CSF is recognized as an important factor for stimulating hematopoiesis and prolonging eosinophil survival (Ruef and Coleman, 1990). It also enhances $LTC_4$ release (Silberstein *et al.,* 1986) and eosinophil cytotoxicity (Lopez *et al.,* 1986). At high concentrations (produced locally during inflammation), GM-CSF can act as a true chemotaxin for eosinophils and can mediate eosinophil migration directly (Warringa *et al.,* 1991). Although IL-8 is primarily considered to be a neutrophil-activating factor, under certain conditions IL-8 may have actions on eosinophils. Intraperitoneal injection of IL-8 in the guinea pig causes a T cell and eosinophil infiltrate in the lung (Burrows *et al.,* 1991), and induces bronchial hyperresponsiveness (Warringa *et al.,* 1991). Eosinophils express functional IL-8 receptors, as shown by changes in $[Ca^{2+}]_1$ after IL-8 stimulation (Kernen *et al.,* 1991). Furthermore, eosinophils from normal donors respond chemotactically to IL-8 if preincubated with GM-CSF or IL-3 (Warringa *et al.,* 1991). Other chemokines can activate lymphocytes and, in particular, basophil and eosinophil leukocytes. Among them RANTES, MCP-3, and MIP-1$\alpha$ induce migration and activation of human eosinophils (Rot *et al.,* 1992). Finally, many of the specific biologic effects attributable to IL-1 share the common feature of promoting inflammation. Indeed, IL-1 can induce cytokine genes, protein synthesis and secretion in a wide variety of cell types, increases the expression of adhesion molecules on endothelial cells, and modulates other cell surface molecules which are critical for cell–cell interaction (reviewed in Dinarello, 1992).

## V. TRANSENDOTHELIAL MIGRATION OF EOSINOPHILS

The movement of leukocytes from blood into tissue is a characteristic feature of inflammation (Rot, 1992). For neutrophils, endothelial-dependent adherence represents the initial step in the emigration process that is governed by the endothelial barrier (Moser *et al.,* 1989). Adherence of human eosinophils to cultured endothelial cells has many of the same functional and molecular characteristics as neutrophil–endothelial cell adherence. With respect to the repertoire of adhesion molecules involved, eosinophil adherence requires expression and/or functional activation of CD11b/CD18 (Lamas *et al.,* 1988), which is known to bind to the intercellular adhesion molecule-1 (ICAM-1) expressed on the endothelium. ICAM-1 has been shown to be crucial for eosinophilic infiltration in a primate model of asthma (Wegner *et al.,* 1990). Blood eosinophils can also bind to endothelial leukocyte adhesion molecule-1 (ELAM-1) (Weller *et al.,* 1991). Recently, the involvement of vascular cell adhesion molecule-1 (VCAM-1) was shown for eosinophil adherence. On the endothelial surface, VCAM-1 (Dobrina *et al.,* 1991) interacts with the $\beta_1$-integrin VLA-4, which is expressed on eosinophils but not on neutrophils. In addition, some attractants molecules have been shown to exert their effect while being expressed on the endothelial cell surface ("signaling" molecules). IL-8 expressed on the endothelial surface have been shown to induce neutrophil transmigration (Huber *et al.,* 1991).

A model of events that lead to virus-induced asthma can be hypothesized as follows: (1) the airway epithelium is infected by viruses, (2) cytokines and other proinflammatory mediators are released, and (3) these factors upregulate adhesion molecules and signaling molecules on vascular endothelial cells; these induce (4) extravasation of inflammatory cells such as eosinophils and (5) their functional activation.

Thus, to understand the relevance of cytokines to the mucosal inflammation that characterizes virus-induced asthma, we have investigated the expression and release of chemokines, colony-stimulating factors and of IL-1, IL-6, and TNF by airway epithelial cells infected with RSV. The biological function of these cytokines for blood eosinophil migration, survival, and cytotoxycity will be discussed.

## VI. CYTOKINE PRODUCTION BY RSV-INFECTED AIRWAY EPITHELIAL CELLS

Chemokines are a recently discovered class of small cytokines (92–99 amino acids) which have a common structure with four conserved cysteines, a short amino-terminal and a longer carboxy-terminal sequence (reviewed in Baggiolini and Dahinden, 1994). Two subfamilies are distinguished by the arrangement of the fist two cysteines, either separated by one amino acid (CXC) or adjacent (CC). CXC chemokines have biological activities similar to those of IL-8. Other members of this subfamily are the three closely related proteins GRO$\alpha$, GRO$\beta$, and GRO$\gamma$, epithelial-cell-derived neutrophil-activating protein (ENA-78), and granulocyte chemotactic protein 2 (GCP-2). Prototype members of the CC chemokine subfamily, once identified as histamine-releasing factors, are the macrophage inflammatory protein-1$\alpha$ (MIP-1$\alpha$), the monocyte chemotactic protein 1 (MCP-1), and RANTES. The CC chemokines have a selective effect on basophil and eosinophil chemotaxis and activation, and we hypothesized that they may play a central role in the pathogenesis of RSV-induced bronchiolitis. To investigate the expression and release of chemokines by RSV-infected airway epithelium, Hep-2 (larynx), A549 (alveolar type II), BEAS-2B (bronchial), and normal human bronchial epithelial cells (NHBC) were employed in these studies. Confluent monolayers of epithelial cells were infected with sucrose density-gradient-purified RSV and the conditioned media were tested for the presence of immunoreactive chemokines by ELISA. Results of these experiments are summarized in Table I. Negligible levels of IL-8 were detected in uninfected monolayers. Following RSV infection high levels of IL-8 were produced by all of the epithelial cell lines and by NHBC. The IL-8 concentrations peaked at 48 hr postinfection, when the monolayers of showed >90% cytopathic effect (CPE) (Garofalo *et al.*, 1993). These results have been corroborated by other investigators (Arnold *et al.*, 1994; Noah and Becker, 1993). Steady-state mRNA levels of IL-8 gene following RSV infection have also been investigated using reverse transcriptase-polymerase chain technique (RT-PCR). A549 epithelial cells were infected with RSV and at specific time intervals RNA was extracted and RT-PCR was performed using primers specific for human IL-8. RSV caused a rapid rise in IL-8 mRNA levels by 4 hr, and continued IL-8 mRNA expression was observed at 24 and 48 hr postinfection. In preliminary experiments we have also shown that $GRO\alpha$ is produced by RSV-infected A549 and NHBC.

Two members of the CC chemokine subfamily, MIP-$1\alpha$ and MCP-1, were not detected in uninfected or RSV-infected BEAS-2B and NHBC. On the other hand, A549 released significant amounts of both chemokines starting at 24–36 hr postinfection. RANTES was strongly induced in both bronchial cells and A549 cells by RSV infection, reaching levels greater than 3000 pg/ml at 48 hr postinfection. The levels of RANTES production were greater than those obtained by exposing A549 cells to optimal concentrations of IL-1 and TNF$\alpha$, two potent agonists of epithelial cell function. Viral replication seems to be essential for RANTES generation because the inactivation of RSV by UV-light treatment completely blocked the release of this chemokine.

Cytokines with important proinflammatory and immunoregulatory activity were also investigated using the A549 cell model. Cytokine mRNA signals were sought using the RT-PCR technique. Uninfected A549 showed small quantities of IL-$1\alpha$ and TNF$\alpha$ mRNA, whereas the mRNA for IL-$1_\beta$ was detected in somewhat greater

*TABLE I*

CHEMOKINES PRODUCED BY RSV-INFECTED EPITHELIAL CELLS

| Cell source | IL-8 (ng/ml) | GRO$\alpha$ (ng/ml) | RANTES (pg/ml) | MIP-$1\alpha$ (pg/ml) | MCP-1 (pg/ml) |
|---|---|---|---|---|---|
| A549 | $13.6 \pm 4.6$ | 2.2 | $3268 \pm 406$ | $641 \pm 83$ | 2025 |
| Hep-2 | $9.56 \pm 1.6$ | NT | NT | NT | NT |
| BEAS-2B | $1.65 \pm 0.16$ | NT | $4141 \pm 758$ | – | – |
| NHBC | $1.05 \pm 0.06$ | 2.1 | $3039 \pm 293$ | – | – |

*Note.* NT, Not tested; – not detected.

quantity. Within 4 hr of RSV infection, however, the amounts of mRNA for all three cytokines was increased, which continued over the next 48 hr (Patel *et al.,* 1995). Supernatants from 48-hr RSV-infected cells were also screened for the presence of immunoreactive IL-1 ($\alpha$ and $\beta$ forms), TNF$\alpha$, and IL-6 by ELISA (Table II). Mean concentrations of 121 pg/ml of IL-1$\alpha$, 19pg/ml of IL-1$_\beta$, and 77 pg/ml of TNF$\alpha$ were measured in the supernatants. IL-6 was undetectable in uninfected cells but RSV infection induced the release of more than 500 pg/ml.

Colony-stimulating factors (CSF) are growth factors which control proliferation of stem cells and differentiation along the granulocyte pathway. The CSF are further defined by the types of granulocyte colonies they induce in culture and include neutrophil colony-stimulating factor (G-CSF), macrophage colony-stimulating factor (M-CSF), and granulocyte-macrophage colony-stimulating factors (GM-CSF). These colony-stimulating factors are known to be released from stromal cells and airway epithelial cells (Ohtoshi *et al.,* 1991). As previously discussed, GM-CSF modulates the function of eosinophils and therefore can play a profound role in regulating the presence and survival of these cells in the airway mucosa. As shown in Table III, infection with RSV induced the release of significant amounts of GM-CSF and G-CSF from A549 and from bronchial epithelial cells. Detectable levels of GM-CSF were present in the supernatant starting at 12 hr postinfection.

## VII. Biological Function of RSV-Induced Epithelial Cell Cytokines

The evidence of a profound biological activity of cytokines released by RSV-infected respiratory epithelium comes from recent studies in which the effect of RSV infection on expression of ICAM-1 in A549 cells was evaluated (Patel *et al.,* 1995). Conditioned RSV media (cRSV), produced from growth of RSV in A549 cells, induced a significant increase in the expression of ICAM-1. Treatment of the cells with noninfectious cRSV prepared by UV irradiation (UV-cRSV) resulted in expression of ICAM-1 to a similar extent as the infectious cRSV. These results

*TABLE II*

INFLAMMATORY/IMMUNOMODULATORY CYTOKINES
IN A549 CELLS

| Cytokines (pg/ml) | Uninfected | RSV-infected |
| --- | --- | --- |
| IL-1$\alpha$ | $10.1 \pm 1.4$ | $121.3 \pm 42.4$ |
| IL-1$\beta$ | $0.9 \pm 0.1$ | $18.7 \pm 13$ |
| IL-6 | — | $597 \pm 51$ |
| TNF$\alpha$ | $7.5 \pm 0.7$ | $76.6 \pm 18.4$ |

*Note.* —, not detected.

TABLE III
GROWTH FACTORS PRODUCED BY RSV-INFECTED
EPITHELIAL CELLS

| Cell source | GM-CSF (pg/ml) | G-CSF (pg/ml) |
|---|---|---|
| A549 | 12 ± 5.6 | 2345 |
| Hep-2 | 103 ± 10 | NT |
| NHBC | 157 ± 64 | 141 |
| BEAS-2B | NT | — |

*Note.* NT, not tested; –, not detected.

suggested that RSV induces the synthesis of a soluble mediator(s) which regulates the expression of ICAM-1. Preincubation of UV-cRSV with soluble IL-1 receptor almost completely blocked the enhancement of ICAM-1 expression. Preincubation with neutralizing antibodies to IL-1$\alpha$ and -$\beta$ and TNF$\alpha$ showed that the predominant ICAM-1-enhancing soluble mediator in UV-cRSV was IL-1$\alpha$. These experiments provide direct evidence for an autocrine mechanism of enhanced ICAM-1 expression in RSV-infected epithelial cells that is mediated primarily by IL-1$\alpha$. In addition, these findings may explain why neutrophils attach more avidly to and induce cytotoxicity in RSV-infected epithelial cells (Faden *et al.,* 1984). It is likely that this neutrophil–epithelial interaction occurs in part due to attachment of $\beta$2 integrin molecules on neutrophils with their ligand, ICAM-1, on epithelial cells. The expression of accessory molecules such as ICAM-1 on respiratory cells may also be required for directed cell-mediated cytotoxicity by RSV-specific cytotoxic T lymphocytes which could result both in the elimination of infected cells and in the concomitant damage to the uninfected respiratory mucosa.

In other studies, human microvascular lung endothelial cells (HMVEC) and human umbilical vein endothelial cells (HUVEC) were grown to confluence and tested for the expression of cell-adhesion molecules using cell-based ELISA and flow cytometry. HMVEC expressed about 5-fold higher levels of ICAM-1 compared with HUVEC, whereas we found minimal basal expression of E-selectin on either HMVEC or HUVEC. Basal expression of VCAM-1 was also very low on both endothelial cells. ICAM-1 and E-selectin were increased significantly on both HMVEC and HUVEC after treatment with IL-1$\alpha$ (100 U/ml) and TNF$\alpha$ (250 U/ml) or with IFN$\gamma$ (100 U/ml) (Fig. 1). The expression of E-selectin on cytokine-stimulated endothelial cells was transient with maximal expression at 4–6 hr, whereas the expression of ICAM-1 was strongly induced and sustained for 24–48 hr after stimulation. We could not demonstrate a strong induction of VCAM-1 after cytokine stimulation. When monolayers of HMVEC and HUVEC were exposed to UV-treated conditioned media (20%) obtained from RSV-infected normal human bronchial epithelial cells or A549, expression of ICAM-1 and E-selectin was augmented compared to resting cells. As shown in Fig. 1, HUVEC expressed about 10-fold higher levels of ICAM-1 and 11-fold higher levels of E-selectin after exposure to RSV-conditioned epithelial cell supernatant for 4–6 hr (ICAM-1 and E-selectin) and 24–40 hr (ICAM-1). Similar results were obtained in experiments employing HMVEC. Following exposure to RSV-conditioned supernatant the expression of E-selectin was transient, whereas the expression of ICAM-1 was sustained for 24–40 hr on both endothelial cell types, as we observed in cytokine stimulation. VCAM-1 expression was slightly increased on HUVEC after 24 hr exposure to RSV-conditioned supernatant. Based on the observation that exogenous IL-1$\alpha$ increases ICAM-1 and E-selectin expression on HMVEC and HUVEC and that immunoreactive and bioactive IL-1$\alpha$ activity is present in the supernatant of RSV-infected airway epithelial cells, we postulated that IL-1$\alpha$ was responsible for the enhanced adhesion molecule expression following exposure to RSV-conditioned media. Therefore, the effect of neutralization of IL-1$\alpha$ was examined. Incubation of RSV-conditioned media with a monoclonal Ab anti-IL-1$\alpha$ (5 $\mu$g/ml), prior to the addition to endothelial cell monolayers, completely blocked the upregulation of E-selectin on both HMVEC and HUVEC. Furthermore, monoclonal Ab anti-IL-1$\alpha$ blocked >90% of ICAM-1 upregulation on HUVEC (HMVEC not tested) following exposure for 24 hr to RSV-conditioned media (Fig. 1).

These investigations have established an *in vitro* model to address the role of RSV-infected respiratory epithelial cells in modulating expression of pivotal adhesion molecules on endothelial cells. Following a respiratory viral infection, cytokines produced and released by the airway epithelial cells can induce or enhance the expression of ICAM-1 and E-selectin molecules on endothelial cells, events which may lead to the transendothelial migration of blood leukocytes by a T-cell-independent mechanism.

Evidence of biological function of cytokines released by RSV-infected respiratory epithelium comes also from recent studies in which we have investigated the *in vitro* survival of human eosinophils (Garofalo *et al.*, 1995). Blood eosinophils were isolated from healthy donors by discontinuous Percoll gradients, and both normodense and hypodense populations were further purified (≥98%) by immunomagnetic selection (MACS). Eosinophils were then cultured for 9 days in the presence of medium alone (RPMI with fetal calf serum), conditioned medium of uninfected normal human bronchial cells (20%), UV-irradiated conditioned medium of RSV-infected NHBC (20%) (RSV-epi), or granulocyte macrophage-colony stimulating factor (rhGM-CSF) (40 pg/ml) (Fig. 2). Starting from Day 3 and then at Days 4 and 5 postisolation, the number of viable eosinophils (expressed as mean percent survival of cultured eosinophils) was significantly higher in cultures with RSV-epi (86, 79, and 73, respectively) then in those containing either medium alone (44, 16, 5) or uninfected NHBC supernatant (62, 23, 13) ($P < 0.01$). By Day 7, 72% of eosinophils cultured with RSV-epi were still viable vs only 5% of the eosinophils cultured with medium alone or with uninfected NHBC cell supernatant. Polyclonal anti-GM-CSF antibody (4 $\mu$g/ml) completely neutralized

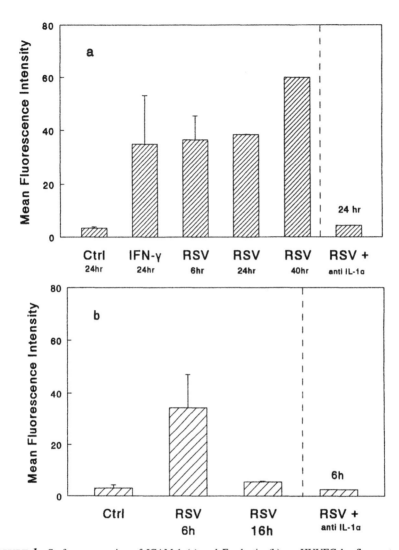

**FIGURE 1.** Surface expression of ICAM-1 (a) and E-selectin (b) on HUVEC by flow cytometry. Composite quantitative fluorescence values expressed as mean ± SEM. Ctrl, resting cells; IFN γ, cells stimulated for 24 hr with 100 U/ml of IFNγ; RSV, cells exposed to UV-irradiated conditioned medium of RSV-infected NHBC for 6, 16, 24, or 40 hr; RSV + anti-IL-1α, cells exposed to UV-irradiated conditioned medium of RSV-infected NHBC which was preincubated with a neutralizing monoclonal anti-IL-1α antibody.

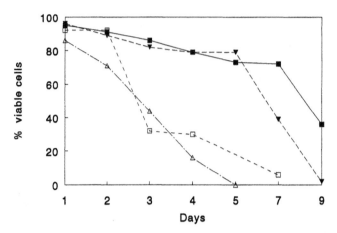

**FIGURE 2.** Eosinophil survival assay by trypan blue exclusion. Eosinophils were cultured for 9 days in the presence of medium alone (open triangles), UV-irradiated conditioned medium of RSV-infected NHBC (filled squares), recombinant human GM-CSF (filled triangles), or UV-irradiated conditioned medium of RSV-infected NHBC which was preincubated with a polyclonal-neutralizing anti-GM-CSF antibody (open squares).

the effect of RSV-epi on eosinophil survival. The results of this study demonstrate that eosinophil survival is sustained by GM-CSF released by RSV-infected epithelial cells.

## VIII. CONCLUDING REMARKS

Airway inflammation is a characteristic feature of RSV infection. Infiltration of the respiratory mucosa by activated mononuclear leukocyte, basophils, and eosinophils has been demonstrated by histological studies and by the presence of cell-specific inflammatory mediators in nasopharyngeal secretions of children with more severe forms of RSV-induced respiratory disease. Studies *in vitro* have also shown that RSV can modulate the biological function of basophils and eosinophils by inducing release from infected respiratory epithelial cells of chemokines (i.e., RANTES) with discrete target-cell selectivity. Although the mechanisms that lead to the accumulation of circulating blood leukocytes within the airway mucosa are still incompletely understood, our investigations suggest that IL-1, generated by respiratory epithelium following RSV infection, may regulate eosinophil extravasation by modulating expression of pivotal endothelial cell adhesion molecules (ICAM-1 and E-selectin). Growth factors such as GM-CSF released by RSV-infected epithelial cells may also promote survival and activation of eosinophils in the airway mucosa and induce the maturation of tissue-resident progenitor cells. Furthermore epithelial cell-driven mucosal inflammation induced by RSV infection may provide an explanation for the increased permeability of the respiratory epithelium to concurrently available antigens, well beyond the apparent histological damage induced by the virus itself. In this way, antigen processing and presentation and type of secretory/cellular local and systemic immune responses ultimately could be altered at the time of an acute viral infection. In conclusion, respiratory epithelial cells, through the expression and release of chemokines, immunomodulatory cytokines, and growth factors in response to infection with RSV, may control the selective concentration and activation of leukocytes and the type of antigen-specific immune response, thus contributing to the initiation and maintenance of harmful inflammatory processes within the airways.

## References

Adams, R. B., Planchon, S. M., and Roche, J. K. (1993). IFN-$\gamma$ modulation of epithelial barrier function: time course, reversibility, and site of cytokine binding. *J. Immunol.* **150,** 2356–2363.

Arnold, R., Scheffer, J., Konig, B., and Konig, W. (1993). Effects of *Listeria monocytogenes* and *Yersinia enterocolitica* on cytokine gene expression and release from human polymorphonuclear granulocytes and epithelial (HEp-2) cells. *Infect. Immun.* **61,** 2545–2552.

Arnold, B., Humbert, H., Werchau, H., Gallati, H., and König, W. (1994). Interleukin-8, interleukin-6, and soluble tumor necrosis factor receptor type I release from a human pulmonary epithelial cell line (A549) exposed to respiratory syncytial virus. *Immunology* **82,** 126–133.

Baggiolini, M., and Dahinden, C. A. (1994). CC chemokines in allergic inflammation. *Immunol. Today* **15,** 127–33.

Björkstén, B. (1994). Inhalant allergy and hypersensitivity disorders. *In* "Handbook of Mucosal Immunology" (P. L. Ogra, W. Strober, J. Mestecky, J. R. McGhee, M. E. Lamm, and J. Bienenstock, eds.), pp. 561–566. Academic Press, San Diego.

Braley, J. F., Peterson, L. B., Dawson, C. A., and Moore, V. L. (1979). Effect of hypersensitivity on protein uptake across the air–blood barrier of isolated rabbit lungs. *J. Clin. Invest.* **63,** 1103–1109.

Bromander, A. K., Kjerrulf, M., Holmgren, J., and Lycke, N. (1993). Cholera toxin enhances alloantigen presentation by cultured intestinal epithelial cells. *Scand. J. Immunol.* **37,** 452–458.

Burrows, L. J., Piper, P. J., Lindley, I. D., and Westwick, J. (1991). Intra-peritoneal injection of human recombinant neutrophil-activity factor/interleukin-8 (hr NAF/IL-8) produces a T-cell and eosinophil infiltrate in the guinea pig lung. Effect of PAF antagonist WEB2086. *Ann. N.Y. Acad. Sci.* **629,** 422–424.

Busse, W. W., Swenson, C. A., Borden, E. C., Treuhaft, M. W., and Dick, E. C. (1983). Effect of influenza A virus on leukocyte histamine release. *J. Allergy Clin. Immunol.* **71,** 382–388.

Chin, J., Maggoffin, R. L., Shearer, L. A., Schieble, J. H., and Lennette, E. H. (1969) Field evaluation of a respiratory syncytial virus vaccine and a trivalent parainfluenza virus vaccine in a pediatric population. *Am. J. Epidemiol.* **89,** 449–463.

Chonmaitree, T., Lett-Brown, M. A., Tsong, Y., Goldman, A. S., and Baron, S. (1988). Role of interferon in leukocyte histamine release caused by common respiratory viruses. *J. Infect. Dis.* **157,** 127–132.

Churchill, L., Friedman, B., Schleimer, R. P., and Proud, D. (1992). Production of granulocyte-macrophage colony-stimulating factor by cultured human tracheal epithelial cells. *Immunology* **75,** 189–195.

Cromwell, O., Hamid, Q., Corrigan, C. J., Barkans, J., Meng, Q., and Collins, P. D. (1992). Expression and generation of interleukin-8, IL-6 and granulocyte-macrophage colony-stimulating factor by bronchial epithelial cells and enhancement by IL-1$_\beta$ and tumour necrosis factor-$\alpha$. *Immunology* **77,** 330–337.

Dinarello, C. A. (1992). Role of Interleukin-1 in infectious diseases. *Immunol. Rev.* **127,** 119–146.

Dobrina, A., Menegazzi, R., Carlos, T. M., Nardon, E., Cramer, R., Zacchi, T., Harlan, J. M., and Patriarca, P. (1991). Mechanisms of eosinophil adherence to cultured vascular endothelial cells. Eosinophils bind to the cytokin-induced endothelial ligand vascular cell adhesion molecule-1 via the very late activation antigen-4 integrin receptor. *J. Clin. Invest.* **88,** 20–26.

Faden, H., Hong, J. J., and Ogra, P. L. (1984). Interaction of polymorphonuclear leukocytes and viruses in humans: Adherence of polymorphonuclear leukocytes to respiratory syncytial virus-infected cells. *J. Virol.* **52,** 16–23.

Freihorst, J., Piedra, P. A., Okamoto, Y., and Ogra, P. L. (1988). Effect of respiratory syncytial virus infection on the uptake of and immune response to other inhaled antigens. *Proc. Soc. Exp. Biol. Med.* **188,** 191–197.

Garofalo, R., Welliver, R. C., and Ogra, P. L. (1991). Concentrations of LTB4, LTC4, LTD4, and LTE4 in bronchiolitis due to respiratory syncytial virus. *Pediatr. Allergy Immunol.* **2,** 30–37.

Garofalo, R., Kimpen, J. L. L., Welliver, R. C., and Ogra, P. L. (1992). Eosinophil degranulation in the respiratory tract during naturally acquired respiratory syncytial virus infection. *J. Pediatr.* **120,** 28–32.

Garofalo, R., Patel, J. A., Sim, T. C., Schmalstieg, F. C., Goldman, A. S., and Ogra, P. L. (1993). Production of cytokines by virus-infected human respiratory epithelial cells. *J. Allergy Clin. Immun.* **91,** 177.

Garofalo, R., Olszewska, B., Pazdrak, K., Alam, R., Mei, F., and Ogra, P. L. (1995). Respiratory syncytial virus (RSV)-infected airway epithelial cells enhance eosinophil survival. *Pediatr. Res.* **37,** 8A.

Gordon, R. E., Case, B. W., and Kleinerman, J. (1983). Acute $NO_2$ effects on penetration and transport of horseradish peroxidase in hamster respiratory epithelium. *Am. Rev. Respir. Dis.* **128,** 528–533.

Groothuis, J. R., Gutierrez, K. M., and Lauer, B. A. (1988). Respiratory syncytial virus infection in children with bronchopulmonary dysplasia. *Pediatrics* **82,** 199–203.

Hall, C. B. (1992). Respiratory syncytial virus. *In* "Textbook of Pediatric Infectious Disease" (D. Feigin and J. D. Cherry, eds.), pp. 1633–1656. Saunders, Philadelphia, Pennsylvania.

Hall, C. B., Douglas, R. G., Jr., Schnabel, K. C., and Geiman, J. M. (1981). Infectivity of respiratory syncytial virus by various routes of inoculation. *Infect. Immunol.* **33,** 779–783.

Hall, C. B., Hall, W. J., Gala, C. L., McGill, F. B., and Leddy, J. P. (1984). A long term prospective study of children following respiratory syncytial virus infection. *J. Pediatr.* **105,** 358–364.

Heiss, L. N., Moser, S. A., Unanue, E. R., and Goldman, W. E. (1993). Interleukin-1 is linked to the respiratory epithelial cytopathology of pertussis. *Infect. Immun.* **61,** 3123–3128.

Holberg, C. J., Wright, A. L., Martinez, F. D., Ray, C. G., Taussig, L. M., and Lebowitz, M. D. (1991). Risk factors for respiratory syncytial virus-associated lower respiratory illnesses in the first year of life. *Am. J. Epidemiol.* **133,** 1135–1151.

Horn, M. E. C., Brain, E., Gregg, I., Yealland, S. J., and Taylor, P. (1975). Respiratory viral infection in children: A survey in general practice, Roehampton 1967–1972. *J. Hyg.* **74,** 157–168.

Horn, M. E. C., Brain, E. A., Gregg, I., Inglis, J. M., Yealland, S. J., and Taylor, P. (1979). Respiratory viral infection and wheezing bronchitis in childhood. *Thorax* **34,** 23–28.

Huber, A. R., Kunkel, S. L., Todd III, R. F., and Weiss, S. (1991). Regulation of transendothelial neutrophil migration by endogenous interleukin-8. *Science* **254,** 99–102.

Ida, S., Hooks, J. J., Siraganian, R. P., and Notkins, A. L. (1977). Enhancement of IgE-mediated histamine release from human basophils by viruses: Role of interferon. *J. Exp. Med.* **145,** 892–906.

Kernen, P., Wymann, M. P., and vonTscharner (1991). Shape changes, exocytosis and cytosolic free calcium changes in stiumulated human eosinophils. *J. Clin. Invest.* **87,** 2012–2017.

Kim, H. W., Canchola, J. G., Brandt, C. D., Pyles, G., Chanock, R. M., Jensen, K., and Parrot, R. H. (1969). Respiratory syncytial virus disease in infants despite prior administration of antigenic inactivated vaccine. *Am. J. Epidemiol.* **89,** 422–433.

Kimpen, J. L. L., Garofalo, R., Welliver, R. C., and Ogra, P. L. (1992). Activation of human eosinophils *in vitro* by respiratory syncytial virus. *Pediatr. Res.* **32,** 160–164.

Laitinen, L. A., Laitinen, A., Haahtela, T., Vikka, V., Spur, B. W., and Lee, T. H. (1993). Leukotriene E4 and granulocytic infiltration into asthmatic airways. *Lancet* **341,** 989–990.

Lamas, A. M., Mulroney, C. M., and Schleimer, R. P. (1988). Studies on the adhesive interaction between purified human eosinophils and cultured vascular endothelial cells. *J. Immunol.* **140,** 1500–1505.

Leibovitz, E., Freihorst, J., Piedra, P. A., and Ogra, P. L. (1988). Modulation of systemic and mucosal immune responses to inhaled ragweed antigen in experimentally induced infection with respiratory syncytial virus implication in virally induced allergy. *Int. Arch. Allergy Appl. Immunol.* **86,** 112–116.

Lett-Brown, M. A., Aelvoet, M., Hooks, J. J., Georgiades, J. A., Thueson, D. O., and Grant, J. A. (1981). Enhancement of basophil chemotaxis *in vitro* by virus-induced interferon. *J. Clin. Invest.* **67,** 547–52.

Lopez, A. F., Williamson, D. J., Gamble, J. R., Begley, C. G., Harlan, J. M., Klebanoff, S. J., Waltersdorph, A., Wong, G., Clark, S. C., and Vadas, M. A. (1986). Recombinant human granulocyte-macrophage colony-stimulating factor stimulants *in vitro* mature human neutrophil and eosinophil function, surface receptor expression, and survival. *J. Clin. Invest.* **78,** 1220–1228.

MacDonald, N. E., Hall, C. B., Suffin, S. C., Alexson, C., Harris, P. J., and Manning, J. A. (1982). Respiratory syncytial viral infection in infants with congenital heart disease. *N. Engl. J. Med.* **307,** 397–400.

Marini, M., Vittori, E., Hollemborg, J., and Mattol, S. (1992). Expression of the potent inflammatory cytokines, granulocyte-macrophage-colony-stimulating factor and interleukin-6 and interleukin-8, in bronchial epithelial cells of patients with asthma. *J. Allergy Clin. Immunol.* **89,** 1001–1009.

Medhurst, A. D., Westwick, J., and Piper, P. J. (1991). hr IL-8-induced hyperresponsiveness in guinea pig perfused lungs. *Ann. N.Y. Acad. Sci.* **629,** 419–421.

Moser, R., Schleiffenbaum, B., Groscurth, P., and Fehr, J. (1989). Interleukin 1 and tumor necrosis factor stimulate human vascular endothelial cell to promote transendothelial neutrophil passage. *J. Clin. Invest.* **83,** 444–455.

Noah, T. L., and Becker, S. (1993). Respiratory syncytial virus-induced cytokine production by a human bronchial epithelial cell line. *Am. J. Physiol.* L 472–478.

Ogra, P. L., Welliver, R. C., Riepenhoff-Talty, M., and Faden, H. S. (1984). Interaction of mucosal immune system and infections in infacy: Implications in allergy. *Ann. Allergy* **53,** 523–534.

Ohtoshi, T., Vancheri, C., Cox, G., Gauldie, J., Dolovich, J., Denburg, J. A., and Jordana, M. (1991). Monocyte–macrophage differentiation induced by human upper airway epithelial cells. *Am. J. Respir. Cell Mol. Biol.* **4,** 255–263.

Otsuka, H., Dolovich, J., Bienenstock, J., and Denburg, J. A. (1987). Metachromatic cell progenitors and specific growth and differentiation factors in human nasal mucosa and polyps. *Am. Rev. Respir. Dis.* **136,** 710–717.

Patel, J. A., Kunimoto, M., Sim., T. C., Garofalo, R., Eliott, T., Baron, S., Ruuskanen, O., Chonmaitree, T., Ogra., P. L., and Schmalstieg, F. C., Jr. (1995). IL-1$\alpha$ mediates enhanced expression of ICAM-1 in pulmonary epithelial cells infected with respiratory syncytial virus. *Am. J. Respir. Cell Mol. Biol.* **13,** 602–609.

Rot, A. (1992). Endothelial cell binding of NAP-1/IL-8: role in neutrophil emigration. *Immunol. Today* **13,** 291–294.

Rot, A., Kreiger, M., Brunner, S. C., Bischoff, S. C., Schall, T. J., and Dahinden, C. A. (1992). RANTES and macrophage inflammatory protein 1$\alpha$ induce the migration and activation of normal human eosinophil granulocytes. *J. Exp. Med.* **176,** 1489–1495.

Ruef, C. and Coleman, D. L. (1990). Granulocyte-macrophage colony-stimulating factor: Pleiotropic cytokine with potential clinical usefulness. *Rev. Infect. Dis.* **12,** 41–62.

Silberstein, D. S., Owen, W. F., Gasson, J. C., DiPersio, J. F., Gold, D. W., Bina, J. C., Soberman, R.,

Austen, K. F., and David, J. R. (1986). Enhancement of human eosinophil cytotoxicity and leuko-triene synthesis by biosynthetic (recombinant) granulocyte-macrophage colony-stimulating factor. *J. Immunol.* **137,** 3290–3294.

Sly, P. D., and Hibbert, M. D. (1989). Childhood asthma following hospitalization with acute viral bronchiolitis in infancy. *Pediatr. Pulmonol.* **7,** 153–158.

Standiford, T. J., Kunkel, S., Basha, M. A., Chensue, S. W., Lynch III, J. P., Toews, G. B., Westwick, R. M., and Strieter, R. M. (1990). Interleukin-8 gene expression by a pulmonary epithelial cell line. *J. Clin. Invest.* **86,** 1945–1953.

Standiford, T., Kunkel, S., Phan, S., Rollins, B., and Strieter, R. M. (1991). Alveolar macrophage-derived cytokines induce monocyte chemoattractant protein expression from human pulmonary type II: like epithelial cells. *J. Biol. Chem.* **266,** 9912–9918.

Tenner-Ràez, K., Racz, P., Myrvik, Q. N., Ockers, J. R., and Geister, R. (1979). Uptake and transport of horseradish peroxidase by lymphoepithelium of the bronchus-associated lymphoid tissue in nor-mal and *Bacillus* Calmette-Guérin-immunized and challenged rabbits. *Lab. Invest.* **41,** 106–115.

Volovitz, B., Welliver, R. C., De Castro, G., Krystofik, D. A., and Ogra, P. L. (1988). The release of leukotriene in the respiratory tract during infection with respiratory syncytial virus: Role in obstruc-tive airway disease. *Pediatr. Res.* **24,** 504–507.

Warringa, R. A. J., Koenderman, L., Kok, P. T. M., Kreukniet, J., and Bruijnzeel, P. L. B. (1991). Modulation and induction of eosinophil chemotaxis by granulocyte-macrophage colony-stimulating factor and interleukin-3. *Blood* **77,** 2694–2700.

Wegner, C. D., Gundel, R. H., Reilly, P., Haynes, N., Letts, L. G., and Rothlein, R. (1990). Intercellular adhesion molecule-1(ICAM-1) in the pathogenesis of asthma. *Science* **247,** 456–459.

Weller, P. F., Rand, T. H., Goelz, S. E., Chi-Rosso, G., and Lobb, R. R. (1991). Human eosinophil adherence to vascular endothelium mediated by binding to vascular cell adhesion molecule 1 and endothelial leukocyte adhesion molecule 1. *Proc. Natl. Acad. Sci. U.S.A.* **88,** 7430–7433.

Welliver, R. C., Wong, D. T., Sun, M., Middleton, E., Jr., Vaughan, R. S., and Ogra, P. L. (1981). The development of respiratory syncytial virus-specific IgE and the release of histamine in nasopharyn-geal secretions after infection. *N. Engl. J. Med.* **305,** 841–846.

# Chapter 30

# Mucosal HIV Infection: A Paradigm for Dysregulation of the Mucosal Immune System

Martin Zeitz,* Thomas Schneider,* and Reiner Ullrich†

*Medical Clinic II, University of the Saarland, 66421 Homburg/Saar, Germany; and †Department of Gastroenterology, Medical Clinic, Klinikum Benjamin Franklin, Free University of Berlin, 12200 Berlin, Germany

## I. INTRODUCTION

The gut-associated lymphoid tissue (GALT) comprises an enormous amount of immune cells and the rectal mucosa is most likely the portal of entry of human immunodeficiency virus (HIV) in the major risk group for HIV infection in industrialized countries, namely, homosexual and bisexual men. In addition, the gastrointestinal tract is a common site of opportunistic infections and malignancies defining acquired immunodeficiency syndrome (AIDS). During the course of HIV infection most patients develop gastrointestinal symptoms. In Europe and North America about 18–50% of HIV-infected patients suffer from diarrhea (Quinn *et al.*, 1987; Heise *et al.*, 1988; René *et al.*, 1989); in developing countries like Zaire or Haiti the percentage of AIDS patients with diarrhea is about 90% (Malebranche *et al.*, 1983; Colebunders *et al.*, 1988). Thus, the intestinal immune system is substantially involved in the course of HIV infection.

Most of our current knowledge on the immunopathogenesis of HIV infection comes from *in vivo* and *in vitro* studies of circulating immune cells. From these studies, a common pattern of the development from HIV infection to the outbreak of full-blown AIDS can be recognized. HIV may enter the host by direct inoculation in the blood stream or by close contact with mucosal surfaces. In the peripheral blood HIV infects the helper/inducer subset of T lymphocytes by the high-affinity binding of its envelope glycoprotein, gp120, to the CD4 molecule (Dagleish *et al.*, 1984). The CD4 receptor is present in high density on the helper T lymphocyte subset, in a lower density on many cells of the monocyte-macrophage lineage, and on certain other cell types. CD4$^+$ memory T cells appear to be prefentially infected (Schnittman *et al.*, 1990). Because most mucosal T cells are memory T cells (Schieferdecker *et al.*, 1992) they may be likely targets for infection. After entry of HIV into the target cell, infection may remain latent. However, as shown recently in this so-called latent phase an enormous struggle takes place between the virus and the immune system (Ho *et al.*, 1995; Wain-Hobson, 1995; Wei *et al.*, 1995). T-cell activation is thought to be a crucial event in the enhancement of viral replication mediated by the interaction of cellular regulatory proteins (e.g., the transcription factor NFκB) with specific DNA sequences of the HIV long-terminal repeat (Nabel and Baltimore, 1987; Nabel, 1991). Thus, replication of HIV is dependent on the state of activation of T cells. Recent studies have demonstrated that during the clinical latent phase of HIV infection, when only minor amounts of HIV can be detected in the peripheral blood, a high virus load and an accelerated virus replication can be observed in the lymph nodes (Pantaleo *et al.*, 1991, 1993a; Embretson *et al.*, 1993). During this period of HIV infection which usually lasts about 10 years CD4 depletion continues and is more pronounced in the intestinal mucosa than in the peripheral blood (Lim *et al.*, 1993a; Schneider *et al.*, 1995). Due to the central role of CD4$^+$ lymphocytes in both cellular and humoral immunity the depletion or functional impairment of this T-cell subset by HIV leads to the severe immunodeficiency seen in patients with AIDS (Dagleish *et al.*, 1984; Rosenberg and Fauci, 1989; Pantaleo *et al.*, 1993b; Weiss, 1993). Disturbed function and loss of CD4$^+$ T cells may also be of special importance for immunoregulation at mucosal surfaces, since activated CD4$^+$ memory T cells predominate in this compartment of the immune system (Zeitz *et al.*, 1988, 1989; Schieferdecker *et al.*, 1992).

In this chapter, data on mucosal HIV load in comparison to the peripheral blood will be given. Then, consequences of HIV infection on the mucosal T-cell response and the humoral immune response will be discussed. Finally, data will be presented which indicate that intestinal mucosal structure and function are disturbed in HIV-infected patients.

## II. HIV-INFECTION OF THE INTESTINAL MUCOSA

Several studies using different methods have demonstrated the presence of HIV proteins or nucleic acids in the intestinal mucosa (Nelson *et al.*, 1988; Fox *et al.*, 1989; Ullrich *et al.*, 1989; Jarry *et al.*, 1990; Kotler *et al.*, 1991, 1993; Clayton *et al.*, 1992; Ehrenpreis *et al.*, 1992; Gill *et al.*, 1992; Becker *et al.*, 1994) (Fig. 1). The infected cells are not definitely characterized. However, most authors agree that mononuclear cells in the lamina propria (morphologically assessed as lymphocytes or macrophages) are infected by HIV. In some studies HIV-infected epithelial cells or enterochromaffine cells were identified as well. The role of epithelial cells as targets of HIV infection *in vitro* is still controversial. *In vitro* studies have shown that epithelial cells can be infected by HIV (Adachi *et al.*, 1987; Bourinbaiar and Phillips, 1990, 1991; Fantini *et al.*, 1991), even in the absence of CD4 expression (Yahi *et al.*, 1992). Two early studies, both employing DNA probes and *in situ* hybridization, reported a preponderance of HIV-infected epithelial compared with lamina propria cells (Mathijs *et al.*, 1988; Nelson *et al.*, 1991), while

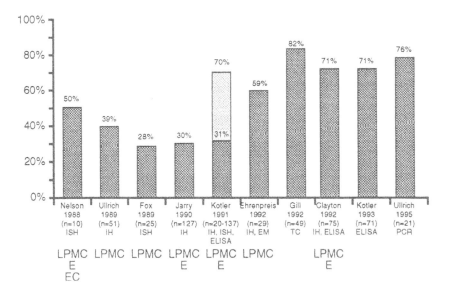

*FIGURE 1.* Summary of the studies investigating intestinal jucosal HIV infection in humans. The *y* axis gives the percentage of HIV-positive tissue samples of HIV-infected patients. (Methods for detection of HIV in the mucosa: ISH, *in situ* hybridization; IH, immunohistology; ELISA, enzyme-linked immunosorbent assay for p24; EM, electron microscopy; TC, tissue culture; PCR, polymerase chain reaction. Identification of HIV-infected cells: LPMC, lamina propria mononuclear cells; E, enterochromaffin cells; EC, epithelial cells.)

in another small series HIV RNA was found in enterocytes of only one of eight patients and in considerably smaller quantity compared with infected lamina propria cells (Heise *et al.*, 1991). Larger studies very rarely (if at all) detected HIV-infected cells in the epithelial layer by different methods (Fox *et al.*, 1989; Ullrich *et al.*, 1989; Jarry *et al.*, 1990). Thus, HIV infection of epithelial cells seems to be scarce *in vivo*. HIV infection of follicular dendritic cells in intestinal lymph follicles has also been reported (Jarry *et al.*, 1990; Racz, 1990). The role of these cells in the afferent part of the intestinal immune system makes them likely candidates for very early and persistent infection with HIV during anal intercourse which could lead to a continuing infection of T cells in the lymphoid follicles. In a recent study on the lamina propria of esophageal mucosa from AIDS patients HIV could be detected in macrophages but not in lymphocytes by *in situ* hybridization methods combined with immunohistology (Smith *et al.*, 1994). In rhesus macaques intravenously infected with the simian immunodeficiency virus (SIV), SIV could be detected in macrophages and T lymphocytes of the intestinal lamina propria as early as 1 week after infection (Heise *et al.*, 1994). This indicates a very fast invasion of the virus in the intestinal mucosa even in the case of parenteral infection.

Direct *in vitro* infection of human fetal small- and large-intestinal explants was demonstrated recently (Fleming *et al.*, 1992). In these experiments it was shown that normal fetal intestinal mucosa can be productively infected by HIV-1, and that only cells of the intestinal immune system like macrophages and T cells are targets of infection when a T-cell tropic HIV strain was used. Interestingly, colonic tissue showed a smaller increase in reverse transcriptase activity and p24 antigen production than the corresponding small-intestinal explants, suggesting that viral replication may be accelerated in the small intestine (Fleming *et al.*, 1992). This is in good agreement with our observation that there is a massive and early loss of CD4$^+$ T cells in the small intestine of HIV-infected humans (Schneider *et al.*, 1995) as discussed later.

The high virus load and accelerated virus replication in lymph nodes during the clinical latent phase of HIV infection (Pantaleo *et al.*, 1991, 1993a; Embretson *et al.*, 1993) is probably also true for the intestinal mucosa. Studies comparing the amount of HIV in the intestinal mucosa with the peripheral blood using a p24 capture assay (Kotler *et al.*, 1991), *in situ* hybridization (Smith *et al.*, 1994), or polymerase chain reaction (PCR) (Becker *et al.*, 1994) have clearly shown a higher virus load in the intestine. In addition, Smith and co-workers found a higher prevalence of HIV-1 mRNA-expressing cells in esophageal mucosa of AIDS patients than in lymph notes from AIDS patients (Smith *et al.*, 1994). Thus, the intestinal mucosa is heavily infected by HIV and may represent an important reservoir for HIV.

It is unclear, so far, how HIV infects cells in the intestinal mucosa. HIV enters the host by direct inoculation in the blood stream or via mucosal surfaces. If the infection takes place in the rectal or vaginal mucosa the virus has to pass the epithelial layer. Several posibilities have been proposed by *in vitro* studies. Like other antigens HIV may be taken up by the specialized dome epithelial cells of Peyer's patches and lymphoid follicles in the colon and rectum, the microfolded (M) cells. These cells are adapted to transport luminal antigens including viruses, bacteria, and even small parasites (Owen and Jones, 1974). M-cell uptake of HIV has been shown in an electromicroscopic *in vitro* study using rabbit intestine (Amerongen *et al.*, 1991). HIV infection of T cells may then occur in the follicle and the infected T cell may pass through the mesenteric lymph node, the thoracic duct, and the peripheral blood, migrating back to the lamina propria (Fig. 2). By this route HIV infection even of distant mucosal sites as the duodenal mucosa could be explained.

Another posibility is the uptake of HIV–anti-HIV antibody complexes via Fc receptors, which are present on the rectal mucosal epithelium (Hussain *et al.*, 1991; Lehner *et al.*, 1991). Furthermore, *in vitro* data suggest an alternative HIV receptor of the galactosyl ceramide type on enterocytes (Fantini *et al.*, 1991; Yahi *et al.*, 1992). From the infected epithelial cells the virus may reach lamina propria T cells by basal budding (Fantini *et al.*, 1991). Finally, the high risk of HIV transmission during anal intercourse might be due in part to traumatic lesions of the rectal mucosa (Kingsley *et al.*, 1987).

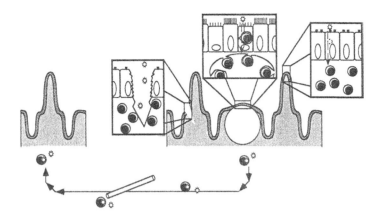

FIGURE 2. Hypothetic model of mucosal HIV infection and accumulation. HIV may be transported by M cells in the follicular-associated epithelium into the Peyer's patches or other organized lymphoid follicles where follicular dentridic cells may be infected. These cells transmit HIV to T cells which migrate back like the uninfected T cells to mucosal surfaces after circulation through the peripheral blood. Since the T cells coming from the mucosa are mainly activated memory T cells, they may be preferentially infected with HIV and an accumulation of HIV-infected T cells may occur in the intestine after homing. Furthermore HIV may directly enter the lamina propria through epithelial cells and infect the lamina propria lymphocytes or enter this compartment through traumatic lesions of the surface.

## III. MUCOSAL IMMUNE SYSTEM IN HIV INFECTION

### A. Intestinal Cellular Immunity

Immunological abnormalities of the intestinal mucosa in HIV infection have been studied mainly by phenotypical analysis of cryostat sections by immunohistology (Rodgers *et al.*, 1986; Budhraja *et al.*, 1987; Ellakany *et al.*, 1987; Jarry *et al.*, 1990; Ullrich *et al.*, 1990; Lim *et al.*, 1993a,b) or on isolated lymphocytes by flow cytometry (Schneider *et al.*, 1994, 1995). A decreased CD4/CD8 ratio and a proportional increase in CD8$^+$ cells were consistently found. However, there was a large variation in the degree of the CD4$^+$ T-cell depletion in the lamina propria, especially in the immunohistological studies which might be due to small numbers of patients studied and technical difficulties. Downregulation of CD4 is well documented in HIV infection, especially in the absence of cytopathic effects (McDougal *et al.*, 1985; Stevenson *et al.*, 1987). *In vitro* studies have shown that CD4 in HIV-infected T cells is trapped intracellularly and not transported to the cell surface (Schneider *et al.*, 1992). Therefore the variable decrease in mucosal CD4$^+$ cells reported by different groups using immunhistology might be explained partially by a variable detection of intracellular CD4 depending on the sensitivity of the method used. On the other hand, in some studies CD4$^+$ macrophages might have been mistaken for CD4$^+$ T cells since immunohistology was performed without double staining as discussed by Lim and co-workers (Lim et al., 1993a).

An intraindividual comparison of lymphocytes isolated simultaneously from the peripheral blood and duodenal mucosa of HIV-infected patients employing three-color flow cytometry revealed a pronounced depletion of mucosal CD4$^+$ T cells even in early stages of the disease not correlating with the peripheral blood (Schneider et al., 1995) (Fig. 3). In this study nearly all HIV-infected patients had CD4 levels of T cells in the duodenal mucosa below 5%. Some patients with relatively preserved CD4$^+$ T cells in the peripheral blood and a CD4$^+$ T-cell depletion of about 1% in the duodenal mucosa already had opportunistic agents like microsporidia or CMV, indicating that peripheral blood CD4$^+$ T-cell counts may be misleading in assessment and prediction of intestinal HIV disease.

Memory T cells have been defined by their high expression of CD45R0 and CD29 and the absence of CD45RA (Sanders et al., 1988). Intestinal T cells which are virtually all CD45RO$^+$ and CD45RA$^-$ differ from circulating memory T cells as they do not express CD29 in high density (Schieferdecker et al., 1992). The reduced expression of CD45RO and CD29 on intestinal T cells in HIV infection (Schneider et al., 1994) (Table I) could result from a preferential loss of differentiated CD4$^+$ memory T cells as described in the peripheral blood (Van Noesel et al., 1990). The decreased proportion of intestinal CD4 T cells expressing CD29 in AIDS patients is in accordance with this hypothesis; however, the proportion of CD45RO, CD45RA, and HML-1 was not altered on the remaining intestinal CD4 T cells in HIV infection (Schneider et al., 1994) (Table I). Thus, depletion of intestinal CD4 T cells seems to be the predominant effect of HIV infection.

CD8$^+$ T cells are consistently increased in the intestinal mucosa of HIV-infected patients compared to controls. Within the CD8 population, activated HLA-DR$^+$ CD8$^+$ T cells and cytotoxic CD11a$^+$ CD8$^+$ T cells are elevated (Schneider et al., 1994) (Table I). These activated cytotoxic CD8$^+$ T cells may recognize HIV antigens (Walker et al., 1988; Culmann et al., 1989; Nixon and McMichael, 1991; Kundu and Merigan, 1992) and play a role in the control of HIV infection, but they could also be harmful by damaging the intestinal epithelium as in HIV-associated alveolitis (Autran et al., 1988).

Natural killer cells which can eliminate virally infected and tumor cells are reduced in the intestinal mucosa of AIDS patients, which may further facilitate infections and malignancies in the intestine (Schneider et al., 1994). Macrophages of the intestinal mucosa in HIV-infected patients are also impaired, as shown by the reduction of the antigen-presenting subset (Lim et al., 1993b). Thus, it is obvious that the cellular mucosal immune response in HIV-infected patients is severely disturbed and is unable to control effectively malignancies and infections in the gastrointestinal tract of AIDS patients.

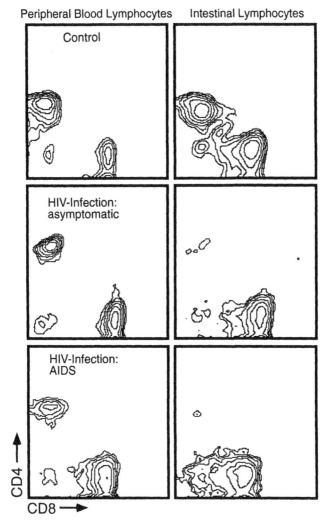

FIGURE 3. Flow cytometric analysis of peripheral blood and duodenal T cells in a control person, an asymptomatic HIV-infected patient, and an AIDS patient. T cells were isolated simultaneously from peripheral blood and uodenal biopsies and stained with fluoresccinated antibodies to CD4, CD8, and CD3. The proportion of CD3[+] T cells expressing CD4 (y axis) and CD8 (x axis) was determined by three-color flow cytometry. The decrease in CD4[+] T cells was more pronounced in the duodenum than in the peripheral blood even in the asymptomatic HIV-infected patient (modified from Schneider et al., 1995).

TABLE I
PHENOTYPICAL CHARACTERISTICS OF ISOLATED DUODENAL
INTESTINAL LYMPHOCYTES OF HIV-INFECTED PATIENTS COMPARED
WITH CONTROLS BY THREE-COLOR CYTOFLUOROMETRY

| Proportion of lymphocytes | HIV vs Controls |
|---|---|
| CD3 (pan T-cell marker) | ≈ |
| $\gamma\delta^+$/CD3 | ≈ |
| CD8$^-$CD4$^-$/CD3 | ≈ |
| CD8$^+$/CD3 | ↑↑ |
| CD8$^+$CD45RA/CD3 (CD8$^+$ naive T cells) | ↑ |
| CD8$^+$CD11a$^+$/CD3 (cytotoxic T cells) | ↑ |
| CD8$^+$CD11b$^+$/CD3 (suppressor T cells) | ≈ |
| CD8$^+$HLA-DR$^+$/CD3 (activated CD8$^+$ T cells) | ↑↑ |
| CD8$^+$CD25$^+$/CD3 (activated CD8$^+$ T cells) | ≈ |
| CD4$^+$/CD3 | ↓↓ |
| CD4$^+$CD45R0$^+$/CD3 (CD4$^+$ memory T cells) | ↓↓ |
| CD4$^+$HLA-DR$^+$/CD3 (activated CD4$^+$ T cells) | ↓↓ |
| CD4$^+$CD25$^+$/CD3 (activated CD4$^+$ T cells) | ↓↓ |
| CD16$^+$CD57$^+$ (natural killer cells) | ↓ |

*Note.* ≈ similar, ↑ increased, ↓ decreased compared with controls. Relative proportions were calculated after gating for CD3$^+$ lymphocytes. From Schneider *et al.* (1995), Ullrich *et al.*, submitted.

## B. Intestinal Humoral Immunity

Insufficient helper function of intestinal CD4 T cells is also indicated by the reduced proportion of IgA plasma cells in the large intestine of AIDS patients reported by Kotler *et al.* (1987) since terminal IgA B-cell differentiation is CD4 T-cell dependent (Kiyono *et al.*, 1984; Kunimoto *et al.*, 1988). A marked decrease in salivary IgA levels was found in AIDS patients, which was due to a selective decrease in IgA2 with normal IgA1 levels (Jackson, 1990). However, divergent results exist concerning the Ig concentrations in the saliva of HIV-infected patients. In contrast to Jackson and co-workers (Jackson, 1990), one group found no difference between IgA in the saliva of controls and HIV-infected patients (Kotler *et al.*, 1987), and another group reported a reduction of both IgA subclasses (Müller *et al.*, 1991).

In the intestinal fluid of HIV-infected patients a reduced level of IgA compared with controls was found, while IgG was increased in the HIV-infected group (Janoff *et al.*, 1994) (Table II). In this study a significantly reduced level of IgA2 and polymeric IgA was demonstrated in duodenal fluid while IgA1 was not altered. The predominance of IgG and monomeric IgA1 in mucosal fluid samples from HIV-infected patients may be explained by exudation of serum immunoglobulins into the intestine, probably due to increased epithelial permeability.

The presence of secretory IgA against HIV in the stool (Mathewson *et al.*,

TABLE II

INTESTINAL MUCOSAL IMMUNGLOBULINS AND PLASMA CELLS IN THE INTESTINAL LAMINA
PROPRIA IN HIV-INFECTED PATIENTS COMPARED WITH CONTROLS

| Ig measured in intestinal fluid[a] | | | | | Immunohistology of plasma cells[b] | | | | |
| --- | --- | --- | --- | --- | --- | --- | --- | --- | --- |
| IgG | IgM | IgA | IgA1 | IgA2 | IgG | IgM | IgA | Iga1 | IgA2 |
| ↑ | ≈ | ↓ | ↑ | ↓ | ≈ | ↑ | ↓ | ≈ | ↓ |

Note. ≈ similar, ↑ increased, ↓ decreased compared with controls.
[a] Janoff et al. (1994).
[b] Kotler et al. (1987); Janoff et al. (1994).

1994), rectal secretions (Mohamed et al., 1994), and intestinal fluid (Janoff et al., 1994) of HIV-infected patients has been demonstrated. The frequency in the detection of secretory IgA against HIV in the stool by an ELISA was higher in HIV-infected patients with diarrhea than in patients without diarrhea (Mathewson et al., 1994). In the study by Janoff et al. (1994) intestinal IgG reacted with most HIV antigens, while intestinal IgA mainly recognized HIV envelope proteins. These studies show that a disturbed mucosal antibody response is present in HIV-infected patients, which may further contribute to the breakdown of the mucosal barrier function in these patients.

## IV. INFLUENCE OF THE ALTERED INTESTINAL IMMUNE SYSTEM ON SMALL-INTESTINAL STRUCTURE AND FUNCTION IN HIV INFECTION

There is growing evidence that functional interrelations exist between the gut epithelium and the mucosal immune system (MacDonald and Spencer, 1988, 1990). The observation that mucosal T-cell activation both in vitro (MacDonald and Spencer, 1988) and in vivo (Griffiths et al., 1988) lead to villous atrophy with increased proliferation of crypt cells further supports this concept. Thus, changes in mucosal architecture might reflect alterations in mucosal immunity (Riecken et al., 1989).

Partial villous atrophy has been found in the small intestine of HIV-infected patients independent of the presence of secondary infections in several studies (Malebranche et al., 1983; Kotler et al., 1984, 1990; Batman et al., 1989; Ullrich et al., 1989, 1990; Cummins et al., 1990; Greenson et al., 1991). Villous atrophy is a nonspecific reaction of the intestinal mucosa to various afflictions. It either is associated with a hyperregenerative increase in crypt cell mitoses leading to crypt elongation (as seen in gluten-sensitive enteropathy), or it results from hyporegeneration, i.e., reduced mitotic rate with shortened crypts (as seen in bowel rest or excluded intestinal loops). Although minor differences in morphometric parameters exist in the available studies in HIV-infected patients, it is clear that the impressive increase in mitoses with strikingly elongated crypts characteristic of gluten enteropathy is not found in HIV-infected patients. Even in the presence of secondary intestinal infections there is an inadequate elongation of crypts and, notably, no increase in crypt mitoses (Anonymous, 1989; Ullrich *et al.,* 1991).

Several studies demonstrated that the specific type of mucosal transformation in HIV infection depends both on the presence of secondary pathogens and on mucosal HIV infection (Ullrich *et al.,* 1989, 1990; Kotler *et al.,* 1990). In patients with HIV-infected cells in the mucosa villous atrophy was accompanied by reduced crypt cell proliferation. In the presence of secondary infections the number of mitotic figures per crypt was slightly increased but inappropriately to the villous atrophy resulting in impaired crypt hyperplasia. Thus, HIV infection is associated with epithelial hypoproliferation (Ullrich *et al.,* 1989).

A recent study on human fetal intestinal explant cultures infected with HIV *in vitro* demonstrated a stimulation of epithelial cell proliferation, which supports the theory of hyperplastic villous atrophy suggested by Batman and co-workers (Batman *et al.,* 1994). These apparently conflicting data may be explained by the completely different conditions: in the fetal explant model early effects of HIV were observed, where HIV infection might lead to T-cell activation with mucosal hyperregeneration. In the human *in vivo* situation long-term effects of HIV infection with loss of activated mucosal T cells were studied.

Not only an altered epithelial proliferation in HIV-infected patients but also an even more pronounced impaired enterocyte maturation was demonstrated in HIV-infected patients by measuring activities of brush-border enzymes (Ullrich *et al.,* 1989) (Fig. 4). Lactase deficiency, the prevalence of which is about 10–20% in whites, was found in nearly 50% of white HIV-infected patients, and was significantly more common in patients with mucosal HIV infection, secondary intestinal infections, or both as compared with controls (Ullrich *et al.,* 1992). In addition, zidovudine therapy was significantly associated with higher activities of brush-border enzymes, indicating improved enterocyte maturation under anti-retroviral therapy (Ullrich *et al.,* 1992).

*In vitro* studies on HIV-infected colonic epithelial tumor cell lines using transmission electromicroscopy also revealed cytopathic effects including an unusual number of secretion bodies, the appearance of intracellular lumina, and disorganized microvilli, indicating a defect in brush-border assembly and differentiation (Fantini *et al.,* 1992). Further studies on intestinal epithelial cell lines infected by HIV *in vitro* demonstrated an exaggerated increase in intracellular calcium after stimulation with a calcium ionophore in infected cultures compared with uninfected cultures (Asmuth *et al.,* 1994). These experiments also suggest that absorptive and secretory functions of enterocytes may be altered by HIV infection.

The morphologic and functional disturbances of the intestinal mucosa in HIV infection might fit into a concept of immune-mediated mucosal transformation: crypt cell proliferation is induced by T-cell activation, therefore the activated CD4$^+$ T cells present in the normal lamina propria might be involved in the maintenance of the normal mucosal architecture. The epithelial hypoproliferation

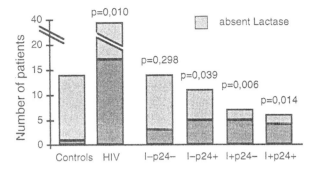

**FIGURE 4.** Lactase deficiency in HIV-infected patients. Duodenal biopsies of control persons and HIV-infected patients were analyzed by quantitative enzyme histochemistry *in situ*. Compared to controls, lactase deficiency was observed in a significantly higher percentage of HIV-infected patients (I-p24⁻: no secondary infections, no p24 antigen in the mucosal; I-p24⁺: no secondary infections, p24 antigen present in the mucosal; I + p24⁻: additional secondary infection, no p24 antigen in the mucosa; I + p24⁺: additional secondary infection, p24 antigen present in the mucosa. Modified from Ullrich *et al.* (1989).

seen in HIV-infected patients could be explained by the early and nearly complete loss of CD4$^+$ T cells in the intestinal lamina proria of HIV-infected patients. Impairment or depletion of activated regulatory CD4$^+$ T cells in the lamina propria by HIV might thus lead not only to a breakdown of the mucosal immune barrier resulting in a variety of opportunistic infections, but also to malabsorption due to mucosal atrophy or enterocyte dysfunction.

## V. SUMMARY

The intestinal (in particular rectal) mucosa is an important portal of entry of HIV in homosexual men, who represent the vast majority of HIV-infected patients in Europe and North America. There are several possibilities for HIV to reach the CD4$^+$ T cells, macrophages, and follicular dendritic cells in the intestinal mucosa. HIV may be transported through M cells directly to mucosal lymphoid follicles. Alternatively, HIV may infect enterocytes via Fc-receptor by antibody-bound HIV or via a CD4-independent receptor. By successive budding on the basal side of enterocytes HIV may be released into the lamina propria. Trauma of the mucosa gives direct access for HIV to the lymphoid compartment of the mucosa. Furthermore, in patients not infected by the intestinal route HIV may also rapidly enter the intestinal mucosa by other mechanisms; intestinal T-lymphocytes are mainly activated memory T cells reentering the mucosal surfaces after circulating through the peripheral blood. In the periphery they may be preferentially infected by HIV. Accumulation of infected T cells could thus occur in the intestinal mucosa. The special phenotypical and functional characteristics of intestinal T lymphocytes may affect the replication and cytopathicity of HIV resulting in an accelerated loss of

CD4$^+$ T cells in the lamina propria. CD4$^+$ T cells play a critical role in antigen-dependent B-cell differentiation, and thus the pronounced CD4$^+$ T-cell depletion in the intestinal mucosa may be responsible for the observed decrease of IgA plasma cells and a reduced secretion of IgA$_2$. Depletion and functional impairment of activated mucosal lamina propria lymphocytes by HIV infection could explain the breakdown of the mucosal immune barrier leading to secondary opportunistic or nonopportunistic infections and secondary malignancies. In addition, due to the interrelation between the mucosal immune system and epithelium, these changes might be responsible for the partial small-intestinal mucosal atrophy and maturational defects in enterocytes observed in HIV-infected patients.

## ACKNOWLEDGMENT

This work was supported by grants II-008-91 and 01 KI 9468 from the BMBF.

## REFERENCES

Adachi, A., Koenig, S., Gendelman, H. E., Daugherty, D., Gattoni, C. S., Fauci, A. S., and Martin, M. A. (1987). Productive, persistent infection of human colorectal cell lines with human immunodeficiency virus. *J. Virol.* **61**, 209–213.

Amerongen, H. M., Weltzin, R., Farnet, C. M., Michetti, P., Haseltine, W. A., and Neutra, M. R. (1991). Transepithelial transport of HIV-1 by intestinal M cells: A mechanism for transmission of AIDS. *J Acquired Immune Defic. Syndr.* **4**, 760–765.

Anonymous. (1989). HIV-associated enteropathy. *Lancet* **2**, 777–778.

Asmuth, D. M., Hammer, S. M., and Wanke, C. A. (1994). Physiological effects of HIV infection on human intestinal epithelial cells: An *in vitro* model for HIV enteropathy. *AIDS* **8**, 205–211.

Autran, B., Mayaud, C. M., Raphael, M., and *et al.* (1988). Evidence for a cytotoxic T-lymphocyte alveolitis in human immunodeficiency virus-infected patients. *AIDS* **2**, 179–183.

Batman, P. A., Fleming, S. C., Sedgwick, P. M., MacDonald, T. T., and Griffin, G. E. (1994). HIV infection of human fetal intestinal explant cultures induces epithelial cell proliferation. *AIDS* **8**, 161–167.

Batman, P. A., Miller, A. R., Forster, S. M., Harris, J. R., Pinching, A. J., and Griffin, G. E. (1989). Jejunal enteropathy associated with human immunodeficiency virus infection: quantitative histology. *J. Clin. Pathol.* **42**, 275–281.

Becker, A., Schneider, T., Schmidt, W., Habermehl, K. O., Zeitz, M., Riecken, E. O., and Ullrich, R. (1994). Die duodenale Mukosa ist im Vergleich zum peripheren Blut ein bevorzugtes Reservoir der HIV-Infektion. *Z. Gastroenterol.* **32**, 545.

Bourinbaiar, A. S., and Phillips, D. M. (1990). HIV transmission across intact epithelia. VIIIth International Congress of Virology, Berlin.

Bourinbaiar, A. S., and Phillips, D. M. (1991). Transmission of human immunodeficiency virus from monocytes to epithelia. *J. Acquired Immune Defic. Syndr.* **4**, 56–63.

Budhraja, M., Levendoglu, H., Kocka, F., Mangkornkanok, M., and Sherer, R. (1987). Duodenal mucosal T cell subpopulation and bacterial cultures in acquired immune deficiency syndrome. *Am. J. Gastroenterol.* **82**, 427–431.

Clayton, F., Reka, S., Gronin, W. J., Torlakovic, E., Sigal, S. H., and Kotler, D. P. (1992). Rectal mucosal pathology varies with human immunodeficiency virus antigen content and disease stage. *Gastroenterology* **103**, 919–933.

Colebunders, R., Lusakumuni, K., Nelson, A. M., Gigase, P., Lebughe, I., van Marck, E., Kapita, B., Francis, H., Salaun, J. J., Quinn, T. C., and et al. (1988). Persistent diarrhoea in Zairian AIDS patients: An endoscopic and histological study. Gut 29, 1687–1691.

Culmann, B., Gomard, E., Kieny, M.-P., Guy, B., Dreyfus, F., Saimot, A.-G., Sereni, D., and Levy, J.-P. (1989). An antigenic peptide of the HIV-1 nef protein recognized by cytotoxic T lymphocytes of seropositive individuals in association with different HLA-B molecules. Eur. J. Immunol. 19, 2383–2386.

Cummins, A. G., LaBrooy, J. T., Stanley, D. P., Rowland, R., and Shearman, D. J. (1990). Quantitative histological study of enteropathy associated with HIV infection. Gut 31, 317–21.

Dagleish, A. G., Beverly, P. C. L., Clapham, P. R., Crawford, D. H., Greaves, M. F., and Weiss, R. A. (1984). The CD4 (T4) antigen is an essential component of the receptor for the AIDS retrovirus. Nature (London) 312, 763–766.

Ehrenpreis, E. D., Patterson, B. K., Brainer, J. A., Yokoo, H., Rademaker, A. W., Glogowski, W., Noskin, G. A., and Craig, R. M. (1992). Histopathologic findings of duodenal biopsy specimens in HIV-infected patients with and without diarrhea and malabsorption. Am. J. Clin. Pathol. 97, 21–28.

Ellakany, S., Whiteside, T. L., Schade, R. R., and vanThiel, D. H. (1987). Analysis of intestinal lymphocyte subpopulations in patients with acquired immunodeficiency syndrome (AIDS) and AIDS-related complex. Am. J. Clin. Pathol. 87, 356–364.

Embretson, J., Zupanic, M., Ribas, J. L., Burke, A., Racz, P., Tenner-Racz, K., and Haase, A. T. (1993). Massive covert infection of helper T lymphocytes and macrophages by HIV during the incubation period of AIDS. Nature (London) 362, 359–362.

Fantini, J., Yahi, N., and Chermann, J.-C. (1991). Human immunodeficiency virus can infect the apical and basolateral surface of human colonic epithelial cells. Proc. Natl. Acad. Sci. U.S.A. 88, 9297–9301.

Fantini, J., Yahi, N., Baghdiguian, S., and Chermann, J.-C. (1992). Human colon epithelial cells productively infected with human immunodeficiency virus show impaired differentiation and altered secretion. J. Virol. 66, 580–585.

Fleming, S. C., Kapembwa, M. S., MacDonald, T. T., and Griffin, G. E. (1992). Direct in vitro infection of human intestine with HIV-1. AIDS 6, 1099–1104.

Fox, C. H., Kotler, D., Tierney, A., Wilson, C. S., and Fauci, A. S. (1989). Detection of HIV-1 RNA in the lamina propria of patients with AIDS and gastrointestinal disease. J Infect. Dis. 159, 467–471.

Gill, J. M., Sutherland, L. R., and Church, D. L. (1992). Gastrointestinal tissue cultures for HIV in HIV-infected/AIDS patients. AIDS 6, 553–556.

Greenson, J. K., Belitsos, P. C., Yardley, J. H., and Bartlett, J. G. (1991). AIDS enteropathy: Occult enteric infections and duodenal mucosal alterations in chronic diarrhea. Ann. Intern. Med. 114, 366–72.

Griffiths, C. E., Barrison, I. G., Leonard, J. N., Caun, K., Valdimarsson, H., and Fry, L. (1988). Preferential activation of CD4 T lymphocytes in the lamina propria of gluten-sensitive enteropathy. Clin. Exp. Immunol. 72, 280–283.

Heise, W., Mostertz, P., Skörde, J., and L'Age, M. (1988). Gastrointestinale Befunde bei der HIV-Infektion. Dtsch. Med. Wochenschr. 113, 1588–1593.

Heise, C., Dandekar, S., Kumar, P., Duplantier, R., Donovan, R. M., and Halsted, C. H. (1991). Human immunodeficiency virus infection of enterocytes and mononuclear cells in human jejunal mucosa. Gastroenterology 100, 1521–1527.

Heise, C., Miller, C. J., Lackner, A., and Dandekar, S. (1994). Primary acute simian immunodeficiency virus infection of intestinal lymphoid tissue is associated with gastrointestinal dysfunction. J. Infect. Dis. 169, 1116–1120.

Ho, D. D., Neumann, A. U., Perelson, A. S., Chen, W., Leonard, J. M., and Markowitz, M. (1995). Rapid turnover of plasma virions and CD4 lympocytes in HIV-1 infection. Nature (London) 373, 123–126.

Hussain, L. A., Kelly, C. G., Hecht, E.-M., Fellowes, R., Jourdan, M., and Lehner, T. (1991). The expression of Fc receptors for immunoglobulin G in human rectal epithelium. *AIDS* **5**, 1089–1094.

Jackson, S. (1990). Secretory and serum IgA are inversely altered in AIDS patients. *In* "Advances in Mucosal Immunology (Proceedings of the Fifth International Congress of Mucosal Immunology)" (T. T. Mac Donald, S. J. Challacombe, P. W. Bland, C. R. Stokes, R. V. Heatley, and A. M. Mowat, eds.), pp. 665–668. Kluwer, Dordrecht, Boston, and London.

Janoff, E. N., Jackson, S., Wahl, S. M., Thomas, K., Peterman, J. H., and Smith, P. D. (1994). Intestinal mucosa immunoglobulins during Human Immunodeficiency Virus Type 1 infection. *J. Infect. Dis.* **170**, 299–307.

Jarry, A., Cortez, A., René, E., Muzeau, F., and Brousse, N. (1990). Infected cells and immune cells in the gastrointestinal tract of AIDS patients. An immunohistochemical study of 127 cases. *Histopathology* **16**, 133–140.

Kingsley, L. A., Deles, R., Kaslow, R., *et al.* (1987). Risk factors for seroconversion to human immunodeficiency virus among male homosexuals. *Lancet* **1**, 345–348.

Kiyono, H., Cooper, M. D., Kearney, J. F., Mosteller, L. M., Michalek, S. M., Koopman, W. J., and McGhee, J. R. (1984). Isotype specificitiy of helper T cell clones: Peyer's patch Th cells preferentially collaborate with mature IgA B cells for IgA responses. *J. Exp. Med.* **159**, 798–811.

Kotler, D. P., Francisco, A., Clayton, F., Scholes, J. V., and Orenstein, J. M. (1990). Small intestinal injury and parasitic disease in AIDS. *Ann. Intern. Med.* **113**, 444–449.

Kotler, D. P., Gaetz, H. P., Lange, M., Klein, E. B., and Holt, P. R. (1984). Enteropathy associated with the acquired immunodeficiency syndrome. *Ann. Intern. Med.* **101**, 421–428.

Kotler, D. P., Reka, S., Borcich, A., and Cronin, W. J. (1991). Detection, localization and quantitation of HIV-assosiated antigens in the intestinal biopsies from patients with HIV. *Am. J. Pathol.* **139**, 823–830.

Kotler, D. P., Scholes, J. V., and Tierney, A. R. (1987). Intestinal plasma cell alterations in the acquired immunodeficiency syndrome. *Dig. Dis. Sci.* **32**, 129–138.

Kotler, D. P., Reka, S., and Clayton, F. (1993). Intestinal mucosal inflammation associated with human immunodeficiency virus infection. *Dig. Dis. Sci.* **38**, 1119–1127.

Kundu, S. K., and Merigan, T. C. (1992). Equivalent recognition of HIV proteins, Env, Gag and Pol by CD4+ and CD8+ cytotoxic T-lymphocytes. *AIDS* **6**, 643–649.

Kunimoto, D. Y., Harriman, G. R., and Strober, W. (1988). Regulation of IgA differentiation in CH12LX B cells by lymphokines: IL-4 induces membrane IgM-positive CH12LX cells to express membrane IgA and IL-5 induces membrane IgA-positive CH12LX cells to secrete IgA. *J. Immunol.* **141**, 713–720.

Lehner, T., Hussain, L., Wilson, J., and Chapman, M. (1991). Mucosal transmission of HIV. *Nature (London)* **353**, 709.

Lim, S. G., Condez, A., Lee, C. A., Johnson, M. A., Elia, C., and Poulter, L. W. (1993a). Loss of mucosal CD4 lymphocytes is an early feature of HIV infection. *Clin. Exp. Immunol.* **92**, 448–454.

Lim, S. G., Condez, A., and Poulter, L. W. (1993b). Mucosal macrophage subset of the gut in HIV: Decrease in antigen-presenting cell phenotype. *Clin. Exp. Immunol.* **92**, 442–447.

MacDonald, T. T., and Spencer, J. (1988). Evidence that activated mucosal T cells play a role in the pathogenesis of enteropathy in human small intestine. *J. Exp. Med.* **167**, 1341–1349.

MacDonald, T. T., and Spencer, J. (1990). Gut immunology. *Bailliere's Clin. Gastroenterol.* **4**, 291–313.

Malebranche, R., Arnoux, E., Guerin, J. M., Pierre, G. D., Laroche, A. C., Elie, R., Morisset, P. H., Spira, T., Mandeville, R., Drotman, P., Seemayer, T., and Dupuy, J. M. (1983). Acquired immunodeficiency syndrome with severe gastrointestinal manifestations in Haiti. *Lancet* **2**, 873–877.

Mathewson, J. J., Jiang, Z. D., DuPont, H. L., Chintu, C., Luo, N., and Zumala, A. (1994). Intestinal secretory IgA immune response against human immunodeficiency virus among infected patients with acute and chronic diarrhea. *J. Infect. Dis.* **169**, 614–617.

Mathijs, J. M., Hing, M., Grierson, J., Dwyer, D. E., Goldschmidt, C., Cooper, D. A., and Cunningham, A. L. (1988). HIV infection of rectal mucosa. *Lancet* **1**, 1111.

McDougal, J. S., Mawle, A., Cort, S. P., Nicholson, J. K., Cross, G. D., Scheppler, C. J., Hicks, D., and Sligh, J. (1985). Cellular tropism of the human retrovirus HTLV-III/LAV. I. Role of T cell activation and expression of the T4 antigen. *J. Immunol.* **135**, 3151–3162.

Mohamed, O. A., Ashley, R., Goldstein, A., McElrath, J., Dalessio, J., and Corey, L. (1994). Detection of rectal antibodies to HIV-1 by a sensitive chemiluminescent Western blot immunodetection method. *J. Acquired Immune Defic. Syndr.* **7**, 375–380.

Müller, F., Froland, S. S., Hvatum, M., Radl, J., and Brandtzaeg, P. (1991). Both IgA subclasses are reduced in parotid saliva from patients with AIDS. *Clin. Exp. Immunol.* **83**, 203–209.

Nabel, G., and Baltimore, D. (1987). An inducible transcription factor activates expression of human immunodeficiency virus in T cells. *Nature (London)* **326**, 711–713.

Nabel, G. J. (1991). Tampering with transcription. *Nature (London)* **350**, 658.

Nelson, J. A., Wiley, C. A., Reynolds-Kohler, C., Reese, C. E., Margaretten, W., and Levy, J. A. (1988). Human immunodeficiency virus detected in bowel epithelium from patients with gastrointestinal symptoms. *Lancet* **1**, 259–262.

Nelson, M. R., Shanson, D. C., Hawkins, D., and Gazzard, B. G. (1991). Shigella in HIV infection. *AIDS* **5**, 1031–1032.

Nixon, D. F., and McMichael, A. J. (1991). Cytotoxic T-cell recognition of HIV proteins and peptides. *AIDS* **5**, 1049–1059.

Owen, R. L., and Jones, A. L. (1974). Epithelial cell specialization within human Peyer's patch: An ultrastructural study of intestinal lymphoid follicles. *Gastroenterology* **66**, 189–203.

Pantaleo, G., Graziosi, C., Butini, L., Pizzo, P. A., Schnittman, S. M., Kotler, D. P., and Fauci, A. S. (1991). Lymphoid organs function as major reservoirs for human immunodeficiency virus. *Proc. Natl. Acad. Sci. U.S.A.* **88**, 9838–9842.

Pantaleo, G., Graziosi, C., Demarest, J. F., Butini, L., Montroni, M., Fox, C. H., Orenstein, J. M., Kotler, D. P., and Fauci, A. S. (1993a). HIV infection is active and progressive in lymphoid tissue during the clinically latent stage of disease. *Nature (London)* **362**, 355–358.

Pantaleo, G., Graziosi, C., and Fauci, A. (1993b). The immunopathogenesis of human immunodeficiency virus infection. *N. Engl. J. Med.* **328**, 327–335.

Quinn, T. C., Piot, P., McCormick, J. B., Feinsod, F. M., Taelman, H., Kapita, B., Stevens, W., and Fauci, A. S. (1987). Serologic and immunologic studies in patients with AIDS in North America and Africa. *JAMA, J. Am. Med. Assoc.* **252**, 2617–2621.

Racz, P. (1990). Pathomorphologie des intestinalen Immunsystems. Presented at the *3rd German AIDS-Congress* November 24–17, Hamburg.

René, E., Marche, C., Regnier, B., Saimot, A. G., Vilde, J. L., Perrone, C., Michon, C., Wolf, M., Chevalier, T., Vallot, T., *et al.* (1989). Intestinal infections in patients with acquired immunodeficiency syndrome. *Dig. Dis. Sci.* **34**, 773–780.

Riecken, E. O., Stallmach, A., Zeitz, M., Schulzke, J. D., Menge, H., and Gregor, M. (1989). Growth and transformation of the small intestinal mucosa—importance of connective tissue, gut associated lymphoid tissue and gastrointestinal regulatory peptides. *Gut* **30**, 1630–1640.

Rodgers, V. D., Fassett, R., and Kagnoff, M. F. (1986). Abnormalities in intestinal mucosal T cells in homosexual populations including those with the lymphadenopathy syndrome and acquired immunodeficiency syndrome. *Gastroenterology* **90**, 552–558.

Rosenberg, Z. F., and Fauci, A. S. (1989). The immunopathogenesis of HIV infection. *Adv. Immunol.* **47**, 377–431.

Sanders, M. E., Makgoba, M., and Shaw, S. (1988). Human naive and memory T cells: reinterpretation of helper-inducer and suppressor-inducer subsets. *Immunol. Today* **9**, 195–9.

Schieferdecker, H. L., Ullrich, R., Hirseland, H., and Zeitz, M. (1992). T cell differentiation antigens on lymphocytes in the human intestinal lamina propria. *J. Immunol.* **149**, 2816–2822.

Schneider, T., Hildebrandt, P., Rokos, K., Schubert, U., Rönspeck, W., Grund, C., Beck, A., Blesken,

R. Kulins, G., Oldenburg, H., and Pauli, G. (1992). Expression of nef, vpu, CA and CD4 during the infection of lymphoid and monocytic cell lines with HIV-1. *Arch. Virol.* **125**, 161–176.

Schneider, T., Jahn, H.-U., Schmidt, W., Riecken, E.-O., Zeitz, M., and Ullrich, R. (1995). Loss of CD4 T lymphocytes in patients infected with human immunodeficiency virus type 1 is more pronounced in the duodenal mucosa than in the peripheral blood. *Gut* **37**, 524–529.

Schneider, T., Ullrich, R., Bergs, C., Schmidt, W., Riecken, E. O., and Zeitz, M. (1994). Abnormalities in subset distribution, activation, and differentiation of T cells isolated from large intestine biopsies in HIV infection. *Clin. Exp. Immunol.* **95**, 430–435.

Schnittman, S. M., Lane, H. C., Greenhouse, J., Justement, J. S., Baseler, M., and Fauci, A. S. (1990). Preferential infection of CD4+ memory T cells by human immunodeficiency virus type 1: Evidence for a role in the selective T-cell functional defects observed in infected individuals. *Proc. Natl. Acad. Sci. U.S.A.* **87**, 6058–6062.

Smith, P. D., Fox, C. H., Masur, H., Winter, H. S., and Alling, D. W. (1994). Quantitative analysis of mononuclear cells expressing human immunodeficiency virus type 1 RNA in esophageal mucosa. *J. Exp. Med.* **180**, 1541–1546.

Stevenson, M., Zhang, X., and Volsky, D. J. (1987). Downregulation of cell surface molecules during noncytopathic infection of T cells with human immunodeficiency virus. *J. Virol.* **61**, 3741–3748.

Ullrich, R., Zeitz, M., Heise, W., L'Age, M., Höffken, G., and Riecken, E. O. (1989). Small intestinal structure and function in patients infected with human immunodeficiency virus (HIV): Evidence for HIV-induced enteropathy. *Ann. Intern. Med.* **111**, 15–21.

Ullrich, R., Zeitz, M., Heise, W., L'Age, M., Ziegler, K., Bergs, C., and Riecken, E. O. (1990). Mucosal atrophy is associated with loss of activated T cells in the duodenal mucosa of human immunodeficiency virus (HIV)-infected patients. *Digestion* **46**(Suppl. 2), 302–307.

Ullrich, R., Riecken, E. O., and Zeitz, M. (1991). HIV-induced enteropathy. *Immunol. Res.* **10**, 456–464.

Ullrich, R., Heise, W., Bergs, C., L'Age, M., Riecken, E.-O., and Zeitz, M. (1992). Effects of zidovudine treatment on the small intestinal mucosa in patients infected with HIV. *Gastroenterology* **102**, 1483–1492.

Ullrich, R., Schneider, T., Bergs, C., Jahn, H. U., Heise, W., L'Age, M., Riecken, E. O., Zeitz, M., and the Berlin Diarrhea/Wasting Syndrome Study Group (1996). Cytofluorometric analysis of T cells isolated from duodenal biopsies of HIV-infected patients and controls. submitted.

Van Noesel, C. J., Gruters, R. A., Terpstra, F. G., Schellekens, P. T., van Lier, R. A., and Miedema, F. (1990). Functional and phenotypic evidence for a selective loss of memory T cells in asymptomatic human immunodeficiency virus-infected men. *J. Clin. Invest.* **86**, 293–299.

Wain-Hobson, S. (1995). AIDS: Virological mayhem. *Nature (London)* **373**, 102.

Walker, B. D., Flexner, C., Paradis, T. J., Fuller, T. C., Hirsch, M. S., Schooley, R. T., and Moss, B. (1988). HIV-1 reverse transcriptase is a target for cytotoxic T lymphocytes in infected individuals. *Science* **240**, 64–66.

Wei, X., Ghosh, S. K., Taylor, M. E., Johson, V. A., Emini, E. A., Deutsch, P., Lifson, J. D., Bonhoeffer, S., Nowak, M. A., Hahn, B. H., Saag, M. S., and Shaw, G. M. (1995). Viral dynamics in human immunodeficiency virus type 1 infection. *Nature (London)* **373**, 117–122.

Weiss, R. A. (1993). How does HIV cause AIDS? *Science* **260**, 1273–1279.

Yahi, N., Baghdiguian, S., Moreau, H., and Fantini, J. (1992). Galactosyl ceramide (or a closely related molecule) is the receptor for human immunodeficiency virus type 1 on human colon epithelial HT29 cells. *J. Virol.* **66**, 4848–4854.

Zeitz, M., Greene, W. C., Peffer, N. J., and James, S. P. (1988). Lymphocytes isolated from the intestinal lamina propria of normal nonhuman primates have increased expression of genes associated with T cell activation. *Gastroenterology* **94**, 647–655.

Zeitz, M., James, S. P., Ullrich, R., and Riecken, E. O. (1989). Characteristics of intestinal T lymphocytes as potential target cells of HIV. *In* "AIDS in Gastroenterology and Hepatology" (M. Classen and H. Dancygier, eds.), p. 14–7. Demeter Verlag, Gräfelfing.

# Chapter 31

# Genital and Rectal Mucosal Immunity against Transmission of SIV/HIV

T. Lehner, L. A. Bergmeier, R. Brookes, L. Hussain, L. Klavinskis,
E. Mitchell, and L. Tao

*Department of Immunology, United Medical and Dental Schools at Guy's Hospital,
London Bridge, London SE1 9RT, England*

Human immunodeficiency virus (HIV) infection is transmitted predominantly through heterosexual intercourse in developing countries and through homosexual intercourse in developed countries (Curran *et al.,* 1985; Winkelstein *et al.,* 1986; European Study Group, 1992). Mucosal transmission through the genitourinary and rectal mucosa constitutes the principal mode of HIV infection. It is important to appreciate that mucosal transmission of HIV differs from vascular transmission, as occurs in intravenous drug abusers or with infected blood products. In vascular transmission HIV is directly disseminated in the circulating blood to lymphoid and other tissues. In mucosal transmission there are a number of barriers or hurdles which need to be passed before the infection is disseminated by blood (Lehner *et al.,* 1996). These barriers are the epithelial tissues and draining lymph nodes, subject to the mucosa being intact.

The aims of this review are to present the potential cells and receptors that bind HIV in the female and male genitourinary, rectal, and oral mucosa, and in foreskin (Hussain *et al.,* 1991, 1992; Hussain and Lehner, 1995). This will be followed by discussion of five immune barriers which have been identified during investigations of genital or rectal immunity (Lehner *et al.,* 1992a, 1993, 1994a, 1996; Brookes *et al.,* 1995).

## I. MUCOSAL CELLS AND RECEPTORS BINDING HIV

### A. CD4 Glycoprotein

CD4 glycoprotein is the principal receptor for HIV and was not found in vaginal, rectal, urethral, oral, or foreskin epithelial cells, although CD4$^+$ mononuclear cells were present in the lamina propria of each epithelium (Hussain *et al.,* 1991, 1992). Nevertheless, CD4 is expressed by Langerhans cells which are present in cervicovaginal, foreskin, and oral epithelia but these cells are not found in the rectum or urethra (Hussain and Lehner, 1995). There were significantly more Langerhans cells in the upper third of vaginal or foreskin epithelium than found in oral epithelium. This may be one factor in determining the high risk factor in uncircumsized males contracting HIV infection (Kreiss and Hopkins, 1992), as compared with the very low risk of transmission of HIV through the normal oral mucosa during oral sex (Dassey, 1988; Detels and Visscher, 1988). Although HIV has been detected in Langerhans' cells of patients with AIDS (Jarry et al., 1990; Tenner-Racz et al., 1987) others have been unable to confirm this (Kanitakis et al., 1989; Kalter et al., 1990).

## B. M Cells

M cells are found among the epithelial cells covering Peyer's patches in the intestine (Owen and Nemanic, 1978). Lymphoid follicles with M cells have been reported in the rectal mucosa (O'Leary and Sweeny, 1986). Rodent M cells are capable of transmitting HIV to lymphoid cells (Amerongen et al., 1991). However, HIV has not yet been identified in human M cells, though HIV nucleic acid has been detected in rectal epithelium (Nelson et al., 1988; Mathijs et al., 1988).

## C. Galactosyl Cerebroside or Sulfatide

Galactosyl cerebroside or sulfatide has been postulated to serve as an alternative receptor for HIV-1 in human colonic epithelial cells which do not express CD4 (Yahi et al., 1992). The envelope gp120 of HIV-1 binds to galactosyl cerebroside and two regions within gp120 have been suggested: the V3 loop is one possible region (van der Berg et al., 1992) and the C2 region (AA 206–275) is another site of gp120 binding CD4 (Bhat et al., 1993). The presence of lactosyl ceramide has been similarly implicated in human vaginal epithelial cells to bind HIV-1 gp120 (Furuta et al., 1994). Binding of HIV-1 to galactosyl or lactosyl ceramide might result in direct infection by HIV-1 or adhesion of infected cells expressing gp120 on their surface.

## D. Fc Receptors for IgG (FcγR)

Fc receptors for IgG (FcγR) offers an alternative mechanism for cell-free HIV infection, by enhancement of HIV–antibody complexes to bind via Fcγ receptors to epithelial cells (Takeda et al., 1988). Indeed, infected seminal fluid contains HIV and IgG antibodies (Wolff et al., 1991), so immune complexes can be formed. FcγII and FcγIII receptors were detected in rectal, endocervical, and urethral epithelia (Hussain and Lehner, 1995; Hussain et al., 1991, 1992) and FcγIII and FcγI receptors in the foreskin epithelium (Hussain and Lehner, 1995), which may enable HIV–antibody complexes to bind to these epithelial cells. However, FcγI and FcγII receptors were not found in oral epithelium and FcγIII receptors were confined to gingival epithelium (Hussain and Lehner, 1995). This would diminish the chances of oral HIV infection by means of HIV-antibody complexes.

### E. HLA Class II Expression on Epithelial Cells

HLA class II expression on epithelial cells may enable HIV-bound $CD4^+$ cells to gain access to the cells. We studied the expression of HLA-DR in cervicovaginal, rectal, urethral, and oral epithelia and foreskin, as HIV in seminal and cervicovaginal fluid might be CD4 cell-associated, and CD4 glycoprotein binds HLA class II antigen (Doyle and Strominger, 1987). It is noteworthy that the epithelial cells lining the endocervical but not vaginal or rectal tract (Hussain et al., 1991, 1992) and male genitourinary tract can express HLA class II (DR) antigen (Ritchie et al., 1984). This may be associated with T-cell activation, especially during infection. Whether HLA class II might enable CD4 cell-associated HIV to bind and facilitate infection of these epithelial cells needs to be explored.

### F. Nonspecific Entry into Epithelial Cells

$CD4^-$ cervical and intestinal cells can be infected directly by HIV-infected monocytes (Bourinbaiar and Phillips, 1991). The mode of entry of HIV appears to be primarily by the phagocytic pathway, through membrane invagination enclosing virions, or through receptor-mediated endocytosis. Direct fusion between viral envelope and epithelial membrane has also been observed by electron microscopy (Bourinbaiar and Phillips, 1991).

### G. Trauma and Infection of the Rectal Mucosa and Cervix

Trauma and infection of the rectal mucosa and cervix have been generally assumed to facilitate transmission of HIV on account of the thin columnar epithelium of the rectum, compared with the thick stratified squamous epithelium of vaginal or oral mucosa. In order to establish this quantitatively, we have measured the thickness of these epithelia by means of video image analysis. Indeed, the mean thickness ($\pm$ SD) of vaginal ($215.5 \pm 89.2$ $\mu$m) or oral ($263 \pm 1.6$ $\mu$m) epithelium is about 9 to 12 times greater than that of rectal epithelium ($24.6 \pm 9.7$ $\mu$m) (Hussain and Lehner, 1995). These results are consistent with the view that rectal mucosa is more vulnerable to be breached during rectal intercourse than vaginal or oral epithelium during vaginal or oral sex. This is compounded by the trauma that can be inflicted to the rectal mucosa during intercourse, and the rich vascular bed of the rectal mucosa which may facilitate entrance of infected seminal fluid to the traumatized blood vessels. Quite apart from the purely morphological features, there is evidence that recurrent infections of the rectum or the cervix and the high incidence of cervical erosions, especially in high-risk groups, facilitate rectal or cervicovaginal transmission of HIV (European Study Group, 1992; Felman, 1990), probably by providing a breach in mucosal integrity.

## II. Mucosal Immunity in Protection against Mucosal Challenge by Live SIV

Systemic immunization with inactivated SIV grown in human cells has failed to protect macaques from vaginal challenge with the live SIV (Marthas *et al.*, 1992). However, a mucosal strategy augmented by systemic immunization has been used more successfully, in which inactivated SIV grown in human cells was prepared in microcapsules administered first IM and then by either the oral or intratracheal route (Marx *et al.*, 1993). Indeed, five out of six macaques were protected when challenged by the vaginal route, and this was associated with vaginal IgA and IgG antibodies. However, rectal transmission with SIV was prevented by intramuscular immunization alone with inactivated SIV grown in human T cells (Cranage *et al.*, 1992). Furthermore, intravenous exposure to low subinfectious doses of live SIV in *Macacca fascicularis* and *Macacca nemestrina* appeared to elicit T-cell-proliferative responses, in the absence of detectable antibodies, and the macaques were protected against an infectious rectal challenge by SIV (Clerici *et al.*, 1994). However, the SIV was grown in human T cells, so that anti-cell antibodies are likely to have been involved in the protection. These experiments suggest that at least xenogeneic anti-cell antibodies (Stott *et al.*, 1991; Langlois *et al.*, 1992; Chan *et al.*, 1992; Arthur *et al.*, 1992) can protect vaginal or rectal transmission of SIV by augmented mucosal–systemic or systemic immunization, respectively (Marx *et al.*, 1993; Clerici *et al.*, 1994).

Recently, recombinant SIV envelope gp120 and core p27 were administered by the novel targeted lymph node immunization strategy (Lehner *et al.*, 1996). This elicited sIgA and IgG antibodies to gp120 and p27 in rectal fluid, rectal and iliac lymph node antibody-secreting B cells, and T-cell-proliferative responses to these antigens. Rectal challenge with an SIV molecular clone showed either total prevention of SIV infection or decreased viral load by more than 90%. If these results were readily reproducible, a subunit vaccine strategy might be pursued by the mucosal route.

## III. Immune Barriers in Mucosal Infections

A fundamental problem in vaccination against SIV/HIV is that the mechanism preventing infection has not been identified. Both B- and T-cell immunity have been reported, with neutralizing IgG antibodies to gp120 (Javaherian *et al.*, 1992; Moore *et al.*, 1994) and CD8[+] MHC class I-restricted cytotoxic cells to gp120 and p27 antigens (Walker *et al.*, 1987; Nixon *et al.*, 1988; Koenig *et al.*, 1988). A working hypothesis has been postulated that sexual transmission of HIV/SIV might be controlled by five successive immune barriers, with each barrier in turn either preventing infection or progressively decreasing the viral load (Table I). Barrier 1 viral adhesion to mucosal surface may be prevented by sIgA (and IgG) antibodies to gp120. If this proves ineffective, Barrier 2, consisting of intraepithelial polymeric IgA to p27 (or gp120), may prevent viral assembly. However, any virus that crosses the epithelium will encounter the subepithelial immune barrier (Barrier 3), consisting of SIV-specific B cells secreting antibodies, CD4 cells producing cytokines, and CD8 cytotoxic cells. If the rectal epithelium is not intact or is breached through trauma, there remains the third immune barrier in the submucosa, the fourth barrier in the draining lymph nodes, and the fifth barrier in the circulation and spleen.

The three different immune mechanisms involved in the first three barriers seem to offer the best chance of preventing viral transmission at the site of mucosal entry. The regional lymph nodes to which any virus that has successfully breached the mucosal and submucosal barriers is carried by macrophages, Langerhans cells, or dendritic cells may not permit the formation of a viral reservoir, on account of the potent CD8, CD4, and B-cell responses. Indeed, IgG-p27-C3d immune complexes may localize on the surface of follicular dendritic cells in lymphoid follicles (Armstrong and Horne, 1984; Tenner-Racz et al., 1987; Biberfeld et al., 1986), activate T and B cells, and prevent or decrease viral load in these lymph nodes. Dissemination of any residual live virus might be arrested by the circulating serum antibodies and T-cell functions. The evidence for the five

*TABLE I*

IMMUNE BARRIERS IN THE PROTECTION AGAINST MUCOSAL
TRANSMISSION OF SIV/HIV

| Barrier | Site | Immunity |
| --- | --- | --- |
| I | Epithelial surface | sIgA and IgG to gp 120 ↓ |
| II | Intraepithelial | polymeric IgA to p27 or gp 120 ↓ |
| III | Subepithelial | Homing of SIV-specific B, CD8, and CD4 (Th1, Th2) cells ↓ |
| IV | Regional lymph nodes | SIV-specific B, CD8, and CD4 (Th1, Th2) cells ↓ |
| V | Central circulating, and splenic cells | SIV-specific B, CD8, and CD4 cells, IgA and IgG antibodies |

potential barriers has been elicited mostly in mucosal immunization studies in macaques.

## A. Epithelial Surface Barrier

Epithelial surface barrier has been characterized by sIgA antibodies to SIV gag p27 and gp120 in rectal and vaginal epithelia and in male urethral washings, urine, and ejaculates (Lehner et al., 1992b, 1993, 1994a; Marx et al., 1993). The function of specific sIgA antibodies at the mucosal surface against SIV/HIV has not been elucidated but they may either prevent viral adhesion to CD4$^+$ cells or epithelial cerebrosides or neutralize the virus. It is also noteworthy that the mucosal surface antibodies contain specific IgG antibodies to SIV gag p27 and gp120, which probably represent mucosal transudates originating from serum. However, finding Fc receptors for IgG in rectal, endocervical, and urethral epithelia offer a receptor-mediated passage of IgG antibodies to those mucosal surfaces. Indeed, cervicovaginal secretions are especially rich in IgG antibodies (Lehner et al., 1992b; Marx et al., 1993).

## B. Intraepithelial Barrier

Intraepithelial barrier applies to rectal and endocervical columnar epithelial cells, which express the poly-immunoglobulin receptors at the basolateral surface of these cells (Brandtzaeg and Krajci, 1992; Kutteh et al., 1988). Polymeric IgA undergoes transcytosis via the receptors, and any virus which may have crossed the epithelial surface barrier might be prevented from assembly by these antibodies (Mazanec et al., 1992). However, this neutralizing sIgA antibody mechanism has so far been demonstrated only in vitro with Sendai virus.

## C. Subepithelial Barrier

Subepithelial barrier consists of homing of specific B, CD4 and CD8 cells, as well as macrophages and dendritic cells. Recently, antibody-secreting IgA and IgG B cells to SIV gag p27 and gp120 have been eluted from rectal and cervicovaginal epithelia of macaques immunized by the subcutaneous targeted iliac lymph node route (Bergmeier and Lehner, 1995; Lehner et al., 1996). We have also eluted CD4$^+$ T cells and macrophages from rectal and cervicovaginal epithelia. These are likely to function as inducer cells, but their Th1- or Th2-type cytokine activity has so far not been tested. It is particularly significant that specific CD8$^+$ cytotoxic T cells to SIV have now been demonstrated formally in cervicovaginal (Lohman et al., 1995) and rectal epithelia (Klavinskis et al., 1996). It is therefore evident that the four principal immune cells—B, CD4, and CD8 cells and macrophages—are present in the subepithelial barrier, and that these can mount both antibody and cellular immune responses against SIV/HIV infection.

## D. Regional Lymph Node Barrier

Regional lymph node barrier consists predominantly of the internal and external, as well as inferior mesenteric lymph nodes. We have demonstrated in macaques after rectal, vaginal, male genital, and targeted lymph node immunization that at least the internal iliac lymph node cells tested show B-cell antibody responses $CD4^+$ T-cell help in antibody synthesis, $CD4^+$ T-cell proliferation, and $CD8^+$ cytotoxic cells to the immunizing SIV antigen (Lehner et al., 1992b, 1993, 1994a,b, 1996; Klavinskis et al., 1995). Furthermore, a hierarchy of T-cell epitopes to SIV gag p27 has been demonstrated (Brookes et al., 1995) and this may vary with the mucosal route of immunization. Hence, in addition to B-cell antibody and CD8 cytototoxic cell responses, the $CD4^+$ T-cell response can be finely tuned to respond to some peptide epitopes with a higher frequency than to others. This may be especially significant, as the lymph nodes may function as reservoirs for SIV replication (Pantaleo et al., 1993; Embretson et al., 1993).

## E. Central Circulating Barrier

Central circulating barrier consists of similar $CD4^+$ T-cell proliferative and $CD8^+$ cytotoxic cells as those described for the lymph nodes. However, the hierarchy of T-cell epitopes differs in circulating T cells from those in the lymph nodes and varies with the route of immunization (Brookes et al., 1995). Serum IgA and IgG antibodies should function in the same way as after systemic immunization, except that the IgG antibody titres are lower and the IgA antibody titres are higher after mucosal immunization (Lehner et al., 1994b).

The concept of five immune barriers being mounted against mucosal SIV/HIV transmission is consistent with recent findings of the crucial role played by regional lymph nodes as reservoirs of infection (Ho et al., 1995; Wei et al., 1995), and as putative inductive sites of specific antibody-forming B cells (Lehner et al., 1996) and cytotoxic CD8 cells to the vaginal (Lohman et al., 1995) or rectal mucosa (Klavinskis et al., 1996). Furthermore, the intraepithelial mechanism of virus-neutralizing IgA antibodies (Mazanec et al., 1992) and the hierarchy of T-cell epitope expression to SIV gag antigen being related to the mucosal route of immunization (Brookes et al., 1995) suggest a wealth of epithelial–lymphoid cell interactions which may be involved in viral infection and protection. The five successive immune barriers may utilize a fail-safe defense strategy, with site-directed differences in isotype (IgA or IgG), subunit antigen (envelope or core protein), and recognition of defined T-and B-cell epitopes. Each of these barriers may in turn either prevent viral transmission or decrease the viral load.

## REFERENCES

Amerongen, H. M., Weltzin, R., Farnet, C. M., Michetti, P., Haseltine, W. A., and Neutra, M. R. (1991). Transepithelial transport of HIV-1 by intestinal M cells: A mechanism for transmission of AIDS. *J. Acquired Immune Defic. Syndr.* **4,** 760–765.

Armstrong, J. A., and Horne, R. (1984). Follicular dendritic cells and virus-like particles in AIDS-related lymphadenopathy. *Lancet* **1,** 370–372.

Arthur, L. O., Bess, J. W., Jr., Sowder II, R. C., *et al.* (1992). Cellular proteins bound to immunodeficiency viruses: Implications for pathogenesis and vaccines. *Science* **258,** 1935–1938.

Bergmeier, L., and Lehner, T. (1995) In preparation.

Bhat, S., Mettus, R. V., Reddy, E. P., Ugen, K. E., Srikanthan, V., Williams, W. V., and Weiner, D. B. (1993). The galactosyl ceramide/sulfatide receptor binding region of HIV-1 gp120 maps to amino acids 206–275. *AIDS Res. Hum. Retro.* **9,** 175–181.

Biberfeld, P., Chayt, K. J., Marselle, L. M., Biberfeld, G., Gallo, R. C., and Haper, M. E. (1986). HTLVIII expression in infected lymph nodes and relevance to pathogenesis of lymphadenopathy. *Am. J. Pathol.* **125,** 436–442.

Bourinbaiar, A. S., and Phillips, D. M. (1991). Transmission of human immunodeficiency virus from monocytes to epithelia. *J. Acquired Immune Defic. Syndr.* **4,** 56–63.

Brandtzaeg, P., and Krajci, P. (1992). Secretory component (the poly-IgA receptor). *In* "Encyclopaedia of Immunology" (I. M. Roitt and P. J. Delves eds.), pp. 1360–1364. Academic Press, London.

Brookes, R., Bergmeier, L. A., Mitchell, E., Walker, J., Tao, L., Klavinskis, L., Meyers, N. J., Layton, G., Adams, S. E., and Lehner, T. (1995). Generation and diversity in the hierarchy of T-cell epitope responses following different routes of immunization with simian immunodeficiency virus protein. *AIDS* **9,** 1017–1024.

Chan, W. L., Rodgers, A., Hancock, R. D., *et al.* (1992). Protection of simian immunodeficiency virus-vaccinated monkeys correlates with anti-HLA class I antibody response. *J. Exp. Med.* **176,** 1203–1207.

Clerici, M., and Shearer, G. M. (1993). A TH1→TH2 switch is a critical step in the etiology of HIV infection. *Immunol. Today* **14,** 107–111.

Clerici, M., Clark, E. A., Polacino, P., Axberg, I., Kuller, L., Casey, N. I., Morton, W. R., Shearer, G. M., and Benveniste, R. E. (1994). T-cell proliferation to subinfectious SIV correlates with lack of infection after challenge of macaques. *AIDS* **8,** 1391–1395.

Cranage, M. P., Baskerville, A., Ashworth, L. A. E., Dennis, M., Cook, N., Sharpe, S., Farrar, G., Rose, J., Kitchin, P. A., and Greenaway, P. J. (1992). Intrarectal challenge of macaques vaccinated with formalin-inactivated simian immunodeficiency virus. *Lancet* **339,** 273–274.

Curran, J. W., Morgan, W. M., Hardy, A. M., Jaffe, H. W., Darrow, W. W., and Dowdle, W. R. (1985). The epidemiology of AIDS: Current status and future prospects. *Science* **229,** 1352–1357.

Dassey, D. E. (1988). HIV and orogenital transmission. *Lancet* **2,** 1023.

Detels, R., and Visscher, B. (1988). HIV and orogenital transmission. *Lancet* **2,** 1023.

Doyle, C., and Strominger, J. L. (1987). Interaction between CD4 and class II MHC molecules mediating cell adhesion. *Nature (London)* **330,** 256–259.

Embretson, J. E., Zupancic, M., Ribas, J. L., Burke, A., Racz, P., Tenner-Racz, K., and Haase, A. T. (1993). Massive covert infection of helper T lymphocytes and macrophages by HIV during the incubation period of AIDS. *Nature (London)* **362,** 359–361.

European Study Group on Heterosexual Transmission of HIV. (1992). Comparison of female to male and male to female transmission of HIV in 563 stable couples. *Br. Med. J.* **304,** 809.

Felman, Y. M. (1990). Recent developments in sexually transmitted diseases: Is heterosexual transmission of HIV a major epidemiologic factor in the spread of AIDS? New York City's experience. *Sexually Transmitted Diseases* **46,** 204–206.

Furuta, Y., Eriksson, K., Svennerholm, B., Fredman, P., Horal, P., Jeansson, S., Vahlne, A., Holmgren,

J., and Czerkinsky, C. (1994). Infection of vaginal and colonic epithelial cells by the human immunodeficiency virus type 1 is neutralized by antibodies raised against conserved epitopes in the envelope glycoprotein gp120. *Proc. Natl. Acad. Sci. U.S.A.* **91,** 12559–12563.

Ho, D. D., Neumann, A. U., Perelson, A. S., Chen, W., Leonard, J. M., and Markowitz, M. (1995). Rapid turnover of plasma virions and CD4 lymphocytes in HIV-1 infection. *Nature (London)* **373,** 123–126.

Homsy, J., Meyer, M., Tateno, M., Clarkson, S., and Levy, J. A. (1989). The Fc and not CD4 receptor mediates antibody enhancement of HIV infection in human cells. *Science* **244,** 1357–1360.

Hussain, L. A., Kelly, C. G., Hecht, E.-M., Fellowes, R., Jourdan, M., and Lehner, T. (1991). The expression of Fc receptors for immunoglobulin G in human rectal epithelium. *AIDS* **5,** 1089–1094.

Hussain, L. A., Kelly, C. G., Fellowes, R., Hecht, E.-M., Wilson, J., Chapman, M., and Lehner, T. (1992). Expression and gene transcript of Fc receptors for IgG, HLA class II antigens and Langerhans cells in human cervico-vaginal epithelium. *Clin. Exp. Immunol.* **90,** 530–538.

Hussain, L. A., and Lehner, T. (1995). Comparative investigation of Langerhans cells and potential receptors for HIV in oral, genitourinary and rectal epithelia. *Immunol.* **85,** 475–484.

Jarry, A., Cortez, A., Rene, E., Muzeau, F., and Brousse, N. (1990). Infected cells and immune cells in the gastrointestinal tract of AIDS patients. An immunohistochemical study of 127 cases. *Histopathology* **16,** 133–140.

Javaherian, K., Langlois, A. J., Schmidt, S., Kaufman, M., Cates, N., Langeduk, J. P. M., Meleon, R. H., Desrosiers, R. C., Burns, D. P., Bolognesi, D. P., LaRose, and Putney, S. D. (1992). The principal neutralization determinant of simian immunodeficiency virus from that of human immunodeficiency virus type 1. *Proc. Natl. Acad. Sci. U.S.A.* **89,** 1418–1422.

Kalter, D. C., Gendelman, H. E., and Meltzer, M. S. (1990). Infection of human epidermal Langerhans' cells by HIV. *AIDS* **4,** 266–268.

Kanitakis, J., Marchand, C., Su, H., Thivolet, J., Zambruno, G., Schmitt, D., and Gazzolo, L. (1989). Immunohistochemical study of normal skin of HIV-1 infected patients shows no evidence of infection of epidermal Langerhans cells by HIV. *AIDS Res. Hum. Retrovir.* **5,** 293–302.

Klavinskis, L. S., Brookes, R., Bergmeier, L. A., Mitchell, E., Tao, L., and Lehner, T. (1996). Cytotoxic T lymphocytes after rectal, vaginal, oral or targeted lymph node immunization in macaques. Submitted for publication.

Koenig, S., Earl, P., Powell, D., Pantaleo, G., Merli, S., Moss, B., and Fauci, A. S. (1988). Group-specific, major histocompatibility complex class-I restricted cytotoxic responses to human immunodeficiency virus 1 (HIV-1) envelope proteins by cloned peripheral blood T cells from an HIV-1 infected individual. *Proc. Natl. Acad. Sci. U.S.A.* **85,** 8638–8642.

Kreiss, J. K., and Hopkins, S. G. (1992). The association between circumcision status and human immunodeficiency virus infection among homosexual men. *J. Infect. Dis.* **168,** 1404–1408.

Kutteh, W. H., Hatch, K. D., Blackwell, R. E., and Mestecky, J. (1988). Secretory immune system of the female reproductive tract. I. Immunoglobulin and secretory component-containing cells. *Obstet. Gynecol.* **71,** 56–60.

Langlois, A. J., Weinhold, K. J., Matthews, T. J., Greenberg, M. L., and Bolognesi, D. P. (1992). The ability of certain SIV vaccines to provoke reactions against normal cells. *Science* **255,** 292–293.

Lehner, T., Panagiotidi, C., Bergmeier, L. A., Tao, L., Brookes, R., and Adams, S. (1992a). A comparison of the immune responses following oral, vaginal or rectal route of immunization with SIV antigens in non-human primates. *Vaccine Res.* **1,** 319.

Lehner, T., Bergmeier, L. A., Panagiotidi, C., Tao, L., Brookes, R., Klavinskis, L. S., Walker, P., Walker, J., Ward, R. G., Hussain, L., Gearing, A. J. H., and Adams, S. E. (1992b). Induction of mucosal and systemic immunity to a recombinant simian immunodeficiency viral protein. *Science* **258,** 1365–1369.

Lehner, T., Brookes, R., Panagiotidi, C., Tao, L., Bergmeier, L. A., Klavinskis, L. S., Walker, J., Walker, P., Ward, R., Hussain, L., Gearing, A. J. H., and Adams, S. E. (1993). T and B cell functions and epitope expression in non-human primates immunized with SIV by the rectal route. *Proc. Natl. Acad. Sci. U.S.A.* **90,** 8638–8642.

Lehner, T., Tao, L., Panagiotidi, C., Klavinskis, L. S., Brookes, R., Hussain, L., Meyers, N., Adams, S. E., Gearing, A. J. H., and Bergmeier, L. A. (1994a). Mucosal model of genital immunization in male rhesus macaques with a recombinant simian immunodeficiency virus p27 antigen. *J. Virol.* **68,** 1624–1632.

Lehner, T., Bergmeier, L. A., Tao, L., *et al.* (1994b). Targeted lymph node immunization with simian immunodeficiency virus p27 antigen to elicit genital, rectal and urinary immune responses in non-human primates. *J. Immunol.* **153,** 1858–1868.

Lehner, T., Wang, Y., Cranage, M., Bergmeier, L. A., Mitchell, E., Tao, L., Hall, G., Dennis, M., Cook, N., Brookes, R., Klavinskis, L., Jones, I., Doyle, C., and Ward, R. (1996). Protective mucosal immunity elicited by targeted lymph node immunization with a subunit SIV envelope and core vaccine in macaques. Submitted for publication.

Lohman, B. L., Miller, C. J., and McChesney, M. B. (1995). Antiviral cytotoxic T lymphocytes in the vaginal mucosa of simian immunodeficiency virus infected rhesus macaques. *J. Immunol.* (in press).

Marthas, M., Sutjipto, S., Miller, C., Higgins, J., Torten, J., Unger, R., Kiyono, H., McGhee, J., Marx, P., and Pedersen, N. (1992). Efficacy of live-attenuated and whole-inactivated simian immunodeficiency virus vaccines against intravenous and intravaginal challenge. "Vaccines 1992" (F. Brown, R. M. Chanock, H. S. Ginsberg, R. A. Lerner, eds.), pp. 117–122. Cold Spring Harbor Laboratory, Cold Spring Harbor, NY.

Marx, P. A., Compans, R. W., Getie, A., Staas, J. K., Gilley, R. M., Muligan, M. J., Yamshchikov, G. V., Chen, D., and Eldridge, J. H. (1993). Protection against vaginal SIV transmission with microencapsulated vaccine. *Science* **260,** 1323–1327.

Mathijs, J. M., Hing, M., Grierson, J., Dwyer, D. E., Goldschmidt, C., Cooper, D. A., and Cunningham, A. L. (1988). HIV infection of the rectal mucosa. *Lancet* **1,** 1111.

Mazanec, M. B., Kaetzel, C. S., Lamm, M. E., Fletcher, D., and Nedrud, J. G. (1992). *Proc. Natl. Acad. Sci. U.S.A.* **89,** 6901–6905.

Moore, J. P., Cao, Y., Ho, D. D., and Koup, R. J. (1994). Development of anti-gp120 antibody response during seroconversion to human immunodeficiency virus type 1 *J. Virol.* **68,** 5142–5155.

Nelson, J. A., Wiley, C. A., Reynolds-Kohler, C., Reese, C. E., Margaretten, W., and Levy, J., (1988). Human immunodeficiency virus detected in bowel epithelium from patients with gastrointestinal symptoms. *Lancet.* **1,** 259–262.

Nixon, D. F., Townsend, A. R. M., Elvin, J. G., Rizza, C. R., Gallwey, J., and McMichael, A. J. (1988). HIV-1 gag specific cytotoxic T lymphocytes defined with recombinant vaccinia virus and synthetic peptides. *Nature (London)* **336,** 484–487.

O'Leary, A. D., and Sweeny, E. C. (1986). Lymphoglandular complexes of the colon: Structure and distribution. *Histopathology* **10,** 267–283.

Owen, R. L., and Nemanic, P. (1978). Antigen processing structures of the mammalian intestinal tract: An SEM study of lymphoepithelial orans. *Scanning Electron Microsc.* **2,** 367–378.

Pantaleo, G., Graziosi, C., Demarest, J. F., Butini, L., Montroni, M., Fox, C. H., Orenstein, J. M., Kotler, D. P., and Fauci, A. S. (1993). HIV infection is active and progressive in lymphoid tissue during the clinically latent stage of disease. *Nature (London)* **362,** 355–357.

Ritchie, A. W. S., Hargreave, B., James, K., and Chisholm, G. D. (1984). Intra-Epithelial lymphocytes in the normal epididymis. A mechanism for tolerance to sperm auto-antigens. *Br. J. Urol.* **56,** 79–83.

Stott, E. J. (1991). Anti-cell antibody in macaques. *Nature (London)* **353,** 393.

Takeda, A., Tuazon, C. U., and Ennis, F. A. (1988). Antibody-enhanced infection by HIV-1 via Fc receptor-mediated entry. *Science* **242,** 580–583.

Tenner-Racz, K., Racz, P., Bofil, M., Schultz-Meyer, A., Dietrich, M., Kern, P., Weber, J., Pinching, A. J., DiMarzo-Veronese, F., Popovic, M., Klatzmann, D., Gluckman, J. C., Tschachler, E., Groh,

U., Popovic, M., Mann, D., Konrad, K., Safai, B., Eron, L., Veronese, F., Wolff, K., and Stingl, G. (1987). Epidermal Langerhans cells—a target for HTLV-III/LAV infection *J. Invest. Dermatol.* **88,** 233–237.

van der Berg, L. H., Sadiq, S., Lederman, S., and Latov, N. (1992). The gp120 glycoprotein of HIV-1 binds to sulfatide and to the myelin associated glycoprotein. *J. Neurosci. Res.* **33,** 513–518.

Walker, B. D., Chakrabarti, S., Moss, B., Paradis, T. J., Flynn, T., Durno, A. G., Blumberg, R., Kaplan, J. C., Hirsch, M. S., and Scholley. (1987). HIV-specific cytotoxic T lymphocytes in seropositive individuals. *Nature (London)* **328,** 345–348.

Wei, X., Ghosh, S. K., Taylor, M. E., Johnson, V. A., Emini, E. A., Deutsch, P., Lifson, J. D., Bonheoffer, S., Nowak, M. A., Hahn, B. H., Saag, M. S., and Shaw, G. M. (1995). Viral dynamics in human immunodeficiency virus type 1 infection. *Nature (London)* **373,** 117–122.

Winkelstein, W., Wiley, J. A., Padian, N., and Levy, J. (1986). Potential for transmission of AIDS-associated retrovirus from bisexual men in San Francisco to their female sexual contacts. *JAMA, J. Am. Med. Assoc.* **255,** 901.

Wolff, H., Mayer, K., Seage, G., Politch, J., Horsburgh, C. R., and Anderson, D. J. (1991). A comparison of HIV-1 antibody classes, titers and specificities in paired semen and blood samples from HIV-1 seropositive men. *J. Acquired Immune Defic. Syndr.* **5,** 65–69.

Yahi, N., Baghdiguian, S., Moreau, H., and Fantini, J. (1992). Galactosyl ceramide (or a closely related molecule) is the receptor for human immunodeficiency virus type 1 on human colon epithelial HT29 cells. *J. Virol.* **66,** 4848–4854.

# Chapter 32

# Beneficial and Harmful Immune Responses in the Respiratory Tract

Peter J. M. Openshaw, Lindsay C. Spender, and Tracy Hussell

*Respiratory Medicine, St. Mary's Hospital Medical School, Imperial College of Science, Technology and Medicine, London W2 1PG, United Kingdom*

Infections of the respiratory and intestinal tract constitute major threats to worldwide health. Together, these mucosal infections are the leading causes of morbidity and mortality in children. Respiratory syncytial virus (RSV) is a major worldwide childhood respiratory pathogen and an unsolved challenge for vaccine development. Clinically, infection is characterized by symptoms and signs of bronchial narrowing, and many children who recover from bronchiolitis are subsequently diagnosed as asthmatic. The mouse model of RSV lung disease has been very successful in reproducing many aspects of the human disease. In this species, some types of vaccination (particularly sensitization to the major surface glycoprotein G) induce virus-specific T helper 2 cells. During subsequent RSV infection, lung eosinophilia develops. These and other studies have shown the dual role of anti-viral T cells in both eliminating virus and causing enhanced disease. This immunopathological paradox is now more clearly understood for RSV disease than for that caused by any other common human infection. This chapter presents a selection of current knowledge about the characteristics, functions, benefit, and harm of antiviral immune responses to RSV.

## I. INTRODUCTION

Mucosal defenses are primarily directed to prevention and elimination of infection. The gastrointestinal tract has proved a very productive site for the study of mucosal immune responses, but in global terms far more lethal infections enter via the respiratory than the gastrointestinal route. WHO estimates indicate that approximately 14 million people die each year from infections that are transmitted via the respiratory tract, compared to 5 million from diseases transmitted by the gastrointestinal route. Most of these deaths occur in childhood. Although many are caused by bacteria, a foothold for bacterial infections of the lung is often gained during acute viral infections. Respiratory viral infections of childhood are therefore of key importance to the development of serious respiratory disease throughout the world.

The threat of respiratory and intestinal infections to world health is, to a degree,

449

inevitable. Breathing, drinking, and eating are unavoidable processes. The prime function at either site depends on providing a large surface area for the exchange of materials with the environment. Any well-adapted pathogen is prone to exploit this necessity to gain access to the internal milieu.

The respiratory and intestinal tracts not only are ideal sites of invasion, but also are well suited to the process of spreading pathogens to other hosts. Irritation of the nasal mucosa causes mucus which contains abundant infectious virus to be secreted. Sneezing and coughing cause secretions to be expelled as droplets. Fine particles of mucus rapidly dry in the air, and can go on to settle on the mucous membranes of new hosts. The cycle of infection does not require the virus to spread to other tissues outside the respiratory tract. Transmission may indeed be most effective if the infected person is not made so ill as to prevent normal social contact. Agents that cause diarrhea and vomiting similarly assist their own spread by inducing local symptoms.

## A. Respiratory Infections in Childhood

Viral bronchiolitis is the single most common cause of hospitalization of infants in the Western World, but the development of effective preventative or therapeutic stratagems has been hampered by lack of information about its pathogenesis. The majority of cases are caused by respiratory syncytial virus (RSV), the annual hospitalization costs of which were estimated to be $300,000,000 in 1988 in the United States alone, with 91,000 children admitted (Heilman, 1990). Antiviral immunity appears not only to protect against infection but also to contribute to lung pathology. The first evidence that specific immunity could be harmful came in the 1960s, when children were vaccinated with formalin-inactivated RSV. Vaccine recipients developed strong serological responses, but were not protected against infection. Most vaccinees who subsequently became infected with RSV developed severe lower respiratory tract disease, and some died as a result. The reasons for vaccine-augmented disease have been studied (e.g., McIntosh and Fishaut, 1980; Murphy et al., 1990; Connors et al., 1992), but no safe, effective vaccine has yet been produced. For a more detailed discussion of immune responses to RSV, see Openshaw (1995).

## B. RSV Virology

RSV belongs to the genus *Pneumovirus* in the family paramyxoviridae, bearing close similarity to measles, canine distemper virus, mumps, and parainfluenza viruses. Electron microscopy shows irregularly shaped and often clumped virions, with a lipid envelope bearing surface glycoproteins G, F, and SH. The nucleocapsid contains a single-strand negative-sense RNA genome of $5 \times 10^6$ kDa, which is nonsegmented. There are 10 genes, with 12 potential gene products. Sequential transcription occurs from $3'$ to $5'$; the first genes to be transcribed are 1c and

1b, which encode nonstructural proteins of unknown function. Then follows the nucleoprotein (N), which is relatively well conserved between natural isolates. The phosphoprotein (P) and SH are next, then the attachment protein (G) and the fusion protein (F). These two proteins are the major surface glycoproteins, against which neutralizing antibody is directed and which show the most natural variability between different natural isolates of RSV. The last two proteins are the M2 (second matrix or 22-kDa protein) and the large protein L, the latter being the RNA polymerase. Both of these are thought to be relatively well conserved.

## III. MOUSE MODEL OF RSV DISEASE

Arguably, the mouse has contributed more to our knowledge of immunology than any other single species. After intranasal (in) infection with human RSV grown in tissue culture, lung virus titres vary by as much as 100-fold between the most and least susceptible inbred strains (Prince et al., 1979). Taylor et al. (1984) showed that RSV reaches a peak virus titre in the lungs of BALB/c mice on Days 4–6, being largely eliminated by Day 9. Pulmonary infection is accompanied by histological changes which bear some resemblance to human RSV-induced bronchiolitis. Transient alveolar lymphocytic influx is followed by focal inflammation (initially comprising mononuclear cells) often sandwiched between bronchioles and small blood vessels.

### A. Local Cellular Response to RSV Infection

Our work with the mouse model of RSV disease has used bronchoalveolar lavage (BAL) as a convenient method of following pathological changes in the lungs following RSV infection (Openshaw, 1989). We find that results from this technique correlate well with those from histological analysis. To recover BAL cells, mice are anesthetized and exsanguinated and the lungs inflated with dilute lignocaine. Cytocentrifuge preparations of BAL cells from uninfected mice largely show macrophages, but after infection the proportion of lymphocytes increases from Day 4, reaching a plateau between Days 6 and 14 (at about 20–40% of recovered cells), thereafter gradually returning to normal. The degree of lymphocytosis correlates with the severity of histological change rated on a subjective scale. Bronchial lavage has the advantage of sampling cells from all areas of the lung, allowing easy quantification of severity of pathological responses and providing cells in an ideal form for further studies.

Using this method, we performed extensive flow cytometric analysis of local cellular responses during primary and secondary infections. The majority of lymphocytes recovered during the first 5 days of primary infection are $CD4^-8^-$ (null) in phenotype. Few are B cells, but most have characteristics of NK cells (T. Hussell and P. J. M. Openshaw, unpublished), and NK activity peaks at about this time. During elimination of the virus from the lungs (Days 6–9), the main single subset is CD8$^+$, although CD4$^+$ cells are also found. It has been proposed that epithelial T cells most frequently exhibit T-cell receptors of the $\gamma\delta$ (rather than $\alpha\beta$) type. Our studies, however (Openshaw, 1991), have shown that almost all the single-positive (CD4 or CD8) T cells, which form the majority of all CD3$^+$ cells recoverable from the lung, bear the $\alpha\beta$ form of T-cell receptor; $\gamma\delta$ T cells are exceedingly rare. Interestingly, a small subset of double-negative cells bear CD3 and the $\alpha\beta$ T-cell receptor, although the total number of these cells is small.

### B. Immunopathology Due to Sensitisation to Specific RSV Proteins

Immunization with recombinant vaccinia viruses (rVV) allows individual RSV proteins to be tested for their ability to protect against RSV infection. If groups of BALB/c mice are sensitized with a panel of rVVs expressing different RSV proteins by dermal scarification and challenged 3–4 weeks later with live RSV intranasal protection against RSV replication is seen in mice immunized to F, G, N, and M2. This protection is, however, associated with an increase in pathology in most cases. Mice primed with rVV-G or -F develop lung hemorrhage by Day 5 of challenge. Mice sensitized with rVV-G, -F, or -N develop polymorph efflux, while only those sensitized with rVV-G develop eosinophilic efflux (14–25% of BAL cells compared to less than 3% in other groups). Interestingly, T cells recovered from the lungs of sensitized mice contain a minor subset of CD4$^-$CD8$^-$ T cells which bear the $\gamma\delta$ form of T-cell receptor (TCR).

Helper T cells can be classified into different types that produce characteristic cytokine profiles, some directing cell-mediated immune responses and others enhancing antibody production by B cells (Fiorentino *et al.*, 1989; Street *et al.*, 1990). These two functional subsets (Th1 and Th2), are known to be differentially induced by some antigens and modes of priming and may reciprocally inhibit. It seemed possible that differential induction of forms of immunopathology could be explained by production of IL-4 and IL-5 from Th2 cells that recognize G, and the introduction of Th1 cells (producing IFN$\gamma$ and IL-2 among other cytokines) by other proteins, including F.

### C. Intracellular Cytokine Responses

Although polarized cytokine production has been seen in mouse and, more recently, in human T-cell clones, detailed analysis of cytokine production by large numbers of individual cells during polyclonal responses to viral infection has not previously been possible. From the studies described above, it seemed that different rVV may prime for T cells with different cytokine production profiles. In order to study intracellular cytokine production directly, a collaboration was established with Dr. Anne O'Garra's laboratory at DNAX in California. A method of intracellular staining for cytokine production developed by Dr. Radbruch's team in Germany (Assenmacher *et al.*, 1994) was developed to the point that it became useful for analysis of mixed natural populations of cells. In essence, populations of T cells are restimulated either specifically with antigen or nonspecifically with mitogen. Naive T cells do not produce cytokines under these conditions, but cells destined to produce specific cytokines will do so. The secretion of cytokine is then blocked by adding brefeldin A and, after a suitable period (typically 2–24 hr), cells are fixed. These fixed cells are permeablized with saponin, a reversible detergent. Anti-cytokine antibodies (conjugated or unconjugated) can then be used to determine the presence of intracellular cytokine. The saponin can be washed away and the cells stained for surface proteins, if these are stable to fixation and permeablization. In the mouse, we have succeeded in staining several surface proteins, including CD4, CD8, B220, and $\gamma\delta$ TCR on such fixed cells. We routinely stain with three fluorophores. Two (e.g., PE and FITC) are used for cytokines, and the third (Quantum red) for the surface protein of choice. It is then possible to look at cytokine coexpression in cells of defined surface phenotype (Openshaw *et al.,* 1995).

To apply this method to cells obtained *ex vivo,* we sampled BAL and mediastinal lymph node (MLN) cells before and after intranasal infection of mice with RSV. Reverse-transcriptase PCR and flow cytometric analysis of intracellular cytokine production showed little or no mRNA or intracellular IFN$\gamma$, IL-4, IL-5, or IL-10 from uninfected mice. After infection, MLN enlarged rapidly and BAL T-cell lymphocytosis peaked on Day 10. mRNA for IFN$\gamma$ peaked on Day 1 postinfection in MLN and on Days 2 to 4 in the BAL. Only low levels of IL-2, IL-4, and IL-5 mRNA were detected at any time at either site, whereas IL-10 mRNA was easily detected in both the MLN and BAL cells. Immunofluorescent staining for IL-4, IL-5, or IL-10 and IFN$\gamma$ in either CD4 or CD8 showed that most CD8$^+$ cells became IFN$\gamma^+$, compared to about one-third of CD4$^+$ cells. Although the numbers of T cells fell between Days 10 and 21, the proportion that were IFN$\gamma^+$ increased with time. Less than 1% of BAL or MLN CD4$^+$ or CD8$^+$ cells were IL-4$^+$ or IL-5$^+$ at any time. Intracellular IL-10 was observed in BAL lymphocytes at early time points, some of which coexpressed IFN$\gamma$. Cytokine mRNA and intracellular protein analysis produced concordant results and both indicated a predominant Th1 cytokine profile in local T cells during primary infection with RSV (T. Hussell, L. C. Spender, and P. J. M. Openshaw, unpublished).

It is to be hoped that the introduction of novel methods to study cytokine production at the single-cell level will help us understand the complex functional relationships between subsets of normal primed T cells. Our ability to look at large populations of T cells recovered from complex and real immune responses *in vivo* will allow concepts of helper T cell subdivisions to move on from the simple division into Th1, Th2, and Th0 to a functional description of cells based on actual production, simultaneous or sequential, of a range of cytokines. Some generalizations will remain, others will emerge or fall. We, for example, have not yet seen coproduction of IL-4 and IFN$\gamma$ in any cells obtained from sites of inflammation, and it may well be that these cytokines are mutually exclusive; IL-10 and IFN$\gamma$

can sometimes be seen within the same cells at the same time, showing that coproduction can be a normal event in nonclonal cells (Hussell, Spender, and Openshaw, unpublished). Bearing in mind that subsets can reciprocally inhibit each other's function and growth, it is possible that a site which is infiltrated by a phenotypic mixture of cells may be functionally dominated by the effects of one subset. With these new techniques, we can watch the emergence of a new field of understanding with excitement and anticipation.

### D. Disease Augmentation by Passive Transfer of T Cells

The effects of potent, activated, specific T cells have been tested by cell-transfer experiments. $CD4^+$ and $CD8^+$ cells have been isolated from polyclonal RSV-specific T-cell lines by immunomagnetic methods. Mice infected with RSV alone showed only mild illness, but more severe disease occurred in mice receiving $CD4^+$ cells. Such mice developed respiratory distress, and lost up to 30% of their body weight. BAL showed a rich efflux of eosinophils. In these studies, $CD8^+$ cells were less pathogenic, producing mild "shock lung" with PMN efflux and lung hemorrhage. Cell for cell, $CD4^+$ cells are therefore more antiviral and more immunopathogenic than $CD8^+$ cells in RSV-infected mice. In these studies, there was evidence that coinjection of $CD4^+$ and $CD8^+$ cells may reduce the severity of pathology, compared to the effects of either subset alone, although this effect was not dramatic (Alwan *et al.*, 1992).

In influenza virus-infected mice, intravenous injection of virus-specific cytotoxic T lymphocytes can reduce severity of lung pathology, reduce the lung virus titre, and prevent death in otherwise lethally infected mice. About 7 million cells need to be injected into each mouse in order to achieve these effects. To show whether similar effects could be demonstrated in RSV-infected mice, T cells from the spleens of BALB/c mice infected intranasally with RSV were stimulated by cycles of antigen and IL-2 *in vitro*. The resulting lines and clones were all $CD8^+$ and cytolytic for class I MHC-matched targets, although they varied in the protein recognized. Congenic mice were persistently infected with RSV and injected with CTL intravenously. As few as $10^6$ of such cells cause complete virus clearance by Day 10, with uninjected mice showing little change in lung virus titer at this time. Remarkably, mice injected with CTL became sick, and some (with more than 1 million cells) died. With 10 million cells, more than half the mice were dead by Day 5. Injection of cells or infection alone was insufficient to cause any appreciable illness. Bronchoalveolar lavage of mice with augmented disease showed a hemorrhagic neutrophilic pneumonitis. Analysis of the T-cell subsets recovered from the lung showed an increase of $CD8^+$ T cells, but an even more striking increase in the number of $CD4^+$, $CD4^-CD8^-$, and B-cell subsets. These studies show that RSV-specific CTL, when injected in a highly activated state, can eliminate virus from the lungs but also cause acute lung injury. It is important to note that the cells recovered by BAL do not give a clear indication that CTL had initiated the immunopathology, and that BAL CD8$^+$ T cells show no specific increase (Cannon *et al.*, 1988). Subsequent studies in C57Bl/6 mice show that CTL of lower potency are able to eliminate virus without causing overt signs of disease if injected later during infection (Muñoz *et al.*, 1991). Signs of illness are not easily appreciated in mice, and some objective measure of lung pathology is essential in studies of this type. A series of excellent studies from Dr. Graham's group have clarified the roles of various T- and B-cell subsets in primary and secondary mouse infection and in challenged mice previously vaccinated in various ways (Tang and Graham, 1994; Graham *et al.*, 1993, 1991).

In further experiments, T-cell lines from mice primed with rVV-G, rVV-M2, or rVV-F were expanded *in vitro* and injected into RSV-infected mice. Mice infected with RSV showed mild illness, recovered fully, and were unaffected by iv injection of control (inactive) lymphocytes. After injection of RSV-specific cell lines, RSV-infected mice developed augmented lung disease with respiratory distress. Dose for dose, the most severe (sometimes fatal) illness was seen in mice receiving G-specific cells. Injection of G-specific cells into RSV-infected mice induced lung hemorrhage, pulmonary neutrophil recruitment (shock lung), and intense pulmonary eosinophilia. Disease was further enhanced by coinjection of M2-specific cells, which alone caused mild shock lung without eosinophilia. F-specific cells alone caused minimal enhancement of pathology, and did not affect the disease caused by G-specific cells. Each cell line reduced lung RSV titre and combined injections eliminated infection completely. Transfer of protein-specific T-cells into naive RSV-infected mice therefore reproduces the patterns of enhanced disease seen in mice sensitized to individual RSV proteins (Alwan *et al.*, 1994). Subsequent studies from other groups have suggested that Th2 phenomena may account for the disease augmentation seen in mice vaccinated with formalin-inactivated RSV (Graham *et al.*, 1993b; Connors *et al.*, 1994).

## III. CONCLUSIONS

The mouse has proven to be a valuable model for the study of human RSV. Virus replicates in the lungs causing nonfatal bronchiolitis and cells can be injected into mice, thereby demonstrating the function of individual T-cell subsets. T cells appear to be the main cause of pathology in this model of lung inflammation, a conclusion broadly supported by studies of animal models by other groups and consistent with the information from human studies. The potential roles of different T-cell subsets are strikingly illustrated by the model. Although the functional separation of T cells into Th1 and Th2 subsets was known to be relevant to protection and disease induction in parasitic infections, these studies were the first to indicate that such factors may also be relevant to disease induced by viruses. Further studies in mice may show how protective immunity can be induced without inducing harmful secondary responses to RSV infection. Although the results from mouse studies should not be interpreted too literally in relation to human disease, they illustrate the types of mechanism that may operate and suggest key studies that should be performed in man.

## ACKNOWLEDGMENTS

We thank Professor Ite Askonas, Professor Gail Wertz and her co-workers in Alabama, and our current and past co-workers in the Respiratory Unit for their invaluable contributions and The Wellcome Trust for their continued support.

## REFERENCES

Alwan, W. H., Record, F. M., and Openshaw, P. J. M. (1992). CD4+ T cells clear virus but augment disease in mice infected with respiratory syncytial virus: Comparison with the effects of CD8+ cells. *Clin. Exp. Immunol.* **88,** 527–536.

Alwan, W. H., Kozlowska, W., and Openshaw, P. J. M. (1994). Distinct types of lung disease caused by functional subsets of antiviral T cells. *J. Exp. Med.* **179,** 81–87.

Assenmacher, M., Schmitz, J., and Radbruch, A. (1994). Flow cytometric determination of cytokines in activated murine T helper lymphocytes: Expression of interleukin-10 in interferon-gamma and in interleukin-4-expressing cells. *Eur. J. Immunol.* **24,** 1097–1101.

Cannon, M. J., Openshaw, P. J. M., and Askonas, B. A. (1988). Cytotoxic T cells clear virus but augment lung pathology in mice infected with respiratory syncytial virus. *J. Exp. Med.* **168,** 1163–1168.

Connors, M., Kulkarni, A. B., Firestone, C. Y., Holmes, K. L., Morse, H. C., Sotnikov, A. V., and Murphy, B. R. (1992). Pulmonary histopathology induced by respiratory syncytial virus (RSV) challenge of formalin-inactivated RSV-immunized BALB/c mice is abrogated by depletion of CD4+ T cells. *J. Virol.* **66,** 7444–7451.

Connors, M., Giese, N. A., Kulkarni, A. B., Firestone, C.-Y., Morse III, H. C., and Murphy, B. R. (1994). Enhanced pulmonary histopathology induced by respiratory syncytial virus (RSV) challenge of formalin-inactivated RSV-immunized BALB/c mice is abrogated by depletion of interleukin-4 (IL-4) and IL-10. *J. Virol.* **68,** 5321–5325.

Fiorentino, D. F., Bond, M. W., and Mosmann, T. R. (1989). Two types of mouse T helper cell. IV. Th2 clones secrete a factor that inhibits cytokine production by Th1 clones. *J. Exp. Med.* **170,** 2081–2095.

Graham, B. S., Bunton, L. A., Wright, P. F., and Karzon, D. T. (1991). Role of T lymphocyte subsets in the pathogenesis of primary infection and rechallenge with respiratory syncytial virus in mice. *J. Clin. Invest.* **88,** 1026–1033.

Graham, B. S., Henderson, G. S., Tang, Y.-W., Lu, X., Neuzil, K. M., and Colley, D. G. (1993). Priming immunization determines T helper cytokine mRNA expression patterns in lungs of mice challenged with respiratory syncytial virus. *J. Immunol.* **151,** 2032–2040.

Heilman, C. A. (1990). Respiratory syncytial and parainfluenza viruses. *J. Infect. Dis.* **161,** 402–406.

McIntosh, K., and Fishaut, J. M. (1980). Immunopathologic mechanisms in lower respiratory tract disease of infants due to respiratory syncytial virus. *Prog. Med. Virol.* **26,** 94–118.

Muñoz, J. L., McCarthy, C. A., Clark, M. E., and Hall, C. B. (1991). Respiratory syncytial virus infection in C57BL/6 mice: Clearance of virus from the lungs with virus-specific cytotoxic T cells. *J. Virol.* **65,** 4494–4497.

Murphy, B. R., Sotnikov, A. V., Lawrence, L. A., Banks, S. M., and Prince, G. A. (1990). Enhanced pulmonary histopathology is observed in cotton rats immunized with formalin-inactivated respiratory syncytial virus (RSV) or purified F glycoprotein and challenged with RSV 3–6 months after immunization. *Vaccine* **8,** 497–502.

Openshaw, P. J. M. (1989). Flow cytometric analysis of pulmonary lymphocytes from mice infected with respiratory syncytial virus. *Clin. Exp. Immunol.* **75**, 324–328.

Openshaw, P. J. M. (1991). Pulmonary epithelial T cells induced by viral infection express T cell receptors α/β. *Eur. J. Immunol.* **21**, 803–806.

Openshaw, P. J. M. (1995). Immunopathological mechanisms in respiratory syncytial virus disease. *Springer Semin. Immunopathol.* **17**, 187–201.

Openshaw, P. J. M., Murphy, E. E., Hosken, N. A., Manio, V., Davis, K., and O'Garra, A. (1995). Heterogeneity of intracellular cytokine synthesis at the single cell level in polarised T helper 1 and T helper 2 populations. *J. Exp. Med.* **182**, 1357–1367.

Prince, G. A., Horswood, R. L., Berndt, J. A., Suffin, S. C., and Chanock, R. M. (1979). Respiratory syncytial virus infection in inbred mice. *Infect. Immun.* **26**, 764–766.

Street, N. E., Schumacher, J. H., Fong, T. A. T., Bass, H., Fiorentino, D. F., Leverah, J. A., and Mosmann, T. R. (1990). Heterogeneity of mouse helper T cells: Evidence from bulk cultures and limiting dilution cloning for precursors of Th1 and Th2 cells. *J. Immunol.* **144**, 1629–1639.

Tang, Y.-W., and Graham, B. S. (1994). Anti-IL-4 treatment at immunization modulates cytokine expression, reduces illness, and increases cytotoxic T lymphocyte activity in mice challenged with respiratory syncytial virus. *J. Clin. Invest.* **94**, 1953–1958.

Taylor, G., Stott, E. J., Hughes, M., and Collins, A. P. (1984). Respiratory syncytial virus infection in mice. *Infect. Immun.* **43**, 649–655.

# part
# VI

# MUCOSAL VACCINES

# Chapter 33

# Vaccines for Selective Induction of Th1- and Th2-Cell Responses and Their Roles in Mucosal Immunity

Mariarosaria Marinaro,* Hiroshi Kiyono,*·† John L. VanCott,* Nobuo Okahashi,* Frederik W. van Ginkel,* David W. Pascual,* Elisabeth Ban,* Raymond J. Jackson,* Herman F. Staats,‡ and Jerry R. McGhee*·†

*Departments of Microbiology and Oral Biology, Immunobiology Vaccine Center,
University of Alabama at Birmingham Medical Center, Birmingham, Alabama 35294;
†Department of Mucosal Immunology, Research Institute for Microbial Diseases, Osaka University,
Osaka 565, Japan; and ‡Center for AIDS Research, Department of Medicine,
Duke University Medical Center, Durham, North Carolina 27710

## I. INTRODUCTION

Mucosal surfaces serve as portals of entry for many infectious agents and at the same time constitute an elaborate defense system which includes the mucosa-associated lymphoreticular tissue (MALT). The induction of protective mucosal immune responses that would serve as a first line of defense for the host represents a considerable scientific and technological challenge and extensive efforts are currently underway worldwide to design vaccines able to confer protection at these vulnerable sites (Staats *et al.,* 1994). In fact, the interaction between pathogens and MALT has piqued the interest of many scientists since the development of effective mucosal vaccines relies almost entirely on our understanding of the mucosal immune system (Ogra *et al.,* 1980; Mestecky and McGhee, 1987; McGhee and Mestecky, 1990). The introduction of the oral poliovirus vaccine, which will soon result in the worldwide eradication of the disease, represents an excellent example of protection through mucosal vaccination. Mucosal immunization has the major advantage of inducing both secretory and systemic antibody responses and, moreover, the existence of a common mucosal immune system can be exploited to design vaccines able to protect mucosal surfaces that are less accessible to mucosal immunization (Mestecky, 1987; Phillips-Quagliata and Lamm, 1988; Scicchitano *et al.,* 1988).

The site of immunization and the choice of adjuvant and vehicles to deliver vaccines all play important roles in determining the degree of dissemination of secretory IgA (S-IgA) antibodies, the predominant immunoglobulin isotype present in mucosal secretions (Mestecky and McGhee, 1987). In the gastrointestinal (GI) tract, Peyer's patches (PP) are one major source of IgA plasma cell precursors that undergo direct antigen-driven proliferation, migration, and differentiation to repopulate the intestinal lamina propria with specific IgA-producing plasma cells (Robertson and Cebra, 1976; Mestecky and McGhee, 1987). However, T-cell-mediated immune (CMI) responses are also associated with mucosal immunity and the homing of sensitized T cells appears to be similar to that described for IgA plasma cell precursors (Waldman and Ganguly, 1974; Tomasi, 1976; reviewed by Cerf-Bensussan et al., Chap. 20, this volume). Thus, the selective induction of humoral and cellular immune responses by mucosal vaccination is desirable for the prevention of the majority of microbial diseases.

The differentiation pathways which T-helper (Th) cells undergo during mucosal and systemic immune responses is currently receiving extensive study, since it has been suggested that the function of mature Th cells is based upon the types of cytokines produced (Mosmann and Coffman, 1989; Mosmann and Moore, 1991). In particular, Th1 cells, secreting IFN$\gamma$, IL-2, and tumor necrosis factor-$\beta$ (TNF$\beta$), are associated with delayed-type hypersensitivity and are less efficient than the Th2 subset (producing IL-4, IL-5, IL-6, IL-9, IL-10, and IL-13) in providing help for antibody responses. The pattern of antibody isotypes secreted during an immune response is dependent upon the phenotype of the stimulating Th cells. Thus, in the murine system, Th1 cells through the secretion of IFN$\gamma$ are more efficient in stimulating IgG2a production, whereas Th2 cells producing IL-4 induce IgG1 and IgE antibodies (Snapper et al., 1988; Finkelman et al., 1989).

Although the actual molecular basis for the generation of an IgA antibody response in mucosal tissues has not yet been fully elucidated, the identification of cytokines that specifically stimulate IgA synthesis in vitro raises the possibility that specific cytokines are involved in the establishment of a mucosal microenvironment conducive to an IgA response. Both Th2- (e.g., IL-4, IL-5, IL-6 and IL-10) and, to a lesser degree, Th1- (e.g., IL-2) type cytokines have been shown to influence maturation of surface IgA$^+$ B cells into IgA secreting plasma cells (Coffman et al., 1987; Murray et al., 1987; Beagley et al., 1988, 1989; Fujihashi et al., 1991; Ramsay et al., 1994). Antigen-specific B-cell responses to mucosally delivered vaccine proteins are dependent upon CD4$^+$ Th cells, and the frequency of Th1- and Th2-cell responses after mucosal immunization may determine the level and isotype of mucosal as well as systemic antibody responses. Thus, the knowledge of the type of immune responses (e.g., Th1 or Th2) induced by an immunization regimen provides a powerful tool to design and screen candidate vaccines which elicit the desired immune response. For example, CMI responses may be preferable to clear infections due to intracellular pathogens while strong mucosal and serum antibody responses (better sustained by Th2-type cells) may be required to neutralize the effect of soluble antigens such as bacterial toxins and proteolytic enzymes.

In this chapter, we will summarize some of our recent findings on the role of Th1 and Th2 cells and derived cytokines for the induction and regulation of mucosal and systemic immune responses to well-defined vaccines and delivery systems (Fig. 1). In addition, we will briefly discuss additional mucosal immunization approaches including mucosal delivery of soluble proteins, recombinant bacterial and viral vectors, and mucosal DNA (genetic) immunization.

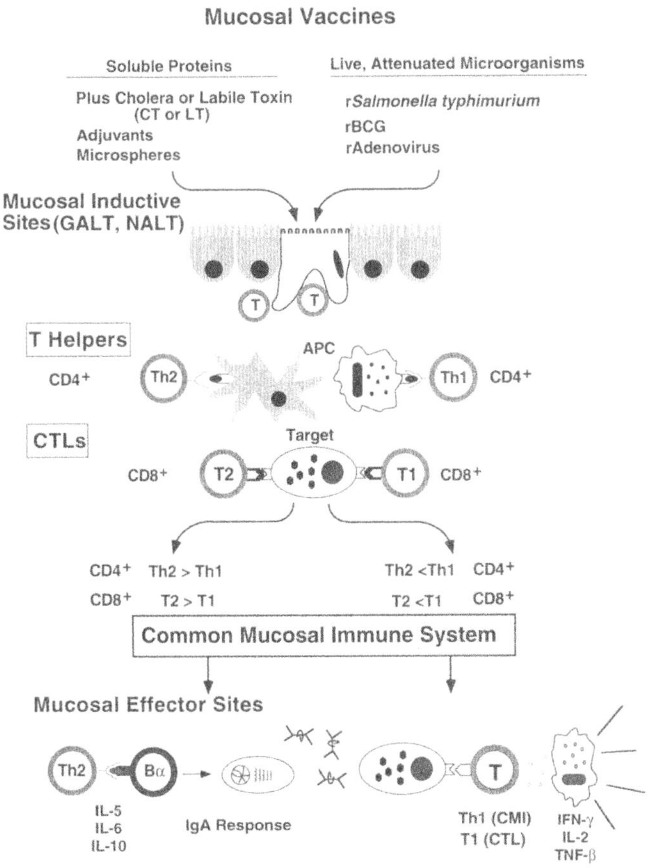

FIGURE 1. Scheme illustrating the principle that the nature of adjuvant or delivery system (including recombinant bacteria or viruses) influences the type of (Th) cells induced with subsequent mucosal or systemic antibody responses. There is also evidence that CD8$^+$ CTLs may exhibit T1-like or T2-like cytokine profiles and would contribute to humoral or CMI-type responses.

## II. T-HELPER SUBSETS AND B-CELL RESPONSES FOLLOWING ORAL IMMUNIZATION WITH CHOLERA TOXIN AS MUCOSAL ADJUVANT

The induction of optimal antigen-specific S-IgA antibodies following oral immunization with soluble protein antigens is often difficult to achieve since these proteins are degraded by proteolytic enzymes present in the GI tract. Moreover, prolonged feeding or the administration of large doses of protein antigens may induce oral tolerance (Tomasi, 1980; Challacombe and Tomasi, 1980; Weiner *et al.*, Chapter 39). However, cholera toxin (CT) is known to be a strong mucosal immunogen and also acts as a mucosal adjuvant when administered orally together with unrelated proteins. Although several studies have shown that CT may have a direct effect on immune cells (Bromander *et al.*, 1991; Woogen *et al.*, 1987; Lycke *et al.*, 1989; Lebman *et al.*, 1988; Lycke and Strober, 1989; Munoz *et al.*, 1990), the molecular mechanisms responsible for CT adjuvanticity have not yet been identified. Defining the molecular basis of the adjuvant effect of CT may allow the development of effective mucosal vaccines, and may contribute to the understanding of mechanisms regulating mucosal immune responses.

We have previously investigated the influence of CT on Th1- and Th2-type $CD4^+$ Th-cell subsets when the toxin was coadministered orally with the well-defined protein antigen tetanus toxoid (TT) (Xu-Amano *et al.*, 1993). Cytokine analysis of antigen-specific $CD4^+$ T cells isolated from both the systemic (spleen; SP) and the mucosal compartments (Peyer's patches; PP) revealed that Th2-type responses were induced. In particular, a high frequency of IL-4- and IL-5-producing cells was observed during peak mucosal S-IgA and serum IgG anti-TT and anti-CT-B antibody responses (Jackson *et al.*, 1993; Xu-Amano *et al.*, 1993), while the frequency of IFN$\gamma$- and IL-2-secreting cells remained at levels observed in unimmunized mice. Comparable cytokine patterns were noted both by the ELISPOT technique and by mRNA analysis. Moreover, using a quantitative reverse-transcriptase PCR for cytokine-specific mRNA, a significant increase in IL-4 but not IFN$\gamma$ mRNA was observed in TT-stimulated $CD4^+$ T cells (Marinaro *et al.*, 1995).

In order to correlate the cytokine profile observed *in vitro* with the antigen-specific antibodies induced *in vivo*, we have recently analyzed the pattern of antibody isotypes and subclasses. Our analysis revealed that mice receiving CT and TT three times at weekly intervals had significant increases in TT-specific IgG1 and IgE, sustained by Th2 cell-derived IL-4. Moreover, using two additional protein antigens [ovalbumin (OVA) and hen egg-white lysozyme (HEL)], we observed a similar isotype and subclass distribution when the proteins were coadministered orally with CT. Thus, anti-OVA or anti-HEL serum IgG1 and IgE as well as S-IgA antibodies were detected. Taken together, the data show that the antibody isotype and IgG subclass response observed *in vivo* was consistent with the Th2-type cytokine profile obtained by quantitative analysis of cytokine message. Thus,

Th2 cells and derived cytokines induced by the adjuvant CT supported serum IgG1, IgE, and mucosal S-IgA antibody responses (Fig. 1 and Table I).

## III. T-HELPER SUBSETS AND B-CELL RESPONSES FOLLOWING ORAL IMMUNIZATION WITH rSALMONELLA

Live attenuated *Salmonella* have been developed as mucosal vaccine delivery vectors for recombinant proteins associated with microbial virulence (Curtiss *et al.*, 1993; Chatfield *et al.*, 1993; Roberts *et al.*, 1994). It has been shown that *Salmonella* vaccines elicit protective antibody and CMI responses in the host after either parenteral or mucosal immunization (Chatfield *et al.*, 1992; Roberts *et al.*, 1994). *Salmonella typhimurium*, like other microorganisms, i.e., *Leishmania major, Listeria monocytogenes*, or *Mycobacterium tuberculosis*, has been shown to induce a Th1-dependent immune response (Ramarathinam *et al.*, 1991; Locksley and Scott, 1991; Scott, 1991; Zhong and de la Maza, 1988; Flesch and Kaufmann, 1987; Muotiala and Makela, 1990). Further, IFNγ, a Th1-type cytokine, is essential for clearing *S. typhimurium* infection *in vivo* in part through the activation of macrophages for intracellular killing (Muotiala and Makela, 1990; Ramarathinam *et al.*, 1991, 1993; Mastroeni *et al.*, 1992).

In our studies, we have used recombinant (r) *Salmonella typhimurium* BRD 847 *(aro A-, aro D-)* expressing the C fragment of tetanus toxin (r*Salmonella*-Tox C) under regulation of a *nir*B promoter. This delivery system was shown to induce long-lasting immune responses and protection against systemic lethal tetanus toxin challenge in mice following a single oral dose of $10^{10}$ CFU (Chatfield *et al.*, 1992; Roberts *et al.*, 1994). Our studies showed that oral administration of r*Salmonella*-Tox C to mice elicited mucosal S-IgA and serum IgG responses, primarily of the IgG2a and IgG2b subclasses. Further, supernatants from both SP and PP CD4$^+$ T-cell cultures showed increases in Th1-type cytokines (e.g., IFNγ and IL-2) as well as the Th2 cytokine IL-10, but not IL-4 or IL-5. To confirm these results, we assessed IFNγ- and IL-2-specific T-cell responses by ELISPOT assay and significant numbers of IFNγ and IL-2 spot-forming cells (SFCs) were noted in CD4$^+$ T-cell cultures stimulated with TT. Analysis of mRNA by quantitative RT-PCR also revealed significant messages for Th1 (IL-2 and IFNγ) and Th2 (IL-10) cytokines (VanCott *et al.*, 1996). These results showed that TT-specific IgA responses were elevated in the GI tract following induction of mainly Th1 cells producing IFNγ and Th2 cells producing IL-10, but not Th2 cells producing IL-4 and IL-5 in GI tract inductive sites (i.e., the PP) (Fig. 1).

Induction of TT-specific IgA responses in a Th1-dominant environment could be explained by the existence of alternate or compensatory Th2 cell pathways. For example, in the absence of traditional Th2 type cells producing IL-4 and IL-5, IL-10-secreting CD4$^+$ Th cells together with Th1 cells may support both mucosal and systemic IgA responses. Moreover, we found that Mac-1$^+$ cells, which are enriched in macrophages, produced high levels of IL-6 in mice orally immunized with r*Salmonella*. IL-6 has been shown to be the most effective terminal differentiation factor for IgA-committed B cells to become IgA-producing cells in both human and murine systems (Beagley *et al.*, 1989; Fujihashi *et al.*, 1991). Further, it has been shown that IL-10 plays an essential role in IgA B cell differentiation in humans (Briere *et al.*, 1994). These results suggested that Th2-derived IL-10, as well as macrophage-derived IL-6, may provide important signals for regulating mucosal S-IgA responses in the absence of Th2 cells producing IL-4 and IL-5 in mice orally immunized with r*Salmonella*-Tox C (Fig. 1).

## IV. MUCOSAL IMMUNITY IN CYTOKINE KNOCKOUT MICE

### A. Studies in IFN$\gamma^{-/-}$ Mice

To examine the importance of IFN$\gamma$ in the development of vaccine-induced mucosal IgA responses, we immunized IFN$\gamma$-deficient (IFN-$\gamma^{-/-}$) mice with live, attenuated r*S. typhimurium* BRD 847 expressing Tox C or with soluble TT with CT as adjuvant. IFN$\gamma^{-/-}$ mice immunized with r*Salmonella*-Tox C showed increased serum titers of TT-specific IgM, IgG, and IgA antibodies when compared with wild-type mice, probably because of the substantial increase in numbers of *Salmonella* organisms in PP and SP of these mice. Analysis of the IgG subclasses revealed a shift from IgG2a in wild-type mice to IgG1 in IFN$\gamma^{-/-}$ mice. However, TT-specific IgE responses were not detected in mice orally immunized with r*Salmonella*. In contrast, wild-type and IFN$\gamma^{-/-}$ mice immunized orally with TT plus CT also exhibited a similar antibody isotype pattern which was characterized by serum IgG1 and IgE responses. Both vaccine regimens were capable of inducing brisk mucosal S-IgA antibody responses in IFN$\gamma^{-/-}$ mice. These results suggested that the lack of IFN$\gamma$, which markedly affected the development of serum IgG2a responses, did not alter mucosal S-IgA responses to either a Th1 (i.e., r*Salmonella*-Tox C vaccine) or a Th2 (i.e., combined TT plus CT vaccine) vaccine regimen.

When cytokine profiles were evaluated by cytokine-specific ELISPOT and ELISA in CD4$^+$ T cells from PP and SP of IFN$\gamma^{-/-}$ mice orally immunized with r*Salmonella*-Tox C, as expected no IFN$\gamma$ production was noted following *in vitro* restimulation of CD4$^+$ T cells with TT antigen in the presence of accessory cells (Table I). However, two Th2-derived cytokines, IL-4 and IL-5, were increased. The increase in IL-4 and IL-5 cytokines was consistent with the induction of serum IgG1 antibodies since this IgG subclass is regulated by IL-4. In this regard, IFN$\gamma^{-/-}$ mice orally immunized with TT plus CT also developed a typical Th2-type response that was similar to that induced in wild-type mice. Thus, the lack of IFN$\gamma$ had profound effects on the type of immune response elicited by an oral r*Salmonella* vaccine, which normally induces strong Th1-type IFN$\gamma$-producing T cells and IgG2a-producing B cells, but had little effect on the development of immune responses to TT delivered with CT adjuvant (Table I). These findings provide additional evidence that delivery of TT by r*Salmonella* vector versus coad-

TABLE I

TT-Specific Th1 and Th2 Cytokine Profiles of CD4$^+$ T Cells from Normal, IL-4$^{-/-}$ and IFN$\gamma^{-/-}$ Mice

| | Th1 type | | Th2 type | | | Mucosal |
|---|---|---|---|---|---|---|
| | IFN$\gamma$ | IL-2 | IL-4 | IL-5 | IL-10 | IgA |
| IL-4$^{-/-}$ | | | | | | |
| rSalmonella | + + | + | − | − | + + | + + |
| TT + CT | + | + | − | − | − | − |
| IFN$\gamma^{-/-}$ | | | | | | |
| rSalmonella | − | − | + | + | + | + + |
| TT + CT | − | − | + | + | + | + + |
| Normal | | | | | | |
| rSalmonella | + | + | − | − | + | + + |
| TT + CT | − | − | + | + | + | + + |

ministration of TT with CT as an adjuvant selectively elicits Th1- versus Th2-type responses to TT, respectively, in normal mice (Fig. 1 and Table I).

## B. Studies in IL-4$^{-/-}$ Mice

IL-4 is a growth and differentiation factor for B cells and induces the differentiation of T cells toward a Th2 phenotype (Le Gros et al., 1990; Sad and Mosmann, 1994; Swain et al., 1990). The original study which described the development of IL-4 gene-disrupted (IL-4$^{-/-}$) mice provided evidence that Th2-type cytokines were not expressed by CD4$^+$ T cells in this strain (Kopf et al., 1993). In order to determine if IL-4 was essential for the induction of antigen-specific mucosal and systemic immune responses, we immunized IL-4$^{-/-}$ mice with rSalmonella-Tox C or with TT coadministered with CT as adjuvant. Oral immunization of IL-4$^{-/-}$ mice with rSalmonella-Tox C resulted in TT-specific mucosal S-IgA and serum IgG responses that were comparable to those seen in wild-type mice. On the other hand, IL-4$^{-/-}$ mice orally immunized with TT and mucosal adjuvant CT showed significantly lower levels of mucosal S-IgA anti-TT antibody responses when compared with wild-type mice; however, serum IgG anti-TT antibody levels were similar in both mouse strains. Of interest was the finding that IgG2a was the major IgG subclass induced in serum of IL-4$^{-/-}$ mice immunized with either oral regimen (Okahashi et al., 1996). Neither total nor TT-specific IgE or IgG1 responses were induced in IL-4$^{-/-}$ mice immunized with either vaccine preparation, confirming the notion that IL-4 plays a necessary role for the induction of antigen-specific IgG1 and IgE responses (Kopf et al., 1993). These results supported the results from normal mice that oral *Salmonella* vaccines potentiate mucosal S-IgA responses to expressed proteins in the absence of IL-4 (Table I).

In order to determine which cytokines contribute to the induction of vaccine antigen-specific mucosal S-IgA antibody responses, PP and SP CD4$^+$ T cells from IL-4$^{-/-}$ mice orally immunized with r*Salmonella*-Tox C or with TT plus CT were restimulated *in vitro* with TT-coated latex beads in the presence of feeder cells. Table I summarizes the cytokine profile of IFN$\gamma^{-/-}$ and IL-4$^{-/-}$ mice orally immunized with *Salmonella* expressing Tox C or with TT plus CT.

Oral r*Salmonella* induced strong IFN$\gamma$ responses in IL-4$^{-/-}$ mice. However, IL-5 was also not induced in CD4$^+$ T cells from IL-4$^{-/-}$ mice given r*Salmonella*, suggesting that IL-4 and IL-5 may be coregulated. The most interesting result was the observation that CD4$^+$ T cells from r*Salmonella*-immunized IL-4$^{-/-}$ mice produced both IL-6 and IL-10 (Okahashi *et al.*, 1996). On the other hand, IL-4$^{-/-}$ mice orally immunized with TT plus CT showed no increase in Th2-type cytokines (IL-5, IL-6, or IL-10). These results indicate that IL-4 is necessary for the development of antigen-specific mucosal IgA responses when TT is coadministered with the mucosal adjuvant CT. In this regard, others have also shown that IL-4$^{-/-}$ mice failed to respond to soluble protein antigens given orally with CT as a mucosal adjuvant (Vajdy *et al.*, 1995). In our studies, IL-4 was not an essential cytokine for the induction of antigen-specific mucosal IgA antibody when the vaccine was delivered to mucosa-associated tissues by a recombinant live vector (e.g., *Salmonella*). Taken together, our findings show that oral immunization with r*Salmonella* expressing a foreign antigen induces antigen-specific mucosal IgA responses without a requirement for either IFN$\gamma$ or IL-4. Our studies provide further evidence that IL-4 from Th2-type cells is involved in mucosal adjuvanticity induced by CT.

## V. LIVE ATTENUATED ADENOVIRUS VECTORS DELIVER TRANSGENES TO THE RESPIRATORY EPITHELIA

Delivery of vaccine antigens to the upper respiratory tract is a promising approach for inducing protective mucosal and systemic immune responses. The ability of some adenoviruses to invade the respiratory tract was exploited for the delivery of recombinant vaccine antigens intranasally. Attenuated adenovirus vectors for expression of heterologous antigen were constructed both for gene therapy and for induction of immunity to transgenes. In this regard, most adenovirus-based delivery vehicles have been derived from group C adenoviruses, initially rendered replication-deficient by deletion of the E1 region (Graham and Prevec, 1992). The E1 region encodes for the immediate early gene products and is required for initiation of viral replication. Further attenuations have been achieved by deletions of other early genes, which include the E3 and E4 regions. An Ade5 double mutant (E1/E3 deleted) carrying the *lacZ* gene (Ade5-*lacZ*) was used in our studies. Although the deletion of the E3 region was not required for rendering the vector replication-deficient, its deletion may increase the vector immunogenicity since the E3 region is associated with persistent infection of group C adenovirus in lymphoid tissues (Wold and Gooding, 1989).

In order to better understand the immune response to adenoviral vectors, CD-1 and C57BL/6N mice were immunized intratracheally (i.t.), intranasally (i.n.), or intraperitoneally (i.p.) with the Ade5-*lacZ* vector. The resulting immune responses were characterized by elevated serum IgA, IgM, and IgG titers to the vector as well as to β-galactosidase (β-gal). These immune antibodies were derived from the mucosal and systemic compartments of the lung, lower respiratory lymph nodes (LRLN), nasal passages (NP), and, to a lesser degree, the systemic compartment of the spleen, when lymphoid cells from these tissues were assessed by the ELISPOT method (van Ginkel *et al.*, 1995). Significant levels of IgA and IgM antibodies were detected in bronchial lavages from these mice. The immune serum IgG antibodies were predominantly composed of the IgG2b subclass, and to a lesser extent consisted of IgG1 and IgG2a antibodies specific for the Ade5 vector and IgG2a antibodies specific for β-gal. This observation differs from what was obtained with immune responses to wild-type Ade5 virus which was characterized by an IgG2a-dominated antibody response (Coutelier *et al.*, 1990).

The lung functions as an effector site for the generation of immune responses by i.t. administration of Ade5-*lacZ*. Antigen-specific mononuclear cells are generated in draining lymph nodes (Bienenstock and Clancy, 1994), which is consistent with our finding that elevated levels of antibody-producing (AFC) were present in the LRLN. Subsequent studies will address the relative importance of IFNγ for immunity to Ade5 vectors and β-gal. To determine the types of cytokines induced following i.t. administration of Ade5-*lacZ* vector, IFNγ knockout (IFNγ$^{-/-}$) mice, and wild-type mice received three i.t. instillations. Following *in vitro* stimulation of splenic lymphocytes with inactivated Ade5 virus, a Th2-cytokine profile was obtained. In contrast, *in vitro* stimulation with β-gal induced low levels of IL-4 secretion in IFNγ$^{-/-}$ mice, whereas a dominant Th1-type response was observed in normal (IFNγ$^{+/+}$) mice. Furthermore, IFNγ$^{-/-}$ mice displayed decreased IgG2a and IgG3 antibody levels to both adenovirus and β-gal when compared to normal mice. This demonstrates the propensity of IFNγ$^{-/-}$ mice to elicit a Th2-mediated IgG antibody profile, while no significant changes in IgA and IgG serum antibody levels were observed. Furthermore, the viral neutralization titers in the serum of normal and IFNγ$^{-/-}$ mice were identical. Virus neutralization titers, an important parameter of protective immunity, were more dependent on the route of Ade5-*lacZ* administration (i.n. gave the lowest and i.p. the highest serum neutralization titers) than on the presence or absence of IFNγ. This demonstrates that anti-Ade5 vector immunity does not require IFNγ for immune protection, and suggests that the manner in which the transgene (vaccine gene) is expressed, i.e., intracellular or secreted, will dictate the type of Th-cell immunity that will be induced.

## VI. Polynucleotide Mucosal Vaccines

A limitation to the development of vaccines against viruses such as influenza is the diversity of viral envelope proteins among different strains. Therefore, efforts in vaccine development have focused on induction of memory cytotoxic T lymphocytes (CTLs) that react to epitopes shared by different strains of virus. Most efforts to generate CTL responses have used replicating vectors either to produce the antigen in the host cell or for delivery of peptides into the cytoplasm. However, the selection of peptide epitopes presented by MHC molecules is dependent on the structure of an individual's MHC molecules, and the peptide approach has shown some limitation in humans. As an alternate method of immunization against influenza, DNA vaccines are a promising approach for protection of mucosal surfaces. Like recombinant vectors, the transfected DNA results in presentation of antigenic epitopes in association with class I MHC. In addition, the significant advantages of using gene transfer technology for mucosal immunization against influenza are that (i) no infectious agents are being used, (ii) combined vaccines are easily and rapidly made, (iii) DNA stability is not affected by high temperature and therefore is more suitable for third-world vaccination.

The feasibility of polynucleotide vaccines was first shown in studies using direct injection of plasmid DNA into the quadriceps of mice (Wolff *et al.*, 1990). In the past year, many studies have shown that protection against mucosal pathogens may be achieved by DNA immunization (Wang *et al.*, 1993; Fynan *et al.*, 1993; Ulmer *et al.*, 1993; Lowrie *et al.*, 1994; Xu and Liew, 1994). Most DNA immunization protocols performed so far have used inoculation of the DNA into muscle cells or by particle bombardment into dermal or epidermal cells (Danko and Wolff, 1994). In natural states, most foreign antigens are first confronted by the mucosae. Thus, gene administration to the mucosae would mimic exposure to most pathogens and may more efficiently induce a protective immune response. In this regard, studies by Robinson *et al.* (unpublished) suggest that intranasal inoculation of a plasmid expression system for influenza hemagglutinin (HA) induces resistance to lethal challenge with live influenza viruses in mice (Fynan *et al.*, 1993). Therefore, we have undertaken studies aimed at targeting DNA encoding HA to the lung in order to induce a protective mucosal immune response against influenza A viruses. We are currently assessing the immune response obtained by introduction of HA plasmid DNA by either intranasal or intramuscular injection. The plasmid construct expressing HA comprises the cytomegalovirus (CMV) immediate early promoter, the complete sequence of HA cDNA from A/PR/8/34 influenza virus, and rat preproinsulin II sequences including eukaryotic enhancer regulatory elements and a polyadenylation site. High titers of serum anti-HA IgG antibodies were detected in mice following intramuscular immunization with HA-encoding plasmid. Since the major IgG subclass was IgG2a followed by IgG2b, it is likely that Th1-type cells producing IFN$\gamma$ were responsible for the induction of those antibody responses. On the other hand, mucosal delivery of the plasmid did not result in detectable titers of antibodies at either the systemic or mucosal level. Thus, our current studies are directed toward defining delivery systems that are optimal for the induction of a protective immune responses by mucosal immunization with the HA encoding plasmid.

## VII. SUMMARY

We have used both normal and cytokine knockout mice to help determine the precise requirements for $CD4^+$ Th-cell regulation of serum IgG subclass and mucosal IgA antibody responses. In these studies, we have used different oral delivery systems to induce mucosal and systemic antibody responses to the vaccine TT and to other vaccine antigens (Fig. 1). In normal mice, oral administration of TT with CT as an adjuvant induced Th2-type cells and cytokines which led to mucosal IgA and serum IgG1, IgA and IgE responses. On the other hand, oral immunization with r*Salmonella*-Tox C results in Th1-type responses as well as Th2-cell-derived IL-10 and macrophage-derived IL-6 which correlated with mucosal IgA and serum IgG2a antibody responses. Intranasal immunization with recombinant adenovirus expressing $\beta$-gal-induced Th1-type responses to $\beta$-gal and Th2-type responses to the adenovirus.

Two major conclusions can be drawn from our studies with the TT antigen in normal, IFN$\gamma^{-/-}$, and IL-4$^{-/-}$ mice. First, oral administration of r*Salmonella*-Tox C, which elicits classical Th1-type responses, also induces significant mucosal S-IgA antibodies when given to mice with defective Th1- (IFN$\gamma^{-/-}$) or Th2 (IL-4$^{-/-}$) cytokine pathways. Interestingly, we detected Th2-type cells producing IL-10 and macrophages secreting IL-6 in both normal and cytokine deficient mice, and we postulate that these two cytokines are of importance for murine S-IgA responses. Second, oral administration of TT plus CT as an adjuvant induces classical Th2-type responses in both normal and IFN$\gamma^{-/-}$ mice. Further, lack of IL-4 results in abrogation of TT-specific mucosal IgA responses. Thus, the IL-4 pathway is necessary for mucosal IgA responses induced after oral immunization with a protein vaccine and the mucosal adjuvant cholera toxin.

We have continued efforts to develop other mucosal delivery systems which would favor induction of protective mucosal immunity to virus infection. Our initial studies with live attenuated adenovirus vector indicated that both serum and mucosal antibody responses were induced following immunization via the respiratory tract. Genetic mucosal immunization with DNA (or mRNA) from pathogenic viruses which exhibit antigenic variation, would offer the possibility for induction of CTL responses to cross-reactive epitopes. We are currently pursuing this approach with an influenza HA DNA vaccine.

## Acknowledgments

This work was supported by NIAID-DMID Contract AI 15128 for the Mucosal Immunization Research Group, by NIH Grants AI 18958, DE 04217, DK 44240, AI 35544, CA 54430, DE 09838, and DE 08228, and by Cystic Fibrosis Foundation Grants P896 and Z946. We thank Ms. Wendy Jackson for the preparation of the manuscript.

## References

Beagley, K. W., Eldridge, J. H., Kiyono, H., Everson, M. P., Koopman, W. J., Honjo, T., and McGhee, J. R. (1988). Recombinant murine IL-5 induces high rate IgA synthesis in cycling IgA-positive Peyer's patch B cells. *J. Immunol.* **141,** 2035–2042.

Beagley, K. W., Eldridge, J. H., Lee, F., Kiyono, H., Everson, M. P., Koopman, W. J., Hirano, T. J., Kishimoto, T., and McGhee, J. R. (1989). Interleukins and IgA synthesis. Human and murine IL-6 induce high rate IgA secretion in IgA-committed B cells. *J. Exp. Med.* **169,** 2133–2148.

Bienenstock, J., and Clancy, J. (1994). Bronchial mucosal lymphoid tissue. *In* "Handbook of Mucosal Immunology," (P. L. Ogra, *et al.,* Eds)., pp. 529–538. Acad. Press, San Diego, CA.

Briere, F., Bridon, J.-M., Chevet, D., Souillet, G., Bienvenu, F., Guret, C., Martinez-Valdez, H., and Banchereau, J. (1994). Interleukin 10 induces B lymphocytes from IgA-deficient patients to secrete IgA. *J. Clin. Invest.* **94,** 97–104.

Bromander, A., Holmgren, J., and Lycke, N. (1991). Cholera toxin stimulates IL-1 production and enhances antigen presentation by macrophages *in vitro. J. Immunol.* **146,** 2908–2914.

Challacombe, S. J., and Tomasi, T. B., Jr. (1980). Systemic tolerance and secretory immunity after oral immunization. *J. Exp. Med.* **152,** 1459–1472.

Chatfield, S. N., Charles, I. G., Makoff, A. J., Oxer, M. D., Dougan, G., Pickard, D., Slater, D., and Fairweather, N. F. (1992). Use of the nirB promoter to direct the stable expression of heterologous antigens in *Salmonella* oral vaccine strains: Development of a single dose oral tetanus vaccine. *Bio/ Technology* **10,** 888–892.

Chatfield, S. N., Roberts, M., London, P., Cropley, I., Douce, G., and Dougan, G. (1993). The development of oral vaccines based on live attenuated *Salmonella* strains. *FEMS Immunol. Med. Microbiol.* **7,** 1–7.

Coffman, R. L., Seymour, B. H. P., Lebman, D. A., Hiraki, D. D., Christiansen, J. A., Shrader, B., Cherwinski, H. M., Savelkoul, H. F. J., Finkelman, F. D., Bond, M. W., and Mosmann, T. R. (1988). The role of helper T cell products in mouse B cell differentiation and isotype regulation. *Immunol. Rev.* **102,** 5–28.

Coffman, R. L., Shrader, B., Carty, J., Mosmann, T. R., and Bond, M. W. (1987). A mouse T cell product that preferentially enhances IgA production. I. Biologic characterization. *J. Immunol.* **139,** 3685–3690.

Coffman, R. L., Varkila, K., Scott, P., and Chatelain, R. (1991). Role of cytokines in the differentiation of CD4+ T-cell subsets *in vivo. Immunol. Rev.* **123,** 189–207.

Coutelier, J.-P., Coulie, P. G., Wauters, P., Heremans, H., and van der Logt, J. T. (1990). *In vivo* polyclonal B-lymphocyte activation elicited by murine viruses. *J. Virol.* **64,** 5383–5388.

Curtiss III, R., Kelly, S. M., and Hassan, J. O. (1993). Live oral avirulent *Salmonella* vaccines. *Vet. Microbiol.* **37,** 397–405.

Danko, I., and Wolff, J. A. (1994). Direct gene transfer into muscle. *Vaccine* **12,** 1499–1502.

Finkelman, F. D., Katona, I. M., Urban, J. F., J., and Paul, W. E. (1989). Control of *in vivo* IgE production in the mouse by IL-4. *Ciba Found. Symp.* **147,** 3–22.

Flesch, I., and Kaufmann, S. H. E. (1987). Mycobacterial growth inhibition by interferon-gamma activated bone marrow macrophages and differential susceptibility among strains of *M. tuberculosis. J. Immunol.* **138,** 4408–4413.

Fujihashi, K., McGhee, J. R., Lue, C., Beagley, K. W., Taga, T., Hirano, T., Kishimoto, T., Mestecky, J., and Kiyono, H. (1991). Human appendix B cells naturally express receptors for and respond to interleukin 6 with selective IgA1 and IgA2 synthesis. *J. Clin. Invest.* **88,** 248–252.

Fynan, E. F., Webster, R. G., Fuller, D. H., Haynes, J. R., Santoro, J. C., and Robinson, H. L. (1993). DNA vaccines: Protective immunization by parental, mucosal and gene-gun inoculations. *Proc. Natl. Acad. Sci. U.S.A.* **90,** 11478–11482.

Graham, F. L., and Prevec, L. (1992). Adenovirus-based expression vectors and recombinant vaccines. *In* "Vaccines: New Approaches to Immunological Problems." (R. W. Ellis, Ed.), pp. 363–390. Butterworth-Heinemann, Boston.

Jackson, R. J., Fujihashi, K., Xu-Amano, J., Kiyono, H., Elson, C. O., and McGhee, J. R. (1993). Optimizing oral vaccines: Induction of systemic and mucosal B-cell and antibody responses to tetanus toxoid by use of cholera toxin as an adjuvant. *Infect. Immun.* **61,** 4272–4279.

Kopf, M., LeGros, G., Bachmann, M., Lamers, M. C., Bluethmann, H., and Kohler, G. (1993). Disruption of the murine IL-4 gene blocks Th2 cytokine responses. *Nature (London)* **362,** 245–248.

Lebman, D. A., Fuhrman, J. A., and Cebra, J. J. (1988). Intraduodenal application of cholera holotoxin increases the potential of clones from Peyer's patch B cells of relevant and unrelated specificities to secrete IgG and IgA. *Reg. Immunol.* **1,** 32–40.

LeGros, G., Ben-Sasson, S. Z., Seder, R., Finkelman, F. D., and Paul, W. E. (1990). Generation of interleukin 4 (IL-4)-producing cells *in vivo* and *in vitro:* IL-2 and IL-4 are required for *in vitro* generation of IL-4-producing cells. *J. Exp. Med.* **172,** 921–929.

Locksley, R. M., and Scott, P. (1991). Helper T-cell subsets in mouse *Leishmaniasis:* Induction, expansion and effector function. *Immunol. Today* **12,** A58–A61.

Lowrie, D. B., Tascon, R. E., Colston, M. J., and Silva, C. L. (1994). Toward a DNA vaccine against tuberculosis. *Vaccine* **12,** 1537–1540.

Lycke, N., and Strober, W. (1989). Cholera toxin promotes B cell isotype differentiation. *J. Immunol.* **142,** 3781–3787.

Lycke, N., Bromander, A. K., Ekman, L., Karlsson, U., and Holmgren, J. (1989). Cellular basis of immunomodulation by cholera toxin *in vitro* with possible association to the adjuvant function *in vivo. J. Immunol.* **142,** 20–27.

Marinaro, M., Staats, H. F., Hiroi, T., Jackson, R. J., Coste, M., Boyaka, P. N., Okahashi, N., Yamamoto, M., Kiyono, H., Bluethmann, H., Fujihashi, K., and McGhee, J. R. (1995). Mucosal adjuvant effect of cholera toxin in mice results from induction of T helper 2 (Th2) cells and IL-4. *J. Immunol.* **155,** 4621–4629.

Mastroeni, P., Villarreal-Ramos, B., and Hormaeche, C. E. (1992). Role of T cells, TNF-α and IFN-γ in recall of immunity to oral challenge with virulent *Salmonella* in mice vaccinated with live attenuated aro-*Salmonella* vaccines. *Microb. Pathog.* **13,** 477–491.

McGhee, J. R., and Mestecky, J. (1990). In defense of mucosal surfaces. Development of novel vaccines for IgA responses protective at the portals of entry of microbial pathogens. *Infect. Dis. Clin. North Am.* **4,** 315–341.

Mestecky, J. (1987). The common mucosal immune and current strategies for induction of immune response in external secretions. *J. Clin. Immunol.* **7,** 265–276.

Mestecky, J., and McGhee, J. R. (1987). Immunoglobulin A (IgA): Molecular and cellular interactions involved in IgA biosynthesis and immune response. *Adv. Immunol.* **40,** 153–245.

Mosmann, T. R., and Coffman, R. L. (1989). Th1 and Th2 cells: Different patterns of lymphokine secretion lead to different functional properties. *Annu. Rev. Immunol.* **7,** 145–173.

Mosmann, T. R., and Moore, K. W. (1991). The role of IL-10 in crossregulation of Th1 and Th2 responses. *Immunol. Today* **12,** A49–A53.

Munoz, E., Zubiaga, A. M., Merrow, M., Sauter, N. P., and Huber, B. T. (1990). Cholera toxin discriminates between T helper 1 and 2 cells in T cell receptor mediated activation: Role of cAMP in T cell proliferation. *J. Exp. Med.* **172,** 95–103.

Muotiala, A., and Makela, H. P. (1990). The role of IFN-$\gamma$ in murine *Salmonella typhimurium* infection. *Microb. Pathog.* **8,** 135–141.

Murray, P. D., McKenzie, D. T., Swain, S. L., and Kagnoff, M. F. (1987). Interleukin 5 and interleukin 4 produced by Peyer's patch T cells selectively enhance immunoglobulin A expression. *J. Immunol.* **149,** 2669–2674.

Ogra, P. L., Fishaut, M., and Gallagher, M. R. (1980). Viral vaccination via the mucosal route. *Rev. Infect. Dis.* **2,** 352–369.

Okahashi, N., Yamamoto, M., VanCott, J. L., Chatfield, S. N., Roberts, M., Bluethmann, H., Hiroi, T., Kiyono, H., and McGhee, J. R. (1996). Oral immunization of interleukin-4 (IL-4) knockout mice with a recombinant *salmonella* strain or cholera toxin revels that CD4$^+$ Th2 cells producing IL-6 and IL-10 are associated with mucosal immunoglobulin A responses. *Infect. Immun.* **64,** 1516–1525.

Phillips-Quagliata, J. M., and Lamm, M. E. (1988). Migration of lymphocytes in the mucosal immune system. *In* "Migration and Homing of Lymphoid Cells" (A. J. Husband, ed.), Vol. 2, pp. 53–75. CRC Press, Boca Raton, Florida.

Ramarathinam, L., Niesel, D. W., and Klimpel, G. R. (1993). *Salmonella typhimurium* induces IFN-$\gamma$ production in murine splenocytes. Role of natural killer cells and macrophages. *J. Immunol.* **150,** 3937–3981.

Ramarathinam, L., Shaban, R. A., Neisel, D. W., and Klimpel, G. R. (1991). Interferon gamma (IFN-$\gamma$) production by gut-associated lymphoid tissue and spleen following oral *Salmonella typhimurium* challenge. *Microb. Pathog.* **11,** 347–356.

Ramsay, A. J., Husband, A. J., Ramshaw, I. A., Bao, S., Mathaei, K. I., Kohler, G., and Kopf, M. (1994). The role of interleukin-6 in mucosal IgA antibody responses *in vivo. Science* **264,** 561–563.

Richman, L. K. (1979). Immunological unresponsiveness after enteric administration of protein antigens. *In* "Immunology of Breast Milk" (P. L. Ogra and D. Dayton, eds.), pp. 49–52. Raven, New York.

Roberts, M., Chatfield, S. N., and Dougan, G. (1994). *Salmonella* carriers of heterologous antigens. *In* "Novel Delivery Systems for Oral Vaccines" (D. T. O'Hagan, ed.), pp. 27–58. CRC Press, Ann Arbor, MI.

Robertson, S. M., and Cebra, J. J. (1976). A model for local immunity. *Ric. Clin. Lab.* **6**(Suppl. 3), 105–119.

Sad, S., and Mosmann, T. R. (1994) Single IL-2-secreting precursor CD4 T cell can develop into either Th1 or Th2 cytokine secretion phenotype. *J. Immunol.* **153,** 3514–3522.

Scicchitano, R., Stanisz, A., Ernst, P., and Bienenstock, J. (1988). A common mucosal immune system revisited. *In* "Migration and Homing of Lymphoid Cells" (A. J. Husband, ed.), Vol. 2, pp. 1–34. CRC Press, Boca Raton, FL.

Scott, P. (1991). IFN-$\gamma$ modulates the early development of Th1 and Th2 responses in a murine model of cutaneous *Leishmaniasis. J. Immunol.* **147,** 3149–3155.

Snapper, C. M., Peschel, C., and Paul, W. E. (1988). IFN-$\gamma$ stimulates IgG2a secretion by murine B lymphocytes stimulated with bacterial lipopolysaccharide. *J. Immunol.* **140,** 2121–2127.

Staats, H. F., Jackson, R. J., Marinaro, M., Takahashi, I., Kiyono, H., and McGhee, J. R. (1994). Mucosal immunity with implications for vaccine development. *Curr. Opin. Immunol.* **6,** 572–583.

Swain, S. L., Weinberg, A. D., English, M., and Huston, G. (1990). IL-4 directs the development of Th2-like helper effectors. *J. Immunol.* **145,** 3796–3806.

Tomasi, T. B. (1976). "The Immune System of Secretions." Prentice-Hall, Englewood Cliffs, New Jersey.

Ulmer, J. B., Donelly, J. J., Parker, S. E., Rhodes, G. H., Felgner, P. L., Dwarki, V. J., Gromkowski, S. H., Deck, R. R., DeWitt, C. M., Friedman, A., Hawe, L. A., Leader, K. R., Martinez, D., Perry, H. C., Shiver, J. W., Montgomery, D. L., and Liu, M. A. (1993). Heterologous protection against influenza by injection of DNA encoding a viral protein. *Science* **259,** 1745–1749.

Vajdy, M., Kosco-Vilbois, M. H., Kopf, M., Kohler, G., and Lycke, N. (1995). Impaired mucosal immune responses in interleukin 4-targeted mice. *J. Exp. Med.* **181,** 41–53.

VanCott, J. L., Staats, H. F., Pascual, D. W., Roberts, M., Chatfield, S. N., Yamamoto, M., Coste, M., Carter, P. N., Kiyono, H., and McGhee, J. R. (1996). Regulation of mucosal and systemic antibody responses by T helper cell subsets, macrophages, and derived cytokines following oral immunization with live recombinant *salmonella*. *J. immunol.* **156,** 1504–1514.

van Ginkel, F. W., Liu, C.-G., Simecka, J. W., Dong, J.-Y., Greenway, T., Frizzell, R. A., Kiyono, H., McGhee, J. R., and Pascual, D. W. (1995). Intratracheal gene delivery with adenoviral vector induces elevated systemic IgG and mucosal IgA antibodies to adenovirus and $\beta$-galactosidase. *Hum. Gene Ther.* **6,** 895–903.

Waldman, R. H., and Ganguly, R. (1974). Immunity to infections on secretory surfaces. *J. Infect. Dis.* **130,** 419–440.

Wang, B., Ugen, E., Srikantan, V., Agadjanyan, M. G., Dang, K., Refaeli, Y., Sata, A. L., Boyer, J., Williams, W. V., and Weiner, D. B. (1993). Gene inoculation generates immune responses against human immunodeficiency virus type I. *Proc. Natl. Acad. Sci. U.S.A.* **90,** 4156–4160.

Wold, W. S. M., and Gooding, L. R. (1989). Adenovirus region E3 proteins that prevent cytolysis by cytotoxic T cells and tumor necrosis factor. *Mol. Biol. Med.* **6,** 433–452.

Wolff, J. A., Malone, R. W., Williams, P., Chong, W., Acsadi, G., Jani, A., and Felgner, P. L. (1990). Direct gene transfer into mouse muscle *in vivo*. *Science* **247,** 1465–1468.

Woogen, S. D., Ealding, W., and Elson, C. O. (1987). Inhibition of murine lymphocyte proliferation by the B subunit of cholera toxin. *J. Immunol.* **139,** 3764–3770.

Xu, D. and Liew F. Y. (1994). Genetic vaccination against *Leishmaniasis*. *Vaccine* **12,** 1534–1536.

Xu-Amano, J., Kiyono, H., Jackson, R. J., Staats, H. F., Fujihashi, K., Burrows, P. D., Elson, C. O., Pillai, S., and McGhee, J. R. (1993). Helper T cell subsets for immunoglobulin A responses: Oral immunization with tetanus toxoid and cholera toxin as adjuvant selectively induces Th2 cells in mucosa associated tissues. *J. Exp. Med.* **178,** 1309–1320.

Zhong, G. M., and de la Maza, L. M. (1988). Activation of mouse peritoneal macrophages *in vitro* or *in vivo* by recombinant murine gamma IFN inhibits the growth of *Chlamydia trachomatis* serotype L1. *Infect. Immun.* **56,** 3322–3325.

# Chapter 34

# Generalized and Compartmentalized Mucosal Immune Responses in Humans: Cellular and Molecular Aspects

Marianne Quiding-Järbrink,* Kristina Eriksson,* Mekuria Lakew,* Eugene Butcher,†
Jacques Banchereau,‡ Andrew Lazarovits,§ Jan Holmgren,* and Cecil Czerkinsky*,¶

*Department of Medical Microbiology and Immunology, University of Göteborg,
S-413 46 Göteborg, Sweden;
†Department of Pathology, Stanford University School of Medicine, Palo Alto, California 94305;
‡Laboratory of Immunology Research, Schering-Plough Corp., 69571 Dardilly, France;
§Department of Medicine, University of Western Ontario, London, Ontario, Canada N6A 5C1;
and ¶INSERM Unit 80, 69437 Lyon, France

Although the immune apparatus is remarkably diverse, there is strong evidence that certain specialized types of immune responses take place and are basically restricted to certain anatomic locations within the body. The gut-associated lymphoid tissue (GALT), the largest mammalian lymphoid organ system, and the broncho-associated lymphoid tissue (BALT) represent well-known examples of such compartmentalized immunological systems as evidenced by (i) the existence of defined lymphoid microcompartments within the gut and the airway mucosae, (ii) phenotypically and functionally distinct B-cell, T-cell, and accessory-cell subpopulations (Brandtzaeg, 1995), and (iii) restrictions imposed on lymphoid cell recirculation potential to (and from) various tissues (Picker and Butcher, 1994). Through the compartmentalization of their afferent and efferent limbs, the GALT and the BALT function essentially independently of the systemic immune apparatus.

Immune responses expressed in mucosal tissues are typified by secretory immunoglobulin A (S-IgA), the predominant Ig class in human external secretions (and by far the most abundant Ig class in the body), and the best known entity providing specific immune protection for the gut and other mucosal tissues (Mestecky *et al.*, 1987). Generation of a protective S-IgA immune response at mucosal surfaces, where many significant infections begin, is thus of paramount importance but is not readily achieved by the conventional route of parenteral injection, although this is usually effective in eliciting circulating antibodies. In contrast, mucosal administration of antigens, such as by ingestion, inhalation, rectal instillation, or topical deposition onto a mucosal surface, may result in the concomitant expression of S-IgA antibody responses in various mucosal tissues and secretions, usually without a pronounced systemic antibody response (Mestecky, 1987). It is generally believed that ingested antigens, once taken up by specialized epithelial cells covering the Peyer's patch dome ("M" cells) and by absorptive epithelial cells of the villi, can be channeled to professional antigen-presenting cells (parenchymal intestinal macrophages and dendritic cells), and/or can be processed and presented directly by those same epithelial cells to underlying B and T lymphocytes. It is also believed that inhaled antigens are uptaken by similar types of cells in the airway epithelium. Following interaction of the antigen with accessory cells and cognate helper T cells and/or B lymphocytes in the local microenvironment of the gut and of the lung mucosae, the sensitized immunocytes, in particular antigen-sensitized B cells but presumably also T cells, leave the patches or their inductive counterpart in the bronchoalveolar mucosa, transit through the draining lymph nodes (mesenteric or bronchial lymph nodes) and the thoracic duct, enter the circulation, and then seed the gut and/or the lungs as well as other mucosal tissues. This latter condition appears to be effected through site-specific receptors ("homing" receptors) on mucosal lymphoid cells plus the presence of complementary structures ("addressins") associated with tissue-specific vascular endothelial cell surfaces (Picker and Butcher, 1994). In their new locations, the committed B cells may further differentiate into plasma cells producing secretory antibodies, mainly S-IgA. The utilization of organ-specific endothelial cell recognition mechanisms by circulating precursors of mucosal IgA immunoblasts and presumably also of mucosal T-cell immunoblasts could explain both the unification of immune responses in diverse mucosal sites and the physiologic segregation of mucosal from nonmucosal immune mechanisms. The notion of a "common mucosal immunological system" that provides immune reactivity not only at the site of antigen deposition but also at remote mucosal sites is especially important when considering strategies of vaccination against mucosal pathogens. Indeed, enteric delivery of immunogens is the most pratical and safe immunization route and may be the most efficient means to achieve protection against mucosal pathogens.

## I. INDUCTION OF GENERALIZED SECRETORY IgA ANTIBODY RESPONSES

The induction of S-IgA responses via ingestion, inhalation, or topical deposition of nonreplicating antigens often requires large amounts of antigen to be delivered repeatedly. The general exceptions to this rule are antigens, soluble and particulate, with the capacity to adhere to intestinal epithelial cells, especially M cells of the PP (de Aizpurua and Russel-Jones, 1988). Among these molecules, cholera toxin (CT) and its nontoxic B subunit (CT-B) are considered the most potent mucosal immunogens in humans.

Induction of mucosal immune responses has been studied mainly following peroral immunization, and the importance of PP in induction of intestinal immune responses and the dissemination of IgA-committed B cell precursors to distant tissues has been demonstrated clearly (Robertson and Cebra, 1976). Animal studies have demonstrated the appearance of specific antibody-secreting cells (ASC) not only in the intestine, but also in secretory glands, following oral immunization (Weisz-Carrington *et al.,* 1979). In addition, many studies performed in orally immunized volunteers have demonstrated the appearance of specific antibodies in external secretions, such as saliva, tears, and milk, from glands anatomically remote from the intestinal inductive site. These responses were often recorded without an accompanying response in serum (Mestecky *et al.,* 1987). Taken together, these studies led to the notion of a common mucosal immune system. According to this generally accepted concept, the generalization of immune responses elicited at mucosal inductive sites is accomplished by migration of lymphocytes from the inductive site, via the circulation, to remote mucosal effector sites. Studies from both our laboratory and others have demonstrated that vaccine-specific ASC can be detected in the circulation during a narrow time-span after peroral immunization of human volunteers (Kantele *et al.,* 1986; Czerkinsky *et al.,* 1987; Fig. 1). Furthermore, such cells could subsequently be detected in minor salivary glands

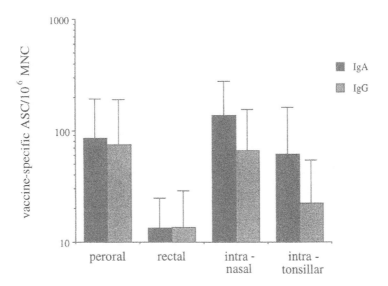

**FIGURE 1.** Mucosal immunization via different routes gives rise to circulating vaccine-specific antibody-secreting cells (ASC). Bars represent the frequencies of circulating IgA (filled bars) and IgG (shaded bars) ASC 1 week after peroral, rectal, intranasal, or intratonsillar immunization of human volunteers with cholera toxin B subunit (CTB). Data are presented as mean ± standard deviation of 6 to 23 individual analyses.

(Czerkinsky *et al.*, 1991), thereby providing a formal demonstration that a common mucosal immune system is operational also in humans.

## II. COMPARTMENTALIZED MUCOSAL IMMUNE RESPONSES IN HUMANS AND SUBHUMAN PRIMATES

Although mucosal immunizations at various inductive sites result in the characteristic dissemination of secretory immune responses, the regions close to the initial site of antigen encounter exhibit a more powerful response than more distant mucosal sites (Ogra and Karzon, 1969, Pierce and Cray, 1982, Haneberg *et al.*, 1994). For instance, results from our laboratory show that oral immunization may induce substantial antibody responses in the small intestine (prominently in the proximal segment), in the ascending colon, and in some distant exocrine glands such as the mammary and salivary glands, whereas it is relatively inefficient at evoking an IgA antibody response in the distal segments of the large intestine, in the tonsils, or in the female genital tract mucosa. Conversely, rectal immunization evokes strong local antibody responses in the rectum but little or no response in the small intestine and colon. Similarly, intranasal or intratonsillar immunization in human volunteers results in antibody responses in the upper airway mucosa and regional secretions, without evoking an immune response in the gut. This compartmentalization of mucosal immune responses seems to be the result mainly of preferential migration of activated cells back to their inductive site. Similar to the situation after peroral immunization, such migrating ASC can be intercepted in the circulation of volunteers immunized with CT-B via the rectal, intranasal, and intratonsillar route (Fig. 1).

Since CTB orally administered to human volunteers is essentially absorbed in the proximal segments of the small intestine, we recently studied the possible redistribution of specific immunocytes to other segments of the gut and to extraintestinal locations after oral immunization with CT. For this purpose, we employed cynomolgus macaques. The characteristics of their intestinal antibody response to orally administered CT are partially compiled in Table I. Thus, intestinal IgA-ASC responses of appreciable magnitude developed in monkeys fed CT; these responses occured as two decreasing gradients, one from the proximal part of the small intestine and the second from the first segment of the large intestine. Another burst of specific IgA-ASC was occasionally observed in the rectum. It could further be noted that strong IgG- and IgM-ASC responses were present in the descending colon, contrasting with the relatively poor IgA response in that segment. It is also interesting to note that large numbers of IgG-ASC were detected in mesenteric lymph nodes of monkeys fed CT, contrasting with a paucity of specific IgG-ASC in spleen and peripheral lymph nodes. The latter observation would suggest that IgG antibodies which contribute the major isotype found in serum of animals fed CT are in fact derived mainly from a mucosal and not a systemic source.

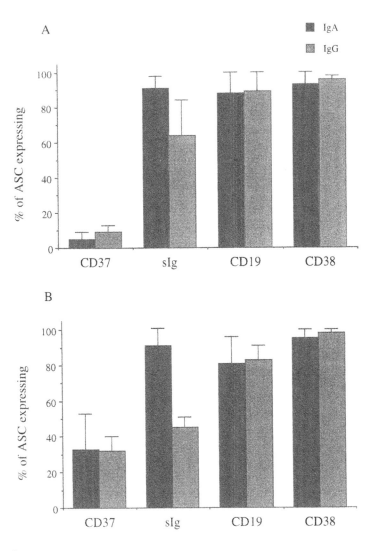

**FIGURE 2.** Cell surface expression of differentiation markers by circulating vaccine-induced antibody-secreting cells (ASC). Bars indicate the percentage of vaccine-specific IgA- (filled bars) and IgG-producing (shaded bars) ASC expressing the indicated cell surface molecule following peroral (A) and subcutaneous (B) immunization of human volunteers. Data are presented as mean ± standard deviation of six individual analyses.

TABLE *I*
ORAL ADMINISTRATION OF CT IN MACAQUES INDUCES ANATOMICALLY SEGMENTED ASC
RESPONSES IN THE INTESTINE

| ASC | Duodenum | Jejunum | Ileum | AC | TC | DC |
|-----|----------|---------|-------|----|----|----|
| IgA | + + + | + + | ± | + + + | + | ± |
| IgG | + | ± | − | − | ± | + + + |

*Note.* Groups of cynomolgus macaques (three or four animals) were fed three doses of CT (25 μg) 3 to 4 weeks apart. One week after the last immunization, the animals were sacrificed and immunocytes were isolated and assayed for ASC numbers by ELISPOT assays. Plus signs denote magnitude of the ASC responses: + + +, over 1000 ASC; + +, 200–1000 ASC; +, 50–200 ASC; ±, 10–50 ASC per million isolated immunocytes. AC, ascending colon; TC, transverse colon; DC, descending colon; MLN, mesenteric lymph nodes.

Another example of compartmentalized immune response within the so-called common mucosal immune system is provided by the results of recent studies involving intratonsillar delivery of immunogens in human volunteers. We examined the capacity of human tonsils to serve as expression sites of locally versus remotely induced immune responses. In these studies we found that peroral cholera vaccination or parenteral tetanus vaccine were at best poorly efficient at inducing an antibody response in tonsils (Quiding-Järbrink *et al.,* 1995a). In contrast, injection of either immunogen into palatine tonsils gave rise to ASC responses that were restricted to the immunized tonsil and comprised both IgA and IgG-secreting cells. Similarly, intranasal immunizations with CTB induced an response that was expressed primarily in the adenoids but poorly in the palatine tonsils. The fact that IgA-ASC would appear in the circulation after either intratonsillar or intranasal immunization (Fig. 1) indicates that the nasal mucosa and the tonsils may well serve important inductive functions as sources of B-cell precursors whose destiny might be elsewhere than the tonsils. One possible destiny for these cells would appear to be the lungs, as suggested by recent studies involving engraftment of human tonsillar B cells in SCID mice (Nadal *et al.,* 1991)

Taken together, the results of these studies demonstrate a high degree of anatomical segmentation within the MALT of primates, with respect to redistribution of IgA- and IgG-secreting ASC. They also lend support to the notion that progenitors of mucosally derived IgA and IgG immunoblasts do indeed exhibit distinct migratory properties.

## III. CHARACTERISTICS OF CIRCULATING ANTIGEN-SPECIFIC MUCOSAL B-CELL IMMUNOBLASTS IN HUMANS

As already mentioned, mucosal immunization via delivery of immunogens by various routes, e.g., rectal, intranasal, and peroral, will almost invariably result in the appearance of circulating B cells capable of spontaneously producing antibodies to the immunizing agent. Though these cells do secrete amounts of immunoglobulins comparable to their plasma cell progenitors, very little is known regarding their phenotypic characteristics, activation stage, and anatomical future.

We have recently developed a simple and general approach to determine the expression of selected cell-surface molecules by specific ASC (Lakew *et al.*, 1995). The technique, which makes use of the combination of immunomagnetic cell separation and ELISPOT techniques, allowed us to compare the phenotypes of vaccine-specific B cells in blood from volunteers immunized with oral cholera vaccine containing CTB and parenteral tetanus vaccine (Quiding-Järbrink *et al.*, 1995b).

From these studies it was evident that the vast majority of ASC originating from either systemic or mucosal sites, although not yet plasma cells, were undergoing final differentiation. Circulating ASC expressed CD38, specifying terminally differentiated B cells and plasma cells, but not the plasma cell marker CD28 (Fig. 2). Furthermore, these cells still expressed HLA-DR, surface Ig, and CD19, all of which are lost immediately before or during the transition of plasmablasts to plasma cells. In addition, several cell surface molecules defining early, mature, and blastic B cells (CD37, CD20, CD22, CD23) were more or less absent from the surface of vaccine-specific ASC (Table II). Generally, systemically derived ASC seemed to be a somewhat more heterogenous population than ASC induced by oral immunization. Furthermore, expression of activation markers (CD25 and CD71, the receptors for IL-2 and transferrin) was always detected on a smaller fraction of CTB-specific ASC than on tetanus toxoid (TT)-specific ASC (Table II). The higher expression of CD25 and CD71 on TT-specific than on CTB-specific ASC suggest that the former population have a higher propencity to proliferate than intestinally derived ASC. Indeed, the ability of specific ASC induced by parenteral immunization to proliferate and give rise to additional ASC has been demonstrated (McHeyzer-Williams *et al.*, 1993).

Taken together, our observations indicate that vaccine-induced, enterically derived ASC constitute one homogenous population with regard to expression of maturation markers. The systemically induced ASC population, on the other hand, was more heterogenous. Furthermore, these results support the theory that circulating ASC induced by immunization at various mucosal and systemic sites represent B-cell immunoblasts en route to their effector sites, in which final differentiation into plasma cells take place.

## IV. ADHESION MOLECULES ON CIRCULATING ASC IN HUMANS: PREDICTIVE MARKERS OF ANATOMICAL FUTURE?

The previously documented compartmentalization and restricted homing within the human mucosal imune system led us to examine the expression of organ-specific adhesion molecules, so-called "homing receptors," on the surface of migrating B cells activated at different mucosal and extramucosal sites.

The process of lymphocyte homing is dependent on binding of adhesion mole-

TABLE II

EXPRESSION OF DIFFERENTIATION MARKERS ON CIRCULATING CT-B- AND TT-SPECIFIC
ASC ISOLATED 1 WEEK AFTER ORAL AND SYSTEMIC IMMUNIZATION

| | Anti-CTB | | Anti-TT | |
| Surface marker | IgA | IgG | IgA | IgG |
| --- | --- | --- | --- | --- |
| CD28 | 7 ± 7 | 4 ± 1 | 20 ± 13 | 23 ± 13 |
| CD20 | 20 ± 8 | 38 ± 16 | 52 ± 29 | 50 ± 13 |
| CD22 | 8 ± 8 | 8 ± 6 | 24 ± 9 | 21 ± 7 |
| CD23 | 11 ± 4 | 19 ± 8 | 46 ± 19 | 46 ± 17 |
| CD25 | 4 ± 3 | 3 ± 3 | 18 ± 18 | 20 ± 2 |
| CD71 | 32 ± 11 | 38 ± 14 | 77 ± 20 | 35 ± 6 |

*Note.* Data are expressed as mean relative percentage ± S. D. of specific ASC expressing the indicated cell surface marker.

cules expressed on lymphocyte to their ligands, "addressins," on postcapillary high-endothelium venules (HEV) in the target organ. According to the generally accepted model of endothelial recognition and extravasation, transient and reversible interactions between selectins and their carbohydrate ligands mediate primary HEV recognition and lymphocyte rolling. These signals, in concert with binding of endothelial surface molecules and/or surface-bound chemokines, induce rapid activation of integrins. Integrin binding to endothelial counterreceptors results in strong adhesion and triggers extravasation (Picker and Butcher, 1994).

In humans, the best-characterized adhesion molecules confering tissue-specificity are integrin $\alpha4\beta7$, L-selectin, and their respective ligands. $\alpha4\beta7$ is a receptor for the mucosal addressin cell adhesion molecule (MAdCAM-1), and is thereby selectively involved in lymphocyte trafficking to mucosal lymphoid tissues and lamina propria. L-selectin has been identified as a lymphocyte homing receptor mediating homing to peripheral lymph nodes, but is also involved in lymphocyte traffic to organized mucosal lymphoid tissues. In addition, it has been shown that the hyaluronate-binding molecule CD44 mediates lymphocyte binding to mucosal HEV *in vitro*. The potential function of CD44, however, has not yet been established *in vivo*.

Using the same approach as in the analyses of differentiation markers described above, we examined the expression of CD44, $\alpha4\beta7$-integrin, and L-selectin on circulating ASC elicited by parenteral, peroral, rectal, and intranasal immunization. The results of these studies showed that almost all (>95%) vaccine-specific ASC, irrespective of immunization route, expressed CD44. Furthermore, virtually all circulating Ig-secreting cells, irrespective of specificity, express CD44, and it is thus not a useful marker of ASC origin or destination.

The expression of L-selectin and $\alpha4\beta7$, on the other hand, varied considerably between ASC populations induced at different sites. Almost all TT-specific ASC activated at systemic sites expressed L-selectin, whereas a smaller but significant proportion of these ASC expressed $\alpha4\beta7$. Oral, as well as rectal, immunization resulted in a reciprocal distribution of $\alpha4\beta7$ and L-selectin compared to parenteral immunization. Thus, almost all circulating ASC activated by intestinal immunization expressed $\alpha4\beta7$, whereas less than half of these cells expressed L-selectin. A third pattern of homing receptor expression was seen among ASC activated by intranasal immunization. In contrast to intestinally derived ASC, the large majority of these cells coexpressed $\alpha4\beta7$ with L-selectin (Fig. 3).

The differential expression of adhesion molecules on circulating ASC, not only from systemic but also from different mucosal sites, may provide a molecular basis for the previously documented compartmentalization of immune responses initiated at different anatomical locations, and for the compartmentalization of mucosal immune systems of the upper versus the lower aerodigestive tract. Interestingly, the distribution of $\alpha4\beta7$ and L-selectin is similar on both IgA- and IgG-secreting cells, irrespective of immunization route. Nevertheless, our earlier studies have shown considerable differences in the distribution of IgA- and IgG-secreting cells induced by peroral immunization. IgA-secreting cells clearly dominate the B-cell responses recorded in some mucosal effector compartments such as the duodenal mucosa and the salivary glands, whereas IgG-secreting cells dominate in the mesenteric lymph nodes and colonic mucosa. Therefore, additional

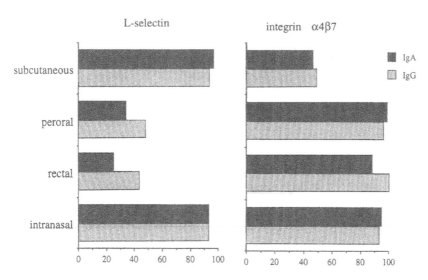

FIGURE 3. Expression of adhesion molecules by circulating vaccine-specific antibody-secreting cells (ASC) induced by different immunization routes. Bars represent the percentage of vaccine-specific IgA- (filled bars) and IgG-producing (shaded bars) ASC induced by subcutaneous, peroral, rectal, or intranasal immunization, expressing the indicated adhesion molecule. Data are presented as mean ± standard deviation of 4 to 10 individual analyses.

recognition events other than $\alpha4\beta7$ and L-selectin binding must take place to succesfully direct a migrating ASC to its particular effector site.

## REFERENCES

de Aizpurua, H. J., and Russel-Jones, G. J. (1988). Oral vaccination. Identification of classes of proteins that provoke an immune response upon oral feeding. *J. Exp. Med.* **167**, 440–451.

Brandtzaeg, P. (1995). Basic mechanisms of mucosal immunity. A major adaptive defense system. *Immunologist* **3**, 89–96.

Czerkinsky, C., Prince, S. J., Michalek, S. M., Jackson, S., Russel, M. W., Moldoveanu, Z., McGhee, J. R., and Mestecky, J. (1987). IgA antibody-producing cells in peripheral blood after antigen ingestion: Evidence for a common mucosal immune system in humans. *Proc. Natl. Acad. Sci. U.S.A.* **84**, 2449–2453.

Czerkinsky, C., Svennerholm, A.-M., Quiding, M., Jonsson, R., and Holmgren, J. (1991). Antibody-producing cells in peripheral blood and salivary glands after oral cholera vaccination of humans. *Infect. Immun.* **59**, 996–1001.

Haneberg, B., Kendall, D., Amerongen, H. M., Apter, F. M., Kraehenbuhl, J.-P., and Neutra, M. (1994). Induction of specific immunoglobulin A in the small intestine, colon-rectum, and vagina measured by a new method for collection of secretions from local mucosal surfaces. *Infect. Immun.* **62**, 15–23.

Hanson, L.-Å., and Brandtzaeg, P. (1989). The mucosal defense system. *In* "Immunological Disorders in Infants and Children" (E. R. Stiehm, Ed.), Vol. 116, pp. 155–168. Saunders, Philadelphia, Pennsylvania.

Kantele, A., Arvilommi, H., and Jokinen, I. (1986). Specific immunoglobulin-secreting human blood cells after peroral vaccination against *Salmonella typhi. J. Infect. Dis.* **153**, 1126–1131.

Lakew, M., Quiding, M., Nordström, I., Holmgren, J., and Czerkinsky, C. (1995). Phenotypic characterization of circulating antibody-secreting cells after enteral and parenteral immunizations in humans. *In* "Advances in Mucosal Immunology" (J. Mestecky *et al.*, Eds.), Part B, pp. 1451–1453. Plenum, New York.

McHeyzer-Williams, M. G., McLean, M. J., Lalor, P. A., and Nossal, G. J. V. (1993). Antigen-driven B cell differentiation *in vivo. J. Exp. Med.* **178**, 295–307.

Mestecky, J. (1987). The common mucosal immune system and current strategies for induction of immune responses in external secretions. *J. Clin. Immunol.* **7**, 265–276.

Mestecky, J., Czerkinsky, C., Russel, M. W., Brown, T. A., Prince, S. J., Moldoveanu, Z., Jackson, S., Michalek, S., and McGhee, J. R. (1987). Induction and molecular properties of secretory and serum IgA antibodies specific for environmental antigens. *Ann. Allergy* **59**, 54–66.

Nadal, D., Albini, B., Schläpfer, E., Chen, C., Brodsky, L., and Ogra, P. L. (1991). Tissue distribution of mucosal antibody-producing cells specific for respiratory cyncytial virus in severe combined immunodeficiency (SCID) mice engrafted with human tonsils. *Clin. Exp. Immunol.* **85**, 358–364.

Ogra, P. L., and Karzon, D. T. (1969). Distribution of poliovirus antibody in serum, nasopharynx and alimentary tract following segmental immunization of lower alimentary tract with polio vaccine. *J. Immunol.* **102**, 1423–1430.

Picker, L. J., and Butcher, E. C. (1994). Physiological and molecular mechanisms of lymphocyte homing. *Annu. Rev. Immunol.* **62**, 561–591.

Pierce, N. F., and Cray, W. C. (1982). Determinants of the localization, magnitude, and duration of a specific mucosal IgA plasma cell response in enterically immunized rats. *J. Immunol.* **128**, 1311–1315.

Quiding-Järbrink, M., Granström, G., Nordström, I., Holmgren, J., and Czerkinsky, C. (1995a). Induction of compartmentalized B-cell responses in human tonsils. *Infect. Immun.* **63**, 853–857.

Quiding-Järbrink, M., Lakew, M., Nordström, I., Banchereau, J., Butcher, E., Holmgren, J., and Czerkinsky, C. (1995b). Human circulating specific antibody-forming cells after systemic and mucosal immunizations: Differential homing commitments and cell surface differentiation markers. *Eur. J. Immunol.* **25,** 322–327.

Robertson, S. M., and Cebra, J. J. (1976). A model for local immunity. *Ric. Clin. Lab.* **6**(Suppl. 3), 105–119.

Weisz-Carrington, P., Roux, M. E., McWilliams, M., Phillips-Quagliata, J. M., and Lamm, M. E. (1979). Organ and isotype distribution of plasma cells producing specific antibody after oral immunization: Evidence for a generalized secretory immune system. *J. Immunol.* **123,** 1705–1708.

# Chapter 35

# Cholera and Oral–Mucosal Anti-infectious and Anti-inflammatory Vaccines

Jan Holmgren,* Cecil Czerkinsky,*·† Michael Lebens,* Marianne Lindblad,*
Jia-Bin Sun,* and Ann-Marie Svennerholm*

*Department of Medical Microbiology and Immunology, Göteborg University,
S-413 46 Göteborg, Sweden; and †INSERM Unit 80, 69437 Lyon, France

We describe the recent development of safe and efficacious oral vaccines against cholera and *Escherichia coli* diarrhea, and current efforts to use the cholera toxin-binding subunit as an immunostimulatory carrier and transmucosal delivery system for inducing mucosal immunity as well as systemic "oral tolerance" against attached foreign antigens. Beyond their implications for the development of anti-infectious vaccines, the findings may have an impact also by providing leads to the development of novel anti-inflammatory vaccines and immunotherapeutics against diseases associated with certain untoward immune responses, e.g., certain chronic infections, autoimmune disorders, allergies, and rejection of allografts.

## I. Introduction

In the last 10 years there has been rapidly growing interest in the development of oral rather than parenteral vaccines. This is based on both logistic and biomedical considerations. Thus, it is now generally recognized that oral vaccines would be easier (and safer) to administer since they do not require medically trained personnel or sterile supplies, and also that oral vaccines generally would be easier to produce and quality-control. It has also become increasingly clear that in order to be efficacious, immunization against the many infections that take place at the mucosal surfaces of the aerodigestive or urogenital tracts usually requires topical–mucosal vaccine application. Since immune-activated lymphocytes from the intestinal mucosa can migrate to various other glandular–mucosal tissues, there is currently much interest in developing oral vaccines not only against enteric infections but also against infections in, e.g., the respiratory and urogenital tracts.

However, to date it has often proved to be difficult in practice to stimulate strong mucosal IgA immune responses by either parenteral or oral–mucosal administration of most nonreplicating antigens, and experience with soluble protein antigens has on the whole been quite disappointing. A notable exception in this regard is cholera toxin (CT) and, in humans better than in other species, its non-toxic B-subunit pentamer moiety (CT-B). Based on this, and as the first of the three themes that will be discussed in this presentation, (i) CT-B has become an important component in recently developed oral vaccines against both cholera and against diarrhea caused by enterotoxigenic *Escherichia coli* (ETEC) bacteria producing CT-like heat-labile enterotoxin(s) (Holmgren and Svennerholm, 1992; Holmgren *et al.*, 1994). (ii) In addition, since the strong immunogenicity of CT and CT-B can to a large extent be explained by their ability to bind to receptors on the intestinal mucosal surface, there has recently been much interest in approaches to use CT-B also as an oral delivery carrier system for other vaccine-relevant antigens; much progress has been made in preparing immunogenic hybrid proteins by coupling various protein or peptide antigens chemically or genetically to CT-B. Indeed, oral administration of such hybrid antigens has in several systems been found to markedly potentiate both intestinal and extraintestinal IgA immune responses against the CT-B-coupled antigens and also to elicit substantial circulating antibody responses (Czerkinsky *et al.*, 1989; Holmgren *et al.*, 1994; Liang *et al.*, 1988). (iii) Finally, recent work in our laboratory has shown that CT-B can also be used as a very efficient carrier protein/transmucosal delivery system for allowing various CT-B-coupled antigens to induce "oral tolerance" systemically against T-cell-mediated delayed-type hypersensitivity (DTH) reactions (Sun *et al.*, 1994). CT-B may therefore be a key component in current efforts to develop "anti-inflammatory vaccines" against diseases associated with, e.g., autoimmune and allergic DTH reactions, as well as to other antigens participating in analogous reactions resulting in the inflammation/immunopathology seen in many chronic infections (Czerkinsky and Holmgren, 1995).

## II. Cholera Vaccines

Two new cholera vaccines, both based on genetic engineering biotechnology, have recently been licensed. The first of these, the "B subunit-whole cell cholera vaccine" (B-WC), uses a two-dose oral administration of a vaccine containing a mixture of recombinantly produced CT-B and killed classical and El Tor cholera vibrios. The B-WC vaccine has proved to be completely safe and to give a high level of short-term protection in field trials (85% for the first 6 months) and also substantial long-term protection (ca. 60% for the first 3 years) which is a marked improvement over previously used parenteral-killed vaccines (Clemens *et al.*, 1990; Holmgren *et al.*, 1992). The recombinant production of the B-subunit component has dramatically simplified and cheapened the production of the vaccine as compared with a first generation of this vaccine in which the CT-B component was prepared from active cholera toxin produced by a wild-type strain (Sanchez and Holmgren, 1989; Lebens *et al.*, 1993); in a recent field trial in Peru, two doses of recombinantly produced vaccine given at 1- to 2-week intervals gave 86% protection (Sanchez *et al.*, 1994).

A second, recently licensed cholera vaccine, CVD 103-HgR, uses a single-dose administration of a genetically engineered, live-attenuated *V. cholerae* strain in which the attenuation has been achieved by genetic deletion of the ctxA gene, which removes the ability of the vaccine strain to make biologically active cholera toxin. By introducing this deletion into a normally poorly colonizing wild-type strain it was possible to overcome the previously notorious problem of residual "toxicity" resulting in mild–moderate diarrhea experienced with other similarly engineered cholera vaccine strains. The CVD 103-HgR vaccine has given similarly good protection as the oral B-WC vaccine in human volunteers against challenge with El Tor cholera vibrios, and the vaccine is currently evaluated for its protective efficacy in a large field trial in Indonesia.

Based on the recent outbreak and spread in Southeast Asia of severe cholera caused by a new serotype, O139, two types of vaccines have recently been developed to cope with this new threat. Since the O139 organism has the same cholera toxin as O1 El Tor and also has the same MSHA and other surface antigens except for the difference in LPS structure, a bivalent oral B-O1/O139 WC vaccine has been developed by us (in collaboration with SBL Vaccine, Stockholm) in which formalin-killed O139 organisms have been added to the previous B-O1 WC vaccine. In a recently completed phase-1 study, the bivalent B-O1/O139 vaccine was found to be both safe and immunogenic for each of its components (Jertborn *et al.*, 1995a). Two alternative experimental O139 vaccines, both of which are live-attenuated vaccines based on genetic engineering to delete both the cholera toxin and several associated genes (zot, ace, cep, RS1, and attRS1), have also been developed by U.S. laboratories and are in clinical testing.

## III. VACCINE AGAINST ETEC DIARRHEA

Infection with ETEC is the most frequent cause of diarrhea both in developing countries and among travellers. Estimates indicate that infections with different types of ETEC account for more than one billion diarrheal episodes and one million deaths annually among children in developing countries. Still, no vaccine for use in humans is available. New knowledge about virulence factors and protective antigens of ETEC, however, specifically the heat-labile (LT) and heat-stable (ST) enterotoxins and various specific colonization factor antigens (CFAs) suggests practical approaches toward development of a useful vaccine against ETEC diarrhea. Such a vaccine should be given orally, and ideally should evoke both anticolonization and antitoxic IgA immune responses in the gut.

The oral B-WC cholera vaccine has been shown to give ca. 70% short-term protection against ETEC diarrhea caused by LT-producing organisms through the B-subunit component. Thus, the results from the cholera vaccine field trial in Bangladesh (Clemens *et al.*, 1988) as well as those from a prospective placebo-controlled study in Finnish travellers to Morocco (Peltola *et al.*, 1991), demonstrated that CT-B, which cross-reacts immunologically with the B subunit of *E. coli* heat-labile toxin, LT-B, induced significant, ca. 70% protection also against *E. coli* LT and LT/ST diarrhea. Our studies in rabbits confirm that immunization with purified

CT-B affords protective immunity against challenge with LT-producing organisms comparable to that of immunization with corresponding doses of purified LT-B (A.-M. Svennerholm and J. Holmgren, unpublished). These findings support the view that CT-B, which can be produced inexpensively and on a large scale through the use of a recombinant production system (Sanchez and Holmgren, 1989; Lebens et al., 1993), can replace LT-B as "toxoid" in an ETEC vaccine.

Adhesion of ETEC to intestinal mucosa represents a critical step in the pathogenesis and is mediated by antigenically distinct fimbriae. In strains pathogenic for humans, three main adhesins have been identified, i.e., the colonization factor antigens CFA/I, CFA/II, and CFA/IV, and since antibodies to each of these antigens were protective in animal models all of them should be included in an oral ETEC vaccine. However, purified CFAs have proved to be sensitive to proteolytic degradation in the human gastrointestinal tract, complicating the use of such a vaccine preparation. Likewise, it would be difficult to construct a vaccine (e.g., a live vaccine) based on the concomitant expression of all these antigens by a single organism, since despite considerable efforts with this goal the different CFAs could not be expressed on the same host strain. A more practical way to construct a vaccine may instead be to prepare killed ETEC bacteria of different strains that express the most important CFAs on their surface and combine these organisms with an appropriate toxoid component. Based on this the recombinantly produced CT-B is used together with formalinized E. coli expressing the most prevalent colonization fimbrial antigens (CFAs I, II, and IV) in a recently developed oral vaccine against ETEC (Åhrén et al., 1993; Svennerholm and Holmgren, 1995). The inactivation of bacteria, which includes mild formalin treatment, causes complete killing of bacteria without significant loss in antigenicity of the different CFAs. Furthermore, the CFAs of these inactivated organisms have been stable during storage for years and during incubation in gastric juice. As in the oral cholera vaccine, the WC component is combined with CT-B to induce antitoxic mucosal immunity, which is known to cooperate synergistically with anti-CFA immunity against experimental ETEC infections in animals. In recent phase-1 and phase-2 trials, this vaccine has been shown to be safe and to stimulate intestinal IgA immune responses both to the CT-B component and to each of the CFA antigens (Åhrén et al., 1993; Jertborn et al., 1995b); based on this the oral B subunit/CFA-ETEC vaccine will now be tested for protective efficacy in phase-3 trials.

## IV. ORAL VACCINES AGAINST OTHER MUCOSAL INFECTIONS

Based on the concept of a common mucosal immune system through which immunity generated by oral vaccination can be disseminated also to extraintestinal mucosal tissues, there is currently intense interest in the development of oral vaccines based largely on genetic engineering against infections in, e.g., the respiratory and urogenital tracts.

The main approaches taken involve either the use of an oral live vector such as attenuated *Salmonella* or adenovirus for expression and delivery of antigens against the target mucosal infection or the construction of gene fusion proteins with CT-B (or *E. coli* LT-B). With regard to the latter systems, studies in animals have shown that oral administration of small amounts of protein antigens (that are not immunogenic per se when given alone by this route) covalently coupled to CT-B can elicit vigorous mucosal as well as extramucosal antibody responses. McKenzie and Halsey (1984) were the first to report that covalent coupling of horseradish peroxidase to CT-B markedly enhanced gut immune responses to the peroxidase antigen after oral administration. More recently, we and others have confirmed and extended those findings to demonstrate also an effective oral delivery potential of CT-B for coupled foreign antigens with regard to stimulation of IgA mucosal responses also outside the intestine, e.g., in salivary glands and in the respiratory and urogenital tracts, as well as for eliciting circulating antibodies. Thus, Czerkinsky *et al.* (1989) demonstrated that oral administration of small amounts of a streptococcal protein antigen covalently linked to CT-B induced both mucosal and extramucosal IgA and IgG antistreptococcal antibody responses in mice. In contrast, equivalent or even 10-fold higher doses of streptococcal antigen given alone or conjugated to a nonbinding protein (bovine serum albumin) were ineffective or, at best, poor in eliciting antibody responses to the streptococcal antigen. Liang *et al.* (1988) found that oral administration of Sendai virus chemically coupled to CT potentiated the IgA immune responses in the upper respiratory tract against Sendai virus in comparison with immunization with other formulations of this antigen. Likewise, in recent studies Drew *et al.* (1992) have shown that chemical conjugates between CT and peptide antigens derived from herpes simplex virus (HSV)-2 glycoprotein D when administered to mice by intraperitoneal (ip) priming followed by either ip or intragastric boosting gave rise to IgA anti-HSV-2 antibodies in vaginal washings and to protection against a lethal intravaginal challenge with HSV-2.

These findings lend support to the notion that peroral immunization with antigens linked (chemically or genetically) with CT-B may be a useful strategy for vaccinating against pathogens encountered not only at enteromucosal surfaces but also at extraintestinal mucosal and nonmucosal sites. With the aid of recombinant DNA engineering, foreign antigens have been linked to either the amino or carboxy ends of the CTB subunit, and a gene overexpression system has been developed to permit production of the hybrid proteins in substantial quantities (Sanchez *et al.,* 1990).

Besides the mucosal immunopotentiating effect of either CT or CT-B (or *E. coli* LT or LT-B) owing perhaps mainly to their similar capacity as oral antigen delivery vehicles, CT (but in most systems tested not CT-B) also has strong adjuvant properties for stimulating mucosal IgA immune responses to admixed (not coupled) unrelated antigens after oral immunization (Elson and Ealding, 1984; Lycke and Holmgren, 1986; Dertzbaugh and Elson, 1991; Holmgren *et al.,* 1993). This adjuvant activity appears to be complex, involving effects on (i) transmucosal antigen uptake, (ii) antigen-presenting cells, (iii) Ig class expression by B cells, and (iv) T helper cell frequency and activity; it also has been closely liked to the ADP-ribosylating action of CT (and specifically of its A subunit) leading to enhanced cyclic AMP formation in the affected cell. It remains unclear whether the enterotoxic activity of orally administered CT or LT can be eliminated without concomitant loss of adjuvanticity.

## V. Oral Vaccination against Autoimmune and Allergic Diseases

Immunization by the oral route not only stimulates IgA and other forms of immunity at the mucosal surfaces associated with moderate-to-high levels of serum antibodies, but also concomitantly induces suppression against certain types of systemic T-cell-mediated immune reactions. This phenomenon is known as "oral tolerance" and is an important physiologic mechanism to avoid harmful allergic and inflammatory reactions in response to inadvertently absorbed undegraded food and environmental antigens. Recently oral tolerance has attracted much renewed interest as a possible mechanism to induce specific immunotherapy in such autoimmune diseases and allergies where the immunopathology characteristically involves a T-cell-mediated DTH immune reaction.

It had been reported that CT as well as CT-B are so exceptionally strong as oral–mucosal immunogens because they do not give rise to any "oral tolerance" and that they indeed could even reverse such tolerance once developed (Elson and Ealding, 1984). We suspected that the tolerance-breaking properties might be selective for CT, and thus, as concerns CT-B, can be explained by low yet significant levels of contamination by CT of CT-B preparations used in previous studies. Consistent with this hypothesis, we have shown that when given by various mucosal (oral, intranasal, vaginal, rectal) routes in the absence of any CT adjuvant, antigens linked chemically or by genetic fusion to CT-B induced the expected mucosal IgA immune response in, e.g., the gut, but instead of abrogating systemic tolerance CT-B strongly stimulated the development of such tolerance (Sun et al., 1994). Based on very similar findings with several soluble protein antigens, including autoantigens such as myelin basic protein (MBP) or collagen II, haptens, and particulate antigens (red blood cells, thymocytes), we have good reason to believe that the CT-B mucosal carrier–delivery system may be extremely advantageous for inducing peripheral tolerance. The system minimizes by several hundred-fold the amount of tolerogen needed and it drastically reduces the number of doses that would otherwise be required by reported protocols of orally induced tolerization. It apparently can also act after initiation of a systemic immune response. Thus single doses of antigens coupled to CT-B were effectively tolerogenic even when given in very minute quantities and could both prevent and reverse T-cell-driven inflammatory reactions (Sun et al., 1994; Czerkinsky and Holmgren, 1995).

Of special interest because of the similarity of this animal model with human multiple sclerosis is the finding that a single dose of oral CT-B conjugated to myelin basic protein (MBP) protects rats against experimental autoimmune encephalomyelitis (EAE), when given either before or after disease induction. We have also seen good effects on autoimmune diabetes in the NOD mouse model by feeding CTB–insulin conjugate (collaboration with C. Thivolet, Lyon) and on collagen II-induced arthritis by feeding CT-B–collagen II conjugate (collaboration with A. Tarkowski, Göteborg) (Czerkinsky *et al.*, 1995). Furthermore, by coupling thymocytes to CT-B and feeding this conjugate to mice we have also been able to significantly prolong the survival of transplanted hearts in allogeneic mouse recipients; again, the effect was superior to that obtained by feeding the cells alone.

Thus, although still at the early stages of animal experimentation, this new tolerization principle may lead to the development of medically useful immunotherapeutic reagents in selected autoimmune and DTH-type allergic diseases.

## VI. CONCLUSIONS AND PROSPECTS

The knowledge summarized here may have profound implications for the design of vaccines aimed on one hand at promoting S-IgA immune responses against the numerous infectious pathogens and other antigens that contact the body through mucous membranes, and on the other hand at protecting the host from potentially harmful cell-mediated immune responses against the same matters. The relative inefficiency of parenteral vaccination to evoke secretory IgA immune responses in mucosal tissues and the fact that it can rather induce DTH reactivity and thereby bystander tissue damage upon subsequent encounter with the corresponding pathogen, constitute two major reasons to encourage the development of strategies to stimulate appropriate immune responses in MALT. Mucosal administration of antigens is certainly a more effective and attractive strategy since, under appropriate conditions, it may efficiently induce expression of antibody responses in various mucosal tissues, and concomitantly lead to specific downregulation of DTH reactivity at local and systemic sites. Our findings as discussed in this article indicate that CT-B may be used as an ultraeffective carrier/vector for antigens linked to it for achieving both of these effects.

These considerations may have an impact beyond the design of anti-infectious vaccines by providing leads to the development of novel anti-inflammatory vaccines and immunotherapeutics against diseases associated with untoward immune responses, e.g., certain chronic infections, autoimmune disorders, allergies, and rejection of allografts.

## REFERENCES

Åhrén, C., Wennarås, C., Holmgren, J., and Svennerholm, A.-M. (1993). Intestinal antibody response after oral immunization with a prototype cholera B subunit-colonization factor antigen enterotoxigenic *Escherichia coli* vaccine. *Vaccine* **11**, 929–934.

Clemens, J. D., Sack, D. A., Harris, J. R., Chakraborty, J., Khan, M. R., Stanton, B. F., Ali, M., Ahmed,

F., Yunus, M., Kay, B. A., Khan, M. U., Rao, M. R., Svennerholm, A.-M., and Holmgren, J. (1988). Impact of B subunit killed whole-cell and killed whole-cell-only oral vaccines against cholera upon treated diarrhoeal illness and mortality in an area endemic for cholera. *Lancet* **1**, 1375–1379.

Clemens, J. D., Sack, D. A, Harris, J. R., Van Loon, F., Chakraborty, J., Ahmed, F., Rao, M. R., Khan, M. R., Yunus, M. D., Huda, N., Stanton, B. F., Kay, B. A., Walter, S., Eckels, R., Svennerholm, A.-M., and Holmgren, J. (1990). Field trial of oral cholera vaccines in Bangladesh: Results from three-year follow-up. *Lancet* **1**, 270–273.

Czerkinsky, C., and Holmgren, J. (1995). The mucosal immune system and prospects for anti-infectious and anti-inflammatory vaccines. *Immunologist* **3**, 97–103.

Czerkinsky, C., Russell, M. W., Lycke, N., Lindblad, M., and Holmgren, J. (1989). Oral administration of a streptococcal antigen coupled to cholera toxin B subunit evokes strong antibody responses in salivary glands and extramucosal tissues. *Infect. Immun.* **57**, 1072–1077.

Czerkinsky, C., Sun, J.-B., Lebens, Michael, Li, B.-L., Rask, C., Lindblad, M., and Holmgren, J. (1995). Cholera toxin B subunit as transmucosal carrier-delivery and immunomodulating system for induction of anti-infectious and anti-pathological immunity. *Ann. New York Acad. Sci.,* in press.

Dertzbaugh, M. T., and Elson, C. O. (1991). Cholera toxin as a mucosal adjuvant. *In* "Topics in Vaccine Adjuvant Research" (D. R. Spriggs and W. C. Koff, Eds.), pp. 119–132.

Drew, M. D., Estrada-Correa, A., Underdown, B. J., and McDermott, M. R. (1992). Vaccination by cholera toxin conjugated to a herpes simplex virus type 2 glycoprotein D peptide. *J. Gen. Virol.* **73**, 2357–2366.

Elson, C. D., and Ealding, W. (1984). Generalized systemic and mucosal immunity in mice after mucosal stimulation with cholera toxin. *J. Immunol.* **132**, 27–36.

Holmgren, J., and Svennerholm, A.-M. (1992). Bacterial enteric infections and vaccine development. *Gastroenterol. Clin. North Am.* **21**, 283–302.

Holmgren, J., Svennerholm, A.-M., Jertborn, M., Clemens, J., Sack, D. A., Salenstedt, R., and Wigzell, H. (1992). An oral B subunit: Whole cell vaccine against cholera. *Vaccine* **10**, 911–914.

Holmgren, J., Lycke, N., and Czerkinsky, C. (1993). Cholera toxin and cholera B subunit as oral–mucosal adjuvant and antigen vector systems. *Vaccine* **11**, 1179–1184.

Holmgren, J., Czerkinsky, C., Lycke, N., and Svennerholm, A.-M. (1994). Strategies for the induction of immune responses at mucosal surfaces making use of cholera toxin B subunit as immunogen, carrier, and adjuvant. *Am. J. Trop. Med. Hyg.* **50**, 42–54.

Jertborn, M., Svennerholm, A.-M., and Holmgren, J. (1995a). Intestinal and systemic immune responses in humans after oral immunization with a bivalent B subunit-O1/O139 whole cell cholera vaccine. *Vaccine,* in press.

Jertborn, M., Åhrén, C., Holmgren, J., and Svennerholm, A.-M. (1995b). Clinical trial of an oral inactivated enterotoxigenic *Escherichia coli* vaccine. Submitted for publication.

Lebens, M., Johansson, S., Osek, J., Lindblad, M., and Holmgren, J. (1993). Large-scale production of *Vibrio cholerae* toxin B subunit for use in oral vaccines. *Bio/Technology* **11**, 1574–1578.

Liang, X., Lamm, M. E., and Nedrud, J. G. (1988). Oral administration of cholera toxin Sendai virus conjugate potentiates gut and respiratory immunity against Sendai virus. *J. Immunol.* **141**, 3781–3787.

Lycke, N., and Holmgren, J. (1986). Strong adjuvant properties of cholera toxin on gut mucosal immune responses to orally presented antigens. *Immunology* **59**, 301–308.

McKenzie, S. J., and Halsey, J. F. (1984). Cholera toxin B subunit as a carrier protein to simulate a mucosal immune response. *J. Immunol.* **133**, 1818–1824.

Peltola, H., Siitonen, A., Kyrönseppä, H., Simula, I., Mattila, L., Oksanen, P. *et al.* (1991). Prevention of travellers' diarrhoea by oral B-subunit/whole cell cholera vaccine. *Lancet,* 1285–1289.

Sanchez, J., and Holmgren, J. (1989). Recombinant system for overexpression of cholera toxin B subunit in *Vibrio cholerae* as a basis for vaccine development. *Proc. Natl. Acad. Sci. U.S.A.* **86**, 481–485.

Sanchez, J., Johansson, S., Lëwenadler, B., Svennerholm, A.-M., and Holmgren, J. (1990). Recombinant cholera toxin B-subunit and gene fusion proteins for oral vaccination. *Res. Microbiol.* **141,** 971–979.

Sanchez, J. L., Vasques, B., Begue, R. E., Meza, R., Castellares, G., Cabezas, C, Watts, D. M., Svennerholm, A.-M., Sadoff, J. C., and Taylor, D. N. (1994). Protective efficacy of the oral, whole cell/ recombinant B subunit cholera vaccine in Peruvian military recruits. *Lancet* **344,** 1273–1276.

Sun, J.-B., Holmgren, J., and Czerkinsky, C. (1994). Cholera toxin B subunit: An efficient transmucosal carrier-delivery system for induction of peripheral immunological tolerance. *Proc. Natl. Acad. Sci. U.S.A.* **91,** 10795–10799.

Svennerholm, A.-M., and Holmgren, J. (1995). Oral B subunit whole cell vaccines against cholera and enterotoxigenic *Escherichia coli. In* "Molecular and Clinical Aspects of Bacterial Vaccine Development" (D. A. Ala'Aldeen and C. E. Hormaeche, eds.), pp. 205–232. Wiley, Chichester, U.K.

# Chapter 36

# Strategies for the Use of Live Recombinant Avirulent Bacterial Vaccines for Mucosal Immunization

Roy Curtiss III, Teresa Doggett, Amiya Nayak, and Jay Srinivasan

*Department of Biology, Washington University, St. Louis, Missouri 63130*

## I. Introduction

Live recombinant avirulent microorganisms can be used as antigen delivery vehicles to especially induce mucosal immune responses following immunization of individuals by oral, intranasal, and intravaginal routes. There are a number of issues of importance in considering the use of live microorganisms for this purpose. One is whether the vaccine induces just a localized mucosal immune response or a generalized response with production of secretory IgA in all secretory glands, and from mucosal tissues throughout the body. An issue that has not been adequately addressed experimentally is the means to induce memory. It is logical to consider that immunizations that only induce local mucosal immune responses are not likely to induce lasting memory, whereas immunization schemes that induce a generalized mucosal immune response are more likely to induce memory. The likelihood of inducing memory may, therefore, depend on the type of bacterial vector used as the antigen delivery vehicle. Some bacterial species used as antigen delivery vehicles do not exhibit well-characterized means of adherence to mucosal tissues or to structures in proximity to inductive sites. These bacterial vectors, following oral administration, more or less pass through the body without adhering to any specific tissues, but nevertheless are randomly taken up by M cells overlying the gut-associated lymphoid tissue (GALT). Other bacterial antigen delivery vectors colonize by a specific adherence mechanism either in the oral cavity or in the intestine. Bacterial vectors in this category can be either noninvasive or invasive, in which case the maintenance of the adherent bacterial population ensures repeat random uptake of the bacterial antigen delivery vector at inductive sites, such as the GALT. In other cases, the adherent microorganism possesses the potential to invade cells lining the mucosal tissue or directly to enter inductive sites, such as the GALT or the bronchus-associated lymphoid tissue (BALT). These or-

*Essentials of Mucosal Immunology*   Copyright © 1996 by Academic Press, Inc. All rights of reproduction in any form reserved.

ganisms may then be killed rapidly by macrophages to release their antigens for processing and presentation. The last group of antigen delivery vectors is derived by attenuation of bacterial pathogens that attach to, invade, and survive within cells present in the mucosal tissue, including the GALT and BALT. Attenuated bacteria then enter other lymphoid tissues within the body to serve as factories to produce foreign antigen(s) in antigen-processing cells. The properties of the bacterial species used as an antigen delivery vector very much influence the size of a dose and the number of repeat doses to achieve a desired level of immune responsiveness.

Bacteria in at least eight genera have been used to achieve immune responses at mucosal sites. It is likely that others will be evaluated in the future. *Lactobacillus fermentum* (Hafner and Timms, 1994) has been used to express foreign antigens, but since these organisms seem not to colonize except in the colon, which may not be the best inductive site for a mucosal immune response. Repetitive oral immunizations of recombinant *L. fermentum* are required to achieve adequate immune responses. *Streptococcus gordonii* has been genetically engineered to express antigens by Fischetti and colleagues (Medaglini *et al.*, 1995). These bacteria attach to and adhere to the tooth surface to produce foreign antigens to stimulate immune responses. Whether the inductive site for the mucosal immune response is in the intestinal tract following swallowing of sluffed-off bacteria and uptake by the M cells overlying the GALT or whether some of the antigen is taken up by inductive sites in the oral cavity is not clearly established. An issue of concern pertains to the possibility of inducing some tolerance to the foreign antigen due to the continued colonization by the genetically engineered *S. gordonii*. On the other hand, increase in immunity rather than tolerance seems to be achieved over time in individuals persistently colonized with oral streptococci.

*Vibrio cholerae* and certain strains of *Escherichia coli* represent microorganisms with the ability to adhere to specific mucosal tissues, but without the ability to survive following uptake into M cells and entry into phagocytic cells in the GALT. Nevertheless, these bacterial species can be rendered avirulent by mutation and endowed with the ability to express foreign antigens that presumably will lead to the induction of mucosal immunity. *Shigella* is an invasive enteropathogen that may transiently colonize the ileum prior to adhering to and invading colonic epithelial cells. Progress is being made in rendering *Shigella* avirulent yet immunogenic (Baron *et al.*, 1987; Viret *et al.*, 1993). Thus the potential exists to genetically modify such strains to express foreign antigens. It is not known, however, whether the ability of *Shigella* to cause apoptosis in macrophages might ameliorate their potential to induce strong immune responses.

*Mycobacterium bovis,* BCG, is being developed as a recombinant antigen delivery vehicle (Jacobs *et al.*, 1990; Connell *et al.*, 1993). Most studies to date have made use of parenteral immunization with recombinant constructs, but BCG is used for oral immunization in some parts of the world; it is likely that oral administration of recombinant BCG constructs will illicit mucosal as well as systemic immune responses. The means by which BCG would invade cells in the intestinal tract has not, to the best of our knowledge, been worked out. *Salmonella* species, like *Listeria,* have the potential after oral inoculation to attach to and invade intestinal epithelial cells (Carter and Collins, 1974), but specifically gain access to visceral organs by invasion into the M cells overlying the gut-associated lymphoid tissue. In this environment, attenuated derivatives of these species have the potential to survive and to produce sufficient foreign antigen to stimulate mucosal as well as systemic and cellular immune responses. Since the *Salmonella*-based antigen delivery vectors are the most readily altered by a diversity of genetic means, and have the potential to induce immune responses with the lowest doses, their attributes which have been most studied will constitute the subject matter for the remainder of this chapter.

## II. AVIRULENT *SALMONELLA* VECTORS

The *Salmonella* vector should be completely avirulent and highly immunogenic. Achieving this balance is not easy, especially when one considers the diversity of the population to be immunized with regard to age, nutritional status, immunocompromised status, coinfection with other pathogens, and immunocompetence. The attenuated *Salmonella* should retain its tissue tropism without causing disease or significant impairment of normal host physiology and growth. For safety, it should have two or more attenuating deletion mutations, so there is no likelihood of reversion. The attenuating phenotype should be unaffected by diet or the host, or other environmental conditions. When used as an antigen delivery vector, the attenuated strain must be capable of giving stable high-level expression of cloned genes in the immunized host. In general, live bacterial vaccines are easy to grow, preserve, and administer at relatively low cost.

Several *Salmonella* serotypes have been rendered avirulent and evaluated for immunogenicity in various animal hosts; *S. typhimurium* has been studied most extensively, especially in the mouse where the model of infection is reasonably analogous to the means by which *S. typhi* infects humans. Avirulent derivatives of *S. typhimurium* have also been studied extensively in chickens, swine, and calves, and to a lesser extent, in monkeys. Attenuated derivatives of *S. choleraesuis* have been studied in mice and swine (Kelly *et al.,* 1992; Stabel *et al.,* 1993) and of *S. dublin* in mice and in calves. For antigen delivery vectors for use in humans, *Salmonella* serotypes that are capable of causing invasive disease are preferable. These include strains of *S. typhi, S. paratyphi A, S. paratyphi B (S. shottmuelleri), S. paratyphi C (S. hirschfeldii), S. dublin,* and *S. choleraesuis.*

Strains of *Salmonella* have been rendered avirulent, yet retain immunogenicity after introduction of a number of different genetically defined mutational lesions. Mutations which render *Salmonella* avirulent yet immunogenic include *galE* (Germanier and Furer, 1971, 1975), *aroA* (Hoiseth and Stocker, 1981), *cya* and *crp* (Curtiss and Kelly, 1987), *phoP* (Galan and Curtiss, 1989), *ompR* (Dorman *et al.,*

1989), *htrA* (Chatfield *et al.,* 1992b), and *cdt* (Kelly *et al.,* 1992). Still additional means to render *Salmonella* avirulent and immunogenic are likely to be discovered and described in the future. It should be noted that each of the listed means of attenuating *Salmonella* works optimally in *S. typhimurium* evaluated for virulence and immunogenicity in mice. When any one of the single attenuating mutational lesions is introduced into *S. typhi,* the constructed candidate vaccine strain usually retains an unacceptable level of virulence when administered to humans at high doses (Hone, *et al.,* 1988a, 1992; Tacket *et al.,* 1992). For this reason, it is more likely that candidate vaccine strains for immunization of humans will possess two or more deletion (Δ) mutations, rendering *Salmonella* avirulent by two or more different mechanisms. This, however, can lead to hyperattenuation and very poor immunogenicity as was observed with *S. typhi* strains with *aroA* and *purA* mutations (Levine and Noriega, 1993).

## III. Recombinant Avirulent *Salmonella* Antigen Delivery Vectors

Avirulent strains of *Salmonella* can be genetically engineered to stably express at high-level colonization and virulence antigens from other bacterial, viral, parasitic, and fungal pathogens (see review by Roberts *et al.,* 1994). When used for oral immunization, these live avirulent recombinant vaccine strains attach to, invade, and colonize the GALT and then pass to other lymphoid tissues, such as mesenteric lymph nodes, liver, and spleen (Curtiss *et al.,* 1988a,b). In these lymphoid tissues, the live avirulent recombinant vaccine strains continue to synthesize the foreign colonization or virulence antigens. Since delivery of antigens to the gut-associated lymphoid tissue stimulates a generalized secretory immune response (Cebra *et al.,* 1976; Bienenstock *et al.,* 1978), oral immunization with these vaccines stimulates mucosal immunity throughout the body (Curtiss *et al.,* 1989). In addition, systemic and cellular immune responses are elicited against the foreign-expressed antigens as well as against *Salmonella* antigens (Stabel *et al.,* 1990; Molina and Parker, 1990; Doggett *et al.,* 1993; Dusek *et al.,* 1994; Roberts *et al.,* 1994). Although oral immunization is the preferred route, live avirulent recombinant *Salmonella* vaccines can also be administered intranasally, intravaginally, and rectally (Srinivasan *et al.,* 1995a; Hopkins *et al.,* 1995).

Recombinant avirulent *Salmonella* antigen delivery systems must be capable of giving stable high-level expression of cloned genes in the immunized host during the period in which the vaccine strain persists in host tissues (Curtiss *et al.,* 1990). Stable expression of foreign antigens has been achieved by integrating a gene encoding a foreign antigen into the chromosome (Hone *et al.,* 1988b; Strugnell *et al.,* 1990; Hohman *et al.,* 1995), in which case a very strong promoter is needed to drive expression. This often does not lead to adequate levels of antigen expression (Cárdenas and Clements, 1993) and so use of plasmid vectors permitting multiple copies of the gene specifying the foreign antigen have been used. Since federal regulatory agencies do not permit expression of antibiotic resistance in live bacterial vaccines, balanced-lethal vector–host systems have been designed to achieve stable high-level expression of foreign antigens in the absence of drug resistance-selective markers (Nakayama *et al.*, 1988; Galan *et al.*, 1990). In one such system, a deletion in the *asd* gene for β-aspartate semialdehyde dehydrogenase is introduced into the chromosome of the avirulent *Salmonella* to impart a requirement for diaminopimelic acid (DAP), an essential constituent of the rigid layer of the bacterial cell wall. Plasmid vectors have the wild-type counterpart to the *asd* gene so that viability of the construct is dependent upon stable maintenance of the plasmid vector (Nakayama *et al.*, 1988; Galan *et al.*, 1990). Since DAP is not present in mammalian tissues, recombinant avirulent *Salmonella* vaccine strains with this balanced-lethal construction are stably maintained with high-level expression of foreign antigen over several weeks. Loss of the Asd$^+$ plasmid vector leads to DAPless death with lysis of the bacterial cell and release of its antigenic contents. *Salmonella* strains attenuated with Δ*cya* and Δ*crp* mutations maintain plasmid cloning vectors more stably and with a higher copy number than *Salmonella* attenuated by other deletion mutations (Curtiss *et al.*, 1988a; Galan *et al.*, 1989). These Δ*cya* and Δ*crp* strains therefore express foreign antigens to a higher level, which enhances the magnitude of the immune responses to the foreign antigens. Various types of promoters can be used to drive expression of foreign antigens *in vivo*. These can be either constitutive or induced to express at high level after entrance of the vaccine strain into the immunized host (Chatfield *et al.*, 1992a). Achieving maximal immune responses to the foreign antigen is dependent upon the amount of the foreign antigen produced by the recombinant avirulent *Salmonella* (Cárdenas and Clements, 1993; Doggett *et al.*, 1993; Srinivasan *et al.*, 1995b) and also upon the inherent immunogenic properties of the foreign antigen. The amount of the antigen can be influenced by the inherent stability of the foreign antigen after synthesis in the avirulent *Salmonella,* the strength of the promoter used to drive expression, and the copy number specified by the origin of replication employed in the plasmid vector. The latter can range from 5 to 10 plasmid copies per chromosome DNA equivalent by use of the pSC101 replicon, 20 to 40 copies per chromosome DNA equivalent for the p15A replicon, 100 to 150 copies per chromosome DNA equivalent by use of the pBR322 replicon, to upward of several hundred copies per chromosome DNA equivalent by using a pUC replicon. Overproduction of the foreign antigen can lead to the formation of inclusion bodies which sometimes are nonimmunogenic or, even worse, are toxic to the bacterial vector leading to hyperattenuation and rendering the construct marginally immunogenic. We have found that constructs that produce between 0.5 and 2.0% of the total protein as the foreign antigen generally give most satisfactory results with regard to stability and immunogenicity. Soon after construction of recombinant avirulent *Salmonella,* studies of comparative growth and stability, for plasmid maintenance and antigen production, should be carried out. Recombinant strains that grow considerably more slowly than the parent strain with the vector alone are less likely to adequately colonize the immunized host and therefore give diminished immune responses. Recombinant strains that grow well, maintain the plasmid vector stably, and give high-level expression of the foreign antigen invariably colonize host tissues very well and induce strong immune responses.

Some foreign antigens may have good B-cell epitopes but lack a strong T-cell epitope. In other cases, the antigen may contain hydrophobic sequences that contribute to toxicity to the recombinant avirulent *Salmonella*. If the foreign antigen is to be expressed and maintained in the cytoplasm of the recombinant avirulent *Salmonella*, it is wise to delete the DNA sequences specifying the hydrophobic regions of the antigen, to engender both less toxicity and greater stability, since these sequences are seldom immunogenic. Considerable work has been carried out to investigate the potential of fusing short sequences including B-cell epitopes of the foreign antigen to other antigenic carriers which provide a strong T-cell epitope. LT-B and CT-B have been used in recombinant avirulent *Salmonella* for this purpose (Schödel *et al.*, 1990; Jagusztyn-Krynicka *et al.*, 1993) as have the Shiga toxin B subunit (Su *et al.*, 1992), hepatitis B virus core (Schödel *et al.*, 1994), and the tetanus toxin fragment C (Fairweather *et al.*, 1990; Khan *et al.*, 1994). Epitopes have also been engineered into flagella (Newton *et al.*, 1989; McEwen *et al.*, 1992) or fimbriae (Verjans *et al.*, 1995), which are exposed on the surface of the recombinant avirulent *Salmonella*. Comparative data to indicate the importance or nonimportance of antigen location in recombinant avirulent *Salmonella* are by and large lacking. There may be some reason to believe that the time of onset, magnitude, and/or duration as well as the type of immune response, might be influenced by antigen localization in the recombinant avirulent *Salmonella* vaccine strain. Thus a number of fusion vectors are being evaluated for surface localization or secretion of foreign antigens by recombinant avirulent *Salmonella*. These vectors have been designed such that fusions are made to all or part of several outer membrane proteins, such as OmpA (Ruppert *et al.*, 1994), Lpp (Matsuyama *et al.*, 1995), TraT (Croft *et al.*, 1991), LamB (Charbit *et al.*, 1993), and PhoE (Janssen *et al.*, 1994). In still other cases, foreign antigens have been secreted by making use of the IgA protease from *Neisseria gonorrhea* (Pohlner *et al.*, 1987). In spite of all of these efforts to alter and possibly optimize the location of foreign antigens expressed by recombinant avirulent *Salmonella*, it has been generally observed that good immune responses are elicited to foreign antigens independent of their site of localization within the recombinant avirulent *Salmonella*. It is thus quite likely that the recombinant avirulent *Salmonella* are disrupted in phagosomes and their antigens processed as the major means of stimulating the immune responses observed.

## IV. IMMUNIZATION WITH RECOMBINANT AVIRULENT *SALMONELLA* VACCINES AND INDUCTION OF MUCOSAL IMMUNE RESPONSES

### A. Vaccines to Prevent Infectious Diseases

Recombinant avirulent *Salmonella* antigen delivery systems have been developed and investigated to express colonization and virulence antigens from various bacterial, viral, and parasitic pathogens with the purpose of inducing protective immunity against the pathogens whose genes are expressed by the recombinant avirulent *Salmonella*. These studies have been reviewed extensively, most recently by Roberts *et al.* (1994). Most of the studies to date have monitored induction of serum antibodies with fewer studies investigating cellular immunity or production of S-IgA and conferring mucosal immunity. Our initial interest in developing the recombinant avirulent *Salmonella* antigen delivery system was to determine whether oral administration of such vaccines might induce adequate titers of S-IgA in saliva against surface antigens of oral pathogenic streptococci in order to prevent dental caries (Curtiss, 1986). Although S-IgA responses against streptococcal surface proteins have been induced to appear in saliva, the immune responses induced (Doggett *et al.*, 1993; Redman *et al.*, 1994) are not likely to be highly protective. Based on our results there is reason to speculate that pathogens that reside continuously in an environment exposed to S-IgA induced due to continual ingestion of antigens from that pathogen are likely to have undergone change due to mutation and selection to eliminate (or at least lessen) the immunogenicity of potential B cell epitopes contained within those surface proteins. This speculation gains further credence when one realizes that there are numerous "normal" flora occupying mucosal niches within the GI tract that do not seem to be affected by the ability of the host to mount mucosal immune responses. Clearly there are some important biological questions that need to be addressed experimentally to resolve these issues. In the meantime, our efforts to construct recombinant avirulent *Salmonella*-expressing surface antigens of oral streptococci are focused on constructing fusions which provide strong T epitope help.

More recently, we have been investigating the mucosal and systemic immune responses to the *Streptococcus pneumoniae* PspA protein (Briles *et al.*, 1988) as expressed by recombinant avirulent *Salmonella* (Nayak *et al.*, in preparation). Prior results have indicated that oral administration of recombinant avirulent *Salmonella* induced much higher SIgA titers against an expressed antigen in the secretions of the intestine and reproductive tract than in the secretions of the upper respiratory tract, including saliva. We therefore investigated the possible use of the intranasal route for immunization with recombinant avirulent *Salmonella* strains expressing immunogenic portions of the PspA protein. Although our results to date indicate that serum antibody titers against either *Salmonella* antigens or an expressed antigen is about the same, whether the route of immunization is peroral, intranasal, intravaginal, or intraperitoneal, the mucosal immune responses seem to be more influenced by the route of immunization. Thus intranasal immunization, although inducing high S-IgA titers in lung secretions, does not induce as high titers of S-IgA in vaginal secretions as were observed following peroral, intravaginal, or intraperitoneal immunizations (Srinivasan *et al.*, 1995b).

## B. Recombinant Avirulent *Salmonella* Contraceptive Vaccines

Several years ago, we commenced to investigate whether recombinant avirulent *Salmonella* expressing gamete-specific antigens could induce immune responses in the reproductive tract that would block fertilization (Curtiss and Tinge, 1993). Our prediction was based upon the discovery by Primakoff *et al.* (1988) that immunization of guinea pigs with the sperm-specific antigen PH-20 induced a long-lasting immunity against fertilization. It was also evident that men and women with significant antibody titers against human sperm were often infertile or had much reduced fertility without other ill effects (Witkin and Chandry, 1989). It was also known that immunization of male and female animals with extracts of whole sperm could induce infertility and the induction of immune responses specifically against sperm autoantigens. The ability of an individual to induce immune responses against gamete-specific antigens is undoubtedly due to the isolation of the reproductive tissues and gamete generation process from the immune surveillance network of the body. It is also due to the fact that these gamete-specific antigens are not expressed in any other tissue which would have led to their recognition as self during embryonic development. To date, much of our work has concentrated on expression of the sperm-specific antigen SP10 (Herr *et al.*, 1990) of macaques and humans and the expression of the murine sperm-specific LDHC4 (Goldberg, 1977) and egg-specific antigen ZP3 (Dean *et al.*, 1989) by recombinant avirulent *Salmonella*. Both systemic and mucosal immune responses are proportional to the amount of antigen expressed by the recombinant avirulent *Salmonella* (Doggett *et al.*, 1993; Srinivasan *et al.*, 1995b). It is also evident that higher and more sustained immune responses are achieved by several immunizations initially within a week to 10 days, rather than spreading doses out over a month or so at weekly or biweekly intervals. Antibody titers persist for 5 to 6 months, and after they have dropped significantly, the mice can be boosted to restimulate rapid increases in S-IgA and serum IgG titers. Thus, it appears that the recombinant avirulent *Salmonella* induces immunological memory with regard to both the systemic and mucosal immune responses to the expressed gamete specific antigen. The recombinant avirulent *S. typhimurium* expressing the human SP-10 sperm antigen induces antibodies which react with proteins in human sperm, as revealed by both indirect immunoflourescence and Western blotting. In experiments with recombinant avirulent *S. typhimurium* expressing murine gamete-specific antigens, reduced fertility has been observed, with regard to both absence of pregnancy over six to eight estrus cycles and delay in time to conception. A reduction in the number of pups per litter in those animals that became pregnant has also been observed. Studies with combinations of recombinant *Salmonella* expressing different murine gamete-specific antigens are in progress. It is evident from all of our experiments that recombinant avirulent *Salmonella* expressing gamete-specific antigens, when used for either oral or intravaginal immunization, induce high antibody titers in the female reproductive tract of mice. Our successes in inducing mucosal immune responses in the reproductive tract lead us to think that the recombinant avirulent *Salmonella* antigen delivery system might be particularly suitable for the development of vaccines against sexually transmitted pathogens.

## V. CONCLUSION

Recombinant avirulent *Salmonella* antigen delivery system technology is continuing to be improved. With each year, discoveries are being made to enhance both the utility and the safety of the system. *Salmonella* are being genetically engineered to enable bacteria to escape the phagosome and thus enhance their potential to produce antigens that will be processed through the MHC class I system. These bacteria are likely to induce better cellular immune responses (Gentschev *et al.,* 1995) than avirulent *Salmonella* that do not escape the phagosome. We are currently attempting to construct avirulent *Salmonella* strains that die if (and soon after) being shed in feces, thus diminishing the possibility of individuals becoming involuntarily immunized. In addition, the bacterial antigen delivery systems offer some safety features not afforded by use of viral vectors. These vaccine strains are all completely sensitive to antibiotics; thus, if an immunized individual experienced fever or other side effects, they could be treated with antibiotics to arrest these adverse symptoms. Recombinant avirulent *Salmonella* already possess their built-in adjuvants, thus eliminating the need for adding such components to vaccine preparations. Although one vaccine strain could be engineered to produce several different antigens, it will be technically easier and probably just as efficacious to make mixtures of several strains, each expressing a different antigen. In this way, there is little likelihood for competition between different expressed antigens, since each would most likely be processed in a different antigen-processing cell. Probably one of the most important features of the recombinant avirulent *Salmonella* antigen delivery system is the potential cost effectiveness. Recombinant avirulent *Salmonella* vaccines can be manufactured with regard to growth, preservation, packaging, and labeling for pennies a dose, with the actual cost per dose influenced most by the number of doses per unit container. In any event, the development of vaccines that do not require refrigeration and that can be reconstituted immediately prior to use, and that can be administered on or into a mucosal surface in the absence of any need for syringes, increases cost efficiency. Both of these considerations enhance safety and efficacy, while further reducing costs for vaccine administration. It is therefore evident that recombinant avirulent *Salmonella* vaccines should have a significant role in preventing infectious diseases in animals, as well as in humans, and possibly in controlling fertility. The latter could be important in vector control or in reducing overexpanding populations of certain animals that have become pests.

## ACKNOWLEDGMENTS

Our research has been funded in part by research grants from the National Institute of Dental Research (DEO6669), the National Institute of Child Health and Human Development (HD29099-05), and the Contraceptive Research and Development (CONRAD) Program, Eastern Virginia Medical School, under a Cooperative Agreement with the United States Agency for International Development (USAID) (DPE-3044-19-00-2015-00).

## REFERENCES

Baron, L. S., Kopecko, D. J., Formal, S. B., Seid, R., Guerry, P., and Powell, C. (1987). Introduction of *Shigella flexneri* 2a type and group antigen genes into oral typhoid vaccine strain *Salmonella typhi* Ty21a. *Infect. Immun.* **55**, 2797–2801.

Bienenstock, J., McDermott, M., Befus, D., and O'Neil, L. M. (1978). A common mucosal immunologic system involving the bronchus, breast, and bowel. *Adv. Exp. Med. Biol.* **107**, 53–59.

Briles, D. E., Yother, J., and McDaniel, L. S. (1988). Role of pneumonococcal surface protein A in the virulence of *Streptococcus pneumoniae*. *Rev. Infect. Dis.* **10**, 5372–5374.

Cárdenas, L., and Clements, J. D. (1993). Stability, immunogenicity and expression of foreign antigens in bacterial vaccine vectors. *Vaccine* **11**, 126–135.

Carter, P. B., and Collins, F. M. (1974). The route of enteric infection in normal mice. *J. Exp. Med.* **139**, 1189–1203.

Cebra, J. J., Gearhart, P. J., Kamat, R., Robertson, S. M., and Tseng, J. (1976). Origin and differentiation of lymphocytes involved in the secretory IgA response. *Cold Spring Harbor Symp. Quant. Biol.* **41**, 201–221.

Chatfield, S. N., Charles, I. G., Makoff, A. J., Oxer, M. D., Dougan, G., Pikard, D., Slater, D., and Fairweather, N. F. (1992a). Use of the *nirB* promoter to direct the stable expression of heterologous antigens in *Salmonella* oral vaccine strains: Development of a single-dose oral tetanus vaccine. *Bio/Technology* **10**, 888–892.

Chatfield, S. N., Strahan, K., Pickard, D., Charles, I. G., Hormaeche, C. E., and Dougan, G. (1992b). Evaluation of *Salmonella typhimurium* strains harbouring defined mutations in *htrA* and *aroA* in the murin salmonellosis model. *Microb. Pathog.* **12**, 145–151.

Charbit, A., Martineau, P., Ronco, J., Leclere, C., Lo-Man, R., Michel, V., O'Callaghan, D., and Hofnung, M. (1993). Expression and immunogenicity of the V3 loop from the envelope of human immunodeficiency virus type 1 in an attenuated *aroA* strain of *Salmonella typhimurium* upon genetic coupling to two *Escherichia coli* carrier proteins. *Vaccine* **11**, 1221–1228.

Connell, N. D., Medina-Acosta, E., McMaster, W. R., Bloom, B. R., and Russell, D. G. (1993). Effective immunization against cutaneous leishmaniasis with recombinant Bacille Calmette-Guérin expressing the *Leishmania* surface proteinase gp63. *Proc. Natl. Acad. Sci. U.S.A.* **90**, 11473–11477.

Croft, S., Walsh, J., Lloyd, W., Russell-Jones, G. J. (1991). TraT: A powerful carrier molecule for the stimulation of immune responses to protein and peptide antigens. *J. Immunol.* **146**, 793–798.

Curtiss III, R. (1986). Genetic analysis of *Streptococcus mutans* virulence and prospects for an anticaries vaccine. *J. Dent. Res.* **65**, 1034–1045.

Curtiss III, R., and Kelly, S. M. (1987). *Salmonella typhimurium* deletion mutants lacking adenylate cyclase and cyclic AMP receptor protein are avirulent and immunogenic. *Infect. Immun.* **55**, 3035–3043.

Curtiss III, R., Goldschmidt, R. M., Fletchall, N. B., and Kelly, S. M. (1988a). Avirulent *Salmonella typhimurium* $\Delta cya$ $\Delta crp$ oral vaccine strains expressing a streptococcal colonization and virulence antigen. *Vaccine* **6**, 155–160.

Curtiss III, R., Kelly, S. M., Gulig, P. A., Gentry-Weeks, C. R., and Galan, J. E. (1988b). Avirulent *Salmonella* expressing virulence antigens from other pathogens for use as orally-administered vaccines. *In* "Virulence Mechanisms of Bacterial Pathogens." (J. Roth, Ed.), pp. 311–328. American Society for Microbiology, Washington, D. C.

Curtiss III, R., Kelly, S. M., Gulig, P. A., and Nakayama, K. (1989). Selective delivery of antigens by recombinant bacteria. *Curr. Top. Microbiol. Immun.* **146**, 35–49.

Curtiss III, R., Galan, J. E., Nakayama, K., and Kelly, S. M. (1990). Stabilization of recombinant avirulent vaccine strains *in vivo. Res. Microbiol.* **141**, 797–805.

Curtiss III, R., and Tinge S. A. (1993). Recombinant avirulent *Salmonella* vaccines and prospects for an antifertility vaccine. *In* "Proceedings of the Symposium on Local Immunity in Reproduction Tract Tissues, New Delhi, India, November, 1990." (P. D. Griffin and P. M. Johnson, Eds.), pp. 459–476. Oxford University Press, London.

Dean, J., Chamberlin, M. E., Millar, S. E., Ringuette, M. J., Philpott, C. C., Baur, A. W., Chamow, S. M. (1989). Developmental expression of ZP3, a mouse zona pellucida gene. *Prog. Clin. Biol. Res.* **294**, 21–32.

Doggett, T. A., Jagusztyn-Krynicka, E. K., and Curtiss III, R. (1993). Immune responses to *Streptococcus sobrinus* surface protein antigen A expressed by recombinant *Salmonella typhimurium. Infect. Immun.* **61**, 1859–1866.

Dorman, C. J., Chatfield, S., Higgins, C. F., Hayward, C., and Dougan, G. (1989). Characterization of porin and *ompR* mutants of a virulent strain of *Salmonella typhimurium* expressing a cloned *Porphyromonas gingivalis* hemagglutinin. *Infect. Immun.* **57**, 2136–2140.

Dusek, D. M., Progulske-Fox, A., and Brown, T. A. (1994). Systemic and mucosal immune responses in mice orally immunized with avirulent *Salmonella typhimurium* expressing a cloned *Porphyromonas gingivalis* hemagglutinin. *Infect. Immun.* **62**, 1652–1657.

Fairweather, N. F., Chatfield, S. N., Makoff, A. J., Strugnell, R. A., Bester, J., Maskell, D. J., and Dougan, G. (1990). Oral vaccination of mice against tetanus by use of a live attenuated *Salmonella* carrier. *Infect. Immun.* **58**, 1323–1326.

Galan, J. E., and Curtiss III, R. (1989). Virulence and vaccine potential of *phoP* mutants of *Salmonella typhimurium. Microb. Pathog.* **6**, 433–443.

Galan, J. E., Timoney, J. F., and Curtiss III, R. (1989). Expression and localization of *Streptococcus equi* M protein in *Escherichia coli* and *Salmonella typhimurium. In* "Equine Infectious Diseases V, Proceedings of the Fifth International Congress" (D. G. Powell, Ed.), pp. 34–40. Univ. Press of Kentucky, Lexington.

Galan, J. E., Nakayama, K., and Curtiss III, R. (1990). Cloning and characterization of the *asd* gene of *Salmonella typhimurium:* Use in stable maintenance of recombinant plasmids in *Salmonella* vaccine strains. *Gene* **94**, 29–35.

Gentschev, I., Sokolovic, Z., Mollenkopf, H.-J., Hess, J., Kaufmann, S. H. E., Kuhn, M., Krohne, G. F., and Goebel, W. (1995). *Salmonella* strain secreting active Listeriolysin changes its intracellular localization. *Infect. Immun.* **63**, 4202–4205.

Germanier, R., and Furer, E. (1971). Immunity in experimental salmonellosis. II. Basis for the virulence and protective capacity of *galE* mutants of *Salmonella typhimurium. Infect. Immun.* **4**, 663–673.

Germanier, R., and Furer, E. (1975). Isolation and characterization of *galE* mutant Ty21a of *Salmonella typhi:* A candidate strain for a live, oral typhoid vaccine. *J. Infect. Dis.* **131**, 553–558.

Goldberg, E. (1977). Isozymes in testis and spermatozoa. *In* "Current Topics in Biology and Medical Research." (M. C. Ratazzi, J. G. Scandalios, and G. S. Whitt, eds.), pp. 79–124. Liss, New York.

Hafner, L. M., and Timms, P. (1994). Genetic manipulation of a vaginal strain of *Lactobacillus fermentum* and its maintenance within the reproductive tract after intravaginal administration. *J. Med. Microbiol.* **41**, 272–278.

Herr, J. C., Flickinger, C. J., Homyk, M., Klotz, K., John, E. (1990). Biochemical and morphological characterization of the intraacrosomal antigen SP10 from human sperm. *Biol. Reprod.* **42**, 181–193.

Hohman, E. L., Oletta, C. A., Loomis, W. P., and Miller, S. I. (1995). Macrophage-inducible expression of a model antigen in *Salmonella typhimurium* enhances immunogenicity. *Proc. Natl. Acad. Sci. U.S.A.* **92**, 2904–2908.

Hoiseth, S. K., and Stocker, B. A. D. (1981). Aromatic-dependent *Salmonella typhimurium* are nonvirulent and effective as live vaccines. *Nature (London)* **291**, 238–239.

Hone, D. M., Attridge, S. R., Forrest, B., Morona, R., Daniels, D., LaBrooy, J. T., Bartholomeusz, R. C. A., Shearman, D. J. C., and Hackett, J. (1988a). A *galE* via (Vi antigen-negative) mutant of *Salmonella typhi* Ty2 retains virulence in humans. *Infect. Immun.* **56**, 1326–1333.

Hone, D., Attridge, S., Vanden Bosch, L., and Hackett, J. (1988b). A chromosomal integration system for stabilization of heterologous genes in *Salmonella* based vaccine strains. *Microb. Pathog.* **5**, 407–418.

Hone, D., Tacket, C. O., Harris, A. M., Kay, B., Losonsky, G., and Levine, M. M. (1992). Evaluation in volunteers of a candidate live oral attenuated *Salmonella typhi* vector vaccine. *J. Clin. Invest.* **90**, 412–420.

Hopkins, S., Kraehenbuhl, J., Schödel, F., Potts, A., Peterson, D., Grandi, P. D., and Nardelli-Haefliger, D. (1995). A recombinant *Salmonella typhimurium* vaccine induces local immunity by four different routes of immunization. *Infect. Immun.* **63**, 3729–3786.

Jacobs, W. R., Jr., Snapper, S. B., Lugosi, L., and Bloom, B. R. (1990). Development of BCG as a recombinant vaccine delivery vehicle. *Curr. Top. Microbiol. Immunol.* **155**, 153–160.

Jagusztyn-Krynicka, E. K., Clark-Curtiss, J. E., and Curtiss III, R. (1993). *Escherichia coli* heat-labile toxin subunit B fusions with *Streptococcus sobrinus* antigens expressed by *Salmonella typhimurium* oral vaccine strains: Importance of the linker for antigenicity and biological activities of the hybrid proteins. *Infect. Immun.* **61**, 1004–1015.

Janssen, R., Wauben, M., van der Zee, R., and Tommassen, J. (1994). Immunogenicity of a mycobacterial T-cell epitope expressed in outer membrane protein PhoE of *Escherichia coli*. *Vaccine* **12**, 406–409.

Kelly, S. M., Bosecker, B. A., and Curtiss III, R. (1992). Characterization and protective properties of attenuated mutants of *Salmonella choleraesuis*. *Infect. Immun.* **60**, 4881–4890.

Khan, C. M. A., Villarreal-Ramos, B., Pierce, R. J., Hormaeche, R. D. D., McNeill, H., Ali, T., Chatfield, S., Capron, A., Dourgan, G., and Hormaeche, C. E. (1994). Construction, expression, and immunogenicity of multiple tandem copies of the *Schistosoma mansoni* peptide 115–131 of the P28 glutathione S-transferase expressed as C-terminal fusions to tetanus toxin fragment C in a live Aro-attenuated vaccine strain of *Salmonella*. *J. Immunol.* **153**, 5634–5642.

Levine, M. M., and Noriega, F. (1993). Vaccines to prevent enteric infections. (Review) *Bailliere's Clin. Gastroent.* **7**, 501–517.

Matsuyama, S., Tajima, T., and Tokuda, H. (1995). A novel periplasmic carrier protein involved in the sorting and transport of *Escherichia coli* lipoproteins destined for the outer membrane. *EMBO J.* **14**, 3365–3372.

McEwen, J., Levi, R., Horwitz, R. J., and Arnon, R. (1992). Synthetic recombinant vaccine expressing influenza haemagglutinin epitope in *Salmonella flagellin* leads to partial protection in mice. *Vaccine* **10**, 405–411.

Medaglini, D., Pozzi, G., King, T. P., and Fischetti, V. A. (1995). Mucosal and systemic immune responses to a recombinant protein expressed on the surface of the oral commensal bacterium *Streptococcus gordonii*. *Proc. Natl. Acad. Sci. U.S.A.* **92**, 6868–6872.

Molina, N. C., and Parker, C. D. (1990). Murine antibody response to oral infection with live *aroA* recombinant *Salmonella dublin* vaccine strains expressing filamentous hemaglutinin antigen from *Bordetella pertussis*. *Infect. Immun.* **58**, 2523–2528.

Nakayama, K., Kelly, S. M., and Curtiss III, R. (1988). Construction of an Asd$^+$ expression-cloning vector: Stable maintenance and high level expression of cloned genes in a *Salmonella* vaccine strain. *Bio/Technology* **6**, 693–697.

Nayak, A. R., Tinge, S. A., McDaniel, L. S., Briles, D. E., and Curtiss, R. Evaluation of a live recombinant avirulent oral *Salmonella* vaccine expressing pneumococcal surface protein A (PspA). In preparation.

Newton, S. M., Jacobs, C. O., and Stocker, B. A. (1989). Immune response to cholera toxin epitope inserted in *Salmonella flagellin. Science* **244,** 70–72.

Pohlner, J., Halter, R., Beyreuther, K., and Meyer, T. T. (1987). Gene structure and extracellular secretion of *Neisseria gonorrhoeae* IgA protease. *Nature (London)* **325,** 458–462.

Primakoff, P., Lathrop, W., Woolman, L., Cowan, A., and Myles, D. (1988). Fully effective contraception in male and female guinea pigs immunized with the sperm protein PH-20. *Nature (London)* **335,** 543–546.

Redman, T. K., Harmon, C. C., and Michalek, S. M. (1994). Oral immunization with recombinant *Salmonella typhimurium* expressing surface protein antigen A of *Streptococcus sobrinus:* Persistence and induction of humoral responses in rats. *Infect. Immun.* **62,** 3162–3171.

Roberts, M., Chatfield, S. N., and Dougan, G. (1994). *Salmonella* as carriers of heterologous antigens. "Novel Delivery Systems for Oral Vaccines" (D. T. O'Hagen, Ed.), pp. 27–58. CRC Press, Ann Arbor, MI.

Ruppert, A., Arnold, N., and Hobom, G. (1994). OmpA-FMDV VP1 fusion proteins: Production, cell surface exposure and immune responses to the major antigenic domain of foot-and-mouth disease virus. *Vaccine* **12,** 492–498.

Schödel, F., Milich, D. R., and Will, H. (1990). Hepatitis B virus nucleocapsid/pre-S2 fusion proteins expressed in attenuated *Salmonella* for oral vaccination. *J. Immunol.* **145,** 4317–4321.

Schödel, F., Kelly, S. M., Peterson, D. L., Milich, D. R., and Curtiss III, R. (1994). Hybrid hepatitis B virus core-pre-S proteins synthesized in avirulent *Salmonella typhimurium* and *Salmonella typhi* for oral vaccination. *Infect. Immun.* **62,** 1669–1676.

Srinivasan, J., Nayak, A., Curtiss III, R., and Rubino, S. (1995a). Effect of the route of immunization using recombinant *Salmonella* on mucosal and humoral immune responses. *In* "Vaccines 95" (R. M. Chanock, R. Brown, H. S. Ginsberg, and E. Norrby, Eds.), pp. 273–280. Cold Spring Harbor Laboratory, Cold Spring Harbor, NY.

Srinivasan, J., Tinge, S., Wright, R., Herr, J. C., and Curtiss III, R. (1995b). Oral immunization with attenuated *Salmonella* expressing human sperm antigen induces antibodies in serum and the reproductive tract. *Biol. Reprod.* **53,** 462–471.

Stabel, J. J., Mayfield, J. E., Tabatabai, L. B., and Wannemuehler, M. J. (1990). Oral immunization of mice with attenuated *Salmonella typhimurium* containing a recombinant plasmid which codes for production of a 31-kilodalton protein of *Brucella abortus. Infect. Immun.* **58,** 2048–2055.

Stabel, T. J., Mayfield, J. E., Morfitt, D. C., and Wannemuehler, M. J. (1993). Oral immunization of mice and swine with an attenuated *Salmonella choleraesuis* [Δcya-12 Δ(crp-cdt)19] mutant containing a recombinant plasmid. *Infect. Immun.* **61,** 610–618.

Strugnell, R. A., Marshall, D., and Fairweather, N. (1990). Stable expression of foreign antigens from the chromosome of *Salmonella typhimurium* vaccine strains. *Gene* **88,** 57–61.

Su, G. F., Brahmbhatt, H. N., Wehland, J., Rohde, M., and Timmis, K. N. (1992). Extracellular export of Shiga toxin B-subunit/haemolysin A (C-terminus) fusion protein expressed in *Salmonella typhimurium aroA*-mutant and stimulation of B-subunit specific antibody responses in mice. *Microb. Pathog.* **13,** 465–476.

Tacket, C. O., Hone, D. M., Curtiss III, R., Kelly, S. M., Losonsky, G., Guers, L., Harris, A. M., Edelman, R., and Levine, M. M. (1992). Comparison of the safety and immunogenicity of ΔaroCΔaroD and ΔcyaΔcrp *Salmonella typhi* strain in adult volunteers. *Infect. Immun.* **60,** 536–541.

Verjans, G. M., Janssen, R., UytdeHaag, F. G., van Doornik, C. E., Tommassen, J. (1995). Intracellular processing and presentation of T cell epitopes, expressed by recombinant *Escherichia coli* and *Salmonella typhimurium,* to human T cells. *Eur. J. Immun.* **25,** 405–410.

Viret, J. F., Cryz, S., Jr., Lang, A. B., and Favre, D. (1993). Molecular cloning and characterization of the genetic determinants that express the complete *Shigella* serotype D *(Shigella sonnei)* lipopolysaccharide in heterologous live attenuated vaccine strains. *Mol. Microbiol.* **7,** 239–252.

Witkin, S. S., and Chandry, A. (1989). Association between recurrent spontaneous abortions and circulating IgG antibodies to sperm tails in women. *J. Reprod. Immunol.* **15,** 151–158.

# Chapter 37

# Use of Attenuated *Salmonella* Vectors for Oral Vaccines

John D. Clements, Celeste Chong, and Kenneth L. Bost

*Department of Microbiology and Immunology,*
*Tulane University School of Medicine,*
*New Orleans, Louisiana 70112*

## I. INTRODUCTION

Microbial pathogens can infect a host by one of several mechanisms. They may enter through a break in the integument induced by trauma, they may be introduced by vector transmission, or they may interact with a mucosal surface. The majority of human pathogens initiate disease by the last mechanism, i.e., following interaction with mucosal surfaces. Bacterial and viral pathogens that act through this mechanism first make contact with the mucosal surface where they may attach and then colonize, or be taken up by specialized absorptive cells (M cells) in the epithelium that overlay Peyer's patches and other lymphoid follicles (Bockman and Cooper, 1973; Owen *et al.*, 1986). Organisms that enter the lymphoid tissues may be readily killed within the lymphoid follicles, thereby provoking a potentially protective immunological response as antigens are delivered to immune cells within the follicles (e.g., *Vibrio cholerae*). Alternatively, pathogenic organisms capable of surviving local defense mechanisms may spread from the follicles and subsequently cause local or systemic disease (i.e., *Salmonella* spp., poliovirus, rotavirus in immunocompromised hosts).

Secretory IgA (S-IgA) antibodies directed against specific virulence determinants of infecting organisms play an important role in overall mucosal immunity (Cebra *et al.*, 1986). In many cases, it is possible to prevent the initial infection of mucosal surfaces by stimulating production of mucosal S-IgA levels directed against relevant virulence determinants of an infecting organism. Secretory IgA may prevent the initial interaction of the pathogen with the mucosal surface by blocking attachment and/or colonization, neutralizing surface-acting toxins, or preventing invasion of the host cells. While extensive research has been conducted to determine the role of cell-mediated immunity and serum antibody in protection against infectious agents, less is known about the regulation, induction, and secretion of S-IgA. Parenterally administered inactivated whole-cell and whole-virus preparations are effective at eliciting protective serum IgG and delayed type hypersensitivity reactions against organisms that have a significant serum phase in their pathogenesis (i.e., *Salmonella typhi*, Hepatitis B). However, parenteral vaccines are not effective at eliciting mucosal S-IgA responses and are ineffective against bacteria that interact with mucosal surfaces and do not invade (e.g., *V. cholerae*).

Oral immunization can be effective for induction of specific S-IgA responses if the antigens are presented to the T and B lymphocytes and accessory cells contained within Peyer's patches where preferential IgA B-cell development is initiated. Peyer's patches contain T-helper (Th)-cells that mediate B-cell isotype switching directly from IgM cells to IgA B cells. The patches also contain T cells that initiate terminal B-cell differentiation. The primed B-cells then migrate to the mesenteric lymph nodes and undergo differentiation, enter the thoracic duct, then the general circulation, and subsequently seed all of the secretory tissues of the body, including the lamina propria of the gut and respiratory tract. IgA is then produced by the mature plasma cells, complexed with membrane-bound secretory component, and transported onto the mucosal surface where it is available to interact with invading pathogens (Strober and Jacobs, 1985; Tomasi and Plaut, 1985). The existence of this common mucosal immune system explains in part the potential of live oral vaccines and oral immunization for protection against pathogenic organisms that initiate infection by first interacting with mucosal surfaces (Fig. 1).

A number of strategies have been developed for oral immunization, including the use of attenuated mutants of bacteria (i.e., *Salmonella* spp.) as carriers of heterologous antigens (Cárdenas and Clements, 1992, 1993a,b; Clements and Cárdenas, 1990; Clements and El-Morshidy, 1984; Clements *et al.*, 1986), encapsulation of antigens into microspheres composed of poly-DL-lactide-glycolide (PGL), protein-like polymers, proteinoids (Santiago *et al.*, 1993), gelatin capsules, different formulations of liposomes (Alving *et al.*, 1986; Garcon and Six, 1993; Gould-Fogerite and Mannino, 1993), adsorption onto nanoparticles, use of lipophilic immune stimulating complexes (ISCOMS) (Mowat and Donachie, 1991), and addition of bacterial products with known adjuvant properties (Clements *et al.*, 1988; Dickinson and Clements, 1995; Douce *et al.*, 1995; Elson, 1989; Lycke and Holmgren, 1986; Lycke *et al.*, 1992).

A number of attenuated mutants of *Salmonella* are able to interact with the lymphoid tissues in Peyer's patches, but not able to cause systemic disease. Some of these mutants are effective as live vaccines (i.e., able to protect against infection with the virulent *Salmonella* parent) and are candidates for use as carriers for other virulence determinants. Different mutants have been employed for this purpose (Fig. 2), including *galE* mutants, which lack the enzyme uridine diphosphate (UDP)-galactose-4-epimerase (Germanier and Fürer, 1975; Gilman *et al.*, 1977; Wahdan *et al.*, 1980), and *aroA* mutants, which have specific nonreverting deletions in the common aromatic biosynthetic pathway leading to chorismic acid

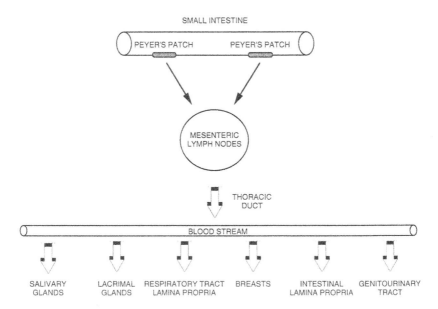

**FIGURE 1.** Generalized pathway for stimulation of specific mucosal immune responses. From Clements (1987, Fig. 1, p. 138).

(Hoiseth and Stocker, 1981; Robertsson *et al.,* 1983; Smith *et al.,* 1984a,b; Stocker *et al.,* 1983). *galE* mutants of *Salmonella* have been used as carriers by: Formal *et al.* (1981), who conjugally transferred the form I plasmid of *Shigella sonnei* to *S. typhi* Ty21a; Clements and El-Morshidy (1984), who utilized *S. typhi* Ty21a as a recipient for a recombinant plasmid containing the gene for production of the nontoxic B subunit of the heat-labile enterotoxin of *Escherichia coli* (LT-B); Yamamoto *et al.* (1985), who transferred a plasmid encoding colonization factor antigen (CFAI) and heat-stable enterotoxin from *E. coli* into *S. typhi* Ty21a; and Manning *et al.* (1986), who introduced molecularly cloned antigenic determinants of Inaba and Ogawa serotypes of *V. cholerae* O1 lipopolysaccharide into derivatives of *S. typhi* Ty21a and an analogous *S. typhimurium* strain for experiments in mice.

*aroA* mutants of *Salmonella* have been used as carriers by Clements *et al.* (1986) to study mucosal and serum antibody responses to both the carrier and LT-B following oral immunization; by Dougan *et al.* (1986) to construct an *aroA S. typhimurium* strain containing a plasmid which codes for the K88 fimbrial antigen of enterotoxigenic *E. coli;* by Maskell *et al.* (1986), who demonstrated that mucosal anti-LT-B IgA increased following immunization with a *S. typhimurium* derivative containing a plasmid coding for production of LT-B; and by Brown *et al.* (1987) to study antibody responses of mice to β-galactosidase (GZ) expressed in *S. typhimurium* strain SL3261.

Attenuated mutants of *Salmonella* have also been examined as carriers for anti-

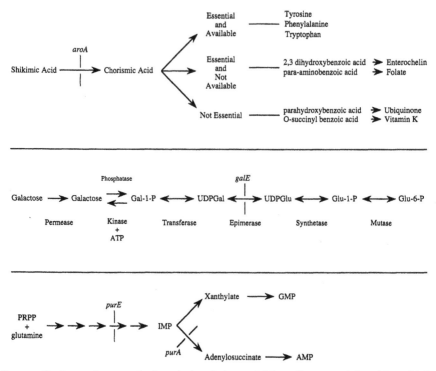

**FIGURE 2.** Attenuation strategies for reducing virulence of *Salmonella* vectors. Adapted from Cárdenas and Clements (1992, Fig. 2, p. 329; Fig. 3, p. 331; Fig. 4, p. 332).

gens of *Streptococcus mutans* in the development of a potential anticaries vaccine (Curtiss, 1986; Curtiss and Kelly, 1987; Curtiss *et al.*, 1987). These researchers have constructed a number of *S. typhimurium* and *S. typhi* strains possessing various deletion mutations and capable of expressing both surface protein antigen A (Spa A) and glucosyltransferase of *S. mutans*. Sadoff *et al.* (1988) reported the construction of a potential anti-malaria vaccine using a nonvirulent *S. typhimurium* strain as a carrier for a plasmid expressing a circumsporozoite protein of *Plasmodium berghei*. The number of reported uses of this system of antigen delivery for the development of both humoral and cell-mediated immunity increases daily. The examples cited are to give the reader an appreciation for the potential of this technique.

## II. USE OF ATTENUATED MUTANTS OF *SALMONELLA* AS VACCINE VECTORS

*Salmonella* becomes an attractive carrier when one considers the natural pathogenesis of the organism and the behavior of appropriately attenuated mutants, which can interact with the lymphoid tissues in Peyer's patches without causing systemic disease. In the context of the mucosal immune system, the immunologically relevant events occur within those Peyer's patches, not on the surface of mucosal epithelial cells. Consequently, live oral vaccines that colonize the proximal small-bowel epithelium (Kaper *et al.*, 1984; Levine *et al.*, 1988) or killed whole-cell vaccines administered with subunits of toxins that bind to the surface of epithelial cells (Clemens *et al.*, 1986; Svennerholm *et al.*, 1984) do not present antigens efficiently. They do work somewhat; efficacy rates of approximately 65% have been reported from the field trials on killed whole-cell cholera vaccines. However, antitoxic immunity was not a significant contributor to long-term ($>1$ year) protection in these studies and there was little or no heterologous protection. Use of *Salmonella* as a carrier allows the placement of appropriate antigens directly into the lymphoid follicles, permitting maximum stimulation of relevant lymphoid cells for production of IgA. This opens the possibility of vaccines which can invoke significant levels of mucosal antibodies beyond those achievable by other means.

This system has been characterized extensively using attenuated mutants of *Salmonella* as a carrier for a recombinant plasmid that codes for production of the B subunit of the heat-labile enterotoxin (LT-B) of *E. coli*. This information is summarized below. In addition, a number of related questions are addressed: (1) the effect of multiple genetic mutations on carrier efficacy, (2) the effect of repeated use on carrier efficacy, and (3) the effect of gene location on stability, expression, cellular location, and immunogenicity of cloned antigens. Data are also presented on the role of persistence, antigen dose, and strain viability in the use of *Salmonella* as a vaccine carrier.

## A. Construction of a Potential Live Oral Bivalent Vaccine for Typhoid Fever and Cholera–*Escherichia coli*-Related Diarrheas

One of the first reported uses of an avirulent *Salmonella* as a carrier for other antigens was by Formal *et al.* (1981). These researchers constructed a potential live oral bivalent vaccine for typhoid fever and shigellosis due to *Shigella sonnei*. The plasmid responsible for production of the form I antigen in *S. sonnei* was conjugally transferred to *S. typhi* Ty21a and recipient strains were shown to produce both form I antigen and normal *S. typhi* somatic antigens. These experiments suggested the possibility of developing a multivalent live oral vaccine that could provide protection against a number of bacterial enteric pathogens, specifically typhoid fever, shigellosis, and, if the appropriate antigens could be expressed in this system, cholera and the cholera-related enteropathies. To further explore this possibility, *S. typhi* Ty21a was utilized to construct a potential live oral vaccine for typhoid fever and the cholera–*E. coli*-related diarrheas (Clements and El-Morshidy, 1984). This study examined the development of antitoxin following immunization with *Salmonella* carrying a cholera-related toxoid antigen. *S. typhi* Ty21a was used as a recipient for a recombinant plasmid containing the gene for production of the nontoxic B subunit of the heat-labile enterotoxin of *E. coli* (LT-B). This protein shares extensive sequence and immunologic homology with the B subunit of the *V. cholerae* enterotoxin (CT-B). The *S. typhi* derivative was shown to contain the recombinant LT-B plasmid and produced LT-B that possessed no demonstrable biological activity and was structurally and immunologically indistinguishable from the LT-B produced by strains of *E. coli* harboring the same plasmid. The derivative strain was rapidly cleared after intraperitoneal injection into mice, caused no diarrhea or other manifestations when inoculated orally into guinea pigs, and retained the galactose sensitivity characteristic of the parent *S. typhi* strain Ty21a.

Since *S. typhi* is not a natural pathogen for animals other than humans, the ability of this strain, when delivered orally, to induce a specific mucosal antitoxin response cannot be tested except in human volunteers. A mouse invasive *aroA* mutant of *S. dublin* was obtained which was capable of producing a transient infection following oral inoculation of mice analogous to the events associated with oral inoculation of humans with Ty21a (Clements *et al.,* 1986). This provided a suitable model for testing this mechanism of antigen delivery as a means of stimulating significant levels of mucosal antibodies. The derivative strain, designated EL23, produced LT-B that was, by all criteria, identical to LT-B produced by *E. coli* or by the *S. typhi* derivative, and the relative distribution of LT-B produced by these different organisms was similar (94–99% remained cell associated).

A number of specific questions were then addressed relative to immunization schedules, the effect of boosting parenterally vice orally, the presence of mucosal memory, and the ability of mucosal antibodies derived by this method of immunization to neutralize the biological activity of the CT and LT *in vitro*. Initial priming studies comparing oral immunization with LT-B to oral immunization with strain EL23 showed that immunization with LT-B produces significantly higher levels of antitoxin serum IgG (Fig. 3A) and initially higher levels of antitoxin mucosal secretory IgA (Fig. 3B). The differences in IgA levels were no longer significant by the fifth week. Mice receiving strain EL23 orally also developed progressively increasing mucosal and serum antibody responses to the LPS of the vaccine strain (not shown). The effect of boosting mice primed orally with strain EL23 was also investigated, and boosting ip with LT-B gave the highest sustained levels of antitoxin serum IgG (Fig. 4A), while boosting ip or po with LT-B gave equivalent mucosal antitoxin IgA responses (Fig. 4B). The mucosal antibody response was also shown to be IgA specific and to be capable of neutralizing the biological activities of both LT and cholera toxin *in vitro* (Table I).

## B. Effect of Multiple Mutations on the Efficacy of *Salmonella* Vectors

In contrast to results obtained with *S. dublin aroA* mutants in mice, Levine *et al.* (1987b) reported that human vaccine recipients receiving *S. typhi* (*aroA, purA155, hisG* 46) mutants (Edwards and Stocker, 1988) developed low humoral responses

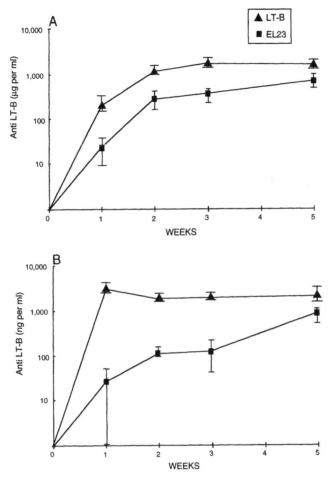

**FIGURE 3.** Serum IgG (A) and mucosal IgA (B) antitoxin responses following oral immunization with either LT-B or *S. dublin* strain EL23. Female BALB/c mice were immunized orally with two doses containing either 64 μg of LT-B or $10^{10}$ CFU each of strain EL23 on Days 0 and 4. Groups of animals were sacrificed at weekly intervals thereafter and analyzed for production of antibodies to LT-B. Serum and mucosal antitoxin levels were zero for control animals throughout the study. Each data point represents the mean of determinations in four to six animals. Standard error bars are shown. From Clements *et al.* (1986, Fig. 4, p. 689).

to the O polysaccharide of the vaccine strain. It is not clear why the *S. typhi* mutants were unable to induce a humoral response; this may have been due to the presence of two nonreverting auxotrophic characters in the *S. typhi* strains, as contrasted with single nonreverting auxotrophic characters in the studies employing *S. dublin* mutants in mice (Clements *et al.,* 1986), or to the single *purA* mutation not present in the oral mouse studies. Use of *Salmonella* as a carrier for delivery of heterologous antigens in humans will likely employ an attenuated *S.*

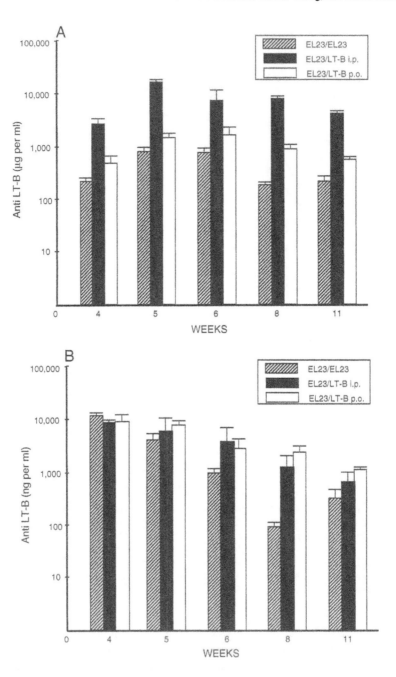

**FIGURE 4.** Serum IgG (A) and mucosal IgA (B) antitoxin responses following oral immunization with *S. dublin* strain EL23. Female BALB/c mice were immunized orally with two doses containing $10^{10}$ CFU each of strain EL23 on Days 0 and 4. At 21 days post-primary immunization, groups of

TABLE I

NEUTRALIZATION OF ADRENAL CELL ACTIVITY[a] OF CHOLERA AND
*E. COLI* ENTEROTOXINS[b,c]

| Antiserum | Cholera toxin | LT |
|---|---|---|
| Pooled mucosa | 128[d] | 256[c] |
| Pooled mucosa + | | |
| goat antiserum against mouse IgA | 6 | 32 |
| Pooled mucosa + | | |
| rabbit antiserum against mouse IgG | 128 | 256 |

[a] The adrenal cell assay was conducted using mouse Y-1 adrenal cells minicul-
ture.
[b] Approximately 10 minimal rounding doses were used.
[c] From Clements *et al.* (1986, Table 2, p. 691).
[d] Reciprocal of highest serum dilution showing complete neutralization of biological activity. Pooled mucosa from control animals had no effect.

*typhi,* perhaps one derived as above. It was therefore of interest to determine if
the failure to induce a humoral response noted above was a function of the double
mutation or of either single mutation. To accomplish this, three strains of *S. dublin*
containing an *aroA* mutation, a *purA* mutation, or both *aroA* and *purA* mutations
were examined for the ability to colonize, invade, persist in tissues, and evoke
serum and mucosal antibody responses to the lipopolysaccharide of the parent
strain following oral feeding of mice (Sigwart *et al.,* 1989). The organisms used
for this study were nalidixic acid-resistant derivatives of *S. dublin* strain SL5608
(wild type) and included *S. dublin* strain SL7163 (*aroA*148), *S. dublin* strain
SL7165 (*purA*155), and *S. dublin* strain SL7164 (*aroA*148, *purA*155). These three
nalidixate resistant auxotrophic strains are referred to below just as *aroA, purA,*
and *aroA purA* instead of by their strain numbers.

## 1. Colonization, Invasion, and Persistence in Mouse Tissues
As shown in Table II, there was evidence for colonization of the small intestines,
invasion, and persistence in mouse tissues only with *aroA,* which was isolated
from the small intestines, Peyer's patches, livers, and spleens of animals up
through the third day postinoculation. Thereafter, only the livers and, beginning at
Day 8 postinoculation, the small intestines were infected. *aroA* could be isolated

animals were boosted with $10^{10}$ CFU of EL23, 100 $\mu$g of LT-B given ip, or 100 $\mu$g of LT-B given po.
Groups of animals were sacrificed at weekly intervals thereafter and analyzed for production of antibodies to LT-B by ELISA. Values shown begin at Week 4 post-primary immunization (i.e., 1 week
following booster immunizations). Serum and mucosal antitoxin levels were zero for control animals
throughout the study. Each data point represents the mean of determinations in four to six animals.
Standard error bars are shown. From Clements *et al.* (1986, Fig. 5, p. 690).

TABLE II

TABLE II

COLONIZATION, INVASION, AND PERSISTENCE IN MOUSE TISSUES[a]

| | Day 1[b] | Day 3 | Day 7 | Day 8 | Day 14 | Day 21 | Total |
|---|---|---|---|---|---|---|---|
| | | | aroA | | | | |
| Small intestine | 3/3 | 3/3 | 0/3 | 1/3 | 1/3 | 1/5 | 9/20 |
| Peyer's patches | 3/3 | 2/3 | 0/3 | 0/3 | 0/3 | 0/5 | 5/20 |
| Liver | 2/3 | 1/3 | 1/3 | 1/3 | 1/3 | 1/5 | 7/20 |
| Spleen | 1/3 | 1/3 | 0/3 | 0/3 | 0/3 | 0/5 | 2/20 |
| Blood | 0/3 | 1/3 | 0/3 | 0/3 | 0/3 | 0/5 | 1/20 |
| | | | purA | | | | |
| Small intestine | 1/3 | 0/3 | 0/3 | 0/3 | 0/3 | 0/4 | 1/19 |
| Peyer's patches | 0/3 | 0/3 | 0/3 | 0/3 | 0/3 | 0/4 | 0/19 |
| Liver | 1/3 | 0/3 | 0/3 | 0/3 | 0/3 | 0/4 | 1/19 |
| Spleen | 0/3 | 0/3 | 0/3 | 0/3 | 0/3 | 0/4 | 0/19 |
| Blood | 1/3 | 0/3 | 0/3 | 0/3 | 0/3 | 0/4 | 1/19 |
| | | | aroA purA | | | | |
| Small intestine | 0/3 | 0/3 | 0/3 | 0/3 | 0/3 | 0/4 | 0/19 |
| Peyer's patches | 1/3 | 0/3 | 0/3 | 0/3 | 0/3 | 0/4 | 1/19 |
| Liver | 0/3 | 0/3 | 0/3 | 0/3 | 0/3 | 0/4 | 0/19 |
| Spleen | 0/3 | 0/3 | 0/3 | 0/3 | 0/3 | 0/4 | 0/19 |
| Blood | 0/3 | 0/3 | 0/3 | 0/3 | 0/3 | 0/4 | 0/19 |

[a]From Sigwart et al. (1989, Table 2, p. 1859).
[b]Number of specimens culture positive/number tested.

only from the blood of one animal on 1 day (Day 3 postinoculation). Of the 20 animals immunized in this group, aroA was isolated from the small intestines of 9, from the Peyer's patches of 5, from the livers of 7, from the spleens of 2, and from the blood of 1. purA was isolated from the small intestine, liver, and blood of only a single animal, and then only on the first day postinoculation. Thereafter, purA was not detected in any tissue throughout the 21 days of the study. Similarly, aroA purA was isolated from the Peyer's patches of a single animal at 1 day postinoculation and not subsequently detected in any tissue throughout the 21 days of the study.

## 2. Humoral Response Following Immunization with the Attenuated Mutants

A major consideration in the selection of an appropriate live-vaccine or carrier organism is the ability of that organism to evoke an appropriate immunologic response. As an indicator of that response, we examined the serum IgG and mucosal IgA responses against the lipopolysaccharide (LPS) of the parent S. dublin strain, SL5608. Mice immunized orally with aroA, purA, and aroA purA developed serum anti-LPS antibodies and maintained them throughout the course of the experiment, 5 weeks post-primary inoculation (Table III). There was, however, great variability between individual animals in all groups; statistical differences between immunized groups and control values from unimmunized animals were not consistent at 1, 2, or 3 weeks following the primary inoculation. By the end of the 5th week, serum anti-LPS IgG had increased from 0 to 14.1 $\mu$g/ml in animals immunized with *aroA*, a value significantly greater than that obtained following immunization with either *purA* (2.89 $\mu$g/ml) or *aroA purA* (2.37 $\mu$g/ml). Also seen in Table III, mucosal anti-LPS IgA was consistently significantly higher in animals immunized with *aroA* than in the other two groups. By the end of the fifth week, mucosal anti-LPS IgA had increased to 27.3 ng/ml in animals immunized with *aroA*, had increased to 1.36 ng/ml in animals immunized with *purA*, and had increased to 0.97 ng/ml in animals immunized with *aroA purA*.

These studies demonstrated that, of the three strains tested, only SL7163, with the single *aroA* mutation, was able to colonize significantly, invade, and persist in tissues. More importantly, this strain was shown to consistently evoke appropriate serum and mucosal antibody responses. Neither the *purA* nor the *aroA purA* mutant demonstrated these characteristics. It is not known if the presence or lack of observed statistical significance, as determined by the Student *t* test, during the 5 weeks of the experiment, correlates with biological significance. Clearly, immunization with SL7163, with the single *aroA* mutation, was more effective at eliciting appropriate antibody responses, especially at the mucosal surface. These observations suggested that the *purA* defect, causing adenine requirement, reduces the live-vaccine efficacy of attenuated *Salmonella*. The impact on the effectiveness of *Salmonella* as a carrier of heterologous antigens is not known.

## C. Effect of Multiple Use on Carrier Efficacy

A major consideration in the proposed use of *Salmonella* as a carrier for heterologous antigens is the consequence of repeated use of the carrier. Specifically, if *Salmonella* is used as a carrier for one antigen, will it be an effective vehicle for

TABLE III

SERUM AND MUCOSAL ANTI-LPS RESPONSES[a]

|  | Week 1 | Week 2 | Week 3 | Week 4 | Week 5 |
|---|---|---|---|---|---|
|  | IgG[b] ($\mu$g/ml) | | | | |
| *aroA* | 1.32 ± 0.30 | 4.83 ± 0.73 | 7.71 ± 2.78 | 7.66 ± 2.00 | 14.1 ± 4.21 |
| *purA* | 0.47 ± 0.25 | 0.85 ± 0.25 | 2.80 ± 1.95 | 0.58 ± 0.22 | 2.89 ± 2.17 |
| *aroA purA* | 8.05 ± 6.6 | 5.35 ± 3.31 | 5.00 ± 1.44 | 1.32 ± 0.91 | 2.37 ± 0.82 |
|  | IgA[c] (ng/ml) | | | | |
| *aroA* | 2.78 ± 0.72 | 45.29 ± 12.72 | 15.28 ± 2.75 | 26.45 ± 7.04 | 27.3 ± 5.19 |
| *purA* | 0.57 ± 0.19 | 1.41 ± 0.17 | 0.40 ± 0.19 | 0.17 ± 0.07 | 1.36 ± 0.85 |
| *aroA purA* | 1.08 ± 0.73 | 0.14 ± 0.05 | 0.39 ± 0.16 | 0.21 ± 0.09 | 0.97 ± 0.75 |

[a]From Sigwart *et al.* (1989, Table 3, p. 1860).
[b]Mean ± S.E.M. as determined by ELISA.
[c]Mean ± S.E.M. as determined by ELISA.

delivery of other antigens? Does prior experience with the carrier limit the immunologic response to a heterologous antigen? Can *Salmonella* be used as a carrier for antigens of enteric bacterial pathogens and then subsequently for caries or malaria? A number of unresolved questions about this system were examined including (i) the nature of the humoral response if two strains of *Salmonella* are employed which are serologically identical or which are serologically different, (ii) the temporal relationship of priming and boosting doses on the subsequent immunological response to the carrier and the foreign antigen, and (iii) differences in serum IgG and mucosal IgA responses between immunologically experienced and immunologically naive animals (Bao and Clements, 1991).

For these studies, groups of mice were orally immunized (primed) with either one or the other of two aromatic dependent mutants of *Salmonella (S. dublin* SL1438 *aro his* or *S. typhimurium* SL1479 *aro his).* These strains were chosen because (i) they are immunologically related but not identical with respect to the O antigen, (ii) the wild-type parents of both strains are pathogens for the mouse and attenuated mutants of both have been shown to be effective carriers of foreign antigens in this model system, and (iii) both strains have been attenuated with an equivalent *aroA* deletion. Animals were then boosted orally with *S. dublin* strain EL23. This strain is the same *S. dublin* SL1438 used above following transformation with a plasmid that codes for production of a foreign antigen. For these studies, the foreign antigen was the B subunit of the heat-labile enterotoxin (LT-B) of *E. coli* since, as mentioned above, antibodies directed against this protein are potentially useful in ameliorating secretory diarrheal disease due to cholera related enterotoxins. *S. dublin* strain EL23 was administered orally by gavage at 2 weeks, 6 weeks, or 9 weeks after the primary immunization. Animals were sacrificed 3 weeks following the boost and assayed for the presence of serum IgG and mucosal IgA directed against the foreign antigen (LT-B) by ELISA. Comparisons were then made between experimental and control groups to determine differences in serum and mucosal antibody responses between animals primed with either the homologous (SL1438) or heterologous (SL1479) strain and boosted with EL23.

As shown in Fig. 5, control animals developed a mean serum anti-LT-B specific IgG response of 29.6 $\mu$g/ml when immunized orally with EL23 with no priming dose. By contrast, mice with prior immunologic experience with a homologous *Salmonella* strain, those having received a primary oral immunization with strain SL1438 2 weeks before administration of EL23, developed a significantly higher mean serum anti-LT-B IgG response following the administration of the boosting dose of EL23. Animals receiving the boosting dose of EL23 at either 6 or 9 weeks post-primary immunization developed significantly higher levels of serum anti-LT-B IgG than did control animals or animals boosted orally with EL23 at 2 weeks post-primary immunization. Mice primed with the heterologous serotype strain, SL1479, also developed significantly higher levels of serum anti-LT-B at all three time points when compared to immunologically naive control mice.

One of the principal advantages of *Salmonella* as a vaccine vector is the poten-

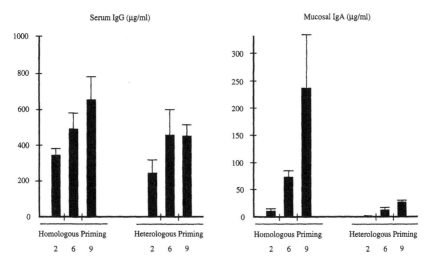

**FIGURE 5.** Effect of primary immunization with homologous or heterologous serotype strains on production of serum IgG and mucosal IgA directed against foreign antigens. Female BALB/c mice having no prior immunological experience with *Salmonella* were primed orally either with *Salmonella* SL1438 or with *Salmonella* SL1479, and then boosted orally with EL23 at 2, 6, or 9 weeks post-primary immunization. Animals were sacrificed 3 weeks following the boost and assayed for the presence of serum IgG and mucosal IGA directed against LT-B by ELISA. Each data point represents the mean of determinations in five to six animals. Standard error bars are shown. Adapted from Bao and Clements (1991, Fig. 1, p. 3842; Fig. 2, p. 3843).

tial to elicit production of significant levels of mucosal IgA directed against a target antigen. It was therefore of interest to determine the ability of animals with prior immunologic experience against the vector, or an immunologically related species, to mount a mucosal IgA response against the target antigen. As shown in Fig. 5, animals with prior immunologic experience with the carrier demonstrated increases in mucosal anti-LT-B specific IgA levels when compared to the levels observed in control groups. The values obtained for the 6- and 9-week groups were statistically significantly different than values obtained for the control and 2-week groups. Mucosal anti-LT-B specific IgA was also determined in groups of animals primed with the heterologous serotype strain and anti-LT-B specific IgA also increased at each of the three boosted time points. The values for animals boosted at 2, 6, or 9 weeks were significantly higher than those values obtained from control animals receiving EL23 only. The 6- and 9-week group values were significantly higher than those of the 2-week or control groups. However, in contrast to the results obtained for serum anti-LT-B IgG, the mucosal anti-LT-B IgA response following experience with a homologous strain was significantly higher than the response obtained following experience with a heterologous strain at all three time points.

These observations demonstrate that prior immunologic experience with a homologous serotype strain of *Salmonella* potentiates the subsequent antibody response when the same strain is used as a carrier of foreign antigens. Both serum and mucosal antibody responses increased over time. Prior immunologic experience with a heterologous serotype of *Salmonella* also potentiates the subsequent serum and mucosal antibody responses directed against the foreign antigen when compared to responses in unprimed control animals. Serum antibody responses in animals primed with either the homologous or the heterologous serotype strain were not statistically significantly different, while animals primed with the homologous serotype strain developed significantly higher mucosal antibody responses against the foreign antigen. These findings demonstrate that prior immunologic experience with *Salmonella* as a vaccine against typhoid fever or as a carrier for one foreign antigen will not preclude its subsequent use as a carrier for antigens of other pathogens. Prior immunologic experience with one strain does not limit the immunologic response to a foreign antigen delivered by the same strain or a second immunologically related strain. In fact, prior immunologic experience with *Salmonella* increases the subsequent humoral response to a foreign antigen when compared to the response seen in animals having no prior experience with the organisms.

### D. Effect of the Nature and Degree of Bacterial Attenuation on the Humoral Immune Response Directed against Foreign Antigens

Overlying the studies on the efficacy of *Salmonella* as a carrier are the studies on alternatives to *S. typhi* Ty21a as a live oral anti-typhoid vaccine. Despite the safety and efficacy of Ty21a, it is not without problems. The organism is difficult to grow and must be given on multiple occasions to be effective, and the nature of the attenuation is not well defined. A number of new candidate anti-typhoid vaccines have been constructed using molecular technologies to create specific, defined mutations. The first of two such strains tested in volunteers (Levine *et al.*, 1987b) each had an *aroA* deletion, expected by itself to cause complete loss of virulence, and as an additional safety factor, a deletion at *purA* (Edwards and Stocker, 1988). Unlike mice given an $\Delta aroA$ mutant of *S. dublin* orally (Sigwart *et al.*, 1989) volunteers who received an oral dose of even $10^{10}$ CFU of either of the two $\Delta aroA$ $\Delta purA$ live vaccine strains, 541Ty (Vi-positive) or 543Ty (Vi-negative), developed no or only very low titers of humoral antibody to the 0 antigen of the vaccine strain and were not colonized by the organisms. More recently, other strains harboring mutations affecting the metabolism of aromatic compounds have been examined. Mutations in *aroC* and *aroD* were associated with reduced virulence of *S. typhi* for humans (Tacket *et al.*, 1992). One strain examined, CVD908, is an *aroC aroD* mutant of *S. typhi* Ty2, and produced no adverse reactions in volunteers receiving up to $5 \times 10^7$ CFU orally. In addition, a single oral dose of $5 \times 10^7$ CFU of CVD908 induced seroconversion in 50% of recipients. Other genetically attenuated mutants of *S. typhi* have also been examined in humans, including CVD906, an *aroC aroD* mutant of *S. typhi* ISPI820, and χ3927, a *cya crp* mutant of Ty2. These latter two strains were shown to cause fevers or vaccine bacteremia in volunteers at relatively low doses.

We evaluated two different attenuated mutants of *S. typhi* for use as vaccine carriers: 543Ty *aroA purA* and 659Ty *aroA aroD*. We transformed each of these strains with plasmid pJC217 (Clements and El-Morshidy, 1984) which codes for production of LT-B and each was fed orally to mice. For this experiment, groups containing 6 BALB/c mice each were immunized orally with $1 \times 10^{10}$ of one or another of these strains on two separate occasions (Days 0 and 4). This regimen was repeated for each animal at 21 and 25 days post-primary immunization. Animals were sacrificed 2 weeks after the final dose. Two control preparations were included in this study: EL23 which is an *aroA S. dublin* transformed with plasmid pJC217, and SE12 which is *S. typhi* Ty21a transformed with the same plasmid. In previous studies, we had demonstrated that EL23 was an effective carrier in mice and had demonstrated that SE12 gave little or no response when fed orally to mice. Our presumption was that the failure of the Ty21a derivative was a reflection of the noted species restriction. However, as shown in Table IV, animals immunized orally with *S. typhi* strains 543Ty(pJC217) and 659Ty(pJC217) developed significant serum and mucosal antibody responses against the foreign antigen. The serum anti-LT-B responses developed following oral immunization with 543Ty(pJC217) and 659Ty(pJC217) were significant, although lower than those developed following oral immunization with strain EL23. By contrast, the differences in mucosal IgA anti-LT-B levels in mice receiving 543Ty(pJC217) and 659Ty(pJC217) were not statistically different than those developed in response to oral immunization with EL23. Mice immunized orally with strain SE12 developed only a marginal serum IgG response and no detectable mucosal IgA response against LT-B.

If host-adaptation is not, a priori, a requirement for an organism to be an efficient carrier, the next obvious question has to do with viability of the carrier strain. In our evolving hypothesis, the nature of the array of antigens present on the bacterial cell surface at the time of oral inoculation would be the most important determinant of carrier efficacy. It may not, in fact, be necessary or desirable for

*TABLE IV*

HUMORAL RESPONSE FOLLOWING IMMUNIZATION WITH DIFFERENT SPECIES OF *SALMONELLA* VARYING IN THE NATURE AND DEGREE OF BACTERIAL ATTENUATION[a]

| Anti-LT-B[a] | S. dublin EL23 | S. typhi 543Ty(pJC217) | S. typhi 659Ty(pJC217) | S. typhi SE12 |
|---|---|---|---|---|
| Serum IgG | 697 ± 180 μg/ml | 152 ± 85 μg/ml | 224 ± 33 μg/ml | 10 ± 3 μg/ml |
| Mucosal IgA | 511 ± 128 ng/ml | 386 ± 187 ng/ml | 306 ± 82 ng/ml | None detected |

[a] From Cárdenas *et al.* (1994, Table 1, p. 836).

the carrier to be viable as long as any necessary bacterial attachment and uptake factors are maintained. It is now accepted that oral, killed typhoid vaccines are not effective at inducing protective anti-typhoid immunity. At this point, it was not known if oral killed *Salmonella* could function as an effective carrier of other antigens to the mucosal immune system. In order to test this hypothesis, we immunized groups of mice with viable and nonviable preparations of EL23 (Cárdenas and Clements, 1993b). Two groups of BALB/c mice consisting of five mice each were immunized with an equal number of organisms harvested from TSA plates. One group received organisms that had been killed by exposure to UV irradiation after overnight growth. The number of viable organisms following treatment was reduced to less than $10^3$ cfu/ml as determined by plate counts. We have previously determined that the minimum number of organisms of this strain necessary to produce an immune response against LT-B in these animals is between $10^9$ and $10^{10}$. Consequently, animals in this group received the same number of total organisms ($10^{10}$), but between six and seven logs fewer viable organisms than required to induce a humoral response. UV killing was chosen as a means of reducing viability while preserving surface structures on the bacteria. Animals were boosted at 21 and 25 days post-primary immunization. As shown in Table V, animals immunized orally with viable EL23 developed serum IgG and mucosal IgA anti-LT-B responses consistent with our previous findings. Significantly, mice immunized orally with UV-killed EL23 developed serum IgG and mucosal IgA antibody responses equivalent to those developed in animals orally immunized with the same number of viable EL23.

We next extended these observations and examined other methods of killing the organisms that may also preserve the ability of these strains to function as carriers. Specifically, EL23 was killed with acetone, ethanol, heat, or formalin and mice were immunized orally as above. As shown in Fig. 6, EL23 rendered nonviable by a variety of chemical means retained the ability to elicit serum and mucosal antibody responses against a foreign antigen. The serum IgG anti-LT-B responses following oral immunization with heat, ethanol, or acetone-killed EL23 were statistically equivalent to one another and also to the serum IgG anti-LT-B response following oral immunization with viable EL23. Likewise, the mucosal IgA anti-LT-B response following oral immunization with heat, ethanol, or acetone-killed

TABLE V

HUMORAL RESPONSE FOLLOWING IMMUNIZATION WITH VIABLE
AND UV-KILLED SALMONELLA[a]

| Anti-LT-B[a] | S. dublin EL23 | S. dublin EL23 (UV-killed) |
|---|---|---|
| Serum IgG | 450 ± 79 μg/ml | 863 ± 356 μg/ml |
| Mucosal IgA | 1676 ± 280 ng/ml | 3064 ± 1320 ng/ml |

[a]From Cárdenas et al. (1994, Table 2, p. 837).

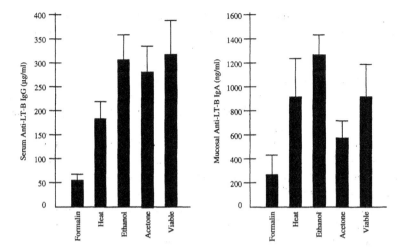

**FIGURE 6.** The effect of strain viability on the humoral response directed against foreign antigens. *S. dublin* EL23 was killed with acetone, ethanol, heat, or formalin. Groups of Balb/c mice were immunized orally with $1 \times 10^{10}$ CFU of one or another of these strains on two separate occasions (Days 0 and 4). This regimen was repeated for each animal at 21 and 25 days post-primary immunization. Animals were sacrificed approximately 2 weeks after the final dose. EL23 rendered nonviable by a variety of chemical means retained the ability to elicit serum and mucosal antibody responses against the foreign antigen. Results are presented from groups containing four or five mice each and from two independent experiments. The standard error of the mean was calculated for all data, and means of variously immunized groups were compared by the Student $t$ test. Statistical significance was considered to be $P \le 0.05$. From Cárdenas *et al.* (1994, Fig. 1, p. 837).

EL23 were statistically equivalent to one another and also to the mucosal IgA anti-LT-B responses following oral immunization with viable EL23. In this study, only formalin-killed EL23 were unable to elicit serum or mucosal antibody responses equivalent to those obtained with viable EL23. The serum IgG anti-LT-B and mucosal IgA anti-LT-B responses following oral immunization with formalin-killed EL23 were statistically significantly lower than levels obtained with all other immunization regimens.

## F. Viability and Antigen Dose as Determinants of the Humoral Immune Response Directed against Foreign Antigens

To address the question of the importance of antigen dose, we prepared three different strains of *galE S. typhimurium* J706 expressing markedly different levels of LT-B (Cárdenas *et al.,* 1994). These strains were designated J1000 (a J706 derivative with a single copy of the LT-B gene on the chromosome utilizing the *lac* promoter), J706(pDF87) (intermediate copy number, pBR322 based LT-B plasmid utilizing the pBR322 *tet* promoter), and J706(pJC217) (high copy number pUC based LT-B plasmid utilizing the *lac* promoter). *S. typhimurium* J706 served as a negative control for these studies. This scheme has a number of features upon which we were able to capitalize. The chromosomal gene in J1000 is a stable integrate that constitutively expresses low but consistent levels of LT-B. The two plasmid-containing strains express higher levels of antigen, but recombinant plasmids are not stable in these constructs. For instance, after overnight growth in TSB, >90% of recovered isolates have lost pUC-based plasmids that code for production of LT-B, even when the strain is grown in the presence of the stabilizing antibiotic (unpublished observation). Since >95% of LT-B is synthesized during the first 8 hr of growth *in vitro,* the majority of these organisms deliver antigen to the GALT but do not synthesize antigen *in situ.* This is analogous to the nonviable organism question with respect to *de novo* synthesis of antigen. For this experiment, groups of BALB/c mice consisting of four mice each were immunized orally with $1 \times 10^{10}$ of one or another of these strains on two separate occasions as indicated above. Three weeks post-primary immunization, mice were sacrificed and examined for serum and mucosal antibodies directed against LT-B by ELISA.

As shown in Fig. 7, mice developed increasing serum and mucosal anti-LT-B responses that correlated with the amount of antigen present within the organisms at the time of immunization. Since all of these strains persist to the same extent (Hone *et al.,* 1989; Sigwart *et al.,* 1989) these findings provide clear evidence that there is a minimum threshold below which significant levels of antibody are not elicited and that persistence does not play a major role in eliciting antibody against the foreign antigen.

In the above studies on the effect of strain viability on the humoral immune response we demonstrated that appropriately prepared nonviable organisms are as effective as viable organisms in eliciting *humoral* immune responses against a foreign antigen. This is clearly a controversial finding and needs to be explored more fully. Viable *Salmonella* that persist within macrophages do not effectively contribute to the host humoral response, especially in the GALT. Within this context, the *Salmonella* must first be taken up by an appropriate antigen presenting cell (APC), killed, and lysed within the phagolysosome, and its antigens processed and exported to the surface of the APC for presentation in context with MHC. As long as the bacterium is viable, antigen not displayed on the surface of the organism or secreted by the organism is not available to the APC and, consequently, not available for immune stimulation. Moreover, viable organisms only remain within the Peyer's patches and mesenteric lymph nodes for a short period of time and these lymphoid tissues are the IgA inductive sites, not the liver and spleen where the organisms eventually persist. In circumstances where induction of an IgA response is an important consideration, the Peyer's patches and mesenteric lymph nodes would be the most relevant sites for antigen presentation. Rendering the organisms nonviable prior to oral administration facilitates antigen processing by the APC in the GALT. It is clear, however, that not all methods of killing are equivalent in terms of preserving the ability of these strains to function as carriers.

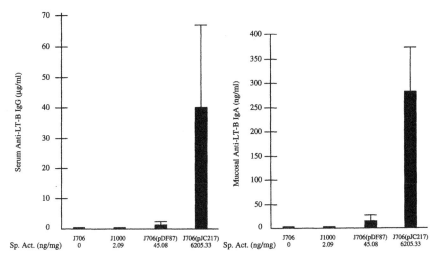

**FIGURE 7.** Effect of varying the antigen dose on the humoral immune response directed against foreign antigens. Groups consisting of four Balb/c mice each were immunized orally with $1 \times 10^{10}$ CFU of one or another of three different strains of *galE S. typhimurium* J706 expressing markedly different levels of LT-B. Expression was quantitated using purified LT-B as a standard and is expressed in terms of specific activity as ng LT-B (based on ELISA) per milligram total protein. Mice were immunized on two separate occasions (Days 0 and 4) and were sacrificed 3 weeks post-primary immunization. *S. typhimurium* J706 served as a negative control for these studies. Mice developed increasing serum and mucosal anti-LT-B responses that correlated with the amount of antigen present within the organisms at the time of immunization. The standard error of the mean was calculated for all data, and means of variously immunized groups were compared by the Student *t* test. Statistical significance was considered to be $P \leq 0.05$. From Cárdenas *et al.* (1994, Fig. 2, p. 838).

Formalin-killed organisms were not as effective as delivery vehicles as were organisms killed by other methods.

The use of nonviable *Salmonella* as carriers for delivery of antigens to the mucosal lymphoid tissues is analogous to the use of liposomes and microspheres for oral antigen delivery. Eldridge *et al.* (1989) demonstrated that biodegradable microspheres containing bacterial antigens were efficiently internalized by M cells and that mice receiving such antigen carrier preparation showed a rise in antigen specific antibodies. If one views killed *Salmonella* as "formerly-viable microspheres," it is logical that they, too, would be efficient delivery vehicles. Two additional points should be noted. The first is that these observations were made using LT-B, which is immunologically and structurally related to cholera toxin B subunit. Both of these molecules are highly immunogenic oral antigens even when delivered as soluble proteins without encapsulation. How broadly our findings apply to other proteins is not yet known. The second point is that we have only determined the ability of these strains to induce humoral immunity; the influence of persistence, viability, and antigen dose on development of cellular immunity is not clear.

The issue of strain viability is one of great concern. Attenuated *Salmonella* have been proposed as carriers for a variety of antigens of eukaryotic, prokaryotic, and viral origin. Certainly, there is great potential benefit if such vaccines can be made safe and effective. However, there is a high risk–benefit ratio associated with administration of a gram-negative organism that causes bacteremia and persists in tissues for extended periods of time, especially in vaccines intended for administration to children, potentially immunosuppressed individuals, or individuals in developing countries where nutrition is not optimum and infectious disease rates are high. Our findings indicate that viability is not a requirement for use of a *Salmonella* strain as a carrier. If this proves to be true in humans as well as in animals, then the approach to carrier selection and safety will change dramatically. Even the most promising alternatives to Ty21a as a live oral anti-typhoid vaccine may cause vaccine bacteremia when administered in doses above $5 \times 10^7$. It is not known if these or other strains will be efficient carriers of heterologous antigens at the relatively low level shown to be completely safe. Our own evidence would indicate that bacteremia and persistence in tissues is not necessary for oral immunization and it may therefore be best to dissociate the question of what makes the best alternative to Ty21a as a live oral anti-typhoid vaccine from the question of what makes a good carrier for heterologous antigens.

## III. Differential Production of IL-12 mRNA by Murine Macrophages in Response to Viable or Killed *Salmonella* spp.

In humans, immunologic protection against typhoid fever, caused by *Salmonella* spp., can be achieved by parenteral immunization with acetone-killed whole cells (Ashcroft *et al.*, 1964) or purified capsular polysaccharide (Robbins and Robbins, 1984). Protection following oral immunization can be achieved with live-attenuated vaccines such as *S. typhi* Ty21a (Germanier and Fürer, 1971, 1975; Levine *et al.*, 1987a; Wahdan *et al.*, 1980). However, killed oral typhoid vaccines are not effective at inducing protective anti-typhoid immunity (Chuttani *et al.*, 1973, 1977). The reason for this difference in the ability of orally administered viable or killed organisms to elicit a protective response against typhoid fever is not known. A reasonable hypothesis is that viable organisms are able to induce some immune function related to T-cell regulation, presumably cell-mediated immunity, not induced by orally administered killed organisms.

T-helper-cell responses are divided into two classifications, Th1 and Th2, which are able to regulate the type of immune response and are characterized by the profile of cytokines secreted (Mosmann *et al.*, 1986; Mosmann and Coffman, 1989). Th1 cells secrete IFN$\gamma$, IL-2, and TNF$\beta$, which provide help for cell-mediated immunity. Th2 cells secrete IL-4, IL-5, IL-6, IL-10, and IL-13 which support the humoral arm of the immune response. Recent evidence indicates a central role for IL-12 in protection against a variety of bacterial and parasitic diseases, based upon the ability of IL-12 to promote the development of Th1 cells from Th0 cells (Hsieh *et al.*, 1993). Since *Salmonella* is a facultative intracellular pathogen, protection against typhoid fever may require development of a predominantly Th1 response related to induction of IL-12. We employed a murine model of salmonellosis to investigate the role of IL-12 in the protection derived from oral immunization with viable organisms (Chong *et al.*, 1996).

## A. Survival of BALB/c Mice Immunized with Viable Attenuated or Killed *Salmonella*

To investigate in an experimental animal model whether viability of the vaccine strain is important for protection against challenge with wild-type *Salmonella*, groups of BALB/c mice were orally immunized with $1 \times 10^{10}$ viable or killed *S. dublin* SL1438 (a nonreverting aromatic-dependent histidine requiring mutant) and subsequently challenged with $1 \times 10^7$ wild-type parent *S. dublin* SL1363 (approximately 100 $LD_{50}$). Groups of mice were orally immunized on Day 0 and Day 7, then challenged with SL1363 on Day 14. By Day 6 postchallenge, all mice immunized with killed SL1438 were moribund with ruffled fur whereas all mice immunized with viable SL1438 were healthy. By Day 9 postchallenge, 6 of 10 mice immunized with killed SL1438 were dead, and the remainder were near death and were sacrificed. In contrast, all mice immunized with viable SL1438 remained healthy. Therefore, mice immunized with viable SL1438 were protected against challenge with wild-type SL1363 whereas those immunized with killed SL1438 were not (Table VI).

## B. Differential Production of IL-12 p40 mRNA by Macrophages from BALB/c Mice

To investigate the cellular basis for immunologic protection against challenge with SL1363, IL-12 p40 mRNA production by macrophages from BALB/c mice was

*TABLE VI*

SURVIVAL OF BALB/c MICE IMMUNIZED WITH VIABLE
ATTENUATED OR KILLED *SALMONELLA*

| Immunogen[a] | No. dead/total[b] | % Survival |
|---|---|---|
| Viable SL1438 | 0/10 | 100 |
| Killed SL1438 | 10/10 | 0 |

[a]Mice were immunized orally with doses containing $1 \times 10^{10}$ CFU each of either viable or ethanol-killed SL1438 on Days 0 and 7. Mice were then challenged orally with $1 \times 10^7$ SL1363 on Day 14.

[b]Day 9 postchallenge. By Day 9 postchallenge, 6 of 10 mice immunized with killed SL1438 were dead; the remainder were near death and were sacrificed. In contrast, all mice immunized with viable SL1438 remained healthy.

examined. Elicited peritoneal macrophages were infected *in vitro* with either viable or killed SL1438; 4 hr postinfection, total RNA was extracted and reverse-transcribed, and the levels of IL-12 p40 mRNA were assessed by PCR. As shown in Fig. 8, macrophages infected with viable SL1438 (V) produced higher amounts of IL-12 p40 mRNA than did macrophages infected with killed SL1438 (K). As a control, macrophages were treated with either LPS or complete medium (Ø).

### C. Differential Production of IL-12 p40 mRNA by Macrophages from C3H Mice 4 hr Postinfection

Since LPS is able to induce the expression of IL-12 from macrophages, it was necessary to determine whether the production of IL-12 p40 mRNA was an LPS-related event or truly a function of strain viability. For this study, mice from the C3H lineage were utilized. C3H/HeN (Lps$^n$) and C3H/HeJ (Lps$^d$) are isogenic except for the Lps allele (Watson *et al.,* 1977, 1978). Elicited peritoneal macrophages from either C3H/HeN (Fig. 9A) or C3H/HeJ (Fig. 9B) mice were infected *in vitro* with either viable or killed SL1438 and 4 hr postinfection total RNA was extracted and reverse-transcribed, and the levels of IL-12 p40 mRNA were assessed by PCR. Macrophages from both strains of mice infected with viable SL1438 (V) produced higher amounts of IL-12 p40 mRNA than did macrophages infected with killed SL1438 (K). PCR products for glyceraldehyde 3-phosphate dehydrogenase (G3PDH) revealed similar efficiencies of reverse transcription and equal amounts of input cDNA between samples. Since macrophages from both LPS-sensitive and LPS-resistant animals produced IL-12 p40 mRNA in response to both viable and killed *Salmonella,* it is unlikely that the observed response is solely an LPS-mediated event.

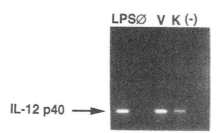

**FIGURE 8.** Induction of IL-12 p40 mRNA by macrophages from BALB/c mice 4 hr following exposure to viable attenuated or killed *Salmonella.* Peritoneal macrophages from BALB/c mice were incubated with LPS, complete medium (Ø) or viable (V) or ethanol-killed (K) SL1438 at a multiplicity of infection of 1:1 for 60 min. The macrophages were washed three times with PBS to remove extracellular bacteria and further incubated in complete medium containing gentamycin to kill any remaining extracellular bacteria. At 4 hr, total RNA was isolated from macrophages and reverse-transcribed, and cDNA from each sample was subjected to PCR for determination of IL-12 p40 mRNA. From Chong *et al.* (1996, Fig. 1, p. 1156).

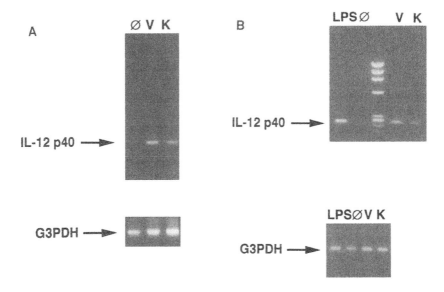

**FIGURE 9.** Induction of IL-12 p40 mRNA by macrophages from C3H mice 4hr following exposure to viable attenuated or killed *Salmonella*. Peritoneal macrophages from C3H/HeN (A) or C3H/HeJ (B) mice were incubated with LPS, complete medium (Ø) or viable (V) or ethanol-killed (K) SL1438 at a multiplicity of infection of 1:1 for 60 min. The macrophages were washed three times with PBS to remove extracellular bacteria and further incubated in complete medium containing gentamycin to kill any remaining extracellular bacteria. At 4 hr, total RNA was isolated from macrophages and reverse-transcribed, and cDNA from each sample was subjected to PCR for determination of IL-12 p40 mRNA. cDNA from each sample was also subjected to PCR amplification for expression of the housekeeping gene, glyceraldehyde 3-phosphate dehydrogenase (G3PDH). From Chong *et al.* (1996, Fig. 2, p. 1156).

## D. Quantification of IL-12 p40 mRNA Production by Macrophages from C3H Mice

In order to quantify the differences observed in IL-12 p40 mRNA between macrophages infected with viable or killed SL1438, QC-RT-PCR was performed. Serial threefold dilutions of IL-12 p40 competitor DNA were added to individual tubes, each containing the same amount of cDNA from a particular sample, and PCR was performed. As the amount of competitor decreased, a point of equivalence was reached in which there were equal amounts of sample cDNA and competitor. The competitor is 78 bp smaller than the 266-bp IL-12 p40 fragment amplified by RT-PCR and is amplified by the same primer pair. Macrophages from both C3H/HeN (Fig. 10A) and C3H/HeJ (Fig. 10B) mice infected with viable SL1438 had a point of equivalence in lane 3 and macrophages infected with killed SL1438 had a point of equivalence threefold lower (lane 4). Compared to control macrophages (not shown), macrophages from both C3H/HeN and C3H/HeJ mice infected with viable SL1438 produced approximately 27-fold more IL-12 p40 mRNA (Table

VII). Macrophages from both strains of mice infected with killed SL1438 produced approximately ninefold more IL-12 p40 mRNA than did control macrophages. Since the relative production of IL-12 p40 mRNA by both groups of macrophages was the same, it can be concluded that the differential production seen as a result of infection with viable or killed SL1438 is also not due to the presence of LPS on these organisms.

### E. Quantification of IL-12 p40 mRNA Produced by Macrophages from C3H mice 24 hr Postinfection

In order to determine whether the observed increase in IL-12 p40 mRNA is sustained over time, macrophages from C3H/HeN or C3H/HeJ mice were infected *in*

*TABLE VII*

INCREASES IN IL-12 P40 MRNA PRODUCTION BY MACROPHAGES FROM C3H MICE EXPOSED
TO VIABLE ATTENUATED OR KILLED *SALMONELLA* AS DETERMINED BY QC-RT-PCR[a]

| Time postexposure (hr) | Strain | Treatment | Relative increase in IL-12 p40 mRNA[b] |
|---|---|---|---|
| 4 | C3H/HeN | Media | 1 |
| | | Viable | 27 |
| | | Killed | 9 |
| | C3H/HeJ | Media | 1 |
| | | Viable | 27 |
| | | Killed | 9 |
| 24 | C3H/HeN | Media | 1 |
| | | Viable | 3 |
| | | Killed | <3 |
| | C3H/HeJ | Media | 1 |
| | | Viable | <3 |
| | | Killed | <3 |

[a]From Chong et al. (1996, Table 1, p. 1158).
[b]Peritoneal macrophages were exposed to complete media, viable attenuated, or killed SL1438 at a multiplicity of infection of 1:1 for 60 min. The macrophages were washed three times with PBS to remove extracellular bacteria and further incubated in complete medium containing gentamycin to kill any remaining extracellular bacteria. At 4 or 24 hr, total RNA was isolated from macrophages and reversed transcribed, and cDNA from each sample was subjected to QC-RT-PCR. Amplification was quantified by visualization. As the amount of competitor decreased, a point of equivalence was reached in which there were equal amounts of sample cDNA and competitor. The point of equivalence was compared between different samples with IL-12 p40 mRNA from macrophages exposed to complete media arbitrarily set at 1.

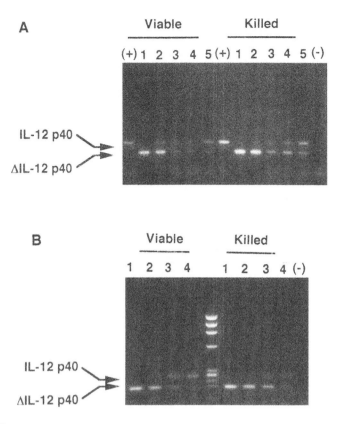

**FIGURE 10.** QC-RT-PCR for the production of IL-12 p40 mRNA by macrophages from C3H mice 4 hr following exposure to viable attenuated or killed *Salmonella.* cDNA samples from C3H/HeN (A) or C3H/HeJ (B) mice remaining after RT-PCR had been performed for Fig. 9 were also analyzed by QC-RT-PCR to quantify IL-12 p40 mRNA production. Serial dilutions (1:3) of IL-12 p40 competitor DNA were added to individual tubes, each containing the same amount of cDNA from a particular sample, and PCR amplified. The location of the 266-bp sample IL-12 p40 mRNA fragment and the 188-bp competitor is shown and a point of equivalence can be determined. Macrophages from both C3H/HeN (A) and C3H/HeJ (B) mice infected with viable Sl1438 had a point of equivalence in lane 3 and macrophages infected with killed SL1438 had a point of equivalence in lane 4. In addition, a negative control is shown ( − ) in which DNA was omitted from the PCR reaction. From Chong *et al.* (1996, Fig. 4, p. 1157).

*vitro* with either viable or killed SL1438; at 24 hr postinfection total RNA was extracted and reverse-transcribed, and the levels of IL-12 p40 were assessed by QC-RT-PCR. Macrophages from C3H/HeN and C3H/HeJ mice infected with viable or killed SL1438 produced quantitatively similar amounts of IL-12 p40 mRNA (Table VII). Compared to control macrophages, there was an approximate three-fold increase in levels of IL-12 p40 mRNA. Therefore, the dramatic and rapid upregulation of IL-12 p40 mRNA observed at 4 hr postexposure is a transient event.

Recently we reported the results of a study in which mice orally immunized with *S. dublin* EL23, a nonreverting aromatic-dependent histidine requiring mutant transformed with a plasmid which carries a gene that codes for production of the B subunit of the heat-labile toxin (LT-B) of enterotoxigenic *E. coli*, were analyzed for their ability to initiate production of IL-12 mRNAs at mucosal sites (Bost and Clements, 1995). Six or 20 hr following oral inoculation, the Peyer's patches and mesenteric lymph nodes were removed and poly A+ mRNA was prepared from each tissue. Constitutive production of an mRNA encoding the p35 subunit of IL-12 was observed in control as well as immunized mice. Conversely, production of an mRNA encoding the p40 subunit of IL-12 was not detected in control animals, but was dramatically upregulated in orally inoculated mice. Using QC-RT-PCR, differences in the magnitude of IL-12 p40 mRNA production were quantified. Six hours after oral inoculation with the *Salmonella* construct, mice had 12.1- and 8.4-fold increases in IL-12 p40 mRNA in the Peyer's patches and mesenteric lymph nodes, respectively, when compared to control mice. By 20 hr, the pattern of increased mRNA production was reversed, showing 2.5- and 17.6-fold increases in the Peyer's patches and mesenteric lymph nodes, respectively.

In the study described above, we focused on the ability *S. dublin* to elicit production of IL-12 p40 mRNA in macrophages from LPS-sensitive and LPS-resistant mice. Exposure of macrophages to either viable or killed organisms resulted in a dramatic and rapid upregulation of IL-12 p40 mRNA when compared to control macrophages. By 4 hr postexposure, viable organisms had induced a 27-fold increase in IL-12 p40 mRNA while killed organisms had induced a 9-fold increase. This was observed in macrophages isolated from both LPS-sensitive and -resistant mice. By 24 hr postexposure, the levels of IL-12 p40 mRNA had decreased to less than 3-fold above control level in macrophages from both strains of mice. The observed increase in IL-12 p40 mRNA is unlikely to be solely LPS-mediated for the following reasons: (i) Infection of murine macrophages with *Listeria monocytogenes* (a gram-positive facultative intracellular pathogen) results in increased production IL-12 (Hsieh *et al.*, 1993), and (ii) IL-12 p40 mRNA increased in macrophages from both C3H/HeN (Lps[n]) and C3H/HeJ (Lps[d]) mice. The temporal shift in production of IL-12 p40 mRNA observed both *in vivo* (from Peyer's patches at 6 hr postinoculation to mesenteric lymph nodes at 20 hr postinoculation) and *in vitro* (elevated expression in macrophages at 4 hr postexposure and near baseline levels by 24 hr postexposure) is consistent with our understanding of the pathogenesis of these organisms. It is most likely that the *Salmonella* first contact macrophages in the Peyer's patches, resulting in an immediate upregulation of IL-12 expression, and subsequently contact macrophages in the mesenteric lymph nodes as they follow their natural progression in disease. Coupled with our previous findings, this study begins to explain at a molecular level how orally administered viable *Salmonella* might stimulate cell-mediated immunity to a greater extent than orally administered killed organisms. Specifically the higher levels of IL-12 induced by viable *Salmonella* may result in the development of a Th1 response and cell-mediated immunity. In contrast, the lower levels of IL-12 induced by killed *Salmonella* may not be sufficient to promote a Th1 response, the result being failure to protect against challange with virulent wild-type organisms. These findings provide insight into a possible mechanism for anti-typhoid immunity induced by oral immunization with viable *Salmonella*.

## REFERENCES

Alving, C. R., Richards, R. L., Moss, J., Alving, L. I., Clements, J. D., Shiba, T., Kotani, S., Wirtz, R. A., and Hockmeyer, W. T. (1986). Effectiveness of liposomes as potential carriers for vaccines. Applications to cholera toxin and human malaria sporozoite antigen. *Vaccine* **4**, 166–172.

Ashcroft, M. T., Ritchie, J. M., and Nicholson, C. C. (1964). Controlled field trial in British Guiana school children of heat-killed-phenolized and acetone-killed lyophilized typhoid vaccines. *Am. J. Hyg.* **79**, 196–206.

Bao, J. X., and Clements, J. D. (1991). Prior immunologic experience potentiates the subsequent antibody response when *Salmonella* is used as a vaccine carrier. *Infect. Immun.* **59**, 3841–3845.

Bockman, D. E., and Cooper, M. D. (1973). Pinocytosis by epithelium associated with lymphoid follicles in the bursa of Fabricius, appendix and Peyer's patches. An electron microscopic study. *Am. J. Anat.* **136**, 455–477.

Bost, K. L., and Clements, J. D. (1995). *In vivo* induction of interleukin-12 mRNA expression after oral immunization with *Salmonella dublin* or the B subunit of *Escherichia coli* heat-labile enterotoxin. *Infect. Immun.* **63**, 1076–1083.

Brown, A., Hormaeche, C. E., de Hormaeche, R. D., Winther, M., Dougan, G., Maskell, D. J., and Stocker, B. A. D. (1987). An attenuated *aroA Salmonella typhimurium* vaccine elicits humoral and cellular immunity to cloned β-galactosidase in mice. *J. Infect. Dis.* **155**, 86–92.

Cárdenas, L., and Clements, J. D. (1992). Oral immunization using live attenuated *Salmonella* spp. as carriers of foreign antigens. *Clin. Microbiol. Rev.* **5**, 328–342.

Cárdenas, L., and Clements, J. D. (1993a). Development of mucosal protection against the heat-stable enterotoxin (ST) of *Escherichia coli* by oral immunization with a genetic fusion delivered by a bacterial vector. *Infect. Immun.* **61**, 4629–4636.

Cárdenas, L., and Clements, J. D. (1993b). Stability, immunogenicity, and expression of foreign antigens in bacterial vaccine vectors. *Vaccine* **11**, 126–135.

Cárdenas, L., Dasgupta, U., and Clements, J. D. (1994). Influence of strain viability and antigen dose on the use of attenuated mutants of *Salmonella* as vaccine carriers. *Vaccine* **12**, 833–840.

Cebra, J. J., Fuhrman, J. A., Lebman, D. A., and London, S. D. (1986). Effective gut mucosal stimulation of IgA-committed B cells by antigen. *In* "Vaccines 86: New Approaches to Immunization. Developing Vaccines against Parasitic, Bacterial, and Viral Diseases" (F. Brown, R. M. Channok, and R. A. Lerner, eds.), pp. 129–133. Cold Spring Harbor Laboratory, Cold Spring Harbor, New York.

Chong, C., Bost, R. L., and Clements, J. D. (1996). Differential production of Interleukin-12 mRNA by murine macrophages in response to viable or killed *Salmonella* spp. *Infect. Immun.* **64**, 1154–1160.

Chuttani, C. S., Prakash, K., Vergese, A., Gupta, P., Chawla, R. K., Grover, V., and Agarwal, D. S. (1973). Ineffectiveness of an oral killed typhoid vaccine in a field trial. *Bull. W.H.O.* **48**, 756–757.

Chuttani, C. S., Prakash, K., Gupta, P., Grover, V., and Kamar, A. (1977). Controlled field trial of a high-dose oral killed typhoid vaccine in India. *Bull. W.H.O.* **55**, 643–644.

Clemens, J. D., Sack, D. A., Harris, J. R., Chakraborty, J., Khan, M. R., Stanton, B. F., Kay, B. A.,

Khan, M. U., Yunus, M., Atkinson, W., Svennerholm, A., and Holmgren, J. (1986). Field trial of oral cholera vaccines in Bangladesh. *Lancet* **2**, 124–127.

Clements, J. D. (1987). Use of attenuated mutants of *Salmonella* as carriers for delivery of heterologous antigens to the secretory immune system. *Pathol. Immunopathol. Res.* **6**, 137–146.

Clements, J. D., and Cárdenas, L. (1990). Vaccines against enterotoxigenic bacterial pathogens based on hybrid *Salmonella* that express heterologous antigens. *Res. Microbiol.* **141**, 981–994.

Clements, J. D., and El-Morshidy, S. (1984). Construction of a potential live oral bivalent vaccine for typhoid fever and cholera—*Escherichia coli*—related diarrheas. *Infect. Immun.* **46**, 564–569.

Clements, J. D., Lyon, F. L., Lowe, K. L., Farrand, A. L., and El-Morshidy, S. (1986). Oral immunization of mice with attenuated *Salmonella enteritidis* containing a recombinant plasmid which codes for production of the B subunit of heat-labile *Escherichia coli* enterotoxin. *Infect. Immun.* **53**, 685–692.

Clements, J. D., Hartzog, N. M., and Lyon, F. L. (1988). Adjuvant activity of *Escherichia coli* heat-labile enterotoxin and effect on the induction of oral tolerance in mice to unrelated protein antigens. *Vaccine* **6**, 269–277.

Curtiss III, R. (1986). Genetic analysis of *Streptococcus mutans* virulence and prospects for an anticaries vaccine. *J. Dent. Res.* **65**, 1034–1045.

Curtiss III, R., and Kelly, S. M. (1987). *Salmonella typhimurium* deletion mutants lacking adenylate cyclase and cyclic AMP receptor protein are avirulent and immunogenic. *Infect. Immun.* **55**, 3035–3043.

Curtiss III, R., Goldschmidt, R., Kelly, S., Lyons, M., Michalek, S., Pastian, R., and Stein, S. (1987). Recombinant avirulent *Salmonella* for oral immunization to induce mucosal immunity to bacterial pathogens. *In* "Vaccines: New Concepts and Developments. Proceedings of the 10th International Convocation on Immunology" (H. Kohler and P. T. LoVerde, Eds.), pp. 261–271. Longman Scientific and Technical, Harlow and Essex, U.K.

Dickinson, B. L., and Clements, J. D. (1995). Dissociation of *Escherichia coli* heat-labile enterotoxin adjuvanticity from ADP-ribosyltransferase activity. *Infect. Immun.* **63**, 1617–1623.

Douce, G., Turcotte, C., Cropley, I., Roberts, M., Pizza, M., Domenghini, M., Rappuoli, R., and Dougan, G. (1995). Mutants of *Escherichia coli* heat-labile toxin lacking ADP-ribosyltransferase activity act as nontoxic, mucosal adjuvants. *Proc. Natl. Acad. Sci. U.S.A.* **92**, 1644–1648.

Dougan, G., Sellwood, R., Maskell, D., Sweeney, K., Liew, F. Y., Beesley, J., and Hormaeche, C. (1986). *In vivo* properties of a cloned K88 adherence antigen determinant. *Infect. Immun.* **52**, 344–347.

Edwards, M. F., and Stocker, B. A. D. (1988). Construction of Δ*aroA his* Δ*pur* strains of *Salmonella typhi*. *J. Bacteriol.* **170**, 3991–3995.

Eldridge, J. H., Gilley, R. M., Staas, J. K., Moldoveanu, Z., Meulbroek, J. A., and Tice, T. R. (1989). Biodegradable microspheres: Vaccine delivery system for oral immunization. *Curr. Top. Microbiol. Immunol.* **146**, 59–66.

Elson, C. O. (1989). Cholera toxin and its subunits as potential oral adjuvants. *Immunol. Today* **146**, 29–33.

Formal, S. B., Baron, L. S., Kopecko, D. J., Washington, O., Powell, C., and Life, C. A. (1981). Construction of a potential bivalent vaccine strain: Introduction of *Shigella sonnei* form I antigen genes into the *galE Salmonella typhi* Ty21a typhoid vaccine strain. *Infect. Immun.* **34**, 746–750.

Garcon, N. M. J., and Six, H. R. (1993). Universal vaccine carrier. Liposomes that provide T-dependent help to weak antigens. *J. Immunol.* **146**, 3697–3702.

Germanier, R., and Fürer, E. (1971). Immunity in experimental salmonellosis. II Basis for the avirulence and protective capacity of *galE* mutants of *S. typhimurium*. *Infect. Immun.* **4**, 663–673.

Germanier, R., and Fürer, E. (1975). Isolation and characterization of *galE* mutant Ty21a of *Salmonella typhi*: A candidate strain for a live, oral typhoid vaccine. *J. Infect. Dis.* **131**, 553–558.

Gilman, R. H., Hornick, R. B., Woodward, W. E., DuPont, H. L., Snyder, M. J., Levine, M. M., and

Libonati, J. P. (1977). Evaluation of a UDP-glucose-4- epimeraseless mutant of *Salmonella typhi* as a live oral vaccine. *J. Infect. Dis.* **136,** 717–723.

Gould-Fogerite, S., and Mannino, R. J. (1993). Targeted fusogenic proteoliposomes: Functional reconstitution of membrane proteins through protein–cochleate intermediates. *In* "Liposome Technology," 2nd ed., Vol. III, "Interaction of Liposomes with the Biological Milieu" (G. Gregoriadis, Ed.), pp. 261–276. CRC Press, Boca Raton, FL.

Hoiseth, S. K., and Stocker, B. A. D. (1981). Aromatic-dependent *Salmonella typhimurium* are non-virulent and effective as live vaccines. *Nature (London)* **291,** 238–239.

Hone, D., Attridge, S., van den Bosch, L., and Hackett, J. (1989). A chromosomal integration system for stabilization of heterologous genes in *Salmonella* based vaccine strains. *Microb. Pathog.* **5,** 407–418.

Hsieh, C. S. S., Macatonia, S. E., Tripp, C. S., Wolf, S. F., O'Garra, A., and Murphy, K. M. (1993). Development of TH1 CD4+ T cells through IL-12 produced by *Listeria*-induced macrophages. *Science* **260,** 547–549.

Kaper, J. B., Lockman, H., and Baldini, M. (1984). Recombinant nontoxigenic *Vibrio cholerae* strains as attenuated cholera vaccine candidates. *Nature (London)* **308,** 655–658.

Levine, M. M., Ferreccio, C., Black, R. E., Germanier, R., and Chilean Typhoid Committee (1987a). Large-scale field trial of Ty21a live oral typhoid vaccine in enteric coated capsule formation. *Lancet* **1,** 1049–1052.

Levine, M. M., Herrington, D., Murphy, J., Morris, J. G., Losonsky, G., Tall, B., Lindberg, A., Svenson, S., Baqar, S., Edwards, M. F., and Stocker, B. A. D. (1987b). Safety, infectivity, immunogenicity and *in vivo* stability of two attenuated auxotrophic mutant strains of *Salmonella typhi,* 541Ty and 543Ty used as oral vaccines in man. *J. Clin. Invest.* **79,** 888–902.

Levine, M. M., Kaper, J. B., Herrington, D., Losonsky, G., Tacket, C. O., Morris, J. G., Tall, B., and Cryz, S. (1988). Safety, immunogenicity, and efficacy of recombinant live oral cholera vaccines CVD 103 and CVD 103-HgR. *Lancet* **2,** 467–470.

Lycke, N., and Holmgren, J. (1986). Strong adjuvant properties of cholera toxin on gut mucosal immune responses to orally presented antigens. *Immunology* **59,** 301–308.

Lycke, N., Tsuji, T., and Holmgren, J. (1992). The adjuvant effect of *Vibrio cholerae* and *Escherichia coli* heat-labile enterotoxins is linked to their ADP-ribosyltransferase activity. *Eur. J. Immunol.* **22,** 2277–2281.

Manning, P. A., Heuzenroeder, M. W., Yeadon, J., Leavesley, D. I., Reeves, P. R., and Rowley, D. (1986). Molecular cloning and expression in *Escherichia coli* K-12 of the O antigens of the Inaba and Ogawa serotypes of the *Vibrio cholerae* O1 lipopolysaccharides and their potential for vaccine development. *Infect. Immun.* **53,** 272–277.

Maskell, D., Liew, F. Y., Sweeney, K., Dougan, G., and Hormaeche, C. E. (1986). Attenuated *Salmonella typhimurium* as live oral vaccines and carriers for delivering antigens to the secretory immune system. *In* "Vaccines 86: New Approaches to Immunization. Developing Vaccines against Parasitic, Bacterial, and Viral Diseases" (F. Brown, R. M. Channok, and R. A. Lerner, Eds.), pp. 213–217. Cold Spring Harbor Laboratory, Cold Spring Harbor, NY.

Mosmann, T. R., and Coffman, R. L. (1989). TH1 and TH2 cells: Different patterns of lymphokine secretion lead to different functional properties. *Annu. Rev. Immunol.* **7,** 145–173.

Mosmann, T. R., Cherwinski, H., Bond, M. W., Giedlin, M. A., and Coffman, R. L. (1986). Two types of murine helper T cell clone. I. Definition according to profiles of lymphokine activities and secreted proteins. *J. Immunol.* **136,** 2348–2357.

Mowat, A. M., and Donachie, A. M. (1991). ISCOMS—a novel strategy for mucosal immunization. *Immunol. Today* **12,** 383–385.

Owen, R. L., Pierce, N. F., Apple, R. T., and Cray, Jr., W. C. (1986). M cell transport of *Vibrio cholerae* from the intestinal lumen into Peyer's patches: A mechanism for antigen sampling and for microbial transepithelial migration. *J. Infect. Dis.* **153,** 1108–1118.

Robbins, J. D., and Robbins, J. B. (1984). Reexamination of the protective role of the capsular polysaccharide (Vi antigen) of *Salmonella typhi*. *J. Infect. Dis.* **150,** 436–449.

Robertsson, J. A., Lindberg, A. A., Hoiseth, S., and Stocker, B. A. D. (1983). *Salmonella typhimurium* infection in calves: Protection and survival of virulent challenge bacteria after immunization with live or inactivated vaccines. *Infect. Immun.* **41,** 742–750.

Sadoff, J. C., Ballou, W. R., Baron, L. S., Majarian, W. R., Brey, R. N., Hockmeyer, W. T., Young, J. F., Cryz, S. J., Ou, J., Lowell, G. H., and Chulay, J. D. (1988). Oral *Salmonella typhimurium* vaccine expressing circumsporozoite protein protects against malaria. *Science* **240,** 336–340.

Santiago, N., Milstein, S., Rivera, T., Garcia, W., Zaidl, T., Hong, H., and Bucher, D. (1993). Oral immunization of rats with proteinoid microspheres encapsulating influenza virus antigens. *Pharm. Res.* **10,** 1243–1247.

Sigwart, D. F., Stocker, B. A. D., and Clements, J. D. (1989). Effect of *purA* mutation on the efficacy of *Salmonella* live vaccine vectors. *Infect. Immun.* **57,** 1858–1861.

Smith, B. P., Reina-Guerra, M., Hoiseth, S. K., Stocker, B. A. D., Habasha, F., Johnson, E., and Merritt, F. (1984a). Aromatic-dependent *Salmonella typhimurium* as modified live vaccines for calves. *Am. J. Vet. Res.* **45,** 59–66.

Smith, B. P., Reina-Guerra, M., Stocker, B. A. D., Hoiseth, S. K., and Johnson, E. (1984b). Aromatic-dependent *Salmonella dublin* as a parenteral modified live vaccine for calves. *Am. J. Vet. Res.* **45,** 2231–2235.

Stocker, B. A. D., Hoiseth, S. K., and Smith, B. P. (1983). Aromatic-dependent *Salmonella* species as live vaccines in mice and calves. In International symposium on enteric infections in man and animals: Standardization of immunological procedures. 1982. *Dev. Biol. Stand.* **53,** 47–54.

Strober, W., and Jacobs, D. (1985). Cellular differentiation, migration, and function in the mucosal immune system. *In* "Advances in Host Defense Mechanisms. Vol. 4. Mucosal Immunity" (J. I. Gallin and A. S. Fauci, Eds.), pp. 1–30. Raven, New York.

Svennerholm, A.-M., Jertborn, M., Gothefors, L., Karim, A. M., Sack, D. A., and Holmgren, J. (1984). Local and systemic antibody responses and immunological memory in humans after cholera disease and after immunization with a combined B subunit-whole cell vaccine. *J. Infect. Dis.* **149,** 884–893.

Tacket, C. O., Hone, D. M., R. Curtiss, I., Kelly, S. M., Losonsky, G., Guers, L., Harris, A. M., Edelman, R., and Levine, M. M. (1992). Comparison of the safety and immunogenicity of ΔaroC ΔaroD and Δcya Δcrp *Salmonella typhi* strains in adult volunteers. *Infect. Immun.* **60,** 536–541.

Tomasi, T. B., and Plaut, A. G. (1985). Cellular differentiation, migration, and function in the mucosal immune system. *In* "Advances in Host Defense Mechanisms. Volume 4. Mucosal Immunity" (J. I. Gallin and A. S. Fauci, Eds.), pp. 31–61. Raven, New York.

Wahdan, M. H., Serie, C., Germanier, R., Lackany, A., Cerisier, Y., Guerin, N., Sallam, S., Geoffroy, P., Tantawi, A. S. E., and Guesry, P. (1980). A controlled field trial of live oral typhoid vaccine Ty21a. *Bull. W.H.O.* **58,** 469–474.

Watson, J., Kelly, K., Largen, M., and Taylor, B. A. (1978). The genetic mapping of a defective LPS response gene. *J. Immunol.* **120,** 422–424.

Watson, J., Riblet, R., and Taylor. B. A. (1977). The response of recombinant inbred strains of mice to bacterial lipopolysaccharides. *J. Immunol.* **118,** 2088–2093.

Yamamoto, T., Tamura, Y., and Yokota, T. (1985). Enteroadhesion fimbriae and enterotoxin of *Escherichia coli:* Genetic transfer to a streptomycin-resistant mutant of the *galE* oral-route live vaccine *Salmonella typhi* Ty21a. *Infect. Immun.* **50,** 925–928.

# Chapter 38

# Oral Tolerance: A Commentary

Charles O. Elson and Jan Zivny

*Department of Medicine,*
*University of Alabama at Birmingham,*
*Birmingham, Alabama 35294*

## I. INTRODUCTION

Oral tolerance is defined as a state of immunological unresponsiveness to an antigen induced by the feeding of that antigen. This term is something of a misnomer in that such tolerance can ensue after the application of antigen to other mucosal membranes such as the respiratory or nasal mucosa. Thus, an argument could be made that the term should be "mucosal tolerance" rather than "oral tolerance." That being said, the bulk of the work in this area has been after the feeding of antigen so most of the information available applies to oral tolerance. This chapter is a brief commentary summarizing the current status of the field, as well as what questions now need to be addressed. The reader is referred elsewhere for detailed reviews (Mowat, 1994; Weiner *et al.*, 1994).

## II. ORAL TOLERANCE IS A CRUCIAL FEATURE OF THE MUCOSAL IMMUNE SYSTEM

The mucosal immune system is constantly exposed to an immense number and variety of food and bacterial antigens. The amount of antigen in or transversing the gut is several orders of magnitude greater than the numbers of cells or quantity of antibody produced per day. Therefore, immunologic nonresponsiveness to lumenal antigens is more common than is immune responsiveness. Another way of viewing this is that oral tolerance allows the mucosal immune system to focus on antigens or pathogens representing a threat to the host. As is true elsewhere in the immune system, the context in which an antigen is encountered largely determines the resulting immune response. The context of infection or invasion by a pathogen receives the highest priority and strongest response. Oral tolerance thus represents one end of the spectrum of response to exogenous antigen and is increasingly being recognized to be an active process, i.e., not simply the absence of a response. The limitation of response to innocuous antigens at mucosal surfaces is as important as the stimulation of immune responses to the antigens of pathogenic microbes.

## III. MAJOR FEATURES OF ORAL TOLERANCE

Work done in the past few decades has defined a number of important features of oral tolerance. First, the tolerance is specific for the antigen that is fed, and this applies to both cellular and humoral immune responses (Miller and Hanson, 1979). Second, the tolerance is partial. In regard to antibody responses, the reduction usually amounts to a one log reduction compared to animals which are parenterally immunized without prior feeding. Third, tolerance is not long-lasting and wanes with time (Melamed and Friedman, 1993b). In mice this generally equates to several months of unresponsiveness which then dissipates. Fourth, the feeding of antigen abrogates the induction of an immune response better than it reduces an established one. There are a number of important parameters for the induction of oral tolerance that are shown in Table I. The types of antigens that have induced oral tolerance include various protein antigens, contact allergens, heterologous red blood cells, and certain killed viruses (Elson, 1985). Although tolerance has been reproducibly demonstrated after the feeding of multiple proteins, most of these have been of eukaryotic origin and it's unclear whether the feeding of bacterial proteins would result in oral tolerance, given the endogenous priming of the mucosal immune system to antigens of the normal bacterial flora. A common feature of tolerogenic antigens is that most induce T-cell-dependent immune responses when given parenterally and most are good immunogens. Oral tolerance does not appear to be induced to T-cell-independent antigens (Titus and Chiller, 1981). The total number of different antigens that have been fed to rodents to induce oral tolerance is fairly limited compared to the large numbers of antigens encountered at mucosal surfaces. Other important parameters for the induction of oral tolerance include the dose of antigen, which usually involves milligram quantities (Friedman and Weiner, 1993), the mucosal route of antigen delivery, and the age (Strobel and Ferguson, 1984; Faria *et al.,* 1993), genetic background, and species of the host (Peri and Rothberg, 1981; Miller and Cook, 1994). Lastly, recent studies have shown that oral tolerance can be enhanced by varying the delivery vehicle or incorporating immunomodulators with the fed antigens as discussed below.

## IV. WHERE IS ORAL TOLERANCE INDUCED?

An antigen delivered into the intestine encounters a very complex environment with many cell types as well as ubiquitous digestive enzymes. The exact site of tolerance induction for any given antigen has not been clearly established. The candidates are Peyer's patches or lymphoid follicles, the epithelial layer, or the

*TABLE I*

IMPORTANT PARAMETERS FOR THE INDUCTION OF
ORAL TOLERANCE

| |
| --- |
| Type of antigen |
| Dose |
| Frequency of feeding |
| Mucosal route |
| Immunogenicity of the antigen |
| Species |
| Genetic background of individual |
| Age |
| Delivery system/adjuvant |

systemic lymphoid compartment (exposed to antigenic fragments generated by digestion in the intestine). Of these possibilities, the data are clearest that the lymphoid follicles or Peyer's patches of the gut represent one site of tolerance induction (Richman *et al.,* 1981; Santos *et al.,* 1993). Interestingly, each of the mucosal surfaces at which tolerance can be induced also contain lymphoid follicles. This does not exclude that there may be other sites of tolerance induction. There has been increasing recognition that the intestinal epithelial cell layer is an active component of the mucosal immune system (Elson and Beagley, 1994). Epithelial cells produce and respond to a wide variety of cytokines and thus communicate with the lymphoid cells in the mucosa (Fig. 1). Moreover, epithelial cells express both MHC class I and class II molecules and have been shown to be able to process soluble antigens. Antigen presentation by gut epithelial cells *in vitro* seems to preferentially induce suppressor cells (Bland and Warren, 1986; Mayer *et al.,* 1988), possibly because epithelial cells lack costimulatory molecules such as B7 (Sanderson *et al.,* 1993). However, most of the data supporting the possible role of epithelial cells in oral tolerance induction come from *in vitro* studies; there is as yet direct no evidence from *in vivo* studies that epithelial cells participate in oral tolerance induction. A third possible site for tolerance induction is the systemic lymphoid compartment through exposure to absorbed antigen fragments. This possibility is suggested by data showing that oral tolerance for DTH responses can be transferred by serum obtained a few hours after feeding antigen to mice (Strobel *et al.,* 1983).

## V. MECHANISMS OF ORAL TOLERANCE

Multiple mechanisms of oral tolerance have been identified, consistent with its importance to the functioning of the mucosal immune system. The most common mechanisms appear to be clonal deletion (Chen *et al.,* 1995), clonal anergy (Mel-

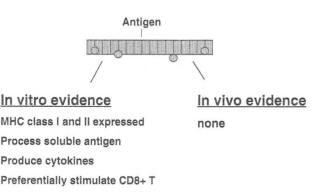

**In vitro evidence**

MHC class I and II expressed

Process soluble antigen

Produce cytokines

Preferentially stimulate CD8+ T

   - gp180 costimulation?

**In vivo evidence**

*FIGURE 1.* The role of epithelial cells in tolerance induction.

amed and Friedman, 1993a), and the induction of suppressor cells (Richman *et al.,* 1978). It must be emphasized that these mechanisms are not mutually exclusive and more than one of them could be operative simultaneously after antigen feeding, e.g., antigen feeding might result in both anergy and suppression. In mice a crucial variable as to which mechanism is triggered appears to be the dose of antigen fed (Table II). Thus, multiple feedings of 1-mg doses have been shown to generate cells producing inhibitory cytokines, whereas large doses of 20 mg or more appear to preferentially induce clonal anergy (Friedman and Weiner, 1994). These two mechanisms can be operationally defined, as shown in Table II, and thus identified in tolerized mice (Friedman and Weiner, 1994). There appears to be a gradient of sensitivity of different cell types to the induction of tolerance with the Th1 CD4$^+$ T cell the most susceptible (Burstein *et al.,* 1992; Melamed and Friedman, 1994) followed by the Th2 CD4$^+$ T cell (Fig. 2). Indeed, T cells appear to be the major target of oral tolerance and the reductions in antibody responses after antigen feeding are more likely due to reductions in helper activity of T cells than they are due to tolerization of B cells directly. There is at present little or no evidence that B cells are tolerized directly by antigen feeding (Titus and Chiller, 1981). The sequence of events immediately following antigen feeding has recently been explored and the picture that is emerging is that there is a stage of cell activation, cell cycling, and cytokine production that occurs in the days after antigen feeding that appears to be necessary for the induction of oral tolerance. This again reinforces the notion that oral tolerance is an active process and not merely the absence of a response. A number of other mechanisms that have been found in peripheral T-cell tolerance in systemic tissues, such as T-cell exhaustion, partial activation of T cells, and downregulation of T-cell receptor expression (Adorini, 1993), have not yet been identified as mechanisms mediating oral tolerance.

TABLE*II*
ORAL TOLERANCE: IMPORTANCE OF DOSE

| Dose | Mechanism |
|---|---|
| Small doses any frequency | No tolerance (threshold effect) |
| Multiple, moderate doses, e.g., 1 mg × 5 | Suppression<br>1. Transferable with cells<br>2. CD4 or CD8<br>3. Candidate cytokines: TGFβ, IL-4, IL-10 |
| Large bolus dose, e.g., 20 mg | Anergy<br>1. Decreased IL-2 on antigen reexposure<br>2. Rescue with exogenous IL-2 |

## VI. ENHANCEMENT OF ORAL TOLERANCE BY DELIVERY SYSTEMS OR ADJUVANTS

In most studies on oral tolerance, soluble antigen is gavaged into mice at various doses. There are very few studies on whether oral tolerance can be enhanced by varying the delivery of antigen or incorporating immunomodulators with the fed antigen. Indeed, there are only three such reports. In one, feeding bacterial lipopolysaccharide along with the protein antigen enhanced oral tolerance to myelin basic protein (Khoury et al., 1990). In the second, antigen was coupled covalently to recombinant cholera toxin B subunit. The oral administration of even single doses of very small amounts of such conjugates resulted in tolerance in delayed-type hypersensitivity responses both to sheep red blood cells and to human gammaglobulin (Sun et al., 1994). The mechanism of the enhancement of tolerance in this system remains unknown. In a third report, oral antigen delivery by way of a multiple emulsion system enhanced oral tolerance induction to bovine serum albumin, ovalbumin, and to a bacterial protein which by itself is a weak inducer of

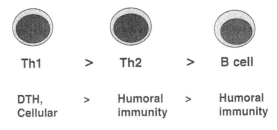

FIGURE 2. Gradient of sensitivity to tolerance induction.

oral tolerance (Elson *et al.*, 1996). These few studies do represent proof of the principle that oral tolerance can be enhanced; moreover these systems may result in a marked reduction in the doses required to induce tolerance which would be of considerable practical benefit. Development of this area will be crucial to the eventual successful application of oral tolerance to the treatment of human disease and is an area begging for further experimental development.

## VII. ORAL TOLERANCE AND ORAL VACCINES

A good deal of effort is being applied to the development of effective oral vaccines. Could oral vaccines generate tolerance instead of immunity? Such an unwanted and potentially deleterious outcome certainly is possible on theoretical grounds and would seem to be a real possibility with some of the approaches being attempted, such as the incorporation of antigen into plants for use as vaccines (Mason *et al.*, 1992). With other approaches, such as the use of living microbial vectors, the induction of oral tolerance would seem to be a more remote possibility. The same is true with approaches using toxin adjuvants such as cholera toxin or *Escherichia coli* heat-labile toxin, which have been shown to abrogate the induction of oral tolerance to coadministered antigen (Elson and Ealding, 1984; Clements *et al.*, 1988). As mentioned above, relatively few antigens of microbial origin have ever been tested in a soluble form for the development of oral tolerance, and there are reasons to believe that these proteins may not be particularly tolerogenic (Dertzbaugh and Elson, 1993). Nevertheless, testing for the induction of tolerance needs to be incorporated into oral vaccine protocols.

## VIII. ORAL TOLERANCE AS A THERAPY FOR EXPERIMENTAL AUTOIMMUNE DISEASE

The feeding of autoantigens has been an effective prevention and treatment of experimental autoimmune diseases in a number of different systems (Thompson and Staines, 1990). These systems tend to have in common the induction of disease by immunization with an autoantigenic protein or peptide and most are mediated by T cells, particularly Th1-type CD4 T cells. Prior feeding of the same antigen that is used to induce the disease can abrogate disease induction or, alternatively, disease can be ameliorated by feeding the antigen to animals with established disease. Some of the diseases and the autoantigens used for feeding are shown in Table III. The best example of the use of oral tolerance to treat experimental autoimmune diseases is experimental allergic encephalomyelitis (EAE) (Bitar and Whitacre, 1988; Higgins and Weiner, 1988). EAE is induced in rodents by immunizing them with myelin basic protein (MBP) in complete Freund's adjuvant. Immunized animals develop a stereotypical paralytic disease that is due to T-cell-mediated autoimmune attack on myelinated neurons in the nervous system. The feeding of MBP to such animals has lowered the incidence and delayed the onset

*TABLE III*
ORAL TOLERANCE AS THERAPY OF EXPERIMENTAL AUTOIMMUNE DISEASE

| Model | Antigen fed |
| --- | --- |
| Arthritis | Type II collagen |
| Experimental allergic encephalomyelitis | Myelin basic protein |
| Nonobese diabetic mouse | Insulin |
| Experimental autoimmune uveoretinitis | Retinal protein S |
| Thyroiditis | Thyroglobulin |

of EAE, diminished its severity, decreased serum IgG anti-MPB, increased salivary IgA anti-MPB, diminished the frequency of anti-MPB antibody-secreting cells and antigen-specific T cells, altered T-cell receptor V gene usage, induced suppression of MPB responses by $CD8^+$ suppressor T cells (Thompson and Staines, 1990), and downregulated inflammatory cytokines in the brain lesions (Khoury *et al.*, 1992). The use of oral tolerance as a therapy is not limited, however, to diseases induced by parenteral immunization with the same antigen because the feeding of insulin to young, prediabetic NOD mice is an effective treatment of this disease (Zhang *et al.*, 1991).

## IX. THE CONCEPT OF BYSTANDER SUPPRESSION

For most human autoimmune or chronic inflammatory diseases, the antigens involved remain unknown. This would seem to be an insurmountable obstacle to the use of oral tolerance as a novel potential therapy. However, this is not necessarily the case as long as the feeding of an autoantigen can be done in such a way as to induce antigen-specific suppressor cells. Once induced in the gut, such cells will circulate widely in the body and, upon reencounter with antigen in lesions, release various inhibitory cytokines (Miller *et al.*, 1992). Such cytokines are themselves nonspecifically inhibitory and thus will downregulate cells in the lesions that recognize other antigens. This phenomenon has been demonstrated experimentally *in vitro* and has been termed "bystander suppression" (Miller *et al.*, 1991). Indeed, bystander suppression has been demonstrated *in vivo* as well in three different models of organ-specific inflammatory disease, including proteolipid protein-induced EAE, which was suppressed by the feeding of a myelin basic protein, virally induced diabetes, which was inhibited by insulin feeding (von Herrath *et al.*, 1995), and adjuvant- or antigen-induced arthritis, which was inhibited by the feeding of collagen type II (Zhang *et al.*, 1990; Yoshino *et al.*, 1995). The various candidate cells and cytokines that might mediate such effects are shown in Fig. 3. These results in experimental animals provide further support for the idea that antigen feeding could become an effective treatment of human autoimmune dis-

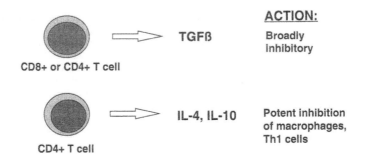

**FIGURE 3.** Candidate cells and cytokines mediating bystander suppression in oral tolerance.

ease. However, almost nothing is known about whether bystander suppression occurs in humans and, if so, how it can be triggered selectively.

## X. Prospects for Oral Tolerance as a Therapy for Human Disease

Attempts to induce oral tolerance in some species, such as rabbits, have been unsuccessful (Peri and Rothberg, 1981) and until recently it's been unclear whether oral tolerance occurred in humans. In a recent study we fed keyhole limpet hemocyanin (KLH) to human volunteers in 10 individual feedings representing a total dose of 0.5 g. The feeding was followed by a subcutaneous immunization with KLH. A control group received only the parenteral immunization. We found a significant reduction in KLH-specific T-cell proliferation and delayed skin-test responses (Husby et al., 1994). Although KLH feeding alone did not induce significant levels of serum antibody, after the parenteral immunization the number of circulating IgG and IgM anti-KLH-producing cells and the titer of serum IgG, IgA, and IgM anti-KLH antibodies and the levels of secretory IgA anti-KLH were significantly greater in the KLH-fed group than in the nonfed group. These data indicate that KLH feeding induced systemic T-cell tolerance but B-cell priming at both systemic and mucosal sites. These results presumably mirror the greater sensitivity of Th1 T cells to oral tolerization that has also been seen in rodents. This study does support the potential usefulness of oral tolerance as a therapy of cellular-mediated but not antibody-mediated human chronic inflammatory or autoimmune diseases.

Phase-I safety trials of oral tolerance in humans have been reported for patients with multiple sclerosis and rheumatoid arthritis. The multiple sclerosis patients with relapsing remitting disease were fed 300 mg per day of bovine myelin or placebo for 1 year in a double-blind fashion (Weiner et al., 1993). Significantly, no toxicity was observed, which was the primary purpose of the study. There did appear to be some reduction in the number of major attacks in patients fed myelin vs those fed placebo but the numbers of patients were quite low. Similarly, the feeding of chicken type-II collagen at 0.1–0.5 mg per day for 3 months to patients with severe active RA did not result in any significant toxicity and did reduce significantly some parameters of arthritis activity (Trentham *et al.,* 1993). Both of these studies involved fairly small numbers of patients and no firm conclusions on efficacy can be derived. Large multicenter dose-ranging trials are underway in the United States in both rheumatoid arthritis and multiple sclerosis patients. Preliminary data coming out of the rheumatoid arthritis study indicate that only the lowest of four doses used had any beneficial effect on the clinical status of the patients. Such trials represent a very expensive way to determine the doses that might be effective in humans. Surrogate assays for bystander suppression in humans are badly needed to help identify doses that might be effective in patients. The patients chosen for testing are also likely to be an important variable in the success or failure of such trials. Oral tolerance may well be an effective treatment early in the disease but not later. In organ-specific autoimmune diseases such as autoimmune diabetes, the number of autoantigens that are recognized and contribute to the disease process expand with time (Lehman *et al.,* 1992; Steinman, 1995) The induction of tolerance early in the disease when only a few autoantigens are driving the process would seem more likely to succeed than at late stages when the reverse is the case. Because antigen feeding has been found to be safe in patients, it would seem more reasonable to target this potential therapy to patients early in their disease course.

## XI. SUMMARY

Oral tolerance can be viewed as a crucial feature of the mucosal immune system allowing mucosal immune focus in the setting of antigen overload. There are multiple variables and parameters that contribute to the induction of oral tolerance, but perhaps the most important of these is the dose of antigen fed. Oral tolerance can be enhanced by manipulation of antigen delivery and probably by various immunomodulators. The development of novel methods to enhance tolerance represents an area of investigation likely to pay rich dividends. Multiple different mechanisms are operative and these may well be present simultaneously. Oral tolerance has been found to be an effective treatment for experimental autoimmune diseases, both induced and spontaneous. Because oral tolerance can be induced in humans, it may well represent an effective therapy for certain chronic inflammatory or autoimmune diseases. The mechanism most likely to be involved in effective therapy of human disease is that of bystander suppression. Thus, methods to induce bystander suppression by antigen feeding in humans should be a high priority for future research.

# REFERENCES

Adorini, L. (1993). Tolerance induction in mature T cells. *Immunologist* 1, 185–190.

Bitar, D. M., and Whitacre, C. C. (1988). Suppression of experimental autoimmune encephalomyelitis by the oral administration of myelin basic protein. *Cell. Immunol.* 112, 364–370.

Bland, P. W., and Warren, L. G. (1986). Antigen presentation by epithelial cells of the rat small intestine. II. Selective induction of suppressor cells. *Immunology* 58, 9–14.

Burstein, H. J., Shea, C. M., and Abbas, A. K. (1992). Aqueous antigens induce *in vivo* tolerance selectively in IL-2- and IFN-gamma-producing (Th1) cells. *J. Immunol.* 148, 3687–3691.

Chen, Y., Inobe, J., Marks, R., Gonnella, P., Kuchroo, V. K., and Weiner, H. L. (1995). Peripheral deletion of antigen-reactive T cells in oral tolerance. *Nature (London)* 376, 177–180.

Clements, J. D., Hartzog, N. M., and Lyon, F. L. (1988). Adjuvant activity of *Escherichia coli* heat-labile enterotoxin and effect on the induction of oral tolerance in mice to unrelated protein antigens. *Vaccine* 6, 269–277.

Dertzbaugh, M. T., and Elson, C. O. (1993). Comparative effectiveness of the cholera toxin B subunit and alkaline phosphatase as carriers for oral vaccines. *Infect. Immun.* 61, 48–55.

Elson, C. O. (1985). Induction and control of the gastrointestinal immune system. *Scand. J. Gastroenterol.* 114S, 1–15.

Elson, C. O., and Beagley, K. W. (1994). Cytokines and immune mediators. "Physiology of the Gastrointestinal Tract," 3rd Ed. Raven, New York.

Elson, C. O., and Ealding, W. (1984). Cholera toxin feeding did not induce oral tolerance in mice and abrogated oral tolerance to an unrelated protein antigen. *J. Immunol.* 133, 2892–2897.

Elson, C. O., Tomasi, T., Dertzbaugh, M. T., Thaggard, G., and Hunter, R. (1996). Oral antigen delivery via a multiple emulsion system enhances oral tolerance. *Ann. N.Y. Acad. Sci.* 778, 156–162.

Faria, A. M., Garcia, G., Rios, M. J., Michalaros, C. L., and Vaz, N. M. (1993). Decrease in susceptibility to oral tolerance induction and occurrence of oral immunization to ovalbumin in 20–38-week-old mice. The effect of interval between oral exposures and rate of antigen intake in the oral immunization. *Immunology* 78, 147–151.

Friedman, A., and Weiner, H. L. (1993). Induction of anergy and/or active suppression in oral tolerance is determined by frequency of feeding and antigen dose. *J. Immunol.* 150, 4A.

Friedman, A., and Weiner, H. L. (1994). Induction of anergy or active suppression following oral tolerance is determined by antigen dosage. *Proc. Natl. Acad. Sci. U.S.A.* 91, 6688–6692.

Higgins, P. J., and Weiner, H. L. (1988). Suppression of experimental autoimmune encephalomyelitis by oral administration of myelin basic protein and its fragments. *J. Immunol.* 140, 440–445.

Husby, S., Mestecky, J., Moldoveanu, Z., Holland, S., and Elson, C. O. (1994). Oral tolerance in humans. T cell but not B cell tolerance after antigen feeding. *J. Immunol.* 152, 4663–4670.

Khoury, S. J., Hancock, W. W., and Weiner, H. L. (1992). Oral tolerance to myelin basic protein and natural recovery from experimental autoimmune encephalomyelitis are associated with downregulation of inflammatory cytokines and differential upregulation of transforming growth factor beta, interleukin 4, and prostaglandin E expression in the brain. *J. Exp. Med.* 176, 1355–1364.

Khoury, S. J., Lider, O., Al-Sabbagh, A., and Weiner, H. L. (1990). Suppression of experimental autoimmune encephalomyelitis by oral administration of myelin basic protein. III. Synergistic effect of lipopolysaccharide. *Cell. Immunol.* 131, 302–310.

Lehman, P. V., Forsthuber, T., Miller, A., and Sercarz, E. E. (1992). Spreading of T-cell autoimmunity to cryptic determinants of an autoantigen. *Nature (London)* 358, 155–157.

Mason, H. S., Lam, D. M., and Arntzen, C. J. (1992). Expression of hepatitis B surface antigen in transgenic plants. *Proc. Natl. Acad. Sci. U.S.A.* 89, 11745–11749.

Mayer, L., Eisenhardt, D., and Shlien, R. (1988). Selective induction of antigen nonspecific suppressor cells with normal gut epithelium as accessory cells. *Monogr. Allergy* 24, 78–80.

Melamed, D., and Friedman, A. (1993a). Direct evidence for anergy in T lymphocytes tolerized by oral administration of ovalbumin. *Eur. J. Immunol.* 23, 935–942.

Melamed, D., and Friedman, A. (1993b). Modification of the immune response by oral tolerance: Antigen requirements and interaction with immunogenic stimuli. *Cell. Immunol.* **146**, 412–420.

Melamed, D., and Friedman, A. (1994). *In vivo* tolerization of Th1 lymphocytes following a single feeding with ovalbumin: Anergy in the absence of suppression. *Eur. J. Immunol.* **24**, 1974–1981.

Miller, A., Lider, O., Roberts, A. B., Sporn, M. B., and Weiner, H. L. (1992). Suppressor T cells generated by oral tolerization to myelin basic protein suppress both *in vitro* and *in vivo* immune responses by the release of transforming growth factor beta after antigen-specific triggering. *Proc. Natl. Acad. Sci. U.S.A.* **89**, 421–425.

Miller, A., Lider, O., and Weiner, H. L. (1991). Antigen-driven bystander suppression after oral administration of antigens. *J. Exp. Med.* **174**, 791–798.

Miller, C. C., and Cook, M. E. (1994). Evidence against the induction of immunological tolerance by feeding antigens to chickens. *Poult. Sci.* **73**, 106–112.

Miller, S. D., and Hanson, D. G. (1979). Inhibition of specific immune responses by feeding protein antigens. IV. Evidence for tolerance and specific active suppression of cell-mediated immune responses to ovalbumin. *J. Immunol.* **123**, 2344–2350.

Mowat, A. M. (1994). Oral tolerance. "Handbook of Mucosal Immunology," pp. 391–402. Academic Press, San Diego.

Peri, B. A., and Rothberg, R. M. (1981). Circulating antitoxin in rabbits after ingestion of diphtheria toxoid. *Infect. Immun.* **32**, 1148–1154.

Richman, L. K., Chiller, J. M., Brown, W. R., Hanson, D. G., and Vaz, N. M. (1978). Enterically induced immunologic tolerance. I. Induction of suppressor T lymphocytes by intragastric administration of soluble proteins. *J. Immunol.* **121**, 2429–2434.

Richman, L. K., Graeff, A. S., Yarchoan, R., and Strober, W. (1981). Simultaneous induction of antigen-specific IgA helper T cells and IgG suppressor T cells in the murine Peyer's patch after protein feeding. *J. Immunol.* **126**, 2079–2083.

Sanderson, I. R., Ouellette, A. J., Carter, E. A., Walker, W. A., and Harmatz, P. R. (1993). Differential regulation of B7 mRNA in enterocytes and lymphoid cells. *Immunology* **79**, 434–438.

Santos, L. M. B., Al-Sabbagh, A., Londono, A., and Weiner, H. L. (1993). Oral tolerance to myelin basic protein induces regulatory TGF-beta secreting T cells in Peyer's patches. *J. Immunol.* **150**, 115A.

Steinman, L. (1995). Escape from "horror autotoxicus": Pathogenesis and treatment of autoimmune disease. *Cell (Cambridge, Mass.)* **80**, 7–10.

Strobel, S., and Ferguson, A. (1984). Immune responses to fed protein antigens in mice. 3. Systemic tolerance or priming is related to age at which antigen is first encountered. *Pediatr. Res.* **18**, 588–594.

Strobel, S., Mowat, A. M., Drummond, H. E., Pickering, M. G., and Ferguson, A. (1983). Immunological responses to fed protein antigens in mice. II. Oral tolerance for CMI is due to activation of cyclophosphamide-sensitive cells by gut processed antigen. *Immunology* **49**, 451–455.

Sun, J. B., Holmgren, J., and Czerkinsky, C. (1994). Cholera toxin B subunit: An efficient transmucosal carrier-delivery system for induction of peripheral immunological tolerance. *Proc. Natl. Acad. Sci. U.S.A.* **91**, 10795–10799.

Thompson, H. S., and Staines, N. A. (1990). Could specific oral tolerance be a therapy for autoimmune disease? *Immunol. Today* **11**, 396–399.

Titus, R. G., and Chiller, J. M. (1981). Orally induced tolerance. Definition at the cellular level. *Int. Arch. Allergy Appl. Immunol.* **65**, 323–338.

Trentham, D. E., Dynesius-Trentham, R. A., Orav, E. J., Combitchi, D., Lorenzo, C., Sewell, K. L., Hafler, D. A., and Weiner, H. L. (1993). Effects of oral administration of type II collagen on rheumatoid arthritis. *Science* **261**, 1727–1730.

von Herrath, M., Dyrberg, T., and Oldstone, M. B. A. (1995). Virus-induced autoimmune diabetes can be prevented by oral tolerance. *Clin. Immunol. Immunopathol.* **76**, S121.

Weiner, H. L., Friedman, A., Miller, A., Khoury, S. J., al-Sabbagh, A., Santos, L., Sayegh, M., Nussenblatt, R. B., Trentham, D. E., and Hafler, D. A. (1994). Oral tolerance: Immunologic mechanisms and treatment of animal and human organ-specific autoimmune diseases by oral administration of autoantigens. *Annu. Rev. Immunol.* **12,** 809–837.

Weiner, H. L., Mackin, G. A., Matsui, M., Orav, E. J., Khoury, S. J., Dawson, D. M., and Hafler, D. A. (1993). Double-blind pilot trial of oral tolerization with myelin antigens in multiple sclerosis. *Science* **259,** 1321–1324.

Yoshino, S., Quattrocchi, E., and Weiner, H. L. (1995). Suppression of antigen-induced arthritis in Lewis rats by oral administration of type II collagen. *Arthritis Rheum.* **38,** 1092–1096.

Zhang, Z. J., Davidson, L., Eisenbarth, G., and Weiner, H. L. (1991). Suppression of diabetes in non-obese diabetic mice by oral administration of porcine insulin. *Proc. Natl. Acad. Sci. U.S.A.* **88,** 10252–10256.

Zhang, Z. Y., Lee, C. S., Lider, O., and Weiner, H. L. (1990). Suppression of adjuvant arthritis in Lewis rats by oral administration of type II collagen. *J. Immunol.* **145,** 2489–2493.

# Chapter 39

# Oral Tolerance: Immunologic Mechanisms and Treatment of Autoimmune Diseases

Howard L. Weiner

*Center for Neurologic Diseases, Brigham and Women's Hospital and Harvard Medical School, Boston, Massachusetts 02115*

Oral tolerance was first described in 1911 when Wells fed hen's egg proteins to guinea pigs and found them resistant to anaphylaxis when challenged (1). Thus, it is a long-recognized method of inducing immune tolerance and refers to the observation that if one feeds a protein and then immunizes with the fed protein, a state of systemic hyporesponsiveness to the fed protein exists. In 1946, Chase fed guinea pigs the contact sensitizing agent, DCNB, and observed that animals had decreased skin reactivity to DCNB (2). Subsequently, numerous investigators have found that animals fed proteins such as ovalbumin or sheep red blood cells do not respond as well to these antigens when subsequently immunized, but do respond normally to other antigens (3). The phenomenon of oral tolerance has also been observed in humans fed and immunized with KLH (4).

In recent years, as more has been learned about the general mechanisms of immune tolerance, investigators have begun to apply oral tolerance as a method to manipulate injurious immune responses, primarily in the area of autoimmune diseases, although its applications appear broader and have included transplantation as well. This area has gained intense interest and is likely to grow since manipulation of systemic immune responses via the mucosal immune system has major practical and theoretical advantages.

Immunologic tolerance is a basic property of the immune system that provides for self/non-self discrimination so that the immune system can protect the host from external pathogens without reacting against self. When the immune system reacts against itself, autoimmune disease results. For a time it was thought that self/non-self discrimination was a simple matter of deleting autoreactive cells in the thymus, but it is now clear that the maintenance of immunologic tolerance is a much more complicated process. Autoreactive cells, such as those reacting with brain, are not deleted and can be found in normal individuals (5,6). Why these cells become activated and cause disease in some individuals whereas in others they remain harmless is a major question in basic immunology. How to control the autoimmune process once it has been initiated is major problem in clinical medicine.

These two areas have come together in recent years as oral tolerance has been used successfully to treat autoimmune diseases in animal models (reviewed in Ref. 7) and is now being applied for the treatment of human disease states (8, 9) Furthermore, an understanding of the basic mechanisms by which orally administered antigens induce immune tolerance is beginning to emerge. As with immunologic tolerance in general, oral tolerance involves multiple mechanisms (10–13). Thus the term oral tolerance is in some ways misleading as it implies that there is one unique mechanism of tolerance induction when antigens are administered orally. This is not the case. Although the gut clearly has unique properties that favor tolerance induction, the type of tolerance induced must now be defined when factors that influence oral tolerance are investigated.

Orally administered antigen encounters the gut-associated lymphoid tissue or GALT, a very well developed immune network that not only evolved to protect the host from ingested pathogens, but also developed the inherent property of preventing the host from reacting to ingested proteins. The GALT consists of villi which contain epithelial cells capable of antigen presentation, intraepithelial lymphocytes, and lamnia propria lymphocytes (14). In addition, there are Peyer's patches, lymphoid nodules interspersed among the villi, which are one of the primary areas in the GALT where specific immune responses are generated. Investigators have attempted to use the GALT to immunize for vaccines but have been hampered by the systemic hyporesponsiveness or oral tolerance that is naturally generated. Nonetheless, as described below, active induction of selected immune responses in the GALT is one of the primary mechanisms by which oral antigen suppresses systemic immunity.

In addition to stimulating the GALT, some oral antigen is absorbed. Although dietary antigens are degraded by the time they reach the small intestine, studies in humans and rodents have indicated that the degradation is partial and that some intact antigen is absorbed (15,16). Absorbed antigen, either undergraded or partially degraded, appears to have an important role in the generation of certain types of oral tolerance.

## I. Mechanisms of Oral Tolerance

It is now known that the mechanisms by which oral tolerance is mediated include the generation of active cellular suppression (regulatory cells), clonal anergy, or clonal deletion; the determining factor is the dose of antigen fed (10–13) (Fig. 1). Low doses favor active suppression, whereas higher doses favor anergy and deletion. Active suppression is mediated by the induction of regulatory T cells in the gut-associated lymphoid tissue such as Peyer's patches. These cells then migrate

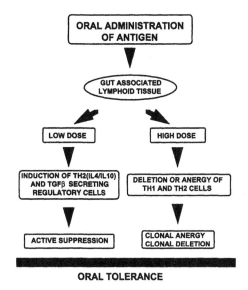

**FIGURE 1.** Mechanisms of oral tolerance.

to the systemic immune system. When higher doses of antigen are fed, clonal anergy results and can be demonstrated by reversal of systemic hyporesponsiveness by culturing with recombinant IL-2 (10,12). Anergy appears to be favored by the passage of antigen into the systemic circulation. When large doses of antigen are fed, clonal deletion occurs (13). Thus, oral tolerance is not a single immunologic event.

Active cellular suppression of immune responses has been studied extensively over the years and has remained ill-defined due to difficulties in cloning suppressor cells and defining their mechanism of action. More recently, it appears that one of the primary mechanisms of active cellular suppression is via the secretion of suppressive cytokines such as TGFβ, IL-4, and IL-10 after antigen-specific triggering (17). In this sense the GALT is unique as it favors the induction of cells which secrete these cytokines, Th2 as opposed Th1 cells and T cells which secrete TGFβ, a potent immunosuppressive cytokine. T cells in lymphoid organs drained by mucosal sites secrete IL-4 as a primary T-cell growth factor whereas those drained by nonmucosal sites secrete IL-2 (18). Oral tolerance has often been demonstrated by a decreased delayed type hypersensitivity (DTH) response to the fed antigen (2, 3, 7) and it is known that DTH is a Th1 response inhibited by IL-4-producing Th2 cells. TGFβ plays an important role in local function of the gut as it serves as a switch factor for IgA production in the mucosa (19) and may also be involved in the homing mechanism of the cells to high endothelial venules

(20). TGF$\beta$ is produced by both CD4$^+$ and CD8$^+$ GALT-derived T cells (17, 21) and is an important mediator of the active component of oral tolerance. TGF$\beta$-secreting MBP-specific CD4$^+$ cells have recently been cloned from the mesenteric lymph nodes of orally tolerized SJL mice (17). These clones were structurally identical to Th1 disease-inducing clones in TCR usage, MHC restriction, and epitope recognition but suppressed rather than induced disease. Thus, mucosally derived CF4$^+$ cells which primarily produce TGF$\beta$ may be a unique T-cell subset with both mucosal T-helper function and downregulatory properties for Th1 and other immune cells.

## II. BYSTANDER SUPPRESSION AND ORAL TOLERANCE

Bystander suppression was discovered during the investigation of regulatory cells induced by oral administration of low doses of MBP (22). It solves a major conceptual problem related to designing antigen- or T-cell specific therapy of inflammatory autoimmune diseases, such as multiple sclerosis, type 1 diabetes, and rheumatoid arthritis, in which the autoantigen is unknown or where there are reactivities to multiple autoantigens in the target tissue. In animal models of autoimmunity, during the course of the chronic inflammatory autoimmune process there is intra- and interantigenic spread of autoreactivity at the target organ (23–27). Similar findings have been observed in human autoimmune disease in which there are reactivities to multiple autoantigens from the target tissue. For example, in multiple sclerosis there is immune reactivity to three myelin antigens, MBP, PLP, and MOG (5, 6). In type 1 diabetes, there are multiple islet-cell antigens that could be the target of autoreactivity including GAD, insulin, and heat-shock proteins (28). Because regulatory cells induced by oral antigen secrete antigen nonspecific cytokines after being triggered by the fed antigen, they suppress inflammation in the microenvironment where the fed antigen is localized. Thus, for an organ-specific inflammatory disease, one need not know the specific antigen that is the target of an autoimmune response but only feed an antigen capable of reducing regulatory cells which then migrate to the target tissue and suppress inflammation. Bystander suppression was demonstrated *in vitro* when it was shown that cells from MBP fed animals suppressed proliferation of an ovalbumin line across a transwell, but only when triggered by the fed antigen (22). The soluble factor was identified as TGF$\beta$. Bystander suppression has also been demonstrated in autoimmune disease models. One can suppress PLP peptide-induced EAE by feeding myelin basic protein (29) and MBP-specific T-cell clones from orally tolerized animals which secrete TGF$\beta$ also suppress PLP-induced disease. Other examples include the suppression of adjuvant (30) and antigen (31) induced arthritis by feeding type II collagen, the suppression of insulitis in the NOD mouse by feeding glucagon (7), and the suppression of LCMV-induced diabetes in mice that have had LCMV proteins expressed via the insulin promoter on the pancreatic islets by feeding insulin (32).

## III. TREATMENT OF AUTOIMMUNE DISEASES IN ANIMALS

A large series of studies have demonstrated that orally administered autoantigens can suppress several experimental models of autoimmunity and transplantation (Table I; reviewed in Ref. 7). The mechanism of suppression in these models depends on dosage administered; in some instances active suppression has been shown and in other instances, clonal anergy. Immunohistochemical studies have demonstrated the upregulation of anti-inflammatory cytokines such as TGF$\beta$ and IL-4 in the target organ of animals fed low dose of autoantigens (33–35). Importantly, for human trials, feeding after immunization (30) and feeding in chronic disease models such as chronic EAE have been successful (36). Thus, it does not appear that feeding an autoantigen to an already sensitized animal necessarily results in further priming. Suppression of disease, however, may be most effective when homologous protein is administered (37) which has important implications for treatment of human autoimmune diseases for which recombinant human proteins would be required. Although one can suppress the generation of antibodies by oral feeding, much larger doses are required and since the gut preferentially induces Th2 responses, the degree to which oral tolerance will be successful in suppressing antibody-mediated diseases is unclear.

## IV. TREATMENT OF AUTOIMMUNE DISEASES IN HUMANS

Investigators have shown that exposure of a contact sensitizing agent via the mucosa prior to subsequent skin challenge led to unresponsiveness in a portion of patients studied (38). Orally administered KLH, 50 mg given daily for 2 weeks

### TABLE I
#### SUPPRESSION OF AUTOIMMUNITY BY ORAL TOLERANCE

| Animal models | Protein fed |
| --- | --- |
| EAE | MBP, PLP |
| Arthritis (CII, AA, Ag, Pris) | Type II collagen |
| Uveitis | S-Antigen, IRBP |
| Diabetes (NOD mouse) | Insulin, glutamate decarboxylase |
| Myasthenia Gravie | AChR |
| Thyroiditis | Thyroglobulin |
| Transplantation | Alloantigen, MHC peptide |

| Human disease trials | Protein |
| --- | --- |
| Multiple sclerosis | Bovine myelin |
| Rheumatoid arthritis | Chicken type II collagen |
| Uveoretinitis | Bovine S-antigen |
| Type I diabetes | Human insulin |

over a 3-week period to human subjects, has been reported to decrease subsequent cell-mediated immune responses, although antibody responses were not affected (4).

Based on the long history of oral tolerance and the apparent safety of the approach, human trials have been initiated in multiple sclerosis (8), rheumatoid arthritis (9), and uveitis (39). These initial phase I/II trials have involved a relatively small number of patients and the clinical efficacy of oral antigen in these diseases must await the results of large-scale trials that are currently in progress (Table I). What can be said from the initial trials is that there was no apparent toxicity or exacerbation of disease. In MS patients, a decrease in MBP reactive cells was observed in the peripheral blood, and in rheumatoid arthritis joint swelling was decreased. In multiple sclerosis there is presently a 500-patient double-blind phase III trial in which patients are randomized by sex and DR type, which may link to the response. In rheumatoid arthritis, a 280-patient double-blind phase II dosing trial has just been completed in which doses ranging from 20 to 2500 $\mu$g were tested. Preliminary analysis of the data suggests a positive effect in patients feed 20 $\mu$g. In uveitis, a double-masked trial of S-antigen and an S-antigen mixture is currently in progress. In addition, trials are being planned both in juvenile and new-onset diabetes in which oral recombinant human insulin will be administered.

## REFERENCES

1. Wells, H. G. (1911). *J. Infect. Dis.* **8,** 147–171.
2. Chase, M. (1946). *Proc. Soc. Exp. Biol. Med.* **61,** 257–259.
3. Mowat, A. M. (1987). *Immunol. Today* **8,** 93–98.
4. Husby, S., Mestecky, J., Moldoveanu, Z., Holland, S., and Elson, C. O. (1994). *J. Immunol.* **152,** 4663.
5. Kerlero de Rosbo, N., Milo, R., Lees, M. B., Burger, D., Bernard, C. C. A., and Ben-Nun, A. (1993). *J. Clin. Invest.* **92,** 2602–2608.
6. Zhang, J., Markovic, S., Raus, J., Lacet, B., Weiner, H. L., and Hafler, D. A. (1993). *J. Exp. Med.* **179,** 973–984.
7. Weiner, H. L., Friedman, A., Miller, A., Khoury, S. J., Al-Sabbagh, A., Santos, L. M. B., Sayegh, M., Nussenblatt, R. B., Trentham, D. E., and Hafler, D. A. (1994). *Annu. Rev. Immunol.* **12,** 809–837.
8. Weiner, H. L., Mackin, G. A., Matsui, M., Orav, E. J., Khoury, S. J., Dawson, D. M., and Hafler, D. A. (1993). *Science* **259,** 1321–1324.
9. Trentham, D. E., Dynesius-Trentham, R. A., Orav, E. J., Combitchi, D., Lorenzo, C., Sewell, K. L., Hafler, D. A., and Weiner, H. L. (1993). *Science* **261,** 1727–1730.
10. Whitacre, C. C., Gienapp, I. E., Orosz, C. G., and Bitar, D. (1991). *J. Immunol.* **147,** 2155–2163.
11. Gregerson, D. S., Obritsch, W. F., and Donoso, L. A. (1993). *J. Immunol.* **151,** 5751–5761.
12. Friedman, A., and Weiner, H. L. (1994). *Proc. Natl. Acad. Sci. U.S.A.* **91,** 6688–6692.
13. Chen, Y., Inobe, J., Marks, R., Gonella, P., Kuchroo, V. J., and Weiner, H. L. (1995). *Nature (London)* **376,** 177–180.
14. Brandtzaeg, P. (1989). *Curr. Top. Microbiol. Immunol.* **146,** 13–28.
15. Husby, S., Jensenius, J. C., and Svehag, S.-E. (1986). *Scand. J. Immunol.* **24,** 447–452.
16. Bruce, M. G., and Ferguson, A. (1986). *Immunology* **59,** 295–300.

17. Chen, Y., Kuchroo, V. K., Inobe, J.-I., Hafler, D. A., and Weiner, H. L. (1994). *Science* **265**, 1237–1240.
18. Daynes, R., Araneo, B., Dowell, T., Huang, K., and Dudley, D. (1990). *J. Exp. Med.* **171**, 979–996.
19. Kim, P.-H., and Kagnoff, M. F. (1990). *J. Immunol.* **144**, 3411–3416.
20. Chin, Y. H., Cai, J. P., and Xu, X. M. (1992). *J. Immunol.* **148**, 1106–1112.
21. Santos, L. M. B., Al-Sabbagh, A., Londono, A., and Weiner, H. L. (1994). *Cell. Immunol.* **157**, 439–447.
22. Miller, A., Lider, O., and Weiner, H. L. (1991). *J. Exp. Med.* **174**, 791–798.
23. McCarron, R., Fallis, R., and McFarlin, D. (1990). *J. Neuroimmunol.* **29**, 73–79.
24. Lehmann, P., Forsthuber, T., Miller, A., and Sercarz, E. (1992). *Nature (London)* **358**, 155.
25. Cross, A. H., Tuohy, V. K., and Raine, C. S. (1993). *Cell. Immunol.* **146**, 261–270.
26. Kaufman, D. L., Clare-Salzier, M., Tian, J., Forsthuber, T., Ting, G. S. P., Robinson, P., Atkinson, M. A., Sercarz, E. E., Tobin, A. J., and Lehmann, P. V. (1993). *Nature (London)* **366**, 72–75.
27. Tisch, R., Yang, X.-D., Singer, S. M., Liblau, R. S., Fugger, L., and McDevitt, H. O. (1993). *Nature (London)* **366**, 72–75.
28. Harrison, L. C. (1992). *Immunol. Today* **13**, 348–352.
29. Al-Sabbagh, A., Miller, A., Santos, L. M. B., and Weiner, H. L. (1994). *Eur. J. Immunol.* **24**, 2104–2109.
30. Zhang, J. Z., Lee,C. S. Y., Lider, O., and Weiner, H. L. (1990). *J. Immunol.* **145**, 2489–2493.
31. Yoshino, S., Wuattrocchi, E., and Weiner, H. L. (1995). *Arthritis Rheum.* **38**, 1092–1096.
32. Herrath, M., Dyrberg, T., and Oldstone, M. B. A. (1995). *Int. Congr. Immunol. Abstr.* **5018**, 846.
33. Khoury, S. J., Hancock, W. W., and Weiner, H. L. (1992). *J. Exp. Med.* **176**, 1355.
34. Hancock, W., Sayegh, M., Kwok, C., Weiner, H. L., and Carpenter, C. (1993). *Transplantation* **55**, 1112–1118.
35. Hancock, W., Polanski, M., Zhang, J., Blogg, N., and Weiner, H. L. (1995). *Am. J. Pathol.* **147**, 1193–1199.
36. Brod, S. A., Al-Sabbgh, A., Sobel, R. A., Hafler, D. A., and Weiner, H. L. (1991). *Ann. Neurol.* **29**, 615–622.
37. Miller, A., Lider, O., Al-Sabbagh, A., and Weiner, H. (1992). *J. Neuroimmunol.* **39**, 243–250.
38. Lowney, E. D. (1968). *J. Invest. Dermatol.* **51**, 411–417.
39. Nussenblatt, R. B., Whitcup, S. M., de Smet, M. D., Caspi, R. R., Kozhich, A. T., Weiner, H. L., Vistica, B., and Gery, I. (1996). Intraocular Inflammatory Disease (Uveitis) and the Use of Oral Tolerance: A Status Report. *N.Y. Acad. Sci.* **778**, 325–337.

# Chapter 40

# A Molecular Approach to the Construction of an Effective Mucosal Vaccine Adjuvant: Studies Based on Cholera Toxin ADP-Ribosylation and Cell Targeting

Nils Lycke

*Department of Medical Microbiology and Immunology,
University of Göteborg, S-413 46 Göteborg, Sweden*

In the present chapter we describe how molecular immunology may be used to better understand regulatory mechanisms in mucosal immunity. With cholera toxin (CT) as the prototype we discuss how current knowledge about the function of a potent mucosal immunoenhancer may be explored to construct compounds that can find general use as future vaccine adjuvants. Two technical achievements were of fundamental importance for the study. The first was the development of gene fusion technology which enabled the linking of genes encoding different properties into a single fusion protein with defined biological functions. Thereby, molecular constructs can be composed that are actively immunomodulating and targeted to a distinct cell population of the immune system. We will present recent data generated in our laboratory that suggest that such targeted adjuvants may, indeed, be constructed and can be made to affect events or cellular subsets that play central roles in the immune response. The second prerequisite for the study was the establishment of transgene and homologous gene recombination technologies which have provided *in vivo* models that greatly facilitate studies of complex regulatory mechanisms such as those controling mucosal immunity. We have taken advantage of these technologies to better understand how an efficient mucosal adjuvant should be constructed. In the gene knock-out mice we have investigated whether a distinct celltype, i.e., $CD8^+$ T cells or $CD4^+$ Th2 cells, or a cytokine is responsible for the adjuvant function of our prototype adjuvant, CT. Our recent findings using these *in vivo* models will be discussed.

There is a growing interest in oral vaccines and the possibility to use such

*Essentials of Mucosal Immunology*   Copyright © 1996 by Academic Press, Inc. All rights of reproduction in any form reserved.

vaccines to protect not only against infectious diseases affecting mucosal surfaces but also against diseases like HIV, chlamydia, and polio (Lycke and Svennerholm, 1990; McGhee *et al.,* 1992; Mestecky *et al.,* 1994). Although live vectors have been found to be efficient delivery systems for oral antigen administration, the clinical use of such vaccines is still unclear (Mestecky *et al.,* 1994; Michalek *et al.,* 1994). This has prompted research with the aim of identifying substances that could find general use as adjuvants in mucosal vaccines. Most soluble protein antigens are normally poor immunogens at mucosal surfaces, and when administered perorally they fail to stimulate significant immune responses (McGhee *et al.,* 1992). By contrast, feeding of most protein antigens will induce oral tolerance, which is characterized by systemic unresponsiveness to a second challenge with the antigen (Mowat, 1994). A powerful mucosal adjuvant should be nontoxic and should greatly improve immunogenicity of the protein antigen and promote the development of long-term immunological memory. Whether it is necessary to break induction of oral tolerance or not is currently a debated issue. It should be noted that all mucosal adjuvant systems described so far have abrogated oral tolerance while promoting gut mucosal IgA immunity (Mowat, 1994). Therefore, it would appear that local IgA immunity and oral tolerance are two mutually exclusive phenomena. Nevertheless, two principally different approaches have been taken to achieve an efficient mucosal adjuvant; the first has focused on constructing powerful delivery systems for oral antigens. Encapsulated microparticles are an example of this research (Eldridge *et al.,* 1989; Challacombe *et al.,* 1992; Michalek *et al.,* 1994). The second approach is to construct an adjuvant that will immunomodulate the response to the oral antigen, thereby evoking strong IgA immunity and immunological memory (Lycke and Svennerholm, 1990). The cholera toxin (CT) system has become a prototype system for this latter approach.

Cholera toxin is an exceptionally potent mucosal immunogen and adjuvant (Elson and Ealding, 1984a,b; Lycke and Holmgren, 1986; Liang *et al.,* 1988). The toxin also breaks induction of oral tolerance and has become the probe used most to understand how an efficient mucosal adjuvant might be constructed (Elson and Ealding, 1984b; Hörnquist *et al.,* 1994). Despite several years of research and many reports on the immunomodulating properties of CT, it is still uncertain which entity of CT is critical for its adjuvant function. For several years we have studied the properties of CT in a mouse model using both *in vivo* and *in vitro* experimental systems (Hörnquist *et al.,* 1994). In our research we have tried to systematically address CT's immunomodulating properties which could affect important events involved in initiating and regulating mucosal immune responses, e.g., antigen-presentation, IgA B-cell differentiation, T-cell regulation, and development of long-term immunological memory.

CT is composed of five enzymatically inactive, nontoxic B subunits (CT-B) held together in a pentamere surrounding a single A subunit that contains a linker to the pentamere via the A2 fragment (CT-A2) and the toxic enzymatically active A1 fragment (CT-A1) of the molecule (Rappuoli and Pizza, 1991). The toxic

CT-A1 has strong ADP-ribosyltransferase activity and is thought to act on several GTP-binding proteins (G-proteins); the activity is strongest on Gs$\alpha$. This results in activation of adenylate cyclase and the subsequent intracellular increase in cAMP. CT-B binds to the ganglioside GM1 receptor, present on most mammalian cells, and thereafter CT-A is translocated into the cell membrane/cytosol of the cell where the CT-A1 and CT-A2 are dissociated. The profuse diarrheal response in cholera is thought to result from CT-A1-induced increased cAMP levels in the intestinal epithelium.

An important issue is, therefore, whether the adjuvant property of CT may be separated from the toxic property. A simple solution to this problem would be to use only the CT-B moiety of the holotoxin. However, most experimental studies using recombinant CT-B agree that this moiety is not acting as a mucosal adjuvant when admixed with a protein antigen and given perorally (Hörnquist et al., 1994). Rather, the principal adjuvant effect has been attributed to the CT-A1-moiety (Lycke et al., 1992). This understanding has prompted research attempting to separate the toxic activity from the adjuvant activity using site-directed mutagenesis of the CT-A-moiety (Burnette et al., 1991). Of note, though, one should bear in mind that there are distinct differences with regard to CT-B's effects in different species and given as an immunoenhancer by different routes. For example, in humans CT-B is highly immunogenic given perorally, whereas it is poorly immunogenic by that route in mice (Lycke and Svennerholm, 1990; Hörnquist et al., 1994). However, in mice CT-B may be used as an effective carrier molecule for oral antigen delivery and in the presence of small doses of holotoxin it may stimulate strong mucosal immune responses (Czerkinsky et al., 1989; Russell and Wu, 1991; Hajishengallis et al., 1995). Used separately as a carrier molecule conjugated to protein antigens, CT-B has been shown recently to greatly facilitate the induction of oral tolerance while having only a poor effect on local intestinal IgA immune responses (Sun et al., 1994). However, in contrast to the peroral administration, an immunoenhancing effect has been documented for CT-B when admixed with protein antigens and given by the intranasal route (Tamura et al., 1988; Wu and Russell, 1993). Thus, the requirements for an immunoenhancing effect of any given adjuvant may differ between species and between different routes of immunization. For the sake of clarity, the rest of the discussion in this chapter will focus on studies in mice and neglect that species differences may exist.

## I. UNDERSTANDING IMMUNOMODULATION BY CT: WHAT DO WE KNOW?

### A. Antigen Uptake and Gut Permeability

One explanation for the potent mucosal adjuvant effect of CT is its ability to bind to the GM1-ganglioside receptor on the gut epithelial cells. Increased uptake of antigen in intestinal follicles may be promoted by CT and it has been found that particles conjugated to CT, in fact, selectively localized to the M cells overlaying the follicles rather than to the normal gut epithelium (Neutra and Kraehenbuhl, 1992). Nevertheless, this cannot be the only effect of CT as a mucosal adjuvant because CT-B, which binds equally well to the GM1-ganglioside receptor on the M cells, is a comparatively poor mucosal adjuvant given perorally (Hörnquist et al., 1994). In addition, CT need not be physically conjugated to the antigen to exert the adjuvant effect, suggesting that the GM1-receptor pathway for antigen-uptake is not the only critical factor for the adjuvant effect (Lycke and Holmgren, 1986). We have investigated whether increased gut permeability for luminal anti-gens could be part of CT's adjuvant function. By comparing the effect on gut permeability to luminal antigens with the adjuvant effect on intestinal immune responses to oral immunizations with CT or CT-B, we found that CT's adjuvant effect on local immunity was linked to an increased gut permeability for luminal antigens whereas CT-B failed to influence any of these events (Lycke et al., 1991c). Thus, CT's gut mucosal adjuvant effect may potentially occur at local sites in the epithelium, lamina propria, or regional lymph nodes and may not be restricted to follicles such as the Peyer's patches (PP).

## B. Does the Adjuvant Effect Require ADP-Ribosyltransferase Activity?

Previous data and the finding of an increased gut permeability for luminal antigens in the presence of CT suggested that the adjuvant effect might depend on the ability of CT, but not CT-B, to activate the adenylate cyclase/cAMP system. Ne-drud and co-workers have shown that glutaraldehyde treatment of CT leads to a 1000-fold reduction in toxicity but preserved capacity to enhance mucosal immune responses after oral immunization (Liang et al., 1989). A concomitant loss of ribo-syltransferase activity occurred such that with a suitable substrate and necessary cofactors (supplied by lysed red cells) 5–10% residual cyclic AMP was generated compared to untreated toxin. To more directly, test the hypothesis that CT-A1 ADP-ribosyltransferase is required for adjuvanticity we compared the adjuvant properties of cholera toxin, the highly homologous E. coli heat-labile toxin (LT), and a mutated form of heat-labile toxin (LTm) which lacks ADP-ribosyltransferase activity. We found that the toxic LT had potent adjuvant properties similar to that of CT. In contrast, the completely nontoxic mutated LT, which had a single amino acid substitution at residue Glu-112 of the A1-subunit, completely lacked adjuvant properties even though it exhibited undiminished binding to the toxin receptor, ganglioside GM1 (Lycke et al., 1992). This finding reinforces the idea that the ADP-ribosyltransferase function of CT is important for the adjuvant effects. Other investigators have reported that additional single amino acid mutations of the A-subunit of CT or LT at Arg7, Asp9, His44, Ser61, His70, Glu79, Arg146, and Arg192 also have diminished or altered ADP-ribosyltransferase activity (Burnette et al., 1991; Grant et al., 1994; Dickinson and Clements, 1995; Douce et al.,

1995); the effects of some of these mutations on the capacity to enhance mucosal immune responses have recently been documented.

The results from these studies, however, are not conclusive. Because of the conflicting findings it is still unclear whether the adjuvant effect of native CT or LT can be ascribed to the enzymatic activities of these toxins: Douce et al reported that the LT mutant LTK-7 with Arg7→Lys acted as a mucosal adjuvant when used for intranasal immunizations despite lacking ADP-ribosyltransferase activity (Douce *et al.*, 1995). However, the LTK-7 mutant was not tested for adjuvant effects after oral administration and the study did not compare the enhancing effect of the nontoxic LTK-7 with that of LT-B in the absence of LTA. Moreover, Grant *et al.* (1994) showed that a mutation in LT-A at position Arg192→Gly reduced, but did not completely block, the ADP-ribosylating ability of LT. This mutation also exerted significant cytotonic activity and was able to stimulate intracellular cAMP increases. By contrast, an exactly identical mutation of LT-A, Arg192→Gly ($LT_{R192G}$), was reported by Dickinson (1995) to have negligible cytotonic effects and be devoid of ADP-ribosylating function but to have retained the ability to act as a mucosal adjuvant. However, a strict mucosal immunization protocol was not employed, because the adjuvant effect was evaluated after oral priming with antigen together with the $LT_{R192G}$ followed by parenteral boosting with antigen alone.

## C. Effects of CT on Antigen Presentation

An important event in immune responses to most soluble protein antigens is the priming of $CD4^+$ T-helper cells. Therefore, we have focused on cognate interactions between antigen-presenting cells (APC) and T cells. In initial studies we used macrophages, freshly isolated or cell lines, as APC to elucidate whether CT affects T-cell activation. These studies demonstrated that CT greatly enhanced APC function leading to increased T-cell proliferation *in vitro*. We found that CT potentiated both allogen- and antigen-specific T-cell proliferation. The mechanism responsible for this effect was an enhanced costimulation by the APC as revealed by increased production of cytokines, IL-1, and upregulated expression of membrane associated molecules such as B-7.1 and B-7.2 (Bromander *et al.*, 1991; Hörnquist *et al.*, 1994). The enhancing effect of CT on surface expression of B-7 molecules was also found with B cells and was mimicked by dibutyryl-cAMP (dBcAMP) but was not observed with the non-ADP-ribosylating CT-B moeity (Fig. 1). Also, gut epithelial cells were found to respond to treatment with CT and demonstrated enhanced allo-antigen activating ability of freshly isolated T cells. CT-treated gut epithelial cells were 50–75% more efficient as APC as compared to untreated cells. Again, the mechanism for this enhancement was due to increased costimulation involving induction of IL-1 and IL-6 production (Bromander *et al.*, 1993). Moreover, APC isolated from MLN or PP of mice orally treated with CT were more effective at presenting antigen relative to such cells from nontreated

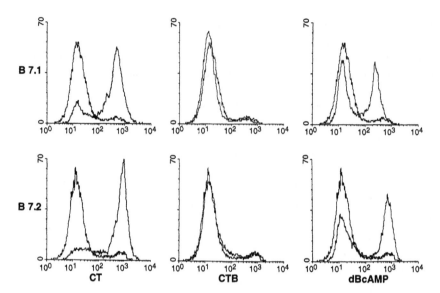

**FIGURE 1.** Surface expression of B-7.1 and B-7.2 molecules on B cells cultured in the presence or absence of CT, rCT-B, or dBcAMP. Enriched spleen B cells were cultured for 24 hr in plain medium or in the presence of 0.1 μg of CT, 1 μg of rCTB, or 100 μM of dibutyryl cAMP (dBcAMP). After washings, cells were double-labeled with anti-Ig PE together with FITC-labeled ant-B7.1 or B-7.2, respectively. FACS profiles showing Ig$^+$ cells from cultures with plain medium are merged with the profiles from indicated cultures. The panels show upregulation of B-7.1 and B-7.2 in cultures with CT or dBcAMP.

animals, indicating that, indeed, the *in vitro* findings reflect the function of CT *in vivo* (Lycke and Svennerholm, 1990). In addition, using limiting dilution analysis we have found that CT increases the frequency of primed antigen-specific CD4$^+$ T cells by 20- to 40-fold as compared to immunizations with antigen alone, without CT-adjuvant (Hörnquist and Lycke, 1993). Accordingly, we believe that the enhancing effect of CT on antigen-presentation and costimulation is one of the most important immunomodulating effects of CT and may, at least in part, explain the adjuvant function of CT *in vivo*.

## D. T-Cell Priming and Differentiation

For long there has been an apparent inconsistency in our understanding of CT's effects on the immune system; while CT has been found to strongly inhibit T-cell functions *in vitro* it has become one of the most frequently used adjuvants to augment immune responses *in vivo*. Both CD4$^+$ and CD8$^+$ T-cell-dependent responses such as IgA antibody production and cytotoxic T-cell effector functions may be strongly augmented by CT adjuvant (Wilson *et al.*, 1991; Hörnquist and Lycke, 1993; Bowen *et al.*, 1994). The adjuvant effect of CT is not restricted to

MHC class I or class II presentation. Although Elson *et al.* have provided evidence to suggest that the immunomodulating effect of CT is genetically restricted by MHC molecules, no mouse strain has yet been reported which is totally unresponsive to the adjuvant effect of CT (Elson, 1992). The data from most studies, rather, seem only to reflect the prevailing MHC restriction in the ability of different mouse strains to respond to a certain antigen and not to the inability to respond to the adjuvant effect of CT.

Studies of CT's effects on T cells *in vitro* have reported mostly inhibitory actions, e.g., that mitogen- or IL-2 dependent T-cell proliferation as well as T-cell receptor mediated activation were all blocked by CT (Imboden *et al.*, 1986; Woogen *et al.*, 1987; Anderson and Tsoukas, 1989; Munoz *et al.*, 1990; Haack *et al.*, 1993; Hörnquist *et al.*, 1994). However, IL-4-driven T-cell proliferation was found less sensitive to CT-inhibition as compared to IL-2 driven proliferation *in vitro* (Anderson and Tsoukas, 1989; Munoz *et al.*, 1990). It was, therefore, proposed that while Th1 cells (IL-2, IFNγ) were blocked by CT, Th2-cell functions (IL-4) were not (Munoz *et al.*, 1990; Lacour *et al.*, 1994). To investigate this hypothesis we established an experimental model for the study of CT's effect on T-cell priming. Mice were given a single dose of KLH with or without the addition of CT-adjuvant and 7 days later T cells were restimulated by recall antigen *in vitro*. CT primarily enhanced CD4$^+$ T-cell priming while CD8$^+$ T cells were not required for the adjuvant effect. No selective effect on either Th1 or Th2 type of CD4$^+$ T cells was evident with CT adjuvant (Hörnquist and Lycke, 1993).

These findings were recently confirmed using gene knockout mice. Such mice are means of choice to explore some of the possible mechanisms for CT's adjuvant effects. We found potent adjuvant effects of CT in CD8$^{-/-}$ mice following oral immunizations with KLH plus CT (Hörnquist *et al.*, 1996). In fact, the CD8$^{-/-}$ mice demonstrated 3- to 5-fold stronger local mucosal B- and T cell responses following oral immunization with KLH and CT-adjuvant as compared to normal C57B1/6 mice (Fig. 2). Also, we found that oral tolerance could be induced in CD8$^{-/-}$ mice and that the development of oral tolerance was abrogated by coadministration of CT to the oral feeding protocol. Both these findings of strong immunomodulating function in CD8$^{-/-}$ mice preclude that CT requires CD8$^+$ T cells to exert its adjuvant effect on the immune system (Woogen *et al.*, 1987; Elson *et al.*, 1995). Thus, although it has been claimed that CT exerts its adjuvant effect through impaired suppresive functions of CD8$^+$ T cells there is currently little experimental support for this notion (Elson *et al.*, 1995). Furthermore, arguing against such a theory is the fact that, whereas CT is a good mucosal adjuvant but CT-B is not, both CT-B and CT have been found to exert similar downregulatory effects on CD8$^+$ T cells (Woogen *et al.*, 1987; Elson *et al.*, 1995).

In the context of soluble protein antigens, CT acts to augment CD4$^+$ T-cell priming as we and others have reported (Wilson *et al.*, 1991; Hörnquist and Lycke, 1993). Whether CT selectively promotes Th1- or Th2-dominated responses has been intensely discussed (Hörnquist and Lycke, 1993; Xu-Amano *et al.*, 1993). In

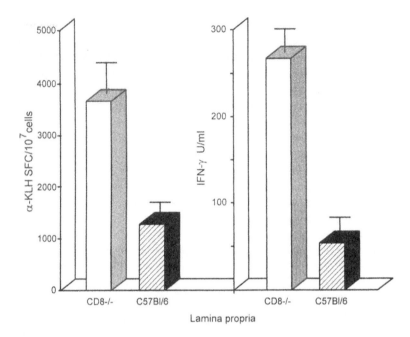

**FIGURE 2.** Mice deficient for CD8[+] T cells show strong adjuvant effects of cholera toxin. Following three oral immunizations with KLH plus CT-adjuvant, local immune responses by lamina propria lymphocytes were evaluated. Antibody production (SFC) was analyzed by the ELISPOT method on freshly isolated cells (left) whereas IFNγ production (right) was detected after *in vitro* culture of isolated T cells in the presence of APC and specific antigen. Figures are from representative experiments showing means ± SD.

collaboration with Manfred Kopf (Basel Institute for Immunology, Basel) and Marie Kosco-Vilbois (Glaxo, Geneva), we found that mucosal immune responses were impaired in IL-4-deficient (IL-4$^{-/-}$) mice (Vajdy *et al.*, 1995). These mice exhibited cytokine profiles and serum IgE and IgG-subclass patterns consistent with no or poor Th2 responses (Kopf *et al.*, 1993; Vajdy *et al.*, 1995). Using the IL-4$^{-/-}$ mice we observed that, although CT failed to promote mucosal immune responses to coadministered proteins following oral immunization, systemic responses after parenteral immunization in the presence of CT were clearly upregulated to the same degree as seen in wild-type mice. In addition, CT exerted an adjuvant effect on intestinal immune responses if antigen was physically conjugated to CT prior to oral administration (M. Vajdy, unpublished observation). Interestingly, CT as an immunogen, contrary to KLH or OVA, was able to stimulate strong gut mucosal anti-CT IgA immune responses following oral immunizations in IL-4$^{-/-}$ mice. Therefore, it may be concluded that the presence of IL-4 or Th2 cells seem not to be required for an adjuvant effect of CT and that CT has the ability to stimulate mucosal immune responses in the gut through an IL-4/Th2-independent pathway. Thus, CT enhances CD4$^+$ T-cell priming *in vivo,* independent of CD8$^+$ T cells, without having any selective effect on the differentiation into Th1- or Th2-type of CD4$^+$ effector cells. The latter point is further supported by the fact that CT does not selectively augment IgG1 responses, influenced by Th2 cells, relative to IgG2a responses, which are under the control of IFN$\gamma$ and Th1 cells (Vajdy *et al.,* 1995).

### E. Direct Effects of CT on B-Cell Isotype-Switch Differentiation

In collaboration with Warren Strober (NIH, Bethesda, MD) and Eva Severinson (Karolinska Institute, Stockholm), we were able to demonstrate that CT causes LPS-stimulated membrane (m)IgM$^+$ B cells to undergo increased isotype-switching to IgG and IgA (Lycke and Strober, 1989; Lycke *et al.,* 1991a,b; Lycke, 1993). Subsequent studies revealed that CT also affected the B-cell responses to T-cell regulatory factors. CT and IL-4 had strong effects on IgG1 switch-differentiation by acting synergistically to induce isotype switching. This effect was manifested at the gene level as demonstrated by enhanced expression of germline $\gamma$1 RNA transcripts (Lycke *et al.,* 1991a,b). The data indicated that CT affected B-cell isotype differentiation at an early stage, prior to final gene recombination, since CT increased Ig constant heavy-chain (CH) RNA transcripts that were in germline configuration. According to current theories on isotype switching the formation of sterile transcripts in germline configuration preceeds the final switching to the transcribed constant heavy-chain gene (Stavnezer *et al.,* 1988). We compared the effect of whole CT with that of CT-B or dBcAMP on IL-4-induced IgG1 switching. We found that CT as well as dBcAMP induced increased expression of sterile germline CH$\gamma$1 RNA transcripts while CT-B failed to do so (Lycke, 1993). Moreover, we found that CT interacted with other lymphokines to affect B-cell differentiation. In spleen B-cell cultures containing IL-5 plus CT we observed greatly enhanced IgA differentiation as compared to cultures containing IL-5 or CT alone (Lycke *et al.,* 1991a). We consider this latter observation important because it supports the idea that CT promotes B-cell isotype switching in the case referred to, from IgM to IgA, since IL-5 only acts to enhance terminal differentiation of B cells already committed to IgA (Harriman *et al.,* 1988). Thus, these results indicate that CT does not act to direct switching in an isotype-specific manner.

### F. Immunological Memory after Mucosal Immunization

A natural aim for vaccination is the generation of a long-standing immunological memory. We have provided evidence to suggest that in mice such memory develops after a single oral vaccination with a protein antigen admixed with CT (Lycke and Holmgren, 1987, 1989; Vajdy and Lycke, 1992, 1993, 1995). Thus, CT may function as a memory-promoting factor in immunization. Recent findings with primed CD4$^+$ T cells from this system revealed that CT promoted a shift in phenotype from the naive, LECAM-1$^+$, Pgp-1$^-$ to a memory phenotype LECAM-1$^-$, Pgp-1$^+$. This shift in phenotype affected 20–30% of the CD4$^+$ T cells following priming with antigen plus CT-adjuvant (Hörnquist and Lycke, 1993; Hörnquist et al., 1996). Moreover, once memory cells have been induced using CT adjuvant our data suggest that there is no need for CT for the elicitation of a secondary type of response. Thus, mucosal memory for KLH can be elicited by challenge with KLH alone without the need for CT (Vajdy and Lycke, 1992). This suggests that a functional memory against infectious organisms may be induced using CT adjuvant.

Our studies now focused on the cellular and molecular characteristics of immunological memory. At the cellular level we found that CT adjuvant promoted the generation of both B- and T-cell memory and these cells demonstrated wide distribution in various tissues (Vajdy and Lycke, 1993). Of particular interest, antigen-specific memory T cells were residing in the lamina propria of the intestine in perorally immunized mice. Moreover, memory T-cell lymphokine repertoires were analyzed and both Th1- and Th2-type of lymphokines were found in response to recall antigen in vitro. This finding further supports the notion that CT does not selectively promote CD4$^+$ Th2 cells, not even in the long-term scale used here (study period of 18–24 months after immunization).

Following systemic immunizations most memory B cells are thought to express surface IgG rather than IgM but little information is available about memory B cells generated by mucosal immunization. At mucosal membranes only isotypes that associate with the poly Ig receptor, i.e., IgM and IgA, may be actively transported and transcytosed, through the epithelial cells from the lamina propria to the gut lumen (Mostov et al., 1984). Since the mucosal surfaces are predominantly protected by secretory IgA (sIgA) antibodies, and little if any IgG can be traced, it is assumed that mucosal memory is carried by B cells that have undergone isotype switch to IgA (Strober and Ehrhardt, 1994; Mestecky et al., 1994). Because isotype-switching to IgA involves deleting out constant heavy chain ($C_H$) genes upstream of the C$\alpha$ gene, such memory B cells would be restricted to mucosal surfaces and have limited usefulness outside the membranes, where instead IgG is required to protect against, e.g., pathogenic microorganisms which evade the mucosal barriers (Stavnezer et al., 1988; Gray, 1993). At variance with this notion, however, B cells isolated many months after oral immunization, in fact, produced IgM antibodies rather than IgA upon reactivation with antigen in vitro (Vajdy and Lycke, 1993, 1995). Thus, it appears that at least some memory B cells following mucosal immunization have not undergone rearrangement of their constant heavy-chain genes with maturational deletion of the CH$\mu$ gene. On reencounter with antigen, these memory B cells may secrete IgM or undergo isotype-switch to whichever downstream isotype is most warranted in the particular microenvironment.

## II. CAN CT'S IMMUNOMODULATING EFFECTS BE MIMICKED IN A POWERFUL NONTOXIC VACCINE ADJUVANT?

Our previous work and that of several other laboratories would suggest that the adjuvant function of CT requires ADP-ribosyltransferase activity and is, therefore, linked to the enzymatically active and toxic subunit, the CTA1. Knowing that a powerful adjuvant derived from the holotoxin structure must include the CT-A1 moiety, this notion most likely precludes any construction of an adjuvant which employs the CT-B binding to the promiscuous ganglioside-GM1 receptor present on a majority of mammalian cells. Since clinical findings with CT have suggested that even small doses of CT ($<5$ $\mu$g) may cause diarrheal responses, it will be difficult to find general acceptance in a vaccine for human use of a toxic molecule which has the potential to bind to and affect any cell in the body. Although promising attempts to reduce toxicity with retained adjuvanticity of CT and LT mutants have been reported, the fact that these constructs lack targeted action will greatly hamper their use.

In collaboration with Björn Löwenadler and Lena Ågren (Pharmacia, Stockholm), we have taken a different and unique approach and constructed a fusion protein that combines the enzymatic property of CT with the targeted action of a carrier protein, namely the *Staphylococcus areus* protein A (Löwenadler and Lycke, 1994). This latter protein is well known for its strong binding to IgG subclasses but can also bind to a significant extent to IgM and IgA (Ljungberg et al., 1993). The rationale for this choice of carrier molecule was that we hoped our fusion protein would target primarily B cells. Potentially, it could also bind other APCs, as dendritic cells and macrophages, via Fc–receptor interactions after complexing with free immunoglobulins. An inherent uncertainty in this high-risk project was whether we could get enzymatic activity of CT-A1 after linking it to a carrier/targeting molecule. Since retained ADP-ribosyltransferase activity of CT-A1 was a prerequisite for the success of the whole strategy, several approaches to the genetic construction were initially tested. Moreover, we did not know whether CT-A1 could affect the immune system at all accessing cells via a pathway separate from the GM1–ganglioside receptor pathway.

### A. Construction of Targeted CT-A1-Fusion Proteins with Adjuvant Action

After much preparatory work we constructed a candidate adjuvant by fusing CT-A1 to DD, a synthetic analogue of a fragment of protein A, which targets the CT-A1 enzyme to B cells primarily and away from the GM1 receptor on, e.g., the gut epithelial cells (Fig. 3). This first fusion protein should be viewed as a model system to answer the critical issues mentioned above. The fusion protein was genetically generated linking CT-A1 to DD in a plasmid vector under the tryptophan promotor (Löwenadler and Lycke, 1994). The CT-A1-DD fusion protein was ex-

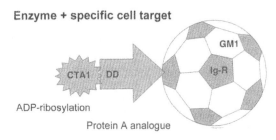

**FIGURE 3.** A novel targeted adjuvant. A gene fusion protein was constructed which has the enzymatic CT-A1-moiety linked to the Ig-binding domain, DD, of *Staphylococcus* protein A. The protein is specifically targeted to B cells and interacts with the cells via the Ig receptor, avoiding the classical CT ganglioside GM1 receptor.

pressed in *E. coli* and recovered from intracellular inclusions. Because of the strong interaction of DD with immunoglobulin, one great advantage of the choice of carrier molecule was the ability to affinity purify the fusion protein on solid-phase IgG-sepharose gel columns (Ljungberg *et al.,* 1993). This highly efficient purification step also allows for industrial exploitation of the CT-A1-DD gene fusion proteins. The chemical characterization of the fusion protein revealed that it was of expected size and reacted with CT-A1 epitope-specific monoclonal antibodies. The solubility of the protein in neutral pH was reduced as compared to that seen in acidic pH.

To test whether the CT-A1-DD fusion protein was enzymatically active and provided adjuvant function on immune responses to unrelated protein antigens, a series of assay systems were established. The ADP-ribosyltransferase activity of the molecule was assessed using the NAD:agmatine assay (Rappuoli and Pizza, 1991). As illustrated in Fig. 4, the construct demonstrated linear dose–response activity in this assay and at best gave 15–25% activity compared to an equimolar dose of whole CT. This result could in part be attributed to the reduced solubility of the CT-A1-DD molecule in neutral or higher pH, which were required for the optimal performance of the NAD:agmatine assay (Tsuji *et al.,* 1990). Nevertheless, the CT-A1-DD molecule exhibited substantial ADP-ribosylating activity. For comparison we introduced a single-amino acid point mutation in the targeted fusion protein at position $Asp_{109}$ of CT-A1. This molecule was found to exert poor ADP-ribosyltransferase activity and was used as a negative control (Fig. 4).

Intravenous or intraperitoneal injections to C57B1/6 mice with KLH together with CT-A1-DD were performed to investigate if the CT-A1-DD construct could enhance the serum anti-KLH response. As shown in Fig. 5, the CT-A1-DD construct significantly increased the serum anti-KLH response as compared to KLH given alone, suggesting that, indeed, CT-A1-DD acted as an adjuvant. The augmentation of anti-KLH serum responses was comparable to that observed with CT adjuvant. By contrast, no effect was seen with the enzymatically inactive mutated

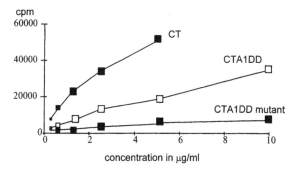

**FIGURE 4.** The ADP-ribosyltransferase activity of CT-A1-DD. The NAD:agmatine assay was used to determine ADP-ribosyltransferase activity. CT, CT-A1-DD, or mutant CT-A1-DD (Asp109) was added in various concentrations as indicated. One representative experiment of five.

CT-A1-DD control (Fig. 3). Subclass analysis of anti-KLH serum antibodies revealed upregulated responses in all IgG-subclasses, similar to that seen with CT adjuvant and no evidence for a selective effect of CT-A1-DD on the Th1 or Th2 $CD4^+$ T-cell subsets. Next we tested intranasal immunizations and found that the CT-A1-DD construct, similar to CT, augmented serum IgG as well as local IgA responses against KLH. These results support our concept of a targeted action of an ADP-ribosylating molecule as a good working hypothesis for an effective vaccine adjuvant. Further studies to explore the cellular and molecular requirements for the action of this novel targeted CT-A1-DD adjuvant are warranted.

Finally, to our satisfaction we noted that CT-A1-DD was nontoxic. Thus, we could inject CT-A1-DD in high doses iv (up to 100 $\mu$g/dose) with no demonstrable

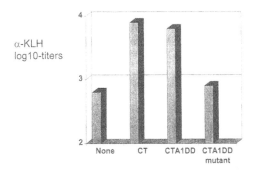

**FIGURE 5.** Serum responses following ip injections with KLH admixed with CT-A1-DD adjuvant. Mice were given two ip doses with 100 $\mu$g of KLH plus adjuvant and 7 days after the last dose serum was collected and analyzed for KLH-specific total Ig-antibody $\log_{10}$ titers. The response to antigen alone, KLH, was compared to that with 1 $\mu$g CT_, 20 $\mu$g CT-A1-DD, or 20 $\mu$g mutant CT-A1-DD added as adjuvant to each dose. This experiment is one of three giving similar results.

effect on the mice, and a negative ligated loop test detecting cAMP-induced fluid accumulation/diarrhea. In contrast to CT the CT-A1-DD molecule did not stimulate cAMP in thymocytes, which were used as indicator cells of the ganglioside GM1–receptor pathway. So far CT-A1-DD appears to be a completely nontoxic, but enzymatically active molecule, which has significant immunoenhancing effects *in vivo*.

## III. Concluding Remarks

We have shown that it is possible to separate the toxic effects of CT from its potent adjuvant effects by genetically constructing fusion proteins with the CT-A1 moiety targeted to primarily B cells but possibly also to other antigen-presenting cells. By avoiding the CT-B–GM1–ganglioside receptor pathway, we now have an adjuvant system which appears to lack completely enterotoxic or other cytotoxic effects. Although having less capacity for ADP ribosylation as compared to CT, it still was able to enhance serum antibody responses to a similar degree as the intact CT. This effect required the ADP-ribosylating property of CT-A1-DD because a mutant CT-A1-DD ($Asp_{109}$) with poor enzymatic activity completely failed to augment the immune response. Thus, our data provide strong evidence to suggest that ADP ribosylation is the key to the adjuvant function of CT. Even mucosal immune responses, i.e., after intranasal immunization, were found to be upregulated in response to CT-A1-DD adjuvant. However, a more critical evaluation of the mucosal adjuvant function after oral administration is still in progress. Also, we are exploring the characteristics of this novel immunomodulator with regard to its actions on the different cytokines and cellular subpopulations that have been found to be affected by intact holotoxin. In particular, more information on the action of CT-A1-DD on B cells and the effect on signal transduction, antigen-presentation, and costimulation due to Ig–receptor interaction is much needed.

   Despite the last few years of intense work describing the immunomodulating function of CT and its B subunit, no study has revealed conclusively a factor or a subpopulation of cells that on its own can be made responsible for the adjuvant effect *in vivo*. Rather, a multifactorial picture emerges of CT as an adjuvant where several events involved in the development and maintenance of an immune response are affected by the toxin. However, we believe that many of the recently debated theories for the adjuvant function have proven wrong. For example, that $CD8^+$ T cells are operational for the adjuvant effect or that CT selectively promotes Th2 cells have clearly been disputed in our recent studies using normal and gene knockout mice. Furthermore, our studies in gene knockout mice have clearly demonstrated that no single cytokine has, as yet, been found indispensible for the adjuvant function. In fact, CT appears to act independently of IL-4 or Th2 cells as shown in $IL-4^{-/-}$ mice. Also, we recently found that neither IFN$\gamma$ nor IL-6 are critically required for an adjuvant function of CT. Information gained in the CT-A1-DD project may be interpreted to suggest that B cells are the crucial target population for CT's adjuvant effect in the context of soluble protein antigens. We, therefore, propose that CT acts as an adjuvant by stimulating B cells to effectively function as antigen-presenting cells for naive as well as secondary CD4$^+$ T cells. The reason why CT-B is not as effective as CT, and does not act as an adjuvant but rather as a carrier molecule, is the fact that it fails to affect costimulation. Upregulation of B-7 molecules, as shown in the present chapter, may be the key factor responsible for the adjuvant function of CT *in vivo*. This hypothesis is currently being investigated in our laboratory.

## ACKNOWLEDGMENTS

I thank past and present members of my group for their invaluable work in the studies described in this chapter. In particular, I thank AnnaKari Bromander, Lena Ekman, Dubravka Grdic, Elisabeth Hörnquist, Ulla Karlsson, Martin Kjerrulf, Karin Schön, and Michael Vajdy Lena Ågren. Also, I thank Greg Harriman, Manfred Kopf, Marie Kosco-Vilbois, Georges Köhler, Björn Lövenadler, John Nedrud, Eva Severinson, and Warren Strober for close and rewarding collaborations. This work was financially supported by The Swedish Medical Research Council, The WHO Transdisease Vaccinology Program, The National Institutes of Health, NUTEK, and The Professor Nanna Svartz Foundation. Finally, I thank my father, Professor Erik Lycke, for critical reading of the manuscript.

## REFERENCES

Anderson, D. L., and Tsoukas, C. D. (1989). Cholera toxin inhibits resting human T cell activation via a cAMP-independent pathway. *J. Immunol.* **143**, 3647–3652.

Bowen, J. C., Nair, S. K., Reddy, R., and Rouse, B. T. (1994). Cholera toxin acts as a potent adjuvant for the induction of cytotoxic T-lymphocyte responses with non-replicating antigens. *Immunology* **81**, 338–342.

Bromander, A. K., Holmgren, J., and Lycke, N. (1991). Cholera toxin stimulates IL-1 production and enhances antigen-presentation by macrophages in vitro. *J. Immunol.* **146**, 2908–2929.

Bromander, A. K., Holmgren, J., and Lycke, N. (1993). Cholera toxin enhances alloantigen-presentation by cultured intestinal epithelial cells. *Scand. J. Immunol.* **37**, 452–458.

Burnette, N., Mar, V. L., Platler, W., Schlotterbeck, D., McGinley, D., Stoney, S., Rhode, S. M. F., and Kaslow, H. R. (1991). Site-specific mutagenisis of the catalytic subunit of cholera toxin: Substituting lysine for arginine 7 causes loss of activity. *Infect. Immun.* **59**, 4266–4270.

Challacombe, S. J., Rahman, D., Jeffrey, J., Davis, S. S., and O'Hagan, D. T. (1992). Enhanced secretory IgA and systemic IgG antibody responses after oral immunization with biodegradable microparticles containing antigen. *Immunology* **76**, 164–170.

Czerkinsky, C., Russell, M. W., Lycke, N., Lindblad, M., and Holmgren, J. (1989). Oral administration of a streptococcal antigen coupled to cholera toxin B subunit evokes strong antibody responses in salivary glands and extramucosal tissues. *Infect. Immun.* **57**, 1072–1077.

Dickinson, B. L., and Clements, J. D. (1995). Dissociation of *Escherichia coli* heat-labile eneterotoxin adjuvanticity from ADP-ribosyltransferase activity. *Infect. Immun.* **63**, 1617–1623.

· Douce, G., Turcotte, C., Cropley, I., Roberts, M., Pizza, M., Domenghini, M., Rappuoli, R., and Dougan, G. (1995). Mutants of *Escherichia coli* heat-labile toxin lacking ADP-ribosyltransferase activity act as nontoxic, mucosal adjuvants. *Proc. Natl. Acad. Sci. U.S.A.* **92**, 1644–1648.

Eldridge, J., Gilley, R. M., Staas, J. R., Moldevanue, Z., Meulbroek, and Tice, T. R. (1989). Biodegradable microspheres: Vaccine delivery system for oral immunization. *Curr. Top. Microbiol. Immunol.* **146**, 59–72.

Elson, C. O. (1992). Cholera toxin as a mucosal adjuvant: Effects of H-2 major histocompatibility complex and *lps* genes. *Infect. Immun.* **60**, 2874–2879.

Elson, D. O., and Ealding, W. (1984a). Generalized systemic and mucosal immunity in mice after mucosal stimulation with cholera toxin. *J. Immunol.* **132**, 2736–2741.

Elson, D. O., and Ealding, W. (1984b). Cholera toxin feeding did not induce oral tolerance and abrogated oral tolerance to an unrelated protein antigen. *J. Immunol.* **133**, 2892–2897.

Elson, C. O., Holland, S. P., Dertzbaugh, M. T., Cuff, C. F., and Anderson, A. O. (1995). Morphologic and functional alterations of mucosal T cells by Cholera toxin and its B subunit. *J. Immunol.* **154**, 1032–1039.

Grant, C. C. R., Messer, R. J., and Cieplak, W. (1994). Role of trypsin-like cleavage at arginine 192 in the enzymatic and cytotonic activities of *Escherichia coli* heat-labile enterotoxin. *Infect. Immun.* **62**, 4270–4278.

Gray, D. (1993). Immunological Memory. *Annu. Rev. Immunol.* **11**, 49–72.

Haack, B. M., Emmrich, F., and Resch, K. (1993). Cholera toxin inhibits T cell receptor signalling by covalent modification of the CD3-$\zeta$ subunit. *J. Immunol.* **150**, 2599–2606.

Hajishengallis, G., Hollingshead, S. K., Koga, T., and Russell, M. W. (1995). Mucosal immunization with a bacterial protein antigen genetically coupled to cholera toxin A2/B Subunits. *J. Immunol.* **154**, 4322–4332.

Harriman, G. R., Kunimoto, D. Y., Elliot, D. Y., Paetkau, V., and Strober, W. (1988). The role of IL-5 in IgA B cell differentiation. *J. Immunol.* **140**, 3033–3039.

Hörnquist, E., and Lycke, N. (1991). Host defense against cholera toxin is strongly CD4[+] T cell dependent. *Infect. Immun.* **59**, 3630–3638.

Hörnqvist, E., and Lycke, N. (1993). Cholera toxin adjuvant strongly promotes T cell priming. *Eur. J. Immunol.* **23**, 2136–2143.

Hörnquist, E., Lycke, N., Czerkinsky, C., and Holmgren, J. (1994). Cholera toxin and cholera B subunit as oral–mucosal adjuvant and antigen carrier systems. *In* "Novel Delivery Systems for Oral Vaccines" (D. O'Hagan, Ed.), Vol. 169, pp. 153–173. CRC Press, Boca Raton, FL.

Hörnquist, E., Grdic, D., Mak, T., and Lycke, N. (1996). CD8-deficient mice exhibit augmented mucosal immune responses following oral immunizations. *Immunology.* **87**, 220–229.

Imboden, J. B., Shoback, D. M., Pattison, G., and Stobo, J. D. (1986). Cholera toxin inhibits the T-cell antigen receptor-mediated increases in inositol trisphospate and cytoplasmic free calcium. *Proc. Natl. Acad. Sci. U.S.A.;* **83**, 5673–5677.

Kopf, M., Le Gros, G., Bachmann, M., Lamers, M. C., Bluethmann, H., and Köhler, G. (1993). Disruption of the murine IL-4 gene blocks Th2 cytokine responses. *Nature (London)* **362**, 245–248.

Lacour, M., Arrighi, J.-F., Muller, K. M., Carlberg, C., Saurat, J.-H., and Hauser, C. (1994). cAMP up-regulates IL-4 and IL-5 production from activated CD4[+] T cells while decreasing IL-2 release and NF-AT induction. *Int. Immunol.* **9**, 1333–1340.

Liang, X., Lamm, M. E., and Nedrud, J. G. (1988). Oral administration of cholera toxin sendai virus conjugate potentiates gut and respiratory immunity against sendai virus. *J. Immunol.* **141**, 1495–1501.

Liang, X., Lamm, M. E., and Nedrud, J. G. (1989). Cholera toxin as a mucosal adjuvant: Glutaraldehyde-treatment dissociates adjuvanticity from toxicity. *J. Immunol.* **143**, 484–490.

Ljungberg, U. K., Jansson, B., Niss, U., Nilsson, R., Sandberg, B., and Nilsson, B. (1993). The interaction between different domains of staphylococcal protein A and human polyclonal IgG, IgA, IgM and F(ab)$_2$: Separation of affinity from specificity. *Mol. Immunol.* **14**, 1279–1285.

Löwenadler, B., and Lycke, N. (1994). Fusion proteins with heterologous T helper epitopes. Recombinant *E. coli* heat-stable enterotoxin proteins. *Int. Rev. Immunol.* **11**, 103–111.

Lycke, N. (1993). Cholera toxin promotes B cell isotype switching by two different mechanisms: cAMP-induction augments germline Ig H-chain RNA transcripts whereas membrane ganglioside GM1-receptor binding enhances later events in differentiation. *J. Immunol.* **150**, 4810–4821.

Lycke, N., and Holmgren, J. (1986). Strong adjuvant properties of cholera toxin on gut mucosal immune responses to orally presented antigens. *Immunology* **59**, 301–308.

Lycke, N., and Holmgren, J. (1987). Long-term cholera antitoxin memory in the gut can be triggered to antibody formation associated with protection within hours after an oral challenge immunization. *Scand. J. Immunol.* **25**, 407–412.

Lycke, N., and Holmgren, J. (1989). Adoptive transfer of gut mucosal antitoxin memory by isolated B cells one year after oral immunization with cholera toxin. *Infect. Immun.* **57**, 1137–1141.

Lycke, N., and Strober, W. (1989). Cholera toxin promotes B cell isotype differentiation. *J. Immunol.* **142**, 3781–3787.

Lycke, N., and Svennerholm, A.-M. (1990). Presentation of immunogens at the gut and other mucosal surfaces. *In* "The Molecular Approach to New and Improved Vaccines" (W. M. Levine, Ed.), pp. 207–227. Dekker, New York.

Lycke, N., Bromander, A. K., Ekman, L., Karlsson, U., and Holmgren, J. (1989). Cellular basis of immunomodulation by cholera toxin *in vitro* with possible association to the adjuvant function *in vivo*. *J. Immunol.* **142**, 20–27.

Lycke, N., Severinson, E., and Strober, W. (1991a). Molecular effects of cholera toxin on isotype differentiation. *Immunol. Res.* **10**, 407–412.

Lycke, N., Severinson, E., and Strober, W. (1991b). Cholera toxin acts synergistically with IL-4 to promote IgG1 switch differentiation. *J. Immunol.* **145**, 3316–3324.

Lycke, N., Karlsson, U., Sjölander, A., and Magnusson, K.-E. (1991c). The adjuvant action of cholera toxin is associated with an increased intestinal permeability for luminal antigens. *Scand. J. Immunol.* **33**, 691–698.

Lycke, N., Tsuji, T., and Holmgren, J. (1992). The adjuvant effect of *Vibrio cholerae* and *E. coli* heat labile enterotoxins is linked to their ADP-ribosyltransferase activity. *Eur. J. Immunol.* **22**, 2277–2281.

McGhee, J. R., Mestecky, J., Dertzbaugh, M. T., Eldridge, J. H., Hirasawa, H., and Kiyono, H. (1992). The mucosal immune system: From fundamental concepts to vaccine development. *Vaccine* **10**, 75–87.

Mestecky, J., Abraham, R., and Ogra, P. L. (1994). Common mucosal immune system and strategies for the development of vaccines effective at the mucosal surfaces. *In* "Handbook of Mucosal Immunology" (P. Ogra, J. Metscky, M. Lamm, W. Strober, J. McGhee, and J. Bienenstock, eds.), pp. 357–372. Academic Press, San Diego.

Michalek, S. M., Eldridge, J. H., Curtiss III, R., and Rosenthal, K. (1994). Antigen delivery systems: New approaches to mucosal immunizations" *In* "Handbook of Mucosal Immunology" (P. Ogra, J. Metscky, M. Lamm, W. Strober, J. McGhee, and J. Bienenstock, eds.), pp. 373–391. Academic Press, San Diego.

Mostov, K. E., Friedlander, M., and Blobel, G. (1984). The receptor for transepithelial transport of IgA and IgM contains multiple immunoglobulin-like domains. *Nature (London)* **308**, 37–40.

Mowat, A. (1994). Oral tolerance and Regulation of Immunity to dietary antigens. *In* "Handbook of Mucosal Immunology" (P. Ogra, J. Metscky, M. Lamm, W. Strober, J. McGhee, and J. Bienenstock, eds.), pp. 185–202. Academic Press, San Diego.

Mowat, A., McI, K., Maloy, J., and Donachie, A. M. (1993). Immune-stimulating complexes as adjuvants for local and systemic immunity after oral immunization with protein antigens. *Immunology* **80**, 527–534.

Munoz, E., Zubiaga, A. M., Merrow, M., Sauter, N. P., and Huber, B. (1990). Cholera toxin discriminates between T helper 1 and 2 cells in T cell receptor-mediated activation: Role of cAMP in T cell proliferation. *J. Exp. Med.* **172**, 95–103.

Neutra, M. R., and Kraehenbuhl, J.-P. (1992). Transepithelial transport and mucosal defence I: The role of M cells. *Trends Cell Biol.* **2**, 134–138.

Rappuoli, R., and Pizza, M. (1991). Structure and evolutionary aspects of ADP-ribosylating toxins. *In*

"Sourcebook of Bacterial Protein Toxins" (J. E. Alouf and J. H. Freer, eds.), pp. 1–21. Academic Press, London.

Russell, M. W., and Wu, H.-Y. (1991). Distribution, persistence and recall of serum and salivary antibody responses to peroral immunization with protein antigen I/II of *Streptococcus mutans* coupled to the cholera toxin B subunit. *Infect. Immun.* **59**, 4061–4070.

Stavnezer, J., Radcliff, G., Lin, Y.-C., Nietupski, J., Berggren, L., Sitia, R., and Severinson, E. (1988). Immunoglobulin heavy-chain switching may be directed by prior induction of transcripts from constant region genes. *Proc. Natl. Acad. Sci. U.S.A.* **85**, 7704–7708.

Strober, W., and Ehrhardt, R. O. (1994). Regulation of IgA B cell development. *In* "Handbook of Mucosal Immunology" (P. L. Ogra, W. Strober, J. Mestecky, J. R. McGhee, M. E. Lamm, and J. Bienenstock, eds.), pp. 159–176. Academic Press, San Diego.

Sun, J.-B., Holmgren, J., and Czerkinsky, C. (1994). Cholera toxin B subunit: An efficient transmucosal carrier-delivery system for induction of peripheral immunological tolerance. *Proc. Natl. Acad. Sci. U.S.A.* **91**, 10795–10799.

Tamura, S., Samegai, Y., Kurata, H., Nagamine, T., Aizawa, C., and Kurata, T. (1988). Protection against influenza virus infection by vaccine inoculated intranasally with cholera toxin B subunit. *Vaccine* **6**, 409–413.

Tsuji, T., Inoue, T., Miyama, A., Okamoto, K., Honda, T., and Miwatani, T. (1990). A single amino acid substitution in the A subunit of *E. coli* enterotoxin results in a loss of its toxic activity. *J. Biol. Chem.* **265**, 22520–22526.

Vajdy, M., and Lycke, N. (1992). Cholera toxin adjuvant promotes long-term immunological memory in the gut mucosa to unrelated immunogens after oral immunization. *Immunology* **75**, 488–492.

Vajdy, M., and Lycke, N. (1993). Stimulation of antigen-specific T and B-cell memory in local as well as systemic lymphoid tissues following oral immunization with cholera toxin adjuvant. *Immunology* **80**, 197–203.

Vajdy, M., and Lycke, N. (1995). Mucosal memory B cells retain the ability to produce IgM antibodies even 2 years after oral immunizations. *Immunology.* **87**, 336–342 .

Vajdy, M., Kosco-Vilbois, M., Kopf, M., Köhler, G., and Lycke, N. (1995). Impaired mucosal immune responses in IL-4 targeted mice. *J. Exp. Med.* **181**, 41–53.

Wilson, A. D., Bailey, M., Williams, N. A., and Stokes, C. R. (1991). The *in vitro* production of cytokines by mucosal lymphocytes immunized by oral administration of keyhole limpet hemocyanin using cholera toxin as an adjuvant. *Eur. J. Immunol.* **21**, 2333–2340.

Woogen, S. D., Ealding, W., and Elson, C. O. (1987). Inhibition of murine lymphocyte proliferation by the B subunit of cholera toxin. *J. Immunol.* **139**, 3764–3770.

Wu, H.-Y., and Russell, M. W. (1993). Induction of mucosal immunity by intranasal application of a streptococcal surface protein antigen with the cholera toxin B subunit. *Infect. Immun.* **61**, 314–320.

Xu-Amano, J., Kiyono, H., Jackson, R. J., Staats, H. F., Fujihashi, K., Burrows, P. D., Elson, C. O., Pillai, S., and McGhee, J. R. (1993). Helper T cell subsets for immunoglobulin A responses: Oral immunization with tetanus toxoid and cholera toxin as adjuvant selectively induces Th2 cells in mucosa-associated tissues. *J. Exp. Med.* **178**, 1309–1320.

# Index

## A

Activation-induced cell death, in IBD, 300

Activation markers
expression by donor-derived lymphocytes in scid mice, 207–208
lamina propria lymphocytes, 229–230

Adenovirus, ADE5-*lacZ* vector, transgene delivery to respiratory epithelia, 468–470

Adhesion molecules
activation
of intraepithelial lymphocytes, 273–274
of lamina propria lymphocytes, 271–273
CD2, 265–266
CD44 (proteoglycan/cartilage-link protein), 270
on circulating antibody-secreting cells, 484–486
expression
on airway epithelial cells after RSV infection, 414–416
on colon epithelial cells after microbial invasion, 69–70
differential, on circulating antibody-secreting cells, 485–486
homing of Peyer's patch-derived blasts, 271
ICAM-1, 266
ICAM-3, 266
immunoglobulin superfamily, 264–265
integrins, 266–267
$\alpha 4 \beta 7$, 268, 485
$\alpha E \beta 7$, 269–270
LFA-1, 267–268
VLA-4, 268
migration of T cells into gut epithelium, 271
selectins, 264, 485
E-selectin, 264
L-selectin, 207–208, 264, 485
P-selectin, 264

in trans-uroepithelial neutrophil migration, 80

Adjuvants
cholera toxin
CTA1-DD fusion protein, 573–576
in *Helicobacter pylori* immunizations, 396–397
recombinant *Salmonella typhimurium* oral immunizations, 465–466
stimulation of mucosal IgA response, 493–494
IL-6, 256–257
oral tolerance enhancement with, 548
tetanus toxoid, 464–465

ADP-ribosyltransferase activity, cholera toxin, 566–567

Antibiotics, prevention of experimental intestinal or systemic inflammation, 310–311

Antibodies, *see also* Autoantibodies; *specific antibody*
anti-asialoglycoprotein receptor, identification and characterization, 357–358
antinuclear, in liver disease, 358–359

Antigen delivery systems, safety concerns, 507–508

Antigen processing and presentation
cholera toxin effects, 567–568
by MHC class I molecules, 4–6
by MHC class Ib molecules
CD1 molecules, 16–17
*H2-M3* region-derived molecules, 15–16
peptide binding, 17–20
*Qa* region-derived molecules, 14
*Tla* region-derived molecules, 14–15
by MHC class II molecules
endosomal targeting, 9–10
invariant chain functions, 7–9

Leukocytes
destructive processes activated by chemokines, 329
intestinal, HPA axis activation effects, 132–133
Leukotrienes
mucosal production in IBD, 326
in respiratory syncytial virus infection, 406
Ligand binding, polymeric immunoglobulin receptor, 154–157
Liver, autoimmune disease, genetics, 362–363
Liver-kidney-microsomal antibody
type 1
cytochrome P450 IID6 antigen, 360
genetics of associated liver diseases, 362–363
identification and characterization, 359
inhibition of cytochrome P450 IID6 function, 360–361
type 2, cytochrome P450 IIC9 antigen, 364–365
type 3, UDP-glucuronosyltransferase antigen, 365–368
Liver-microsomal antibodies
characterization, 359
cytochrome P450 IA2 antigen, 366
LKM, see Liver-kidney-microsomal antibody
L-selectin, see Selectins
Lymph node
immune barrier against HIV, 443
lymphocytes transferred to scid mice, expression of homing receptors and activation markers, 207–208
Lymphocyte activation antigen 4F2, expression on lamina propria lymphocytes, 229
Lymphocyte function-related antigen-1 (LFA-1, CD11a/CD18), 267–268
Lymphocytes, see also Intraepithelial lymphocytes; T cells
homing, adhesion molecule functions, 271
lamina propria
activation markers, 229–230
activation pathways, 234–237
B-cell helper effects, 232
B cell–T cell interactions, 235–237
cytokine production, 231–233
cytokine production under inflammatory bowel conditions, 233–234
homing, 230–231
phenotype, 228–229
regulation by intestinal epithelial cells, 237–239
mucosal, IL-7 receptor expression, 283–285
mucosal, proliferation, regulation by IL-7, 285–286
peripheral blood, phenotypic markers, 228

**M**

Macrophages, see also Pulmonary alveolar macrophages
functions, neuropeptide effects, 131
IL-12 mRNA production after oral immunization with viable attenuated or killed *Salmonella typhimurium*
4 hr postinfection, 534–535
24 hr postinfection, 538–539
quantification, 535–537
survival, 533–534
immune barrier function against HIV, 442–443
intestinal, VIP receptor expression, 129–131
migration in IBD, 324–325
respiratory tract, suppression of T-cell proliferation, 49
Major histocompatibility complex class I molecules
antigen presentation pathway, 4–5
coevolution with transporter associated with antigen processing, 5–6
empty, 6
function, 86
peptide binding, 17–20
peptide transport, 5–6
structure, 86
ubiquitination, 5
Major histocompatibility complex class Ib molecules (nonclassical)
absence of allelic polymorphism, 88
CD1, see CD1 molecules
FcRn, see Fc receptors
function, 88–89
genes for, 85–87
*H2-M* region, 15–16
peptide binding, 17–20
plasticity, 88
*Qa* region-derived molecules, 14
specialization, 88
structure, 87
tissue distribution, 88
TL antigen, structure, 209–210
*Tla* region-derived molecules, 14–15
TL-T10 and T22 recognition by $\gamma\delta$ T-cell clone G8, 175–177

Printed and bound by CPI Group (UK) Ltd, Croydon, CR0 4YY

03/10/2024

01040413-0008